INTRAOPERATIVE CONSULTATION IN SURGICAL PATHOLOGY

CAMBRIDGE ILLUSTRATED SURGICAL PATHOLOGY

Series Editor: Lawrence Weiss, MD
City of Hope National Medical Center, Duarte, California

Other Books in the Series

Modern Immunohistochemistry, Periguo Chu, MD, and Lawrence Weiss, MD

Nervous System, Hannes Vogel, MD

Lymph Nodes, Lawrence Weiss, MD

Head and Neck, Margaret Brandwein-Gensler, MD

Forthcoming

Prostate, Lawrence True, MD

Uterine Pathology, Robert A. Soslow, MD, and Teri Longacre, MD

INTRAOPERATIVE CONSULTATION IN SURGICAL PATHOLOGY

CAMBRIDGE ILLUSTRATED SURGICAL PATHOLOGY

Mahendra Ranchod, MB, ChB, MMed (Path)

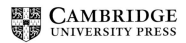
CAMBRIDGE
UNIVERSITY PRESS

CAMBRIDGE UNIVERSITY PRESS
Cambridge, New York, Melbourne, Madrid, Cape Town, Singapore,
São Paulo, Delhi, Dubai, Tokyo, Mexico City

Cambridge University Press
The Edinburgh Building, Cambridge CB2 8RU, UK

Published in the United States of America by Cambridge University Press, New York

www.cambridge.org
Information on this title: www.cambridge.org/9780521897679

First published 2010

Printed in the United Kingdom at the University Press, Cambridge

A catalog record for this publication is available from the British Library

Library of Congress Cataloging-in-Publication Data

Intraoperative consultation in surgical pathology / [edited by] Mahendra Ranchod.
   p. ; cm. – (Cambridge illustrated surgical pathology)
   Includes bibliographical references and index.
   ISBN 978-0-521-89767-9 (Hardback)
   1. Pathology, Surgical.   I. Ranchod, Mahendra, 1942–   II. Series: Cambridge illustrated surgical pathology.
   [DNLM: 1. Pathology, Surgical–methods.   2. Intraoperative Period. WO 142]
   RD57.I58 2010
   617′.07–dc22

                                                                                    2010025713

ISBN 978-0-521-89767-9 Hardback

CONTENTS

CONTRIBUTORS

Reid B Adams, MD
Professor and Chief, Division of Surgical Oncology
Chief, Hepatobiliary and Pancreatic Surgery
University of Virginia Health System
Charlottesville, VA, USA

Syed Ali, MD
Associate Professor of Pathology
The Johns Hopkins University School of Medicine
The Sol Goldman Pancreatic Cancer Research Center
Baltimore, MD, USA

John L. D. Atkinson, MD
Professor of Neurosurgery,
Mayo Clinic,
Rochester, MN, USA

Raffi S. Avedian, MD
Assistant Professor
Department of Orthopaedic Surgery
Stanford University School of Medicine
Stanford, CA, USA

Carl A. Bertelsen, MD, FACS
Department of Surgery,
Good Samaritan Hospital
San Jose, CA, USA

Robert H. Byrd MD
Instructor in Pathology and Immunology
Baylor College of Medicine,
Texas Children's Hospital
Houston, TX, USA

Darrell L. Cass MD
Assistant Professor of Surgery and Pediatrics
Texas Children's Hospital
Houston, TX, USA

John K. C. Chan MBBS, FRCPath, FRCPA
Consultant Pathologist,
Department of Pathology,
Queen Elizabeth Hospital,
Hong Kong, SAR China

Jon M. Davison, MD, PhD
Assistant Professor of Pathology
University of Pittsburgh School of Medicine
Pittsburgh, PA, USA

Megan K. Dishop MD
Associate Professor of Pathology
The Children's Hospital, University of Colorado-Denver,
Denver, CO, USA

Sarah M. Dry
Associate Professor, Department of Pathology,
David Geffen School of Medicine at UCLA
Los Angeles, CA, USA

Umamaheswar Duvvuri MD, PhD
Assistant Professor,
University of Pittsburgh School of Medicine
Staff Surgeon, VA Pittsburgh Health System
Pittsburgh, PA, USA

David W. Eisele, MD, FACS
Professor and Chairman
Department of Otolaryngology-Head and Neck Surgery
University of California, San Francisco
San Francisco, CA, USA

Elliot K. Fishman, MD
Professor of Radiology and Radiological Sciences
The Sol Goldman Pancreatic Cancer Research Center
The Johns Hopkins University School of Medicine
Baltimore, MD, USA

Steven D. Hart, MD
Assistant Clinical Professor,
Department of Pathology,
David Geffen School of Medicine at UCLA,
Santa Monica-UCLA
Santa Monica, CA, USA

Michael R. Hendrickson, MD
Professor of Pathology and
Co-Director of Surgical Pathology
Stanford University School of Medicine
Stanford, CA, USA

Karen M. Horton, MD
Professor of Radiology and Radiological Sciences
The Sol Goldman Pancreatic Cancer Research Center
The Johns Hopkins University School of Medicine
Baltimore, MD, USA

Andrew E. Horvai, MD, PhD
Associate Clinical Professor of Pathology
University of California, San Francisco
San Francisco, CA

Ralph H. Hruban, MD
Professor of Pathology
The Sol Goldman Pancreatic Cancer Research Center
The Johns Hopkins University School of Medicine
Baltimore, MD, USA

Julia C. Iezzoni, MD
Associate Professor
Department of Pathology,
University of Virginia Health System,
Charlottesville, VA, USA

Electron Kebebew, MD
Senior Investigator and
Head of Endocrine Surgery Section
National Cancer Institute,
Surgery Branch CRC,
Bethesda, MD, USA

Richard L. Kempson, MD
Professor Emeritus, Active
Department of Pathology
Stanford University School of Medicine
Stanford, CA, USA

Seth P. Lerner, MD
Professor of Urology,
Beth and Dave Swalm Chair in Urologic Oncology,
Scott Department of Urology,
Baylor College of Medicine,
Houston, TX, USA

Linda W. Martin, MD, MPH
Department of Thoracic Surgery,
The Cancer Institute
St. Joseph Medical Center
Towson, MD, USA

Charles Michael Lombard, MD
Dept. of Pathology, El Camino Hospital,
Mountain View, CA and
Adjunct Associate Clinical Professor of Pathology
Stanford University Medical Center,
Stanford, CA, USA

Teri A. Longacre, MD
Professor and Co-Associate Director of Surgical Pathology,
Department of Pathology,
Stanford University School of Medicine
Stanford, CA, USA

Jesse K. McKenney, MD
Assistant Professor,
Department of Pathology
Stanford University Medical Center
Stanford, CA, USA

Cesar A. Moran, MD
Deputy Chair
Professor of Pathology & Director of Thoracic Pathology
The University of Texas M.D. Anderson Cancer Center
Houston, TX, USA

Michael B. Morgan, MD
Professor of Pathology University of South Florida
College of Medicine
Clinical Professor of Dermatology University of Florida
College of Medicine
Clinical Professor of Dermatology Michigan State
College of Medicine
Chief, Dermatopathology James Haley Veterans
Administration Hospital
Tampa, FL, USA

Isaac M. Neuhaus, MD
Assistant Professor
Department of Dermatology
University of California, San Francisco
San Francisco, CA, USA

Richard J. O'Donnell, MD
Chief, UCSF Orthopaedic Oncology Service
UCSF Helen Diller Family Comprehensive Cancer Center
San Francisco, CA, USA

Mahendra Ranchod, MB, ChB, MMed.
Department of Pathology,
Good Samaritan Hospital, San Jose, CA
Director, Calpath/Gyne-Path Laboratory, Los Gatos, CA
Adjunct Clinical Professor of Pathology,
Stanford University School of Medicine,
Stanford CA, USA

David C. Rice, MB, BCh, FRCSI
Associate Professor,
Department of Thoracic and Cardiovascular Surgery,
The University of Texas M.D. Anderson Cancer Center,
Houston, TX, USA

Jae Y. Ro, MD, PhD
Professor of Pathology and Laboratory Medicine,
The Methodist Hospital and
Weill Medical College of Cornell University
Houston, Texas, USA

Fausto Rodriguez, MD
Assistant Professor
Dept. of Laboratory Medicine and Pathology
Mayo Clinic Rochester, MN, USA

Bernd W. Scheithauer, MD
Professor of Pathology,
Department of Laboratory Medicine and Pathology
Mayo Clinic
Rochester, MN, USA

Timothy M. Schmitt, MD
Assistant Professor
Transplant and Hepatobiliary Surgery
Department of Surgery
University of Virginia Health System
Charlottesville, VA 22908

Richard Schulick, MD
Professor of Surgery
The Sol Goldman Pancreatic Cancer Research Center
The Johns Hopkins University School of Medicine
Baltimore, MD, USA

Raja R. Seethala, MD
Assistant Professor,
Department of Pathology,
University of Pittsburgh School of Medicine,
Presbyterian University Hospital,
Pittsburgh, PA, USA

Steven S. Shen, MD, PhD
Associate Professor of Pathology and Laboratory Medicine
The Methodist Hospital and
Weill Medical College of Cornell University
Houston, TX, USA

Saul Suster, MD
Professor and Chairman
Department of Pathology
Medical College of Wisconsin
Milwaukee, WI, USA

Patrick A. Treseler, MD, PhD
Professor of Pathology
Associate Director of Surgical Pathology
University of California San Francisco
San Francisco, CA, USA

Luan D. Truong, MD
Professor of Pathology and Laboratory Medicine
The Methodist Hospital and
Weill Medical College of Cornell University;
Adjunct Professor of Pathology and
Medicine, Baylor College of Medicine
Houston, TX, USA

Roderick R. Turner, MD
Adjunct Member, John Wayne Cancer Institute at Saint
John's Health Center
Santa Monica, CA, USA

PREFACE

This book is about the pathologist's role as consultant during surgical procedures, a role that requires the pathologist to make a diagnosis that will help the surgeon perform the appropriate surgical procedure. We discuss how intraoperative consultation can be challenging because of time constraints, limited sampling and a restricted repertoire of tests, but proffer that these limitations can be overcome if the pathologist is fully informed of the clinical aspects of the case, is able to extract the maximum amount of information from examination of the specimen, and is aware of what the surgeon needs to perform the correct surgical procedure.

An on-going problem with intraoperative consultation is that specimens are often submitted to the laboratory with minimal clinical history, leaving the pathologist to decide when to seek more information. While many lesions can be correctly interpreted with limited data, there are situations when clinical information is essential to reach the correct diagnosis. Unfortunately, pathologic examination alone will not always reveal the underlying complexity of a case, which is why we recommend a pro-active approach, seeking information before the specimen is sent to the laboratory. The amount of effort expended in gathering this information should be commensurate with the demands of the case, and often the most efficient way to gain this perspective is to talk to the surgeon directly. Our position is that the role of consultant requires the pathologist to take a comprehensive approach to intraoperative diagnosis, gathering relevant clinical information, reviewing imaging studies when appropriate, examining prior biopsy material when necessary, and being familiar with the surgeon's operative plan – because failure to do so may lead to serious errors.

Examination of the surgically excised specimen is the main component of intraoperative consultation, and we discuss the relative merits and shortcomings of gross examination, frozen section and cytologic techniques. Diagnoses rendered intraoperatively are frequently as accurate as final diagnoses, but there are occasions when a specific diagnosis cannot be made, and instead, the pathologist has to offer a provisional diagnosis that is "good enough" for the surgeon to perform the appropriate surgical procedure. We discuss the pragmatism of a "good enough" diagnosis and how its proper use requires an understanding of clinical management and surgical algorithms.

Communication with the surgeon is an important component of intraoperative consultation, a task that pathologists accomplish with variable success. Reporting the diagnosis on a straight-forward case is a simple matter, but is more challenging when handling a complicated case, or when it is not possible to make a specific diagnosis. We discuss strategies for handling these situations, and the benefits of visiting the operating room for direct communication with the surgeon.

Surgical management requires teamwork, and the pathologist is drawn into the team when a surgeon requests an intraoperative consultation. The pathologist now becomes a principal player because the pathologic diagnosis will very likely influence surgical management. The pathologist's contribution is greatest when he is fully engaged as a consultant, and when surgeon and pathologist work co-operatively for the benefit of the patient. This book attempts to capture that spirit of collaboration by having surgeons co-author most of the chapters of this book.

This is not another textbook of surgical pathology. Instead, this book focuses on issues that are relevant to the intraoperative arena, and attempts to address the following questions: What are the indications for intraoperative diagnosis? What information should the pathologist have on hand before rendering a diagnosis? How should specimens be handled intraoperatively? What are the pitfalls in diagnosis, considering the limitations of intraoperative testing? What information should the pathologist provide so that the surgeon may perform the correct surgical procedure? What are the managerial consequences of intraoperative diagnosis? When should the pathologist advise against subjecting a biopsy to frozen section evaluation? How should the pathologist handle an inappropriate request for frozen section diagnosis from a recalcitrant surgeon?

This book is written for surgical pathologists and assumes that the reader has a working knowledge of diagnostic pathology. This text is also meant for pathology residents who are trying to understand the complex role of a consultant during surgical procedures. Residents acquire the skills of intraoperative consultation by an apprenticeship-like process that is variable in quality, a hit-and-miss arrangement that may explain why newly qualified pathologists are often poorly prepared to function in the intraoperative arena. It may be time for residency training programs to adopt a more formal approach to teaching the skills of intraoperative consultation, and perhaps this book will provide a step in that direction.

It is challenging to produce a multi-authored book with a unified voice, and I am grateful to the contributors of this volume for the effort they have made to reach this goal. The contributors should be given credit if this book achieves its goals, but I assume full responsibility for any of this volume's shortcomings.

The ideas and practices espoused in this book are derived from many sources. Some of these contributions are acknowledged in the reference section of each chapter, but many of the subtleties of intraoperative consultation have been passed on from pathologist to pathologist, and from one generation of pathologists to the next, so that their origins are clouded by the passage of time. We honor these contributions by expressing gratitude to our teachers, mentors and colleagues, recognizing that they are part of a lineage of physicians who have helped to shape the field of modern surgical pathology.

MAHENDRA RANCHOD

1 INTRODUCTION

Mahendra Ranchod

Intraoperative consultation (IOC) refers to the pathologist's role as a consultant during surgical procedures. While making a diagnosis is the cornerstone of intraoperative consultation, the role of consultant goes beyond making a diagnosis, and includes discussions about the usefulness, appropriateness and limitations of intraoperative diagnosis, the best specimen to procure for diagnosis, recommendations for ancillary tests, and suggestions for management when the pathologist is unable to make a definite diagnosis. The tools for intraoperative diagnosis (IOD) include some combination of gross examination, frozen sections, and cytologic tests, and at some institutions, a limited number of rapid special stains are also employed.[1] However, the older term "frozen section diagnosis" is so entrenched in our lexicon that we sometimes use it when we mean "intraoperative consultation."

CHANGES IN INTRAOPERATIVE CONSULTATION

The types of specimens submitted for IOD, and the pathologist's role in intraoperative management, have changed significantly over the past two decades. Most of these changes are due to technical innovations in diagnostic imaging, advances in image-guided needle biopsies, changes in surgical management, and advances in medical treatment. The following examples will illustrate these points.

The widespread use of screening mammography, and the shift to tissue-conserving surgery for malignancies, have resulted in a dramatic change in the surgical approach to diseases of the breast. Fine-needle aspiration biopsy (FNA) of palpable lumps and image-directed needle core biopsies are now the favored ways to make an initial diagnosis, and as a result, non-guided open breast biopsies, once the most frequent specimen submitted for frozen section evaluation,[2–4] are now encountered only infrequently.

Similarly, the need for an initial diagnosis by frozen section (FS) has decreased with the widespread use of endoscopic biopsies and image-directed needle biopsies. These procedures frequently yield a tissue or cytologic diagnosis pre-operatively, allowing the surgeon to plan definitive surgery with a firm diagnosis in hand. The resected specimen may be sent for intraoperative evaluation of surgical margins, but not necessarily for diagnosis.

Newer approaches to surgical management, including tissue-conserving surgery, have changed the types of specimens submitted for intraoperative evaluation. Lumpectomies of the breast are now more common than mastectomies, and limb sparing surgical resections of bone and soft tissue malignancies are more common than amputations.

Advances in medical treatment have virtually eliminated some types of surgical procedures. As an example, vagotomy, pyloroplasty, and gastric resections are rarely used to treat peptic ulcers because of the efficacy of anti-microbials, H_2-receptor antagonists and proton pump inhibitors. Consequently, gastric resections for peptic ulcer disease are rarely encountered in modern-day practice.

The pathologist's role in intraoperative management will continue to change as newer approaches to diagnosis and treatment are developed, and it is inevitable that some of the statements made in this book will become dated with time.

DIFFERENCES IN THE USE OF INTRAOPERATIVE DIAGNOSIS

The Mayo Clinic has a unique approach to IOD.[5] Frozen sections are performed on the majority of surgical specimens, and a pathology report is usually available when

Intraoperative Consultation in Surgical Pathology, ed. Mahendra Ranchod. Published by Cambridge University Press.
© Cambridge University Press 2010.

the patient is in the recovery room. This allows for efficient triaging of patient care and is suited to the philosophy of the Mayo Clinic. At virtually all other institutions, IOCs are requested selectively, and they account for approximately 5%–6% of surgical pathology accessions.[6,7] There is a great deal of variation in the utilization of IOC but the common thread is that the test is ordered selectively. This book is written for pathologists who are called upon to render intraoperative diagnoses in selected situations.

INDICATIONS FOR INTRAOPERATIVE DIAGNOSIS

The purpose of IOD is to provide pathologic information that will help the surgeon perform the appropriate surgical procedure as efficiently as possible. The indications for IOD are thus driven by the surgeon's needs. Occasionally there is discordance between what the surgeon would *like* to know and what the surgeon *needs* to know to execute optimal surgical treatment, a situation that may be challenging or frustrating, but one that an experienced pathologist should be able to handle. When performed selectively, there are five main indications for IOD.

1. To establish or confirm a diagnosis that will influence the surgical procedure. Requests for this indication have diminished with the availability of endoscopic procedures and image-directed needle biopsies, but there are still situations when open biopsy or resection are required for initial diagnosis. These include failure to obtain a diagnosis with less invasive methods (e.g., a non-diagnostic FNA of a pulmonary nodule), or when percutaneous needle biopsy is contraindicated (e.g., evaluation of a potentially malignant ovarian mass).

In the College of American Pathologists (CAP) Q-probe study published in 1996,[8] IOD directly influenced the nature of the surgical procedure in approximately 30% of cases. However, IOD is of value even when it does not alter the surgical procedure because it allows the surgeon to undertake a planned surgical procedure with greater conviction.

2. To evaluate margins of resection. When malignant neoplasms are treated by surgical resection, the goal is to remove the neoplasm with adequate clear margins. Requests for evaluation of surgical margins are almost as frequent as requests for initial diagnosis in some series.[9] See "Evaluation of surgical margins" below.

3. To determine the adequacy of an incisional biopsy specimen when the only purpose of the surgical procedure is to obtain tissue for diagnosis, e.g., incisional biopsy of a suspected sarcoma of soft tissue or bone. There are two issues to keep in mind when handling these biopsies: First, if FS is the test of choice, should the entire specimen be submitted for FS or should part of the specimen be spared from potential freezing artifact? This decision depends on the size of the specimen and the surgeon's ability and willingness to obtain more tissue for permanent sections, a question that is easily settled by direct communication with the surgeon. The second issue is to distinguish between *abnormal* tissue and *lesional* tissue. The surgeon's initial biopsy may be from reactive tissue surrounding the target lesion, introducing a risk that the pathologist may interpret these secondary changes as the primary disease. Familiarity with the clinical and imaging data, and discussion with the surgeon, can help to avert this error.

4. To stage malignant neoplasms intraoperatively. Most neoplasms can be successfully staged with diagnostic imaging, but there are situations when surgical staging is necessary to deliver optimal care. There are two main clinical scenarios: In the first situation, FS diagnosis will invoke the "stopping rule," i.e., definitive surgical resection is abandoned because the neoplasm has extended beyond the boundaries of resection; for example, a Whipple's procedure for pancreatic carcinoma will be abandoned if FS confirms the presence of peritoneal metastases. The second is the "go ahead rule." In this situation, IOD gives the surgeon permission to proceed with more extensive surgery; as an example, the surgeon will proceed with surgical staging if a diagnosis of primary carcinoma is rendered on an ovarian mass.*

---

* To the best of my knowledge, the terms "stopping rule," "go ahead rule," and "good enough diagnosis" were coined by Dr. Michael Hendrickson, Department of Pathology, Stanford University School of Medicine.

5. To procure fresh tissue for ancillary studies, such as microbiology, flow cytometry, cytogenetics, molecular diagnostic tests, electron microscopy, and research protocols.

EVALUATION OF SURGICAL MARGINS

Surgical resection is the treatment of choice for many malignant neoplasms, and when the tumor is resectable, the goal is to remove the neoplasm with adequate clear margins. The definition of an adequate margin depends on a variety of factors, including type of neoplasm, stage of disease, anatomic location, and proximity of the tumor to vital structures. The definition of an adequate margin is based on empirical data but there is also an element of arbitrariness, so that an adequate margin may range from 1 mm to 2–3 cm. There is also an increasing realization that, for some malignancies, narrow margins of excision are as good as wide margins.

The only reliable way to evaluate the adequacy of resection is to ink the surgical margins of the specimen, and with more than one color if this will help to localize a positive margin. Inking is best done with a Q-tip, and when the surface area is large, with a cluster of Q-tips or with a small brush. The specimen should not be dipped into a container of ink because this will allow the ink to seep into crevices on the surface of the specimen. Metal staples should be removed before inking because they may be masked by the ink and interfere with sectioning the specimen. Inking is not always as straightforward as one would like to believe. Sometimes, the margins are irregular, making it difficult to decide where to apply the ink. Irregular surfaces occur either because of the nature of the surgical resection (e.g., blunt dissection in partial hepatectomy), the friable nature of the surface tissue (e.g., fatty lumpectomy specimens of the breast) or because the surgeon has created more than one plane of dissection, resulting in flaps of tissue at the margins of the specimen.

A variety of factors determine how well the ink will adhere to the tissue. Ink will not adhere well to desiccated tissue, and the effectiveness of inking will be reduced if the surface is not well dried prior to inking. Adhesion of ink to tissue can be improved by spraying the inked surface with a mordant such as Bouin's solution or dilute acetic acid (white vinegar), but this should be done only after the ink has dried.

There are two main approaches to evaluating surgical margins in complex resections. In the first approach, the pathologist selects tissue from the margins of the excised specimen, whereas in the second approach, the surgeon submits biopsies from the resection bed after definitive excision. The advantage of the latter approach is that the surgeon samples the margins of concern; when these biopsies are small, the entire specimen is embedded for FS so that tumor anywhere in the specimen is interpreted as a positive margin.

Sometimes, the orientation of a specimen is obvious and does not require any specific labeling, e.g., an esophago-gastrectomy. However, when orientation is necessary, the surgeon should submit the specimen with a sketch and/or mark the specimen with sutures. If the orientation is ambiguous, clarification should be obtained before inking and dissecting/sectioning the specimen. If sutures are used for orientation, the surgeon should place them with a loose loop to facilitate easy removal (see Chapter 4, p. 53). Specimens that have been oriented should be marked with at least two colors of ink, and more than two if this will localize a positive margin more precisely (see Chapter 3, p. 27).

When the pathologist samples the margins on an excision specimen, sections can be taken perpendicular or parallel to the margins. The method chosen depends on the type of specimen, the size and shape of the specimen, the type of neoplasm, the distance of the neoplasm from the surgical margin as judged by gross examination, and whether the surgeon is interested in the distance of tumor from the margin. Sections taken parallel to the margin (*en face*) allow for more thorough evaluation, but if the margin is negative, it may not be possible to obtain an accurate measurement of the distance of the tumor from that margin. In contrast, the width of a clear margin can be measured when sections are taken perpendicular to that margin. The latter approach results in partial evaluation of the margin, but thorough sampling and cutting levels into the FS block/s can reduce the risk of false-negative results. As a general guide, sections taken parallel to the margin work well when the neoplasm appears distant from the margin by gross examination (>1–2 cm depending on the anatomic site), whereas sections taken vertical to the margin are preferable when the malignancy is close to the margin by gross examination, e.g., <1 cm from the margin.

When tissue is re-excised from a positive margin, the new margin should be carefully inked to retain orientation during handling. If the re-excised tissue is >5 mm wide, my preference is to make serial sections perpendicular to the new margin, but if the re-excised tissue is a narrow strip <3 mm wide, the entire specimen should be embedded on edge, with the new margin deep in the block.* Sections are thus cut toward the new margin.

Most tissues, especially those that contain muscle, will contract after surgical removal, a phenomenon that is especially noticeable in hollow muscular organs such as esophagus and intestine. This contraction results in a discrepancy between the surgeon's impression of the length of the surgical margin and the pathologist's measurements. As shown by Goldstein et al., the margin in colorectal specimens can shrink to 60% of its in vivo length within 20 minutes of devascularizing the colon.[10] This is important when there are constraints on removing additional normal tissue, as in resections of the esophagus and rectum. Similar discrepancies between in vivo and in vitro measurements have also been reported for excisions from the oral cavity.[11] There is no way to avoid this problem, but the surgeon's measurements naturally take precedence if this comes up for discussion.

Clear margins are not synonymous with adequate margins, and the pathologist should be prepared to report the distance of tumor from the margin if the surgeon is interested in the extent of margin clearance. The width of a margin can be estimated accurately enough by using the diameter of the objectives of a microscope; for example, the diameters of the 2× and 10× objectives of the Olympus BX41 microscope are 10 mm and 2 mm, respectively.

When margins are evaluated with parallel sections, care should be taken to line up all the tissue layers before sampling the margin because some layers retract more than others, leading to incomplete evaluation if the sample is not collected with care; as an example, the mucosa in the upper aerodigestive tract has a tendency to retract from the margin so the sample selected for FS may not include mucosa and lamina propria, tissue layers that are very important to evaluate in resection specimens.

The issue of adequate margins is more complex than is apparent at first glance. One puzzling finding is the absence of residual malignancy in re-excised tissue following a positive margin. When re-excision is delayed, the absence of residual tumor can be explained by tumor ablation as a result of wound healing,[12] but how is the absence of residual carcinoma explained when re-excision is immediate? The corollary is also true: local recurrences may occur after seemingly adequate excision. Some explanations for local recurrence after negative margins are: (a) the reported negative margin was an interpretative error, and the margin was in fact positive; (b) the tumor is multifocal but its multifocality was not appreciated at the time of resection; and (c) the "recurrence" is a new neoplasm that arose in tissue that was normal by conventional histologic examination but abnormal by molecular analysis, and therefore capable of spawning a new malignancy (see Fig. 4.3, p. 46).[12]

Part of the problem with conventional FS evaluation of margins is that histologic sections employ a two-dimensional approach to evaluate lesions that have three dimensions. False-negative margins are more likely when neoplasms have a highly infiltrating pattern of growth and if the leading edge of the tumor happens to be in a plane different from the plane of the histologic sections. Wider margins of resection are therefore necessary for malignancies with an infiltrative pattern of growth. One way to reduce false-negative diagnoses is to prepare more than one FS block when appropriate, and to cut multiple levels when evaluating a malignancy with an infiltrative pattern of growth.

Every attempt should be made to evaluate surgical margins thoroughly during surgery; this includes adequate sampling of the margins, and when appropriate, cutting multiple levels into the block(s). The findings in deeper levels of the same FS block can sometimes be startlingly different, especially for malignancies with an infiltrative pattern of growth. There is no rational argument for intentionally saving tissue for permanent sections if evaluation of the margins is critical to immediate surgical care. The surgeon is interested in having the correct information *during* surgery, not the following day. The reversal of a FS diagnosis from negative to positive margins may require a second surgical procedure, which is unfair to the patient if this could have been averted by more thorough examination intraoperatively.

Sometimes, it is difficult to distinguish a positive margin from a reactive process, particularly with mesenchymal neoplasms such as desmoid fibromatosis, paucicellular dermatofibrosarcoma protuberans and some low-grade

---

* Some pathologists prefer to embed the tissue with the new margin closest to the surface of the block, in which case, the first section represents the true surgical margin. I prefer to embed the tissue with the true margin deep in the FS block for the following reasons: (a) The true margin is still available for evaluation if technical problems are encountered when facing the block; and (b) cutting towards the true margin allows one to determine if any tumor is present in the 3mm thick sample selected for FS, information that may be useful to the surgeon.

sarcomas. This distinction is particularly difficult if the tissue at the margins includes a fibroblastic reaction to previous surgery, leaving the pathologist no option but to defer interpretation of the margins to permanent sections.

Mohs micrographic surgery makes an attempt to evaluate all the surgical margins in a specimen by using a different approach to embedding and sectioning tissue (see Fig. 3.7, p. 29). The Mohs technique is applied mainly to cutaneous malignancies and is especially useful for complex cutaneous malignancies, previously excised malignancies with positive margins, recurrent malignancies, and when tissue conservation is at a premium. Mohs surgery is not subject to the same time constraints as conventional FS; after the first stage has been performed, the patient may leave the surgical suite with an open wound, and because the procedure is performed under local anesthesia, the second stage can be performed later that day after FS results are available. The time between different stages of excision allows the Mohs surgeon to order rapid special stains, including rapid immunohisto-chemical stains, if needed.

UNNECESSARY AND INAPPROPRIATE REQUESTS FOR FROZEN SECTION DIAGNOSIS

Every pathologist encounters unnecessary and inappropriate requests for IOD. *Unnecessary requests* for IOD are those that have no bearing on immediate management. In the study by Weiss et al.,[9] 5% of IODs were considered unnecessary or ambiguous, and this number is probably higher in most hospitals. Sometimes, FS is requested for reasons other than immediate surgical management, and what may appear to be an unnecessary FS can be justified on *non-surgical* grounds. For example, a FS may be ordered to expedite post-operative care, or facilitate post-operative discussion with an anxious patient or family.[8] Sometimes, however, a FS is requested to satisfy the surgeon's curiosity or for reasons that are not clear.[13] We probably all perform unnecessary FSs on occasion but four criteria should be met: (a) There is no risk of compromising the specimen; (b) the specimen has to be sufficient for routine examination as well as all possible ancillary studies; (c) there is a reasonable chance of making a meaningful diagnosis; and (d) there is little risk of providing misleading information. The pathologist should not hesitate to advise the surgeon against

intraoperative evaluation if the test has nothing to offer. There is no reason, for example, to perform random FSs on a diagnostic J-wire directed breast biopsy that lacks a focal lesion. One way to handle requests for unnecessary FS is to re-formulate the request: the surgeon who asks for a FS diagnosis may not want or need the specificity of a FS diagnosis, and gross examination alone may suffice. For example, if FS is requested on a radical orchiectomy specimen, gross examination is usually sufficient to confirm the presence of a malignant neoplasm.

Requests for FS are *inappropriate* when IOD will have no influence on surgical management *and* there is a significant risk of compromising the specimen because of its small size. In this situation, the pathologist should convince the surgeon that nothing will be gained and much may be lost by subjecting the specimen to the artifacts of freezing. If the surgeon is unyielding in her demand, touch or squash cytology preparations may be prepared, as these could yield a good enough diagnosis, thus achieving the dual goals of appeasing the surgeon and preserving the specimen for permanent sections.

THE IMPORTANCE OF CLINICO-PATHOLOGIC CORRELATION

Every surgical pathologist understands the importance of clinico-pathologic correlation. One of the challenges of IOD is the frequent lack of adequate clinical information, a situation that can lead to serious errors. The best approach is to gather relevant clinical information by whatever means necessary, and to be adequately armed before the specimen is submitted for IOD. Failure to do this places the patient at risk and contributes towards tarnishing the pathologist's reputation. In a multi-institutional study by Zarbo et al.,[7] nearly 15% of diagnostic errors were due to lack of familiarity with the clinical history. Both surgeons and pathologists contribute to this unfortunate situation.

Surgeons order clinical laboratory tests without providing clinical information, and it is wrongly assumed that tissue submitted for IOD can be handled in the same way. Sometimes surgeons innocently withhold clinical information, not realizing that this may be crucial for pathologic interpretation. At other times, the surgeon may be focused on the technical challenges of the case and not be fully informed of clinical details that are of interest to the pathologist. Good communication between pathologist and surgeon will limit the impact of these lapses.

A detailed clinical history is not always necessary to render an accurate IOD, and this very fact may lull the pathologist into complacency about the value of clinical data. At many teaching institutions, pathologists or pathologists-in-training routinely pick up specimens from the operating room, allowing familiarity with all aspects of the case before handling the specimen. In the majority of non-teaching hospitals however, specimens are delivered to the laboratory by courier or a mechanical delivery system, and clinical information is limited to what is provided on the pathology requisition form. Pathologists who work under these conditions recognize the fallibility of the system and develop alternative avenues for obtaining clinical information. A quick check of the hospital's electronic information system, and a search for prior pathology reports are helpful first steps. In complex cases, or when the electronic record is deficient, the clinical history should be solicited directly from the surgeon as this may bring about perspectives on the case that cannot be acquired in any other way.

Some types of lesions require correlation with imaging studies. Reading the radiologist's report is often sufficient, but there are situations when it is preferable to review the imaging studies with a radiologist or the surgeon, especially in anatomic locations such as bone, central nervous system and mediastinum. There are situations where serious errors can be made if imaging studies are ignored (see Chapters 6, 17 and 19, on pp. 78, 266, and 306).

There are occasions when it is essential for the pathologist to check on the real-time surgical findings because the surgeon may not volunteer crucial information at the time that the first specimen is submitted for IOD. For example, a mucinous carcinoma of the ovary is more likely to be a metastasis if the malignancy involves both ovaries and other intra-abdominal sites; similarly, carcinoid tumor of the ovary is much more likely to be metastatic if both ovaries are involved. In these two situations, knowledge of the surgical findings should prompt the pathologist to recommend a search for a non-ovarian primary.

Many medical centers require institutional review of outside pathology slides prior to a major surgical procedure. Unfortunately, this practice is not universal so pathologists have to sometimes handle major resection specimens without the benefit of reviewing prior biopsy material. This lack of information places an added burden on the pathologist on FS duty.

It is important to know what is at stake in a particular case, and special attention should be given to high stake cases. This requires full awareness of the clinical issues,

familiarity with relevant imaging and laboratory data, and familiarity with the surgeon's algorithm. When a definitive diagnosis is not possible in a high stake situation, the pathologist should visit the operating room, apprise the surgeon of the problem, and participate in making the best decision for immediate patient care.

LIMITATIONS OF INTRAOPERATIVE DIAGNOSIS

Intraoperative diagnosis often has the specificity of permanent sections, but a definite diagnosis cannot be made in every case. There are good reasons for these limitations:

- Problems may occur when an incisional biopsy is not representative of the lesion. As an example, we encountered an incisional biopsy of an anterior mediastinal mass that showed benign thymic cysts on FS. The pathologist was about to render a diagnosis of benign thymic cyst but was encouraged to first review the chest CT in the operating room, at which time it became clear that the surgeon had sampled the cystic component of a malignant neoplasm. A second biopsy was requested and this showed Hodgkin's lymphoma (Fig. 1.1). It is unlikely that the surgeon would have accepted a diagnosis of benign thymic cyst in this particular case, but failure to review the images, and rendering a diagnosis of benign thymic cyst, may have led the surgeon to conclude that the pathologist did not know how to recognize an obvious malignancy.

- Only a limited number of FS blocks can be prepared on large mass lesions so there is a risk of sampling an area that provides misleading or incomplete information. For example, primary mucinous carcinoma of the ovary may contain a spectrum of changes, including benign-appearing areas, and sampling the wrong area may lead to an incorrect diagnosis. Sampling errors can be minimized by careful gross examination, use of cytoscrape preparations to sample a larger surface area, and careful selection of tissue for FS. This situation underscores the reason why skilled gross examination is so important in the intraoperative arena.

- Some lesions are not amenable to IOD because the diagnosis hinges on focal changes that are identified only after thorough sampling. Minimally invasive follicular carcinoma of the thyroid gland is a case in

(a)

(b)

(c)

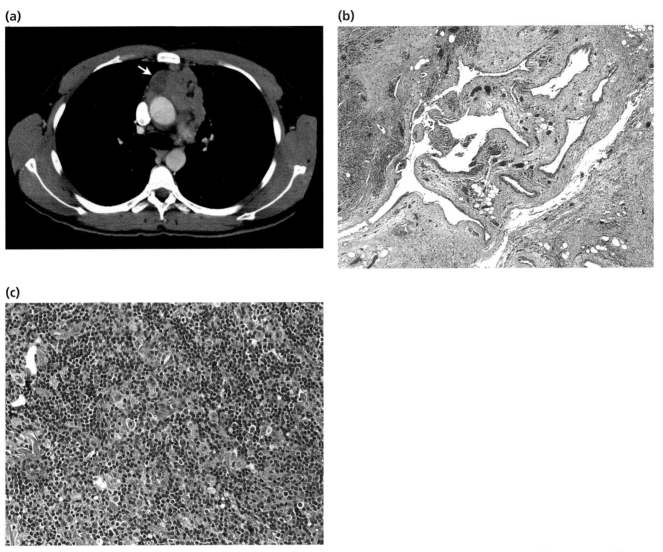

Fig. 1.1. (a) A 33-year-old man with a large anterior mediastinal mass. The surgeon performed an incisional biopsy of the most accessible portion of the lesion, and this happened to be cystic (arrow). (b) The initial FS showed benign thymic cysts. (c) Because the findings on CT scan are those of a malignant neoplasm, a second biopsy was requested and this showed Hodgkin's lymphoma. It is well known that malignancies such as Hodgkin's lymphoma and seminoma evoke the formation of epithelial lined cysts when they involve the thymus gland.

point; capsular and/or vascular invasion are required to make this diagnosis, and it is unlikely that a single FS will detect these changes. Because of the low diagnostic yield, it has been proposed that microscopic examination of an encapsulated solitary thyroid nodule should be deferred to permanent sections (see Chapter 11, p. 168).

- Some neoplasms, including lymphomas, small round cell malignancies of soft tissue and bone, and a variety of neoplasms in other anatomic sites, require ancillary studies for a specific diagnosis, and as a result, only a limited diagnosis can be offered intraoperatively. The pathologist's task is simplified if this limitation is accepted, and if it is understood that all the surgeon needs is a "good enough diagnosis" to facilitate immediate surgical management (see "Good enough diagnosis" below).

THE CONCEPT OF A "GOOD ENOUGH DIAGNOSIS"

Pathologists are programmed to make specific diagnoses, but this is not always possible, nor is it always necessary in the intraoperative setting. Surgical pathologists function on two planes, the scientific and the managerial,[14] and this concept can be modified for the intraoperative setting by positing that a specific diagnosis should be rendered whenever possible, but what the surgeon needs is a "good enough" diagnosis in order to perform the appropriate surgical procedure. For example, when a diagnostic wedge biopsy is performed for a solitary pulmonary nodule, the surgeon's main question is whether the lesion is benign or malignant, and if malignant, if it should resected by lobectomy. If the FS shows a primary, poorly differentiated non-small cell carcinoma, there is no reason to spend an undue amount of time searching for squamous or glandular differentiation, because lobectomy is appropriate regardless of the tumor's differentiation. A diagnosis of "poorly differentiated non-small cell carcinoma, consistent with primary lung carcinoma" is good enough for the purpose of immediate surgical management.

COMMUNICATION DURING INTRAOPERATIVE CONSULTATION

Clear, concise, and skillful communication is essential in the intraoperative setting. Communication is simple when the diagnosis is straightforward, but more challenging when the case is complicated, or when the pathologist is unable to make a definite diagnosis. Pathologists vary in their ability to communicate effectively, but everyone can learn the principles of good communication. The following guidelines should be kept in mind.

- The surgeon is interested in information that will influence immediate surgical management, and she is unlikely to be impressed by histologic details that are of interest to the pathologist, but have no bearing on surgical management. Pathologic information should therefore, be distilled into clinically meaningful information.
- When a firm diagnosis cannot be made, the pathologist should be prepared to discuss management options with the surgeon, because the pathologist is the only person on the management team who understands why a specific diagnosis cannot be made, and who is able to offer a managerial diagnosis. For example, if a thyroid lobectomy specimen contains a neoplasm of uncertain nature, a recommendation could be made to perform no more than a lobectomy, and to wait for permanent sections.

- The way in which the communication is made will naturally depend on a variety of factors, including the complexity of the case, proximity of the frozen section suite to the operating room, communication facilities available, and traditions of the institution. Straightforward diagnoses can be transmitted by telephone or intercom, but there is no substitute for a visit to the operating room when that becomes necessary. Here are a few reasons to visit to the operating room: (a) It allows the pathologist to gather clinical information that may not have been forthcoming prior to surgery; (b) It allows review of diagnostic images that were not available pre-operatively, e.g., images of a bone lesion from another facility; (c) The pathologist can receive an update on the surgical findings when these are different from the surgeon's pre-operative assessment; (d) It allows face-to-face conversation with the surgeon when the diagnosis has to be deferred; (e) Sometimes a visit to the operating room is the only way to obtain a full grasp of the case, and errors are more likely if the pathologist chooses a less direct form of communication. There is one other point: failure to visit the operating room may be interpreted by the surgeon as unwillingness on the part of the pathologist to fully engage in the care of the patient. In my opinion, a pathologist who is unfamiliar with the clinical aspects of a case, and who is reluctant to visit the operating room when the situation calls for direct communication with the surgeon, has failed to discharge his duties as a consultant.

TURN-AROUND TIME OF INTRAOPERATIVE DIAGNOSES

The turn-around time (TAT) for intraoperative diagnosis depends on the test that is performed, the amount of dissection and preparation required, the complexity of the case, and the experience of the pathologist. In a CAP Q-Probe study, the result of a single frozen section was reported within 20 minutes in 90% of cases,[15] and when multiple FSs are performed on a single specimen, each of the additional FSs should take less than 20 minutes. Cytologic preparations (touch, cytoscrape and squash) often take less than 20 minutes, and gross examination can usually be completed within 10–15 minutes of receiving the specimen in the laboratory.

The turn-around time will be longer when there are multiple simultaneous requests for IOD that exceed the laboratory's capacity, or when there are technical problems in obtaining good-quality frozen sections. Delays will also occur in complicated cases that require additional study or when prior biopsy slides have to be reviewed at short notice. I think it is courteous to call the surgeon on the telephone or intercom when there is going to be a delay, with a brief explanation for the delay. Keep in mind that the surgeon is not privy to the goings-on in the frozen section laboratory, and the simple act of making a telephone call may forestall anxiety and irritation that may come from unexplained delays.

Many pathology departments record the arrival of the specimen in the laboratory and the time that the diagnosis is reported to the surgeon. Turn around time for IOD should be recorded if it is required by the institution, and these data should be included in the department's QA report.

DOCUMENTING INTRAOPERATIVE ACTIVITIES

The pathologist who initially handles a fresh specimen for IOD should accurately document the characteristics of the specimen, as well as record the way the specimen was handled, because some gross characteristics are markedly altered after dissection or sectioning, and cannot be reconstructed later. This documentation should be more detailed if the specimen will be "grossed in" by someone else. The following points should be recorded routinely:

- A note should be made if the specimen was received and handled differently from the usual, e.g., if the specimen was received in a sterile container and was initially handled in a sterile fashion.
- The specimen should be weighed when appropriate, and measurements should be recorded in three dimensions. The size and weight of some specimens can change dramatically, e.g., a cystic ovarian neoplasm, so size and weight should be documented before the specimen is sectioned. The weight and/or volume should be recorded for specimens that are received in multiple small pieces.
- It is helpful, and sometimes necessary, to draw a sketch of specimens such as skin and resections of the upper aerodigestive tract submitted for evaluation of margins, as this may be the simplest way to record the way a specimen was inked and sectioned.
- A note should be made if tissue was procured for ancillary studies such as culture, chromosome analysis, flow cytometry, electron microscopy, research etc. and this should include the volume or size of that sample.
- A note should be made of the intraoperative procedures that were performed, e.g., gross examination only, FS, cytologic examination or some combination of these.
- The written version of the IOD should faithfully reflect the verbal communication with the surgeon, and should include any recommendations that were made.
- A note should be made if photographs of the specimen were taken in the fresh state.

There are two main ways to document the real-time intraoperative diagnosis. The first is to have a separate "Intraoperative Diagnosis Requisition/Report Form" that is completed at the time of IOD. This written report is delivered to the operating room immediately after the verbal report has been transmitted, and becomes part of the patient's medical record.[16] This report can be delivered by courier or fax, and, in the future, will no doubt be transmitted electronically. In the second approach, the gross findings and diagnosis are recorded on the pathology requisition form or a separate "Intraoperative Diagnosis Report Form" that is for internal use in the pathology department. The advantage of the first approach is that the surgeon receives a real-time written report, minimizing potential misunderstanding of the pathologist's verbal communication.

ACCURACY OF INTRAOPERATIVE DIAGNOSIS

Intraoperative diagnoses cannot always be as accurate as final diagnoses given the limitations of sampling, time constraints, technical challenges, inability to perform ancillary tests, and restricted access to other opinions. As a result, the diagnosis has to be deferred in a proportion of cases ($<5\%$ in most studies).[4,7,13,17,18] When deferred diagnoses are excluded, intraoperative diagnosis is surprisingly accurate, no doubt because most diagnoses in surgical pathology can be made on H&E stained preparations. Interestingly, the accuracy rates are similar for small hospitals and large hospitals.[7,17] However, errors do occur, and the error rate is $<2\%$ in most series.[4,6,7,13,17,18] Approximately one-third of the discrepancies between IOD and final diagnoses are due to errors in sampling the tissue specimen, one-third to inadequate sectioning of the tissue in the FS block/s, and the remaining one-third are interpretive errors.[6,17] The following guidelines can reduce sampling errors:

- Not enough can be said about the importance of careful gross examination and judicious selection of tissue for IOD. Skilled intraoperative gross examination requires an understanding of the histologic correlates of gross pathology, as well as insight of their significance for immediate surgical management.
- The tissue in the FS block should be adequately sampled. The pathologist who interprets frozen sections should be aware of the amount of tissue in the FS block, and check that the volume of tissue on the slide matches the tissue in the block. This is particularly important when the pathologist who interprets FS slides is different from the person who prepares the FS block, a situation that is common when pathology assistants and histotechnologists assist in the frozen section suite.
- Seasoned pathologists are familiar with the power of examining multiple levels. Multiple levels should be prepared when evaluating high stake biopsies, when the diagnosis is not evident on the first section, when the initial FS slide is suboptimal, when there are disparities between the FS and gross findings, and when evaluating surgical margins in malignancies with an infiltrative pattern of growth.

Approximately 30% of the errors in the 1996 CAP Q-probe studies were interpretive errors.[6,17] For neoplastic disease, false-negative errors (malignancies interpreted as benign) are more frequent than false-positive diagnoses; false-positive diagnoses (benign lesions interpreted as malignant) constitute <1% of the errors.[7] Interpretive errors can be reduced by careful clinico-pathologic correlation and by seeking other opinions when there is uncertainty.

The accuracy rate of IOD has been relatively constant over the past few decades in spite of significant changes in the types of specimens submitted for IOD. This relatively steady rate however, masks the fact that deferral rates are much higher for some types of specimens, but they go unnoticed if they constitute a minority of the cases accessioned (e.g., small volume of pediatric cases in a general hospital). This higher deferral rate however, becomes apparent in selected series, and as pointed out by Coffin et al., error rates (4%) and deferral rates (25%) are higher in pediatric and adolescent populations because of the nature of the specimens encountered in a Children's Hospital.[19]

Two guidelines should be used when evaluating the accuracy of IOD in departmental QA programs: (a) A "good enough diagnosis" should be considered a correct diagnosis when a limited interpretation is all that can be reasonably offered; and (b) the intraoperative diagnosis should be compared to the most specific diagnosis that can be made on H&E stained, paraffin-embedded tissue sections, and not with the final diagnosis, whose specificity relies on ancillary studies such as immunohistochemistry or flow cytometry. When these criteria are applied to the data of Coffin et al., approximately 95% of the deferred diagnoses were appropriate.

QUALITY CONTROL AND QUALITY ASSURANCE

Quality control refers to a process that ensures the highest degree of accuracy and efficiency in the real-time delivery of intraoperative diagnoses, whereas quality assurance refers to a retrospective review of the accuracy of IOD. The two processes are closely related.

Quality control

There are multiple steps between procuring a specimen for intraoperative evaluation and reporting the results to the surgeon. Some of these steps are within the immediate control of the pathologist and others are not, but the pathologist is ultimately responsible for ensuring that the entire process functions smoothly. Pathologists are dependent on the co-operation of the staff in the operating room and the laboratory, and it pays to have periodic educational meetings to reinforce the principles and fine points of specimen handling. Every step is important for a satisfactory outcome, and each participant should understand the importance of her role.

Quality assurance

Intraoperative consultation should be included in every department's quality assurance program. This review can be done monthly or quarterly, depending on the volume of cases. The CAP's multi-institutional Q-Tracks program has shown that regular monitoring of frozen section diagnoses results in improved performance.[20] Only a few points regarding QA will be discussed here.

- Intraoperative diagnoses should be compared with final diagnoses, and for analysis, frozen sections, cytologic examination and gross examination, either alone or in combination, should carry equal weight.
- The original FS slides, cytologic preparations and permanent sections should be reviewed in all cases where the diagnosis was deferred, and all cases where there is a discrepancy between the IOD and final diagnosis.
- As recommended by the Association of Directors of Anatomic and Surgical Pathology (ADASP), deferred diagnoses should be categorized as appropriate and inappropriate, and disagreements between the IOD and final diagnosis should be categorized as minor (with no effect on patient care) and major (with potential adverse outcome).[21] Cases with potential adverse clinical outcome should be evaluated in more detail to see if the error did in fact have an adverse effect on patient care. There is naturally an element of subjectivity in deciding if a deferral is appropriate or not, and whether sampling and interpretive errors are within the standard of care, but these issues can be resolved at departmental QA meetings. Each department should establish acceptable percentages for deferral and errors rates. The ADASP has recommended thresholds of 10% and 5% for deferred diagnoses and discrepancies, respectively[21] and while these percentages are higher than reported in the CAP's multi-institutional Q-probe study (4.2% and 1.7%, respectively),[7] these two sets of data points can be used as guidelines for establishing departmental thresholds.
- It may be useful to categorize deferrals and discrepancies for purposes of analysis. For example, pediatric and adolescent cases could be a separate category because of the higher expected deferral rate. Similarly, IODs on sentinel lymph nodes for breast cancer should be analyzed separately, and these can in turn be divided into sub-categories based on the size of the metastasis; it is obvious that a missed macro-metastasis should be judged differently from a lymph node containing isolated tumor cells detected only by immunohistochemistry.

TELEPATHOLOGY

Robotic telepathology has matured to a level where it can be confidently used for IOD. High-quality resolution, rapid transmission of images, and remote control of the microscope allow for levels of accuracy and convenience similar to viewing the original frozen section slides.[22,23] Telepathology is particularly useful when an opinion is required from a pathologist in a different physical location, as well as for pathologists in training who need support from faculty at night and weekends.

MEDICO-LEGAL ISSUES

As with final diagnoses, errors in the intraoperative arena may lead to litigation. However, it is rare for errors in IOD to reach the stage of litigation and this is probably because: (a) errors are infrequent and only a minority of errors have an adverse effect on patient care;[7] (b) false positive diagnoses for malignancy, where the greatest harm can be done, are rare; (c) the surgeon may not act on an erroneous diagnosis if this is in conflict with the clinical situation; (d) the planned surgical procedure is such that IOD does not significantly affect the extent of surgical resection and; (e) there is an acceptance that IOD has limitations and may not carry the same level of certainty as a final diagnosis.

ACKNOWLEDGMENT

The author would like to thank Ms. Anet James, Digital Imaging Specialist/Photographer, Department of Pathology at Stanford University School of Medicine, for her expert help with the images in Chapters 1, 2, 3, 7, 11, 12, 13, and 16.

REFERENCES

1. Silva EG, Kraemer BB. *Intraoperative Pathologic Diagnosis. Frozen Section and Other Techniques.* Baltimore: Williams & Wilkins, 1987.
2. Ackerman LV, Ramirez GA. The indications for and limitations of frozen section diagnosis. *Brit J Surg* 1959; **46**: 336–350.
3. Nakazawa H, Rosen P, Lane N, Lattes R. Frozen section experience in 3000 cases. *Am J Clin Pathol* 1968; **49**: 41–51.
4. Rogers C, Klatt EC, Chandrasoma P. Accuracy of frozen-section diagnosis in a teaching hospital. *Arch Pathol Lab Med* 1987; **111**: 514–517.
5. Ferreiro JA, Myers JL, Bostwick DG. Accuracy of frozen section diagnoses in surgical pathology: review of a 1-year experience with

24,880 cases at Mayo Clinic Rochester. *Mayo Clin Proc* 1995; **70**: 1137–1141.

6. Gephardt GN, Zarbo RJ. Interinstitutional comparison of frozen section consultations. *Arch Pathol Lab Med* 1996; **120**: 804–809.

7. Zarbo RJ, Hoffman GG, Howanitz PJ. Interinstitutional comparison of frozen–section consultation. *Arch Pathol Lab Med* 1991; **115**: 1187–1194.

8. Zarbo RJ, Schmidt WA, Bachner P *et al.* Indications and immediate patient outcomes of pathology intraoperative consultations. *Arch Path Lab Med* 1996; **120**: 19–25.

9. Weiss SW, Willis J, Jansen J *et al.* Frozen section consultation: utilization patterns and knowledge base of surgical faculty at a university hospital. *Am J Clin Pathol* 1995; **104**: 294–298.

10. Goldstein NS, Soman A, Sacksner J. Disparate surgical margin lengths of colorectal resection specimens between in vivo and in vitro measurements. The effects of surgical resection and formalin fixation on organ shrinkage. *Am J Clin Pathol* 1999; **111**: 349–351.

11. Cheng A, Cox D, Schmidt BL. Oral squamous cell carcinoma margin discrepancy after resection and pathologic processing. *J Oral Maxillofacial Surg* 2008; **66**: 523–529.

12. Wick MR, Mills SE. Evaluation of surgical margins in anatomic pathology: Technical, conceptual and clinical considerations. *Sem Diag Pathol* 2002; **19**: 207–218.

13. Dehner LP, Rosai J. Frozen-section examination in surgical pathology. *Minn Med* 1977; **60**: 83–94.

14. Kempson RL, Fletcher CDM, Evans HL, Hendrickson MR, Sibley RK: Tumors of the Soft Tissues. *AFIP Atlas of Tumor Pathology*. 3rd series. Washington DC, 2001.

15. Novis DA, Zarbo RJ. Interinstitutional comparison of frozen section turnaround time. *Arch Pathol Lab Med* 1997; **121**: 559–567.

16. Nakhleh RE, Fitzgibbons PL. *Quality Improvement Manual in Anatomic Pathology.* 2nd edition, Northfield, Illinois. College of American Pathologists, 2002.

17. Novis DA, Gephardt GN, Zarbo RJ. Interinstitutional comparison of frozen section consultation in small hospitals. *Arch Pathol Lab Med* 1996; **120**: 1087–1093.

18. Oneson RH, Minke JA, Silverberg SG. Intraoperative pathologic consultation. *Am J Surg Pathol* 1989; **13**: 237–243.

19. Coffin CM, Spilker K, Zhou H *et al.* Frozen section diagnosis in pediatric surgical pathology. A decade's experience in a children's hospital. *Arch Pathol Lab Med* 2005; **129**: 1619–1625.

20. Raab SS, Tworek JA, Souers R, Zarbo RJ. The value of monitoring frozen section-permanent section correlation data over time. *Arch Pathol Lab Med* 2006; **130**: 337–342.

21. Association of Directors of Anatomic and Surgical Pathology. Recommendations on quality control and quality assurance in anatomic pathology. *Am J Surg Pathol* 1991; 1007–1009.

22. Frierson HF Jr, Galgano MT. Frozen-section diagnosis by wireless telepathology and ultra portable computer: use in pathology resident/faculty consultation. *Human Pathol* 2007 **38**: 1330–1334.

23. Kaplan KJ, Burgess JR, Sandberg GD *et al.* Use of robotic telepathology for frozen-section diagnosis: a retrospective trial of a telepathology system for intraoperative consultation. *Mod Pathol* 2002; **15**: 1197–1204.

2   TECHNICAL ASPECTS OF INTRAOPERATIVE DIAGNOSIS

Mahendra Ranchod

The techniques used for intraoperative diagnosis (IOD) have undergone relatively few changes during the past two decades. Cryostats have improved, cytologic examination is now a standard part of IOD and a limited number of rapid special stains have been adapted for frozen sections. The absence of major changes confirms the enduring value of standard techniques such as gross examination, frozen section, and cytologic preparations for rendering intraoperative diagnoses.

GROSS EXAMINATION

Gross examination is the starting point for every intraoperative test, and it occurs in two settings: (a) when gross examination is the only test performed, and (b) when gross examination is performed in combination with other tests.

Gross examination as the only test

Gross examination by itself is performed in a minority of cases, and in the CAP Q-probe study published in 1996, 7.8% of cases were subjected to gross examination only.[1] As the only test, gross examination is performed mainly on larger specimens. At times, a diagnosis by gross examination is offered with the understanding that the diagnosis is provisional and may change after routine microscopic examination. Two examples will suffice.

1. When a thyroid lobectomy specimen contains a solitary encapsulated nodule, some pathologists limit intraoperative evaluation to gross examination because of the low yield for detecting minimally invasive follicular carcinoma by FS.[2] The surgeon should therefore, understand that a diagnosis of "follicular neoplasm" is a preliminary diagnosis (see Chapter 11, p. 168).

2. It is appropriate to use gross examination to evaluate the surgical margins on lumpectomy specimens for invasive mammary carcinoma. However, a diagnosis of "clear margins" will be overturned in 10%–15% of cases after routine histologic examination because of margin involvement by DCIS or invasive carcinoma. Fortunately, most surgeons understand the limitations of intraoperative examination on lumpectomy specimens (see Chapter 13, p. 194).

Gross examination performed in combination with other tests

Regardless of the size of the specimen, gross examination is an essential component in all intraoperative diagnoses for the following reasons:

- It determines whether the specimen should be examined by FS, cytologic examination, or both.
- Gross examination will determine whether the specimen should be inked, and if differential inking is necessary.
- The gross appearance of many lesions is characteristic enough that microscopic examination serves mainly to confirm the provisional diagnosis made on gross examination.
- Gross examination will guide sampling of the specimen for histologic examination. For example, an area of softening and necrosis in a large pleomorphic adenoma of the parotid gland may be a clue to carcinoma-ex pleomorphic adenoma, and this area should be included in the FS sample as it may prompt the surgeon to perform more extensive surgery.
- Gross examination provides the context for interpreting microscopic findings, and experienced pathologists

Intraoperative Consultation in Surgical Pathology, ed. Mahendra Ranchod. Published by Cambridge University Press.
© Cambridge University Press 2010.

(a)   **(b)**

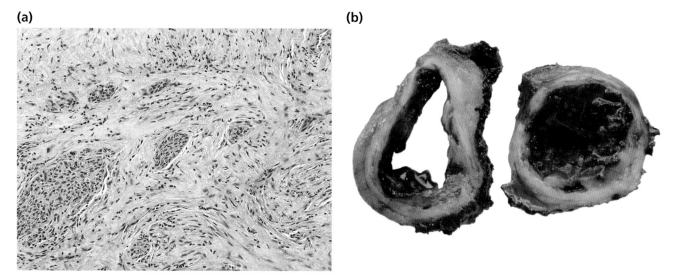

Fig. 2.1. (a) Frozen section of a thyroid lesion showing mildly atypical squamoid cells with an infiltrative pattern. These features raised concern about an unusual thyroid neoplasm when the FS was examined by a pathologist who was unfamiliar with the gross findings. (b) However, the interpretation was promptly revised when the pathologist was informed that the section had been taken from the wall of a large cyst. In the context of a cystic lesion, the spindle cells were interpreted as reactive fibrous tissue and the squamoid cells were correctly interpreted as squamous metaplasia within distorted follicles. This underlines the point that microscopic findings should be correlated with gross pathology.

know the importance of correlating microscopic with gross findings. This point cannot be over-emphasized; it is prudent to re-evaluate the case if there is major discordance between microscopic and gross findings (Fig. 2.1).

■ The gross findings may suggest granulomatous inflammation such as tuberculosis, making cytologic examination preferable to FS, as this will avoid contamination of the work area and exposure of laboratory personnel to an infectious agent.

Additional comments about gross examination

The pathologist who handles a fresh specimen for IOD has the privilege of being the first to handle the specimen, but this privilege comes with the responsibility of handling the specimen properly. While there are protocols for handling large specimens,[3–5] there are qualitative differences in how specimens are dissected and sectioned by different pathologists. Unfortunately, the quality of gross examination is in decline, and there is widespread concern in the pathology community that newly qualified pathologists are not always well trained in gross pathology.[6] There are many reasons why this situation exists and it is unlikely to improve in the foreseeable future. The lack of skill in gross pathology is more than a matter of esthetics; Wiley and Keh re-examined breast specimens that had been initially handled by residents and found major discrepancies

in 5% of cases.[7] In all fairness, the majority of errors occurred in specimens handled by first year residents. However, this paper underscores the fact that gross examination is under-valued in training programs as residents shift their interests to more exotic aspects of surgical pathology.

The following guidelines should be used when performing gross examination, especially on large specimens.

■ It is good practice to be familiar with the clinical aspects of a complex case before sectioning or dissecting the specimen. This includes knowledge of which tissues/ organs are present in the specimen so that sectioning/ dissection can proceed in an informed manner. For example, a small portion of bladder wall may be attached to a colectomy specimen and this could be overlooked if the pathologist is not alerted to its presence.

■ The specimen should be dissected or sectioned in a way that provides information relevant to surgical management.

■ A sharp blade is essential for making clean cuts and for minimizing distortions that are likely to occur with a dull blade. Ideally, the length of the blade should be at least 2–3 times the size of the axis of the specimen. Large solid specimens are best cut with a long straight-edged knife or blade (Fig. 2.2).

■ When a solid or solid/cystic mass is sectioned, the initial sections should be made in a way that preserves

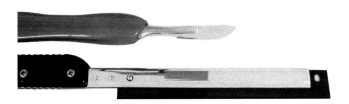

Fig. 2.2. A Bard–Parker blade is excellent for small specimens but large solid specimens should be cut with a long, straight edged blade. Straight-edged blades are excellent for cutting thin parallel sections of tissue that may be otherwise difficult to section, such as breast lumpectomy specimens.

the esthetic quality of the specimen, allowing the specimen to be photographed for conferences and for teaching. Instead of making multiple sections in different planes, parallel sections preserve intact slices of tissue for photography. Sometimes, the uniqueness of a specimen is appreciated only after histologic examination has been completed, and it is frustrating to go back to the specimen to find that it has been mishandled.

- When a hollow muscular organ, such as colon, contains a non-circumferential tumor mass, the specimen should be opened so that the mass is left intact. This can be done quite easily by probing the lumen with a finger in advance of the scissors, and by cutting the wall away from the mass.
- Large mass lesions should be sliced at appropriate intervals, not only to permit optimal fixation but also to detect focal changes that may be different from the dominant lesion (e.g., an area of de-differentiation in a large, well differentiated liposarcoma).
- Tissues vary in their requirement for optimal fixation, and lymphoid neoplasms are amongst the most demanding. If a large lymphoproliferative lesion is encountered in an organ such as spleen, colon or ovary, small, thin samples of the lesion should be placed in a separate container of fixative to optimize fixation of a representative portion of the neoplasm.

FROZEN SECTIONS

The frozen section (FS) technique was first described for clinical use in the late nineteenth century and the first cryostat was developed in the late 1950s.[8] Most laboratories use commercial cryostats for preparing FSs but institutions such as the Mayo Clinic and M.D.

Anderson Hospital use different techniques for freezing tissue.[9,10] Recent advances in cryostat technology include more efficient heat extractors for freezing tissue, improvements in microtome technology and the use of disposable blades. Every step in the preparation of FSs is important and these will be dealt with in turn.

Is frozen section the appropriate test?

When a FS is requested, the first question is whether FS is the appropriate test to perform. The FS technique provides excellent results for most tissues but is less suited for others; for example, cytologic examination is superior to FS for evaluating lymphoproliferative lesions.

Preparing and sampling the specimen

When the specimen contains non-lesional adipose tissue, the fat should be trimmed away because it will interfere with obtaining good frozen sections. Similarly, blood clot does not section well and should be removed when it is admixed with fragments of tissue. However, a distinction should be made between blood clot and hemorrhagic tissue because hemorrhagic tissue may be informative; for example, when chorionic villi are scanty in a D&C specimen, they are often present in the hemorrhagic component of the specimen.

There is no substitute for a sharp blade. Dull blades and knives are the source of many problems and they should be avoided, especially when tissue orientation is critical, as when skin or mucosal tissue has to be cut perpendicular to the surface. A sharp blade also makes it easier to obtain samples of optimal thickness; tissue selected for FS should be no more than 3–4 mm thick because thicker sections may not freeze evenly, resulting in poor quality sections.

Preparation of the frozen section block

Almost all FS techniques involve embedding tissue in a liquid compound that hardens with freezing.* The following points should be kept in mind when embedding tissue:

---

* Liquid embedding compounds are made of a mixture of glycols and resins. The two most popular are Tissue-Tek's optimal cutting temperature (OCT) and the freezing medium made by Triangle Medical Sciences (TBS). The term OCT will be used in this chapter because it is the brand that I am familiar with.

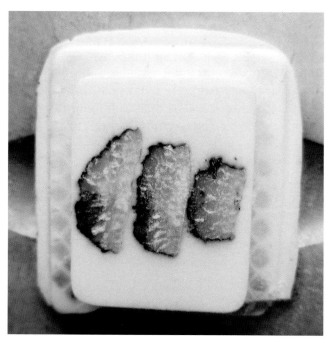

Fig. 2.3. A frozen section block containing strips of skin. It is easier to cut good quality frozen sections when the slices of skin are embedded close together, with unoccupied OCT at the proximal and distal ends of the block.

- When a plastic cryomold is used, it is much better to slightly overfill rather than underfill the cryomold with OCT, to avoid the embarrassment of dislodging a partially adherent frozen block from the chuck.
- When OCT is dispensed hastily, it may result in the formation of air bubbles in the FS block. This can be a problem if a large bubble is in close proximity to a small tissue sample. It is best to remove large air bubbles from the liquid OCT or re-embed the tissue, instead of proceeding with a potentially defective block.
- Tissue density should influence the size of the sample selected for FS because the microtome blade is likely to gouge into the block when it encounters a large volume of dense tissue. For example, ovarian fibromas are dense and the FS sample should measure no more than 1cm in maximum dimension. Similarly, only a limited number of pieces of skin should be embedded if the dermis is thick and dense, as with skin from the back.
- When multiple pieces of tissue, such as skin, are embedded in a block, they should be placed close together instead of separating them with large areas of unoccupied OCT (Fig. 2.3). This will make it easier to control the sections with the tip of a brush if there is a tendency for the tissue to curl on sectioning.
- A strip of unoccupied frozen OCT should be present at the proximal and distal ends of the block to allow for easy manipulation of the section with the tip of a brush. This is particularly important if the tissue at the proximal and distal ends of the block are critical to evaluation of the specimen, as with evaluation of surgical margins in skin specimens (Fig. 2.3).
- Long strips of tissue, such as skin and mucosa, should be embedded with the long axis of the tissue perpendicular to the blade edge (Fig. 2.3). This minimizes folds in the sections.
- When the specimen contains fat and non-fatty tissue, it should be embedded so that the blade first meets the non-fatty component. If fat is encountered first, it may congeal on the edge of the blade and interfere with cutting the remaining non-fatty tissue in the block. When this problem is encountered, the blade should be cleaned with alcohol and the block should be rotated so that the blade first makes contact with the non-fatty part of the tissue.
- Embedding multiple pieces of tissue on the same plane can be a challenge because of displacement that occurs when additional OCT is added. When it is critical to have all the pieces on the same plane, it helps to use a cryomold or to place the tissue fragments on a pre-formed platform of frozen OCT.
- Retaining orientation of a thin walled cystic structure can be achieved in two ways: first, the strips of tissue can be placed on a pre-frozen platform of OCT, and second, preparing a Swiss roll gives the tissue enough bulk to retain its orientation (Fig. 2.4).
- There are two caveats about using pre-formed platforms of frozen OCT: (a) tissue placement should be correct at the outset because the tissue will adhere to the frozen OCT and; (b) the second layer of OCT should go beyond the perimeter of the frozen platform to avoid separation of the two layers of frozen OCT during sectioning. Other techniques have been described for retaining orientation of tissue in frozen section blocks, the most comprehensive of which have been described by Peters et al.[11–16]

Freezing the block

Most tissues cut well at −20 °C but fatty tissue yields better sections at lower temperatures (−40 °C). As a result, partially fatty tissue should be frozen at a lower temperature and this can be done by immersing the block in cold isopentane or by spraying the block with

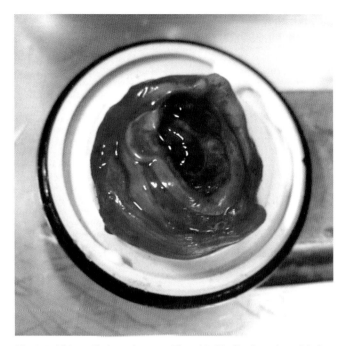

Fig. 2.4. Thin-walled ovarian cyst. The added bulk of a swiss roll helps to retain the vertical orientation of thin walled cystic structures.

a cryospray. Frozen section blocks should be cooled as rapidly as possible to minimize ice crystal formation in the intracellular and extra-cellular compartments of the tissue. This is achieved by using the appropriate cooling method as well as selecting tissue samples that are no more than 3 mm thick.

There are two main methods of producing a frozen block. The most common method is to place the chuck on the cryobar bar of the cryostat. The cryobar bar with attached heat extractor (Peltier effect) will freeze the block to $-20\,°C$ in approximately 1 minute. The advantage of the quick-freeze bar is that it can be set to achieve a temperature of $-20\,°C$ which is ideal for cutting most tissues. If the tissue contains fat, the block can be cooled even further with a cryospray. The second method is to immerse the block in cold liquid. Liquid nitrogen $(-190\,°C)$ was once popular for freezing tissue but it is unwieldy and causes excessive cooling of the block. Isopentane is now the favored liquid medium for freezing tissue, and an electrical cryobath is the most convenient way to cool isopentane $(-40$ to $-60\,°C)$ although dry ice $(-70\,°C)$ is a reasonable alternative. Cold isopentane is particularly useful for freezing partially fatty tissue but if isopentane is used for non-fatty tissue, the block will have to be warmed with the operator's thumb before it will produce good sections. Even if the freezing bar in the cryostat is the main method of preparing FS blocks,

it is useful to have a cryobath in the laboratory to freeze blocks to temperatures colder than $-20\,°C$, as well as for rapid freezing of tissue for other laboratory tests (e.g., gene re-arrangement studies, enzyme analysis or for storing tissue in a tissue bank). A liquid cooling method is necessary of course, when cryomolds are used.

Institutions such as the Mayo Clinic and M.D. Anderson Hospital use different techniques for freezing tissue, mainly because their methods are more efficient for high volumes of frozen sections.[9,10]

Cutting sections

Improvements in cryostats have made it easier to obtain high quality frozen sections for most types of tissue. The temperature in newer cryostats is better controlled, and disposable blades are a boon. However, problems do occur with cutting good-quality sections, and some of the reasons why this may occur are listed below.

- When a liquid coolant is used to freeze FS blocks, the block may be too cold to obtain good sections. A block that is too cold will yield crumbly, shard-like sections, but this is easily corrected by warming the block with one's thumb, and then lightly trimming the block before selecting a section. A block that is not cold enough will yield a very thick section with the first cut, and if the specimen is small, there is a risk of removing most of the specimen from the block with the first section. A soft block can usually be recognized with the naked eye and should be re-cooled before sectioning.

- As stated earlier, only a limited amount of dense tissue should be embedded in a FS block to avoid the blade from gouging into the tissue. With dense tissue, it is even more important to section the block with a smooth continuous motion. If the blade fails to make a smooth cut and leaves ridges in the block, the block should be rotated $90°$ and refaced before attempting to take a section.

- One way to handle partially fatty tissue is to cut sections at different temperatures. The block should be cooled to approximately $-40\,°C$ to obtain a section of the fatty component, and the non-fatty component can be cut at the regular temperature $(-20\,°C)$. It is easier to obtain a section of fatty tissue if the microtome is set at 6–10 microns and if the section is cut with a quick rotation of the microtome wheel.

■ A ripple in the section, or alternating thick and thin sections may mean that there is unwanted movement somewhere in the microtome. The first corrective step is to check that the chuck and blade are securely clamped as these are the most common causes for movement in the microtome.

Lifting the section onto the glass slide

It is tempting to place multiple levels of a small biopsy on one slide but this should be avoided because some of the sections will show air-drying artifacts, and moreover, the sections may slip off the slide during staining if the OCT in the sections overlap. When a section is lifted off the blade, the glass slide should make contact with the entire section to avoid traction distortion that comes from partial contact between glass slide and tissue section.

Other issues regarding frozen sections

At many training institutions, frozen sections are prepared by pathology assistants or histotechnologists. The advantages are that FSs are of consistently higher quality, and residents and fellows are free to pay attention to non-technical aspects of the case. However, the disadvantage is that residents may not learn the nuances of solving technical problems in preparing FSs if they are protected from being on the front line.

CYTOLOGIC EXAMINATION

The use of cytologic preparations is now a standard part of IOD.[10,17–21] This technique was slow in being implemented in the intraoperative setting but was embraced when fine needle aspiration biopsy grew in popularity.

When should cytologic preparations be used?

Cytologic examination may be the sole microscopic test or it may be used to supplement FSs. Cytologic preparations are quick and simple to prepare, they provide cytologic detail that often surpasses that of FSs, they are especially useful for small specimens where tissue conservation is important, and they are superior to FSs for tissues that are fragile and easily distorted

by freezing, such as lymphoid tissue. They are often superior to FSs for tissues that are difficult to section, such as partially fatty tissue and bony tissue (e.g., the cancellous bony margins of major orthopedic resections). In addition, they are safer than FSs for evaluating suspected granulomatous infectious diseases such as tuberculosis.

What are the limitations of cytologic preparations?

Cytologic preparations are inferior to FSs when architectural features are important for distinguishing between different types of carcinomas. For example, a diagnosis of high grade carcinoma of the ovary is easily made on a cytoscrape preparation but FS is more reliable when a distinction has to be made between primary poorly differentiated ovarian carcinoma and poorly differentiated metastatic carcinoma. Because this affects intraoperative management, we recommend the preparation of both cytologic smears and FS when evaluating high grade ovarian malignancies. Cytologic examination is not suitable for evaluating inflammatory processes where architectural features are important, such as determining the adequacy of a thoracoscopic biopsy for interstitial lung disease.

Cytologic preparations of mesenchymal neoplasms are often unsatisfactory, either because of low cellularity or because architectural features are required to make a diagnosis. Cytologic preparations also play a limited role in the evaluation of surgical margins, and this is particularly true when the distance of the neoplasm from the margin has to be measured or estimated.

What are the techniques for making cytologic preparations?

There are three main methods for making cytologic preparations, and since more than one method may work in many situations, the choice depends on the type of specimen and the pathologist's preference.

Touch imprints or touch preparations

In this method, the tissue is touched to the glass slide or the slide is brought into contact with the tissue. This technique works well for very cellular, non-sclerotic neoplasms and for tissue composed of discohesive cells such as lymphoid tissue. They are also suitable for evaluating specimens that are too small to scrape. With alcohol-fixed imprints, only a limited number of impressions should be made on a single slide to avoid air-drying. Touch preparations are preferred for evaluating air-dried, Romanowsky-stained hemato-lymphoid lesions because they produce more consistent monolayer preparations.[*]

Scrape and smear preparations (cytoscrape preparations)

Cytoscrape preparations are made by scraping the cut surface of a specimen with a Bard Parker blade and then smearing the cellular material onto a glass slide. Cytoscrape preparations are suitable for many types of tissue because the amount of material collected can be controlled: soft, cellular neoplasms require gentle scraping, whereas neoplasms with a fibrous component may need more vigorous scraping. It is easy to produce cytoscrape preparations but good quality, esthetically-pleasing smears can be obtained as follows:

- The cellularity of the tissue, judging by its softness or firmness, should guide the force with which the tissue is scraped. Highly cellular lesions, such as a lymph node with suspected lymphoma or a highly cellular malignancy of any type, should be scraped gently, whereas desmoplastic carcinomas may require more assertive scraping. It is always prudent to start gently because over-vigorous scraping of cellular neoplasms will dislodge large tissue fragments and result in thick smears that are difficult to interpret. The goal is to obtain thin, monolayer smears and small tissue fragments.
- After the cellular material has been transferred to a glass slide, it should be spread with a second slide held at right angles to the first (Fig. 2.5). The advantage of this technique is that the second slide can be used to determine the thickness of the smear.
- On naked eye examination, the optimal smear is even, of appropriate thickness and roughly oval in shape, sometimes with a short flare. Large fragments of tissue, fragments of fibrous stroma, flecks of calcium as well as foreign material will interfere with obtaining even smears.

[*] A monolayer of cells is essential for Romanowsky-stained preparations because these stains do not penetrate through multiple layers of cells. Thick, air-dried smears are often uninterpretable.

Squash and smear preparations (squash preparations)

There are variations in the way squash preparations are made but our preference is a two-step technique: squashing the tissue between two glass slides held at right angles to one another, and then smearing the squashed material (squash and smear). Not all tissues lend themselves to this technique because the tissue has to be soft enough to squash. Squash preparations are ideal for lesions of the brain and spinal cord as these specimens are too small to scrape and usually do not yield sufficient cellular material with touch imprints. Squash preparations should therefore, be the first test performed on stereotactic needle core biopsies of the brain. The piece of tissue that is selected should be approximately 1 mm in diameter, because selecting a larger piece leads to undesirably thick smears (Fig 2.6). The ideal squash preparation should be thin enough to allow easy visibility of cellular detail (Fig. 2.7).

When a stereotactic needle biopsy specimen of the CNS consists of multiple cores, the diagnostic yield can be increased by sampling a 1 mm piece from each core; if there are multiple cores, two 1 mm pieces may be placed on a single slide, approximately 1cm apart. The tissue should be squashed with firm pressure, but the smearing should be done as gently as with any other cytologic preparation to avoid mechanical artifacts. The manner in which the material squashes often provides clues to the diagnosis. Glial neoplasms are easy to squash and smear, whereas schwannomas and most meningiomas resist squashing, and smear to a limited extent (Fig. 2.8). Neoplasms with a fibrous component, such as gliosarcomas, squash and spread unevenly, and tumors with abundant calcification spread with streaks.

When a lymphoid neoplasm of the CNS is suspected, one of the slides should be air-dried and stained with Diff–Quik or a Wright–Giemsa stain. This will show the cytoplasmic characteristics to better advantage, as well as show cytoplasmic fragments (so-called lymphoglandular bodies), a very helpful feature in support of a lymphoproliferative lesion (Fig. 2.9).

One more point about cytologic preparations

When cytologic preparations are made on small specimens, the specimen should be placed on a clean, non-absorbent surface such as a telfa pad. This will avoid drying of the specimen (certain to occur with an absorbent paper towel), contamination by other tissue fragments (from the cutting board) and contamination by non-tissue debris (cellulose fragments from a cork cutting board).

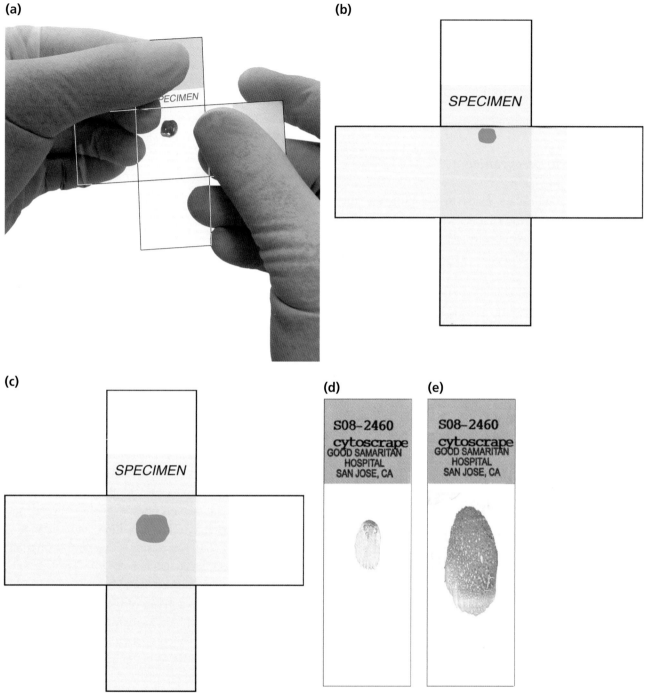

Fig. 2.5. (a) Our approach to making cytoscrape smears, using a two slide technique. The cellular material is deposited near the label end of a slide. A second slide is held at right angles to the first. (b) The placement of the second slide will determine the thickness of the smear; the top edge of the second slide is placed just above the drop of cellular material when the material is scanty, but (c) closer to the label when there is abundant cellular material. (d) With this technique, scanty cellular material will be spread over a smaller area, whereas (e) abundant cellular material will cover a larger surface area. This technique results in smears that are more consistent in thickness.

FIXATION AND STAINING

Most laboratories fix FS and cytology slides in alcohol and stain with hematoxylin and eosin (H&E). There is some variation in the fixatives used for FSs (ethanol, methanol, formaldehyde, ether/methanol, acetone), but our preference is to use 95% ethanol. The H&E stain works well for most laboratories because the stain is familiar and the

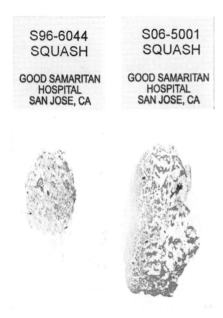

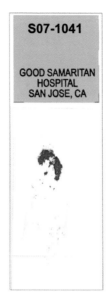

Fig. 2.6. Squash preparations of a glioblastoma. The smear on the left was prepared from a 1mm cube of tissue and is of optimal thickness, whereas the smear on the right was prepared from a 2 mm piece of tissue, and is a little too thick.

Fig. 2.8. Squash preparation of a meningioma. The cellular material resisted squashing, and spread to a limited extent.

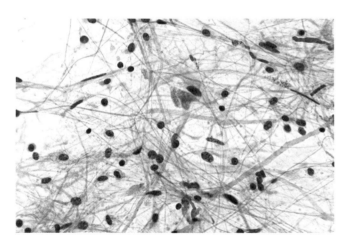

Fig. 2.7. Squash preparation of a pilocytic astrocytoma. Cytoplasmic fibrils and Rosenthal fibers are readily visible.

slides are as permanent as routinely processed tissue, and thus ideal for quality assurance activities and other reviews.

It is difficult to produce high quality FSs on tissues with a low plasma content, such as cartilage and partially cauterized tissue because the sections have a tendency to slip off the slide during staining. Adhesion of tissue to the slide can be improved by using charged or lysine-coated slides, or by allowing the slide to air-dry for a minute after alcohol fixation. It also helps to take the slide through the staining process as gently as possible. If these steps fail, a few drops of toluidine blue or hematoxylin can be placed

onto an unfixed slide and then coverslipped without taking the section through alcohol and xylene.

Some pathologists prefer water-mounted preparations stained with toluidine blue because this stain is quicker to perform and more efficient in laboratories that have high volumes of frozen sections.[9] Toluidine bue-stained sections have their advantages, but as with any stain, the observer should be familiar with the artifacts of this stain. One advantage of water-mounted sections is that lipid droplets are visible, a feature that may be helpful in certain situations, e.g., the recognition of lipid-filled macrophages in a lung biopsy performed for interstitial disease.

SPECIAL STAINS

Rapid stains for mucin are used in some laboratories.[10,22,23] Rapid PAS-diastase, alcian blue and mucicarmine stains may be used for evaluating the margins in resections for signet ring cell carcinomas, and the alcian yellow stain can help evaluate the epidermal margins in Paget's disease. However, these stains are required so infrequently that most laboratories are not set up to perform special stains intraoperatively. The rapid oil-red O stain was in vogue in the 1970s as an ancillary test for distinguishing normal from

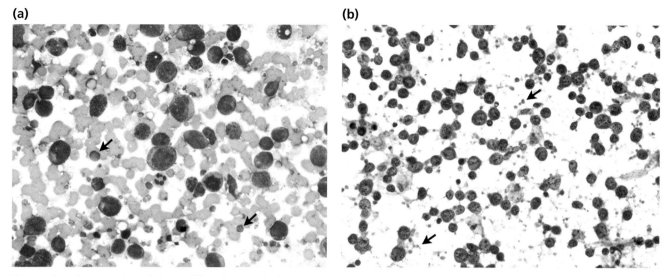

(a) **(b)**

Fig. 2.9. Squash preparation of a large cell lymphoma of the brain stained with Wright–Giemsa and H&E. The discohesiveness of the neoplastic cells, single cell pattern, lack of glial fibrils and the presence cytoplasmic fragments support the diagnosis of large cell lymphoma, and argue against the diagnosis of small cell glioblastoma or metastatic carcinoma. (a) Cytoplasmic fragments, more readily seen in large cell lymphomas, are easily identified on Wright–Giemsa stained preparations as blue blobs but (b) may also be visible on H&E stained smears (arrows).

abnormal parathyroid glands, but there is currently little use for this stain.

A rapid (1 hour) melan-A immunohistochemical stain has been developed for use during Mohs surgery to evaluate the density of atypical melanocytes at the surgical margins of lentigo maligna.[23–25] However, the availability of rapid paraffin processing will very likely eliminate the need for melan-A immunohistochemical stains on frozen sections. A rapid keratin stain has been described for evaluating selected carcinomas of the skin during Mohs surgery but has limited application.[26,27]

REFERENCES

1. Zarbo RJ, Schmidt WA, Bachner P *et al*. Indications and immediate outcomes of pathology intraoperative consultations. *Arch Pathol Lab Med* 1996; **120**: 19–25.
2. Udelsman R, Westra WH, Donovan PI *et al*. Randomized prospective evaluation of frozen-section analysis for follicular neoplasms of the thyroid. *Ann Surg* 2001; **233**: 716–722.
3. Humphrey PA, Dehner LP, Pfeifer JD. *Washington Manual of Surgical Pathology*. Lippincott Williams & Wilkins, 2008.
4. Lester SC. *Manual of Surgical Pathology*, 2nd edition. Saunders, 2005.
5. Schmidt W. *Principles and Techniques of Surgical Pathology*. Menlo Park: Addison Wesley, 1983.
6. Horowitz RE. Expectations and essentials for the community practice of pathology. *Human Pathol* 2006; **37**: 969–973.
7. Wiley EL, Keh P. Diagnostic discrepancies in breast specimens subjected to gross reexamination. *Am J Surg Pathol* 1999; **23**: 876–879.
8. Fechner RE. The birth and evolution of American surgical pathology. In *Guiding the Surgeon's Hand*. Rosai J, ed., Washington DC: American Registry of Pathology, Armed Forces Institute of Pathology, 1997.
9. Ferreiro JA, Myers JL, Bostwick DG. Accuracy of frozen section diagnoses in surgical pathology: review of a 1-year experience with 24,880 cases at Mayo Clinic Rochester. *Mayo Clin Proc.* 1995; **70**: 1137–1141.
10. Silva EG, Kraemer RR. *Intraoperative Pathologic Diagnosis. Frozen Section and other Techniques*. Baltimore, Williams & Wilkins, 1987.
11. Kelley DB, Abt AB. An improved method for mounting frozen-section specimens. *Am J Surg Pathol* 1990; **14**: 186–187.
12. Peters SR. The art of embedding tissue for frozen section. Part I: A system for face down cryoembedding of tissues using freezing temperature embedding wells. *J Histotechnol* 2003; **26**: 11–19.
13. Peters SR. The art of embedding tissue for frozen section. Part II: Frozen block cryoembedding. *J Histotechnol* 2003; **26**: 23–28.
14. Peters SR, Fitzgerald S, Green C *et al*. Paper cryoembedding. *J Histotechnol* 2003; **26**: 173–178.
15. Radivoyevitz MA. Staining method for frozen section. *Am J Surg Pathol* 1989; **13**: 244–245.
16. SooHoo W, Ruebner B, Vogt P *et al*. Orientation of small, flat, frozen-section specimens. *Am J Surg Pathol* 1988; **12**: 573–574.
17. Berger PC. Use of cytologic preparations in the frozen section diagnosis of central nervous system neoplasia. *Am J Surg Pathol* 1985; **9**: 344–354.
18. Folkerth RD. Smears and frozen sections in the intraoperative diagnosis of central nervous system lesions. *Neuropathol Clinics of North America* 1994; **5**: 1–18.
19. Moss TH, Nicoll JAR, Ironside JW. *Intra-operative diagnosis of CNS tumors*. London: Arnold & Oxford University Press, 1997.
20. Nochomovitz L, Sidawy, Janota *et al*. *Intraoperative Consultation. A guide to smears, imprints, and frozen sections*. Chicago: ASCP Press, 1989.
21. Sidawy MK, Silverberg SG. Intraoperative cytology. Back to the future? *Am J Clin Pathol* 1991; **96**: 1–3.
22. Dworak O, Wittekind C. A 30-S PAS stain for frozen sections. *Am J Surg Pathol* 1992; **16**: 87–88.

23. Soans S, Galinda LM, Garcia FU. Mucin stain on frozen sections: a rapid 3-minute method. *Arch Path Lab Med.* 1999; **123**: 378–380.

24. Bricca GM, Brodland DG, Zitelli JA. Immunostaining melanoma frozen sections: the 1-hour protocol. *Dermatol Surg.* 2004; **30**: 403–408.

25. Kelley LC, Starkus L. Immunohistochemical staining of lentigo maligna during Mohs micrographic surgery using MART-1. *J Am Acad Dermatol* 2002; **46**: 78–84.

26. Jimenez FJ, Grichnik JM, Buchanan MD *et al.* Immunohistochemical techniques in Mohs micrographic surgery: their potential use in the detection of neoplastic cells masked by inflammation. *J Am Acad Dermatol* 1995; **32**: 89–94.

27. Zachary CB, Rest EB, Furlong SM *et al.* Rapid cytokeratin stains enhance the sensitivity of Mohs micrographic surgery for squamous cell carcinoma. *J Dermatol Surg Oncol* 1994; **20**: 530–535.

3 SKIN

Mahendra Ranchod, Michael B. Morgan, and Isaac M. Neuhaus

INTRODUCTION

There is great variation in the frequency with which conventional frozen sections are performed on cutaneous malignancies. Many basal carcinomas (BCCs) and squamous cell carcinomas (SCCs) are treated by dermatologists without the aid of frozen section (FS), and many patients with tumors in cosmetically and functionally sensitive anatomic locations, or who have high risk malignancies, are referred for Mohs micrographic surgery. Non-surgical methods of treatment, such as photodynamic therapy and topical immune modulators (e.g., imiquimod) are also beginning to make an impact on the treatment of selected cutaneous malignancies, and these non-surgical approaches will very likely continue to impact the pathologist's role in the intraoperative management of cutaneous malignancies.

INDICATIONS FOR INTRAOPERATIVE DIAGNOSIS

1. To evaluate surgical margins of resection in cutaneous malignancies.
2. To distinguish rapidly progressive, potentially life-threatening medical disorders such as toxic epidermal necrolysis from severe bullous drug eruptions and staphylococcal scalded skin syndrome.

INFORMATION NEEDED BEFORE AND DURING IOD

Cutaneous neoplasms are first evaluated with routinely processed diagnostic biopsies. Issues such as benign versus malignant, and primary versus metastatic malignancy, are resolved before the lesion is subjected to definitive resection, and the pathologist's task at the time of FS is largely limited to evaluating margins of resection. When possible, the prior biopsy slides should be reviewed before performing frozen sections (FSs) on the excisional specimen. Often, however, the original biopsy slides are not available and the FS has to be performed with limited clinical information. Limited information is adequate for most cases but inadequate for others. For example, issues regarding FS evaluation of morpheaform BCC are different from nodular BCC, and the challenges presented by spindle cell squamous carcinoma are different from keratoacanthoma-type SCC.

GENERAL CLINICAL ISSUES

All cutaneous malignancies have a potential for local recurrence, but the capacity to metastasize varies by tumor type. For example, BCC is locally destructive, but rarely metastasizes. Its behavior corresponds to the clinically intermediate group of tumors as defined by Kempson *et al.*[1] In contrast, Merkel cell carcinoma is a true malignancy with a high metastatic rate, even after complete excision.

The treatment of cutaneous malignancies is usually determined by the type of neoplasm. The treatment of BCC is focused on local control, and this can be achieved by local destructive methods, such as curettage with electrocautery, or with surgical excision. In contrast, primary cutaneous melanomas are always treated by surgical resection, with tumor thickness guiding the extent of surgical resection. The optimal treatment of resectable cutaneous malignancies is complete removal with adequate clear margins, and the amount of margin clearance depends on the type of neoplasm and anatomic location. For example, BCC can be excised with a 1–2 mm margin of

Intraoperative Consultation in Surgical Pathology, ed. Mahendra Ranchod. Published by Cambridge University Press.
© Cambridge University Press 2010.

normal tissue, whereas more aggressive malignancies such as deeply invasive melanoma, Merkel cell carcinoma and high grade adnexal carcinomas require wider margins of excision to minimize local recurrence. A margin of 2 cm is arbitrarily used for treating most aggressive malignancies but this is tempered by anatomic location. For example, a 2–3 cm margin is feasible for a Merkel cell carcinoma of the trunk, but a 1 cm margin may be all that is possible for the same neoplasm in a functionally important location.

GENERAL PATHOLOGIC ISSUES

Types of specimens

Skin specimens submitted for FS come in different shapes and sizes, and the size and shape depend on the characteristics of the neoplasm, anatomic location, and the planned technique for closure of the wound. Most skin carcinomas have an approximately round surface outline, and complete excision of the neoplasm with maximum conservation of normal tissue will result in a specimen that is close to round (Fig. 3.1[a]). However, round specimens constitute a minority of specimens submitted for conventional FSs, and they are submitted when the surgeon plans to close the defect with a flap or graft, instead of a linear technique, or when the surgeon plans to defer wound closure until after the initial excision has been evaluated by FS; when clear margins are obtained, the shape of the defect is modified to achieve wound closure.

Most skin specimens submitted for conventional FSs are a combination of an excisional biopsy with a variable amount of surrounding normal skin; normal skin is removed intentionally to create a wound ready for optimal closure. The most common of these specimens is an ellipse (Fig. 3.1[b]), a shape that prevents the formation of cutaneous cones that would occur from primary closure of a round wound. Other specimen shapes that are used much less frequently include triangles and rhomboids, and these and other excisions are sometimes made in preparation for closure of the wound with a local skin flap or graft (Fig. 3.1[c]–[f]). Specimens from anatomic locations with a free margin, such as ear and lip, are usually excised as a wedge (Fig. 3.2).

Orientation of the specimen

Skin excision specimens intended for curative resection of a malignancy should always be oriented. Placement of one or more sutures in the specimen and an accompanying sketch are ideal (Fig. 3.3[a]). The orientation of a specimen to anatomic landmarks may not be clear if the specimen is not accompanied by a sketch, but there are situations when it is reasonable to proceed with FS evaluation and resolve the exact orientation later. For example, when a skin ellipse is submitted with a single suture without more specific orientation, the suture can be taken to be in the 12 o'clock position and the specimen can be inked using an imaginary clock face for orientation (Fig. 3.3[b]). If a surgical margin is positive on FS, the clock face orientation can be matched to anatomic landmarks. However, there is a caveat: if lack of precise orientation carries a risk of compromising FS evaluation, it is prudent to discuss the orientation of the specimen with the surgeon before inking and cutting the specimen.

Precise orientation is essential for complex resection specimens and at times, it is helpful for the pathologist to view the lesion in situ, or to inspect the surgical wound and have the surgeon explain the orientation. The surgeon should place multiple sutures in complex specimens, even if the orientation of the specimen has been explained to the pathologist. This will guard against inadvertent loss of orientation during transport of the specimen to the laboratory. It is also worth asking about the margin/s of greatest concern in complex specimens so that these may be examined first. Surgeons should be encouraged to place sutures in the specimen with a loose loop as these are easier to remove from the specimen (Fig. 3.3[b]), thus avoiding the experience of encountering fragments of suture material when cutting the FS block.

Inking the specimen

All excisional biopsy specimens sent for FS should be inked, and at least two colors should be applied to any specimen that has been oriented. Specimens larger than 2 cm should be inked with three colors as this helps localize an involved margin more precisely (Fig. 3.4). To maximize adhesiveness of the dye, ink should be applied after the specimen has been blotted dry. Inking is best done with a Q-tip, and the ink should be allowed to dry before the specimen is sectioned. A mordant such as Bouin's solution improves adhesiveness of the dye, but this is seldom necessary for skin specimens.

Cutting the specimen

There are standard ways to cut common skin specimens such as a small ellipse, but it is prudent to take a moment

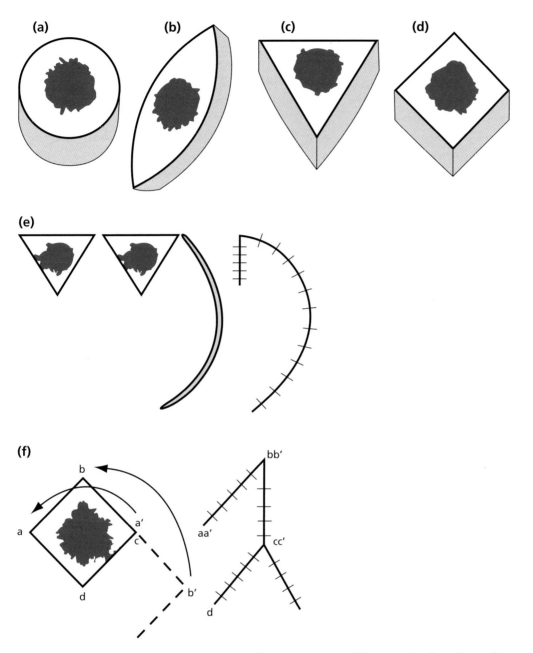

Fig. 3.1. (a) Round specimens represent a minority of specimens submitted for conventional FS. (b) An ellipse is the most common, and it includes trianglular pieces of normal skin at each pole to facilitate closure of the wound. (c) Triangles and (d) rhomboids are removed in preparation for closing the wound with (e) a local flap or (f) graft.

to think about the best way to section an unusually shaped specimen before making the first cut. Unless the specimen is very large, it is best to cut an initial excision specimen perpendicular to the surgical margins. This allows simultaneous evaluation of the peripheral and deep margins, and it also allows the pathologist to report the distance of the neoplasm from the margins. Figure 3.5 illustrates the way to section common skin specimens. When cutting skin

specimens, there is no substitute for a sharp blade because a sharp blade allows more controlled cutting, ensuring vertical sections of even thickness. As a corollary, use of a dull blade runs the risk of making unwanted tangential sections which can confound microscopic interpretation. Figure 3.6 illustrates the way to handle re-excision specimens following positive margins on the initial excision specimen.

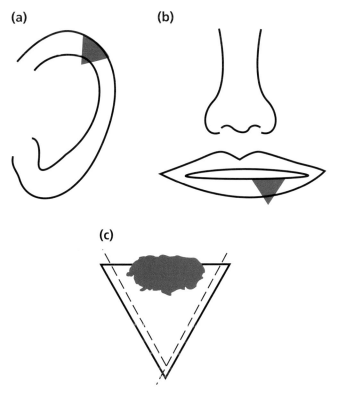

(a) (b)

(c)

Fig. 3.2. (a), (b) Wedge-shaped biopsies are removed from anatomic sites that have a free cutaneous or mucocutaneous margin. (c) When evaluating margins, a 2 mm-wide strip of skin should be cut parallel to each surgical margin and embedded so that the true margin is deepest in the block.

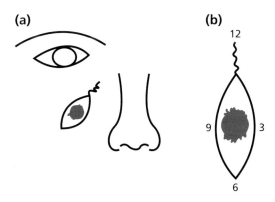

(a) (b)

Fig. 3.3. (a) Orientation of a skin specimen is clear if the specimen is accompanied by a sketch. If there is no sketch, the clock face may be used for initial orientation, with the suture taken as 12 o'clock. (b) The specimen is inked as follows: 12–6 o'clock blue, 6–9 o'clock black, 9–12 o'clock green. If a margin is positive, the clock face can be matched to the patient's anatomic landmarks.

Removing excess fat

Skin specimens with abundant subcutaneous fat are difficult to section. There are two approaches to reducing the amount of fat to improve the quality of frozen sections.

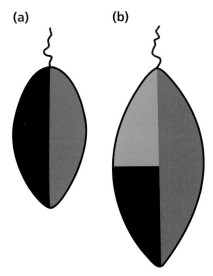

(a) (b)

Fig. 3.4. Inking an ellipse. (a) A small ellipse should be painted with two colors. (b) A large ellipse should be inked with three colors. In example (b), tissue sections from the superior half of the specimen will appear on the slides dyed blue/green, whereas tissue from the inferior half will be dyed blue/black.

If the original biopsy shows a superficially invasive carcinoma, and the subcutaneous fat has been removed to achieve wound closure, the extra fat can be trimmed from the specimen and saved for routine processing if that becomes necessary. Alternatively, the excess fat can be gently scraped with a blade or compressed with a finger to reduce the amount of fat in the sections. Tissue containing fat should be cut at a lower temperature, and this can be achieved by cooling the block in cold isopentane or with a cryospray.

Embedding the specimen

An attempt should be made to embed all the slices of tissue on the same plane, a task that is more easily accomplished when the tissue is embedded in a vinyl cryomold. When a specimen mold is unavailable, the pieces of skin should be placed on a flat platform of frozen OCT; this placement should be done with care because it is difficult to adjust the embedding after the tissue adheres to the frozen OCT. It is tempting to maximize the number of pieces of skin per block, but other factors aside, the thickness of the dermis should be taken into account. Fewer slices of skin should be embedded in a FS block when the dermis is thick to avoid having the blade gouge into the block.

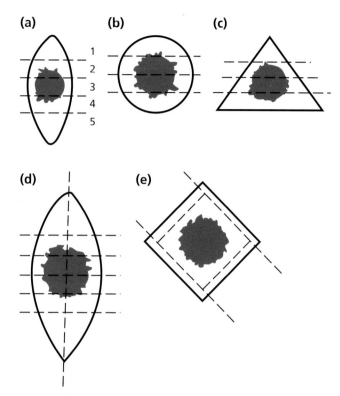

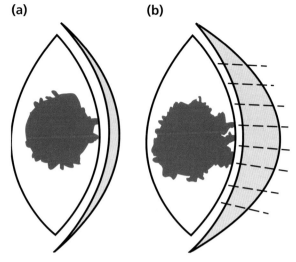

Fig. 3.6. When the initial excision specimen has a positive margin, the approach to the re-excised margins depends on the width of the re-excised tissue. (a) Thin strips of skin are best embedded on edge with the deep margin deepest in the block. (b) If the re-excised skin is wider than 3–4 mm, the new margin should be carefully inked, and sections should be taken at right angles to the new margin.

Fig. 3.5. The size and shape of the excised specimen determines the optimal slicing technique. Some specimens intentionally include normal skin and these areas need not be sampled for FS. (a) For example, there is no reason to include slices 1 and 5 when examining a small ellipse. (b) For small round specimens, slices 1 and 4 should be embedded with the deep margin deepest in the block. This will allow the pathologist to perform multiple levels into the block, with the deepest level of slices 1 and 4 representing the true superior and inferior surgical margins. (c) The same principle applies to triangular and rhomboid specimens. (d) For large specimens, we prefer to bisect the specimen in its long axis and then make sections in the short axis. This allows evaluation of the peripheral and deep margins. (e) If the surgeon is concerned only about the peripheral margins), sections can be made parallel to the margins.

Non-sparing of tissue when evaluating surgical margins

When there is a request for FS evaluation of surgical margins, every effort should be made to render the correct interpretation intraoperatively. This may mean cutting multiple levels, and if necessary, cutting through the block to reach the correct diagnosis. There is no reason to intentionally preserve tissue for permanent sections if this may compromise accurate intraoperative evaluation. A false-negative FS diagnosis may mean a second operative procedure, and this could be complicated if the original wound was closed with a flap or graft (Fig. 3.1[e], [f]).

Mohs micrographic surgery

The goal of Mohs micrographic surgery for malignant neoplasms is complete excision of the tumor, maximum conservation of normal tissue, and FS evaluation of the entire surgical margin.[2] In the original technique, zinc chloride paste was used to fix the tumor tissue in vivo, followed by surgical excision, but this was later modified to a fresh frozen technique. Mohs micrographic surgery is based on the premise that many cutaneous neoplasms grow by direct contiguous extension, and the main threat to the patient is local destructive growth. These tumors

The pieces of skin should be embedded parallel to one another, and they should be oriented in the FS block so that their long axes are perpendicular to the blade. This minimizes folds and compression of the sections. The tissue should be embedded so that a thin strip of unoccupied frozen OCT is present at the proximal and distal ends of the block as this reduces the risk of unwanted folds at the ends of the sections, a factor that is relevant when evaluating margins on skin specimens (see Chapter 2, p. 15). Leaving a free zone of frozen OCT at either end of the FS block is especially important when a brush is used to guide the sections instead of the cryostat's built-in anti-roll device.

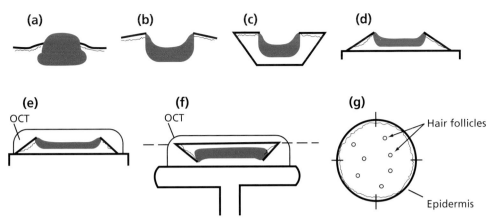

Fig. 3.7. Small skin specimen excised by Mohs technique. (a), (b) The tumor is first debulked with a curet to ease subsequent manipulation. (c) The lesion is then excised with a narrow margin of normal tissue at a 45° angle. (d) The specimen is placed on a cold bar and the edges are manipulated so that the entire peripheral margin adheres to the cold bar. (e) The specimen is covered with OCT compound which is allowed to solidify around the specimen. (f) The specimen and the surrounding frozen OCT are removed from the cold bar, inverted and placed on a specimen holder. The chuck of the microtome is adjusted so that the blade is parallel to the surface of the tissue. Sections are taken close to the surface of the block. (g) Each section includes the deep margin and the entire peripheral margin.

are thus suited to tissue conserving surgery. The manner in which the lesion is excised and the way in which the tissue is embedded for FS are different from conventional FSs. The procedure requires close co-ordination between the Mohs surgeon and the histotechnologist who prepares the frozen sections. The Mohs surgeon removes the lesion, interprets the histologic sections, and in most instances, performs the reconstruction as well. General pathologists are only occasionally involved in the interpretation of these FSs, but the Mohs procedure is summarized here because surgical pathologists should be familiar with this technique. The indications for Mohs surgery are: (a) recurrent or incompletely excised non-melanoma malignancies; (b) highly infiltrative carcinomas or carcinomas with perineural invasion; (c) tumors in functional and cosmetically sensitive areas; (d) large tumors, including tumors on the face that are >1 cm; (e) tumors in immunosuppressed patients; (f) tumors arising in scar or previously irradiated skin; and (g) genetic conditions with increased risk of cutaneous malignancies (e.g., basal cell nevus syndrome and xeroderma pigmentosa).

The first stage of Mohs surgery consists of curettage or excision of any bulky tumor (Fig. 3.7[a], [b]), making the specimen more pliable. The neoplasm is then excised with narrow margins, following the contours of the lesion. The specimen is excised with a 45° angle (Fig. 3.7[c])

because this allows the epidermis at the margin of the specimen to be pushed down to the same plane as the deep margin during the embedding stage (Fig. 3.7[d]). When the peripheral and deep margins are on the same plane, a single histologic section will evaluate all the margins simultaneously (Fig. 3.7[g]). The specimen is embedded in one block if it is small, but large specimens are first cut into quadrants (sectors) and each sector is embedded in a different block. The margins of each piece are inked with a different color, allowing for precise localization of any positive margin. When there is a positive margin, a thin sliver of tissue is excised from just the involved area. Re-excisions, called stages, are performed in a step-wise fashion until the margins are clear. Depending on the size and location of the defect, the wound can be closed primarily or allowed to heal by secondary intention.

The interpretation of histologic sections has to be correlated with the surgeon's mapping procedure, especially when there are multiple stages. Because of the way that tissue is embedded in Mohs surgery, hair follicles are often cut tangentially, and these have to be distinguished from nests of BCC, a distinction that can usually be made with ease but levels are examined if there is any doubt. The cost of Mohs surgery is comparable to conventional excisions with FSs performed in a hospital operating room or an ambulatory care center.

SPECIFIC CLINICO-PATHOLOGIC ISSUES

Basal cell carcinoma (BCC)

Clinical issues

BCCs can be treated in a variety of ways. Optimal treatment is often determined by histologic subtype, size, and anatomic location. Because of their circumscription, superficial and nodular BCCs can be adequately treated by curettage and electrocautery. On the other hand, micronodular and morphea-type BCCs often extend beyond the clinically palpable lesion and are treated with Mohs micrographic surgery or standard surgical excision with FS guidance to achieve clear margins. The surgical procedure selected to treat BCC sometimes depends on the specialist who attends to the patient; general surgeons, plastic surgeons, and ENT surgeons use standard excisions with the aid of conventional FSs, general dermatologists will use curettage

and cautery when possible, and dermatologists skilled in Mohs technique will use this method. While treatment options may vary, Mohs micrographic surgery is the procedure of choice when tissue conversation is at a premium.

A positive margin after initial excision is more likely in the following situations: (a) Neoplasms in anatomic sites such as the nose and ear where the skin is taut, making it more difficult to define the boundaries of the lesion; (b) Certain subtypes of BCC such as infiltrative, morpheaform and micronodular, either because of deep invasion or the infiltrative quality of the tumor; (c) Recurrences arising in scar tissue after prior surgery or radiation treatment because the recurrent carcinoma may be in the deep dermis/subcutaneous tissue and difficult to distinguish from dense scar tissue.

Pathologic issues

Histologically, six patterns of BCC are relevant to the intraoperative setting: nodular, superficial, infiltrative, morpheaform, micronodular, and mixed (Fig. 3.8).[3] Nodular,

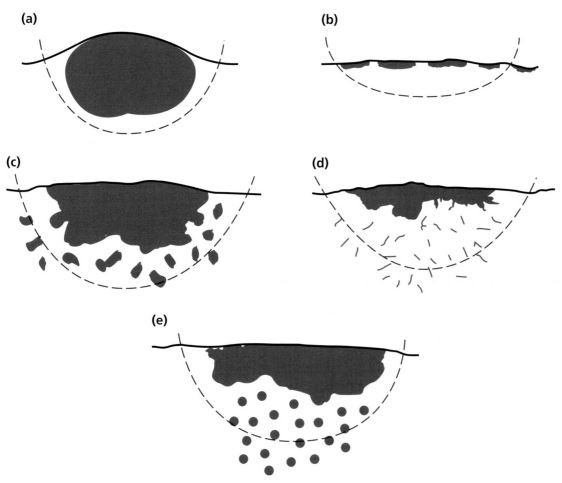

Fig. 3.8. Line drawing showing the common pattens in basal cell carcinoma: (a) nodular, (b) superficial, (c) infiltrating, (d) morphea, (e) micronodular. The dotted lines simulate the surgical excision lines based on clinical examination. These drawings show why some pattens of BCC are more likely to have positive margins on initial excisional biopsy.

(a)

(b)

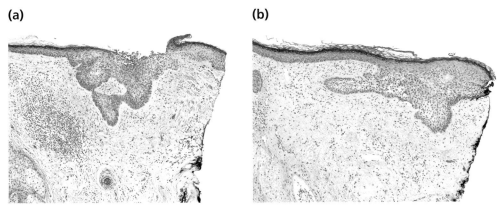

Fig. 3.9. Superficial BCC. (a) The carcinoma was close to, but clear of, the surgical margin in the initial section. (b) A deeper level showed this focus to carcinoma to extend to the surgical margin affirming the point that at least 1mm of normal tissue should be present at the margin in superficial BCC.

infiltrative, and morpheaform BCCs occur mainly in sun-damaged skin such as the face, whereas superficial BCC tends to occur on the trunk. Nodular BCC is the easiest to evaluate on FS because of its circumscription. The characteristic cleft-like spaces between tumor and dermis are absent in FSs, but the distinction between nodular BCC and tangentially sectioned hair follicles is seldom an issue. A narrow margin of normal tissue, even <1 mm, is acceptable for nodular BCCs.

Superficial BCC has an apparent discontinuous pattern of growth when examined in two-dimensional histologic sections, but most of these foci are in continuity. Because of the skip pattern of growth, an interpretation of clear margins should be made with caution if the neoplasm is <1 mm from the margin; evaluation of the margins is even more difficult when the characteristic fibromyxoid stromal reaction is absent (Fig. 3.9). Sometimes, a tangentially sectioned vellous hair follicle may be confused for a bud of BCC but this can usually be resolved by recognizing that superficial BCC has an axis parallel to the epidermis, whereas hair follicles have axes that are perpendicular or oblique to the epidermis. Unfortunately, the characteristic retraction space of superficial BCC may not be present in FSs.

Infiltrative type BCC consists of irregularly-shaped nests of basal cells that frequently invade into the reticular dermis at the time of diagnosis. Because of an apparent skip pattern of growth at the periphery of the lesion, >1 mm of normal tissue should be present before interpreting the margin as negative.

Morphea-type BCC is the most likely subtype to result in false-negative diagnosis on FS. Narrow cords of neoplastic cells infiltrate the dermis and appear discontinuous in two-dimensional sections. The neoplastic cells may be

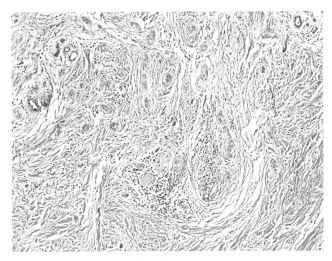

Fig. 3.10. Morphea type BCC. This area was close to a surgical margin. The cords of bland neoplastic cells could be mistaken for reactive endothelial cells or altered sweat ducts.

cytologically bland, and mistaken for eccrine ducts or benign mesenchymal cells (Fig. 3.10). Furthermore, a prominent fibroblastic and chronic inflammatory host reaction may be present and this can mask the tumor. Multiple levels should be prepared routinely, and at least 1–2 mm or normal tissue should be present around the tumor before the margins are declared clear.

Micronodular BCC, an infrequent variant of BCC, grows by forming multiple, separate round tumor nodules in the dermis and subcutaneous fat. The tumor nodules tend to be relatively uniform in size and they may not evoke a significant host reaction. Because the micronodules are separated by relatively normal stroma, a margin of at least 1 mm of normal tissue should be required for a clear margin. BCC with sebaceous differentiation (sebaceous epithelioma) is treated in the same way as conventional BCC.

The main challenge with BCCs on FS is the distinction between BCC and tangentionally sectioned hair follicles. When this becomes an issue at the surgical margins, multiple levels should be examined for clues of normal follicular structures such as a dermal papilla, specialized follicular stroma, sebaceous glands, and arrector pili muscle.

Squamous cell carcinoma

Clinical issues

Actinic keratoses and Bowen's disease (squamous cell carcinoma in situ) are the common precursors of invasive squamous cell carcinoma. The overwhelming majority of actinic keratoses, including bowenoid actinic keratosis, can be treated by cryotherapy, topical medications (such as 5-FU or imiquimod), shave biopsy, or curettage, and do not require surgical resection. On the other hand, Bowen's disease has a high rate of recurrence when treated with cryotherapy or topical 5-FU. Curettage and electrodessication can be used, but the lesion may recur if involved adnexal structures are not eradicated. Surgical excision or Mohs micrographic surgery provide the best cure rates.

Squamous cell CA (SCC), the second most common cutaneous malignancy, has been divided into two main categories based on its metastatic potential.[4,5] Low-risk squamous cell carcinomas arise in sun-damaged skin and have a metastatic potential of <1%, whereas squamous cell carcinomas that arise in non-exposed sites, in immunocompromised patients, and in scars from burns and radiation injury, have a metastatic rate of approximately 10%. Low risk carcinomas are treated by local ablation or surgical excision, depending on size, grade and anatomic location. High risk SCCs are usually treated by surgical excision to ensure that the lesion has been removed with adequate clear margins.

Dermatologists recognize keratoacanthoma (KA) as a distinct entity based on rapid onset, crateriform appearance with a central keratin plug, and spontaneous involution. KAs respond to intralesional injections of 5-FU, bleomycin, or methotrexate. While KA will often involute spontaneously or respond to medical treatment, a subset of patients will have persistent or progressive disease; these patients are assumed to have well differentiated KA-like SCC, and are managed by surgical excision.*

---

* Solitary lesions with a KA pattern probably include two biologically different lesions, but conventional histologic examination does not allow discrimination between lesions that will involute spontaneously and those that will be aggressive. Because of the risk of under-diagnosis, most pathologists consider KA a variant of squamous cell carcinoma.

Verrucous carcinoma of the skin occurs primarily in anogenital locations; this variant of SCC is discussed in more detail on page 46.

Higher grades of SCC vary in their infiltrative capacity. Some poorly differentiated carcinomas are highly infiltrative, invade deeply, and show perineural invasion. They may extend beyond the clinically palpable lesion and require FSs to guide excision. Perineural invasion is clinically silent in the majority of patients, and found only at the time of histologic examination. Rarely however, perineural invasion manifests with nerve palsy (e.g., facial or trigeminal nerve palsy). Perineural invasion is especially serious around the orbit and parotid area, and often requires surgical excision and radiation treatment for control.[6,7] MRI may be used to determine the extent of perineural invasion but this only detects extensive disease.

Pathologic issues

The margins on well-differentiated SCCs are usually easy to evaluate because of the relatively circumscribed nature of the lesion. However, pseudo-epitheliomatous hyperplasia (PEH), which is sometimes prominent in the site of prior biopsy, has to be distinguished from well differentiated invasive SCC. PEH is easily recognized as reactive if it has no resemblance to the original carcinoma, for example, after biopsy of a typical BCC. However, PEH is more difficult to recognize as reactive if it occurs after biopsy of a well differentiated SCC, but the distinction is only relevant if the process involves the margins of excision. Additional tissue should be removed from the involved margin if there is doubt about the nature of the process. PEH also occurs as a reaction to other lesions such as granular cell tumor, deep mycotic infections and chronic ulcers, but these underlying entities should have been identified in the original biopsy and not present as an issue at the time of FS.

Perineural invasion tends to occur more frequently in large, poorly differentiated carcinomas and recurrent carcinomas. It appears as a "skip" lesion on histologic sections and is one of the causes of false negative interpretation of margins. A chronic inflammatory infiltrate around nerves away from the main lesion should prompt careful scrutiny for perineural invasion (Fig. 3.11). Multiple levels of the FS block should be prepared when perineural invasion is identified on the initial FS, and a wide margin of normal tissue should be required before the margin is declared negative. Perineural invasion sometimes extends well beyond the clinical boundaries of the lesion, so there are no simple guidelines for what constitutes an adequate margin.

(a)

(b)

(c)

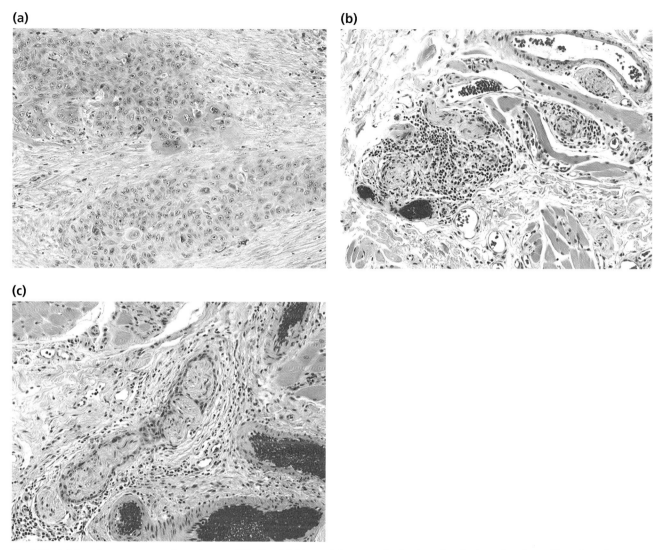

Fig. 3.11. (a) Invasive squamous cell carcinoma of the lip. (b) Many of the nerves in the deep dermis showed perineural lymphocytic aggregates, a finding that should prompt a search for perineural invasion. (c) Further examination showed a few nerves with perineural invasion.

Spindle cell squamous carcinoma can usually be distinguished from scar tissue by its cellularity and atypia, but sometimes it is difficult to make the distinction (Fig. 3.12). Familiarity with the prior biopsy diagnosis is the best way to avoid errors of interpretation. At the time of FS diagnosis, the distinction of carcinoma from fibrosis is relevant only if the spindle cell process approaches or involves a surgical margin.

A minority of invasive SCCs are associated with a wide area of squamous carcinoma in situ. The status of the margin for the in situ carcinoma should be reported because the surgeon's goal will be to remove the entire in situ component as well. In contrast, separate actinic keratoses in the excision specimen should be reported as independent lesions because there is no reason to extend the surgical resection if the actinic keratoses involve the surgical margins.

Sebaceous carcinoma

Clinical issues

Approximately 75% of sebaceous carcinomas occur in peri-ocular locations, followed by scalp and other areas of the face. This tumor has a higher local recurrence rate than BCC and SCC, and a significant tendency to spread to regional lymph nodes and distant sites. Treatment is surgical excision by Mohs micrographic surgery or conventional surgical resection with FS control.

Pathologic issues

The FS approach to sebaceous carcinoma is the same as for infiltrative type BCC and SCC. Frozen sections on grade 3 sebaceous carcinomas in ocular locations are particularly

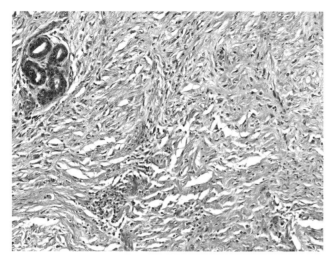

Fig. 3.12. Spindle cell squamous cell carcinoma close to deep margin of the excision. The neoplastic cells are bland and difficult to distinguish from reactive fibroblasts.

challenging because of the highly infiltrative quality of the neoplasm, and the anatomic constraints to wide excision. When an in situ component is present, this should be reported to the surgeon because it may be clinically inapparent; the in situ component requires complete excision with clear margins.

Adnexal neoplasms

Clinical issues

The vast majority of adnexal neoplasms are benign and are excised without the need for FS guidance. Adnexal carcinomas are uncommon and most are recognized as malignant or potentially malignant on clinical examination. Some adnexal carcinomas are highly infiltrative, show perineural invasion and may occur in anatomic sites where wide excision is not possible. If the margins are skimpy or positive, surgical treatment is supplemented with radiation therapy.

Pathologic issues

Cutaneous adnexal carcinomas have a wide range of histologic appearances.[8] Some carcinomas, such as mucinous adenocarcinoma, are distinctive and do not have a benign counterpart. Others, such as papillary digital eccrine adenocarcinoma occur in acral sites and are histologically distinctive. Some carcinomas, such as microcystic adnexal carcinoma, are cytologicaly bland but highly infiltrative, and can be distinguished from similar appearing benign adnexal neoplasms by their infiltrative pattern of growth

(Fig. 3.13). Porocarcinoma, clear cell eccrine carcinoma and malignant spiradenoma resemble their benign counterparts, but have an infiltrative growth pattern, increased mitotic activity, and cytologic atypia. Perineural and lymphovascular invasion provide additional evidence of malignancy, but they are infrequent in low-grade carcinomas.

The diagnosis of carcinoma is usually made on initial biopsy so the purpose of IOD is to evaluate the margins of resection. Occasionally, the original biopsy is non-diagnostic and reported as "atypical adnexal neoplasm," and in this situation, the surgeon may request a diagnosis as well as evaluation of margins. For cytologically low grade carcinomas, the presence of an infiltrative pattern of growth at the interface of tumor with normal tissue is the single most reliable feature for making a diagnosis of carcinoma; the periphery of the neoplasm should be examined if a diagnosis is requested (Fig. 3.14).

The goal of surgical excision is to obtain adequate clear margins. The ideal margin of normal tissue around an adnexal carcinoma is arbitrary, and depends on the anatomic site. A margin of 2 cm is optimal in sites such as the trunk and limbs, but the surgeon will settle for a narrower margin in functionally important sites. Whenever possible, the original biopsy slides should be reviewed because the specimen may be sent for FS with a generic diagnosis of "carcinoma" and it is disconcerting to encounter an unusual adnexal neoplasm in the FS suite when one is mentally prepared to handle a conventional BCC or SCC.

Merkel cell carcinoma

Clinical issues

Merkel cell carcinoma (MCC), a primary endocrine cell carcinoma of skin, occurs mainly in sun-damaged skin of elderly patients. Approximately 50% occur in the head and neck region and 40% on the extremities. MCC is an aggressive malignancy with high rates of local recurrence and nodal spread. About one-third of patients have clinically positive nodes at the time of presentation, and 50% will develop distant metastases during the course of the disease. Five-year survival correlates with stage of disease at the time of diagnosis: 65% for stage I and 47% for stage II. Patients with stage III disease have a median survival of 9 months.

Approximately 40% of Merkel cell carcinomas recur locally. When feasible, the neoplasm is resected widely to minimize local recurrence. A minimum margin of 2 cm is optimal, but this is not always possible. Mohs

(a)

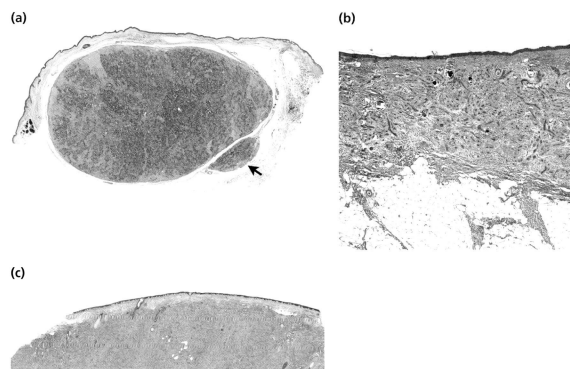

(b)

(c)

Fig. 3.13. (a) Many benign adnexal neoplasms form a circumscribed nodule but satellite nodules, as seen in this cylindroma, may occur. Satellite nodules have a smooth outline and are in close proximity to the main neoplasm. (b) Other benign adnexal neoplasms, such as desmoplastic trichoepithelioma, have an "orderly" and symmetrical infiltrative pattern in the dermis and do not invade the subcutaneous fat. (c) In contrast, microcystic adenexal carcinoma, which shares some features with trichoepithelioma, often involves the subcutaneous fat at the time of diagnosis.

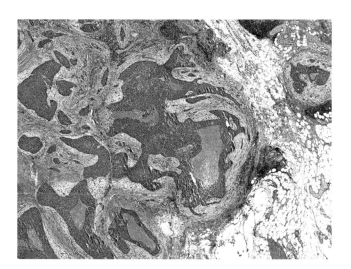

Fig. 3.14. Low grade eccrine carcinoma. The diagnosis can be made with confidence because of the infiltrative pattern of growth and deep invasion.

micrographic surgery is employed for lesions in functionally sensitive locations.[9] Surgical resection is usually followed by post-operative radiation therapy to both the local site and draining lymph nodes. Sentinel lymph node biopsy is currently being explored as an option to evaluate nodal disease, and pathologists may be asked to evaluate lymph nodes intraoperatively. Most Merkel cell carcinomas are resected without FS guidance, but FS may be requested when there are anatomic limitations or when the surgeon is concerned about the margins of resection.

Pathologic issues

The diagnosis of Merkel cell carcinoma is usually made on an initial biopsy specimen. If FS is requested on an excisional specimen, the pathologist's only charge is to evaluate surgical margins. Merkel cell carcinoma is readily recognized on FS; the sheets and trabeculae of neoplastic cells with a high N/C ratio are distinctive, and surgical margins are usually easy to interpret as the neoplasm bears no resemblance to normal cutaneous structures (Fig. 3.15).

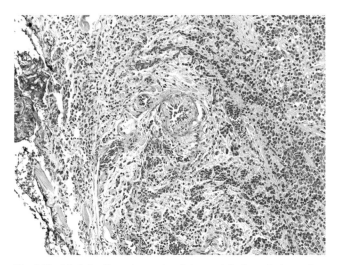

Fig. 3.15. Merkel cell carcinoma involving an inked surgical margin of resection. A positive margin is easy to interpret because the carcinoma does not resemble normal or reactive cutaneous tissue.

Melanocytic neoplasms

Clinical issues

The optimal way to make a diagnosis on a suspected melanoma is to perform an excisional biopsy with a 1 mm margin of normal skin. However, a punch or incisional biopsy may be performed if the lesion is in a functionally important location, or if the lesion is a large, thick, clinically obvious melanoma where an incisional biopsy is likely to provide all the information needed to plan a complex excision. Shave biopsies are performed on melanocytic lesions thought to be benign but, occasionally, a shave biopsy will show an unexpected melanoma.

The definitive treatment of primary cutaneous melanoma is surgical resection with a margin of normal tissue. The margin of tissue around the neoplasm depends on the thickness of the melanoma. Melanoma in situ can be excised with a 5 mm margin of normal skin. Low risk invasive melanomas (<1 mm, and without extensive regression) are usually excised with a 1 cm margin of normal tissue,[10] whereas thicker melanomas are excised with a margin of 2 cm.[11] There is no reason to perform FSs on the margins of resection specimens because the original biopsy findings and the post-biopsy changes are reliable enough to guide the extent of excision.

Unlike other types of melanoma, lentigo maligna (LM) often extends beyond the clinically visible lesion. Most surgeons prefer to excise LM in its entirety even though this often involves wide excision. If the pathologist is uncertain about the status of the margins on FS (either with conventional FSs or Mohs surgery), the surgeon may excise additional tissue and defer closure of the wound until permanent sections are available.[12] In laboratories that have rapid tissue processing, results may be available within 3–4 hours, thus allowing follow-up surgery the same day. There is increasing interest in non-surgical treatment of LM with topical agents such as imiquimod,[13] but to date, the results have been inconsistent, and these modalities are still considered investigational.

Pathologic issues

The initial diagnosis of melanocytic neoplasms is made on paraffin-embedded biopsy specimens. FSs should not be performed to make an initial diagnosis for the following reasons: (a) On occasion, it is difficult to distinguish between nevus and melanoma on optimally processed, paraffin-embedded tissue, and it may be impossible to make the correct diagnosis on FS; (b) definitive surgical treatment for melanoma should not be based on a FS diagnosis; (c) the artifacts produced by performing a FS may compromise the pathologist's ability to subsequently render a firm diagnosis on permanent sections in cases that are diagnostically challenging; and (d) the extent of surgical resection and the need for sentinel node biopsy, are based on risk factors such as tumor thickness, and these prognostic factors are best evaluated on thorough evaluation of optimally processed tissue.

The surgical margins of LM may be difficult to evaluate because the single atypical melanocytes at the periphery of the neoplasm gradually blend with atypical melanocytes of non-neoplastic, sun-damaged skin (Fig. 3.16).[14–16] Non-neoplastic photo-damaged skin may sometimes show confluent growth of single atypical melanocytes in the basal layer of the epidermis so that confluent growth alone is not diagnostic of LM.[15,16] One other limitation is that the artifactual retraction space around atypical melanocytes is absent in FSs, making it difficult to distinguish atypical melanocytes from atypical squamous cells in sun-damaged skin. The margins on lentigo maligna are therefore, difficult to interpret on FS, and surgeons should be encouraged to rely on permanent sections to evaluate the adequacy of excision. Some surgeons however, will request FS evaluation of the margins, Mohs surgeons the most enthusiastic of all. Mohs surgeons sometimes use the rapid melan A immunohistochemical stain to evaluate the margins of lentigo maligna because this stain shows crowded atypical melanocytes to better advantage;[16] however, with the increasing availability of rapid tissue processing,

(a)

(b)

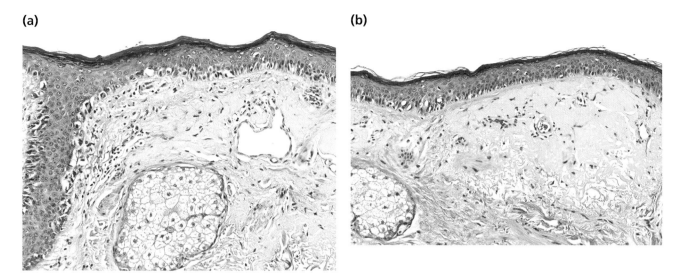

Fig. 3.16. (a) The periphery of a lentigo maligna. The lesion is clearly neoplastic because of the density of atypical melanocytes and involvement of a hair follicle. (b) The epidermis one low power closer to the surgical margin shows scattered atypical melanocytes that we interpret as atypical melanocytes of actinic injury and not LM.

there will no doubt be a move toward evaluating the margins of LM by rapidly processed permanent sections instead of FSs.

Extramammary Paget's disease

Clinical issues

Extramammary Paget's disease typically occurs in apocrine sites, such as the vulva, perianal skin, male genitalia, and axilla. The association with an underlying malignancy varies greatly by anatomic site: less than 5% of vulvar lesions are associated with an organ-based invasive adenocarcinoma, whereas 45% of perianal lesions are associated with an invasive rectal adenocarcinoma.[17,18] Paget's disease often extends beyond the clinically visible lesion resulting in a high frequency of local recurrence. Local recurrence may also be due to multifocality in some cases. Surgical resection, either by wide local excision or Mohs micrographic surgery, is the treatment of choice. Other treatment options include radiation, chemotherapy, topical imiquimod, or photodynamic therapy but these non-surgical modalities have a lower success rate.

Pathologic findings

The initial diagnosis of Paget's disease is made on a routinely processed incisional biopsy. The issue of an underlying or associated invasive adenocarcinoma should also be resolved before definitive excision is undertaken.

Resection of Paget's disease is usually performed with the aid of FS evaluation of the margins, and the recurrence

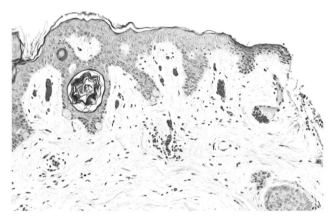

Fig. 3.17. Paget's disease of the vulva. The neoplastic cells near the margin have a signet ring cell appearance with inconspicuous, indented nuclei. The abundant basophilic staining cytoplasm is characteristic of Paget's disease and is a clue to the diagnosis even in the absence of nuclear atypia.

rate is reported to be lower with Mohs surgery than with conventional FSs.[19] It may be difficult to confidently identify isolated Paget cells at the margins of the specimen, especially when the cells have a signet ring cell appearance (Fig. 3.17). Immunostaining with cytokeratin 7 is reported to help in discriminating among Paget cells, squamous cells, and melanocytes, but this immunostain is not widely available as a rapid test. When the FS findings are in doubt, multiple levels should be cut into the block in an attempt to find a cluster of atypical cells. Occasionally, definitive interpretation of the margins has to be deferred to permanent sections and immunohistochemical stains.

(a) **(b)**

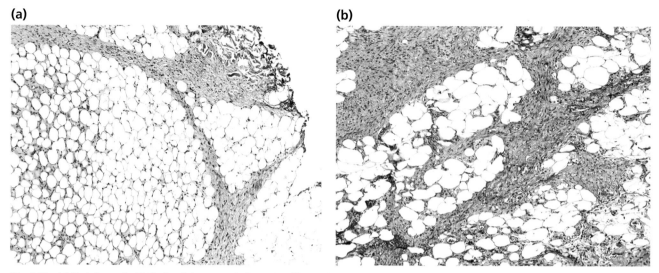

Fig. 3.18. (a) Periphery of a DFSP involving a surgical margin. (b) Another margin in the same case showed similar appearing spindle cells admixed with fat necrosis; the distinction between DFSP and reactive fibroblasts could not be made intraoperatively. The latter area was interpreted as reactive on permanent sections based on a negative CD34 immunohistochemical stain.

Mesenchymal neoplasms

Clinical issues

Atypical fibroxanthoma (AFX), dermatofibrosarcoma protruberans (DFSP) and leiomyosarcoma (LMS) are the three most common potentially aggressive mesenchymal neoplasms of skin.[20–22] All three are capable of local recurrence. While the term sarcoma is appended to two of these neoplasms, metastases occur in <3% of cases.[8,20–22]

AFX typically appears as an ulcerated, erythematous nodule/plaque in heavily sun damaged skin of the head and neck region of older men. The treatment of choice is complete surgical excision with at least a 1cm margin of normal skin, and Mohs surgery is ideal for lesions located on the face.

Approximately 80% of DFSPs occur on the trunk and proximal limbs. DFSP often has extensive subclinical spread, and because of the high incidence of local recurrence, wide excision, with a 2–3 cm margin of normal tissue, is usually necessary. Mohs micrographic surgical excision is reported to have lower recurrence rates.[23]

Cutaneous leiomyosarcoma usually presents as a solitary dermal nodule on the trunk and proximal limbs. Wide surgical excision or Mohs micrographic surgery is the treatment of choice. Dermal leiomyosarcomas rarely metastasize, in contrast to subcutaneous leiomyosarcomas which frequently metastasize to lung, with fatality in approximately 30% of cases.

Pathologic issues

A specific diagnosis would have been established on prior biopsy. Intraoperatively, the pathologist's only task is to evaluate surgical margins. AFX and cutaneous LMS have a limited infiltrative growth pattern beyond the palpable mass and complete surgical resection can usually be performed without the aid of FS. The periphery of DFSP shows variable extension beyond the main lesion. Tumors with limited infiltration are excised without the aid of FS, but FS guidance is needed for DFSPs that are highly infiltrative. If the patient has had a recent attempt at excision, it may be difficult to distinguish DFSP from cellular granulation tissue (Fig. 3.18). When interpretation of the margins is uncertain, the surgeon may delay closure of the wound until results are available with rapid permanent sections, supplemented with CD34 immunohistochemical stains.

Lesions that are fortuitously included in frozen section slides

When evaluating the margins on a malignant neoplasm, a variety of unrelated cutaneous lesions may appear on the FS slides. These are usually easily identified as distinct from the primary malignancy, and should not cause confusion. Actinic keratoses, intradermal nevi, focal acantholytic dyskeratosis, and isolated epidermolytic acanthoma are among the most frequent. If AK is present at the surgical margin, this should be reported with a comment that it is not necessary to re-excise the lesion to achieve clear margins. The other lesions are of no consequence, even if they are the margin.

Frozen sections for medical conditions

Clinical issues

Rarely, life-threatening dermatologic entities may require frozen section diagnosis to facilitate prompt and correct treatment. This is not an intraoperative procedure, but it is discussed here to provide another dimension for the FS test. Among the most important is the distinction between toxic epidermal necrolysis (TEN) and staphylococcal scalded skin syndrome (SSS). Both are potentially fatal, and have characteristic demographic and clinical features. Occasionally, the clinical features are equivocal and a skin biopsy is performed to make the distinction.[24] TEN, which is a hypersensitivity reaction to drugs such as anti-convulsants, penicillins and NSAIDS, and which is mediated by cytotoxic T-lymphocytes, occurs in adults and children. There is widespread, full-thickness dissolution of cutaneous and mucosal surfaces with attendant fluid/electrolyte disturbances and risk of secondary bacterial infection. Treatment includes withdrawal of the causative drug, supportive measures, and sometimes steroids. Antibiotics are given only if there is secondary infection. SSS is an endotoxin-mediated exfoliative dermatitis secondary to a staphylococcal infection. Patients present with widespread cutaneous erosions. SSS occurs mainly in children and the primary site of infection may be relatively trivial. In contrast, adult patients are often immunocompromised and frequently have staphylococcal septicemia. Treatment is with appropriate antibiotics.

Pathologic issues

A punch biopsy of skin will be submitted for FS diagnosis in laboratories that do not have the capability for rapid tissue processing. Histologically, TEN is characterized by variable degrees of epidermal necrosis ranging from scattered dyskeratotic cells to confluent epidermal necrosis resulting in the formation of sub-epidermal vesicles. The underlying dermis usually shows a mild infiltrate of lymphocytes and eosinophils. In contrast, SSS has vesicles in the granular and sub-granular layer, with sparing of deeper epidermis. The dermis does not show any inflammation. The clinician may unroof a bulla and submit this for FS to evaluate the level of the split in the epidermis. The split is subcorneal in SSS and subepidermal in TEN.

REFERENCES

1. Kempson RL, Fletcher CDM, Evans HL, Hendrickson MR, Sibley RK: *Tumors of the Soft Tissues. AFIP Atlas of Tumor Pathology.* 3rd series. Washington DC, 2001.

2. Snow SN, Mikhail GR. *Mohs Micrographic Surgery.* 2nd edition. The University of Wisconsin Press, 2004.

3. Sexton M, Jones D, Maloney M. Histologic pattern analysis of basal cell carcinoma. Study of a series of 1039 consecutive neoplasms. *J Am Acad Derm* 1990; **23**: 1118.

4. Cassarino DS, Derienzo DP, Barr RJ. Cutaneous squamous cell carcinoma: a comprehensive clinico-pathologic classification. Part 1. *J Cut Pathol* 2006; **33**: 191–206.

5. Cassarino DS, Derienzo DP, Barr RJ. Cutaneous squamous cell carcinoma: a comprehensive clinco-pathologic classification. Part 2. *J Cutr Pathol* 2006; **33**: 261–279.

6. Leibovitch I, Huilgol SC, Selva D, Hill D, Richards S, Paver R. Cutaneous squamous carcinoma treated with Mohs micrographic surgery in Australia. II. Perineural invasion. *Dermatol Surg* 2006; **32**: 1369–1374.

7. Mendenhall WM, Amdur RJ, Williams LS, Mancuso AA, Stringer SP, Price-Mendenhall N. Carcinoma of the skin of the head and neck with perineural invasion. *Head Neck* 2002; **24**: 78–83.

8. Patterson JW, Wick MR. *Nonmelanocytic Tumors of the Skin AFIP Atlas of Tumor Pathology, Series 4.* Washington DC, 2006.

9. Gollard R, Weber R, Kosty M, *et al.* Merkel cell carcinoma: a review of 22 cases with surgical, pathologic, and therapeutic considerations. *Cancer* 2000; **88**: 1842–1851.

10. NIH Consensus Development Panel on early melanoma: NIH Consensus Conference. Diagnosis and treatment of early melanoma. *J Am Med Assoc* 1992; **268**: 1314–1319.

11. Balch CM, Urist MM, Karakousis CP, *et al.* Efficacy of 2-cm surgical margins for intermediate-thickness melanomas (1–4 mm). Results of a multi-institutional randomized surgical trial. *Ann Surg* 1993; **218**: 262–269.

12. Cohen LM, McCall MW, Hodge SJ, Freedman JD, Callen JP, Zax RH. Successful treatment of lentigo maligna and lentigo maligna melanoma with Mohs' micrographic surgery aided by rush permanent sections. *Cancer* 1994; **73**: 2964–2970.

13. Wolf IH, Cerroni L, Kodama K, Kerl H. Treatment of lentigo maligna (melanoma in situ) with the immune response modifier imiquimod. *Arch Dermatol* 2005; **141**: 510–514.

14. Barlow RJ, White CR, Swanson NA. Mohs' micrographic surgery using frozen sections alone may be unsuitable for detecting single atypical melanocytes at the margins of melanoma in situ. *Brit J Dermatol* 2002; **146**: 290–294.

15. Hendi A, Brodland DG, Zitelli JA. Melanocytes in long-standing sun-exposed skin: quantitative analysis using the MART-1 immunostain. *Arch Dermatol* 2006; **142**: 871–876.

16. Kelley LC, Starkus L. Immunohistochemical staining of lentigo maligna during Mohs micrographic surgery using MART-1. *J Am Acad Dermatol* 2002; **46**: 78–84.

17. Goldblum JR, Hart WR. Vulvar Paget's disease: a clinicopathologic and immunohistochemical study of 19 cases. *Am J Surg Pathol* 1997; **21**: 1178–1187.

18. Goldblum JR, Hart WR. Perianal Paget's disease. *Am J Surg Pathol* 1998; **22**: 170–179.

19. O'Connor W, Lim K, Zalla M, *et al.* Comparison of Mohs micrographic surgery and wide excision for extramammary Paget's disease. *Dermatol Surg* 2003; **29**: 723–727.

20. Helwig E, May D. Atypical fibroxanthoma of the skin with metastasis. *Cancer* 1986; **57**: 368–376.

21. Kaddu S, Beham A, Cerroni L, *et al.* Cutaneous leiomyosarcoma. *Am J Surg Pathol* 1997; **21**: 979–987.

22. Roses DF, Valensi Q, Latrena G, *et al.* Surgical treatment of dermatofibrosarcoma protuberans. *Surg Gynecol Obstet* 1986; **162**: 449–452.

23. Gloster HM Jr, Harris KR, Roenigk RK. A comparison between Mohs micrographic surgery and wide surgical excision for the treatment of dermatofibrosarcoma protuberans. *J Am Acad Dermatol* 1996; **35**: 82–87.

24. Farmer ER, Hood AF. *Pathology of the Skin*. 2nd edition. New York: McGraw-Hill, 2000.

4 UPPER AERODIGESTIVE TRACT

Raja R. Seethala, Mahendra Ranchod, and Umamaheswar Duvvuri

INTRODUCTION

In the upper aerodigestive tract, malignant neoplasms are responsible for the vast majority of cases that require intraoperative diagnosis. This chapter will focus primarily on squamous cell carcinoma (SCC), the most common malignancy in this site, but the principles espoused for SCC can be applied equally to other resectable epithelial malignancies. The pathologist plays an important role in the intraoperative management of head and neck tumors, a role that can be challenging for the following reasons:

- A wide variety of neoplasms occur in the upper aerodigestive tract (UADT), including a range of squamoproliferative lesions, a wide array of salivary gland neoplasms, as well as endocrine, mesenchymal, melanocytic and hematolymphoid lesions. Intraoperative interpretation is complicated by the fact that disparate neoplasms sometimes have overlapping morphologic features.
- Anatomic structures in the UADT are complex and close collaboration with the surgeon is required to understand the orientation of specimens.
- Most requests for intraoperative diagnosis (IOD) are for evaluation of surgical margins on SCC. This is usually straight forward but there are occasional diagnostic problems and pitfalls, in addition to the challenge of coping with a seemingly unending stream of requests for frozen sections during major resections.

GENERAL CLINICAL ISSUES

The surgeon's approach to malignancies of the UADT is a two-step process: first establish a diagnosis and then institute treatment. A management plan is usually formulated at a multidisciplinary tumor board meeting by a team of physicians interested in diseases of the head and neck, and includes surgeons, radiologists, pathologists, radiation therapists, oncologists, and staff from ancillary services.

Biopsies

An incisional biopsy is the most common approach for superficially located malignancies, while excisional biopsies are performed for clinically benign and small malignant neoplasms. Fine-needle aspiration biopsy (FNA) is performed on submucosal or soft tissue mass lesions but it is rare for this to be done in the intraoperative setting.

Incisional biopsies are submitted for frozen section (FS) evaluation under three main circumstances:

- To determine if the specimen is adequate for diagnosis. The only purpose of the procedure is to obtain sufficient diagnostic tissue, and it is especially important to ensure that sufficient lesional tissue is present for spindle cell lesions and small round cell malignancies where ancillary studies such as immunohistochemistry, flow cytometry, cytogenetics, and electron microscopy may be necessary to make a specific diagnosis.
- To identify the site of a primary carcinoma in a patient who has a known nodal metastasis, because confirmation of a primary malignancy will allow the surgeon to curtail the search elsewhere in the UADT.
- To confirm the diagnosis of malignancy in a patient who has had a biopsy at another institution, and when the original biopsy slides are not available for review. Frozen section confirmation of the diagnosis will allow the surgeon to proceed with immediate definitive surgical resection.

Intraoperative Consultation in Surgical Pathology, ed. Mahendra Ranchod. Published by Cambridge University Press.
© Cambridge University Press 2010.

Surgical resection

Definitive treatment is determined by a variety of factors including type of neoplasm, anatomic location, stage and resectability; while some neoplasms, such as malignant lymphoma, are treated with chemoradiation, the majority of malignancies in the UADT are treated by surgical resection. The goal of surgical resection is complete excision with adequate clear margins because the status of the margins influences outcome; the local recurrence rate for SCC is as high as 80% with positive surgical margins, compared to 25%–45% for negative margins.[1–7] When it is not possible to achieve clear margins because of functional considerations or proximity of the malignancy to vital structures,[8,9] surgical resection may be supplemented with post-operative radiation/chemotherapy. Depending on the anatomic site, a 1–2 cm margin of normal tissue is considered optimal, but a 5 mm margin is acceptable in most anatomic sites; a narrower margin is acceptable in selected situations, such as laser excision of an early stage glottic carcinoma.

The pathologist plays an important role in evaluating surgical margins because the extent of local invasion cannot always be accurately determined by clinical examination and imaging. This may be due to the subtle infiltrative nature of the malignancy, multifocality of the tumor, a skip pattern of growth or perineural invasion beyond the main neoplasm, and this problem is compounded if the patient has had prior radiation therapy, making it difficult to distinguish radiation-induced fibrosis from recurrent malignancy.

Laser excision

Laser excision is used for excising early carcinomas in selected sites such as the vocal cord, where narrow surgical margins are acceptable. Intraoperative evaluation of these specimens is challenging because of their small size and slim margins, calling for close collaboration between surgeon and pathologist. The specimen is carefully oriented, and corresponding areas on the specimen and in the resection bed are marked with one or more dyes to allow for accurate orientation. If further excision is necessary, the dye marks placed in the operative field allow for guided re-excisions. It is difficult to evaluate margins on these specimens because of their small size, thermal injury, and contraction after surgical removal, and whenever possible, the surgeon will submit separate biopsies from the margins of the surgical bed for FS evaluation.

INDICATIONS FOR INTRAOPERATIVE DIAGNOSIS

1. Evaluation of surgical margins on resections for malignancy.
2. Determining the adequacy of an incisional biopsy for initial diagnosis. IOD is requested when anesthesia or sedation are required to perform the biopsy, and when the surgeon's goal is to ensure that an adequate biopsy has been obtained for routine pathologic examination as well as for ancillary tests.
3. Evaluation of a cystic lesion in the neck that the surgeon suspects may be a cystic SCC. If the diagnosis of metastatic SCC is confirmed, the surgeon will undertake a thorough search for a primary carcinoma and save the patient from having to undergo a second operation.
4. To confirm the diagnosis of SCC when prior biopsy slides are not available, and the surgeon wishes to confirm the diagnosis before proceeding with a major resection.
5. Stratification of minor oral salivary gland tumors into high and low risk categories. The low risk category includes benign and low grade malignant tumors, while the high risk category includes intermediate to high grade salivary gland malignancies. The purpose of the FS is to help the surgeon decide on the need for lymph node dissection during the same surgical procedure.
6. For identification and categorization of fungal organisms in an aggressive, acute necrotizing sinusitis. The purpose of the FS is to confirm the diagnosis of invasive fungal sinusitis, which in turn will allow for debridement and prompt institution of antifungal therapy.

INFORMATION NEEDED BEFORE AND DURING SURGERY

At medical centers that have regular head and neck tumor board meetings, the pathologist rendering an IOD is likely to be familiar with the clinical aspects of the case, but when this is not so, the pathologist on FS duty should make every effort to gather relevant information before rendering an IOD.

Clinical history

Familiarity with the clinical aspects of the case will set the stage for correct interpretation of changes encountered on FS; this should include whether the operation is the initial surgical procedure or for a recurrence, and whether the patient had received radiation therapy.

Imaging studies

It is important to be informed about imaging findings when they are relevant, and in complicated cases, it is helpful to review the images with a radiologist.

Previous biopsies

The review of previous biopsies or surgical resections prior to IOD will reduce interpretive errors on FS. For example, the interpretation of changes at the surgical margins are quite different for an excision of a bland spindle cell SCC compared to conventional SCC.

Surgeon's operative plan

It is prudent to be informed of the surgeon's operative plan, and to know what's at stake when making intraoperative diagnoses. The operative plan may change if there are unexpected findings at surgery and the pathologist should find a way to keep track of such changes.

Specimen orientation

It is almost always helpful to see a malignant neoplasm in situ or to have the surgeon orient the specimen in the operating room in relationship to the surgical defect because it is inappropriate to handle a complex specimen without fully understanding its orientation to anatomic landmarks. Even when the orientation of the specimen is clear, the surgeon should place sutures in the specimen to ensure that orientation is retained after the specimen is handled in the laboratory. In addition, if margins are submitted separately from the main specimen, the surgeon should clearly indicate how these are related to the main resection.

HANDLING SPECIMENS AND EVALUATION OF SURGICAL MARGINS

Gross examination is not always reliable for evaluating surgical margins on resections of the UADT because of the "field cancerization" phenomenon, with discontinuous foci of in situ and microinvasive carcinoma away from the main lesion, and the way some carcinomas spread imperceptibly along vessels, nerves and fascial planes well beyond the grossly visible lesion.[1,2] Microscopic examination is therefore, the only certain way to determine if the surgical margins are clear of malignancy.

There are two ways to evaluate surgical margins on resections: (a) the surgeon resects the carcinoma and then submits biopsies from selected areas of the resection bed for FS evaluation; and (b) the resected specimen is submitted to the laboratory, and the pathologist is asked to sample the margins from the resected specimen. Each approach has its advantages and disadvantages, and while there is no clear-cut evidence to show the superiority of one method over the other,[3] we prefer the former whenever feasible.

Submitting separate biopsies from the resection bed

The advantage of this method is that the surgeon identifies areas of concern using the visual and tactile characteristics of the tissue, thereby providing a greater level of assurance that the correct margins are sampled. This is particularly important in the UADT where it is possible to lose precise orientation in a resected specimen when a complex three-dimensional anatomic structure is transformed to a two-dimensional specimen after excision.[4–6] One disadvantage of this approach is that these biopsies are often small, making them difficult to orient. If they are embedded incorrectly, the FS slides may lack a critical layer such as the mucosa, but cutting multiple levels into the block will usually mitigate this situation.

Occasionally, biopsies from the resection bed are wide enough and long enough to be inked for orientation, allowing the pathologist to embed the tissue in a way that will distinguish between the two surfaces of the biopsy, as well as the two halves of the specimen, and with differential inking, permit more precise localization of a positive margin.

There are two ways to embed a specimen when it is wide enough to be oriented and inked, and while pathologists differ in their preference, either method is satisfactory[7] (see Chapter 3, Fig. 3.6).*

---

* The advantage of embedding the tissue with the surgical margin closest to the blade is that the first section represents the true margin; this is an efficient way to evaluate margins in a high volume laboratory. The advantage of embedding the tissue with the surgical margin deep in the block is that the true margin is spared in the event of technical difficulties in preparing frozen sections; in addition, by cutting multiple levels, the pathologist is able to determine if there is any carcinoma in the 3 mm thick piece of tissue embedded for FS evaluation.

Sampling the margins from a resected specimen

Two issues have to be discussed with the surgeon when the entire resected specimen is submitted for margin evaluation: First, the pathologist should be clear about the orientation of the specimen, and this can be done by visualizing the lesion in situ before surgical excision, or by having the surgeon orient the specimen in relation to the surgical resection bed. The surgeon should be asked to place sutures in the specimen, and the location of each suture should be carefully identified to ensure that orientation is retained after transportation to the laboratory. Second, it may not be possible to evaluate all the surgical margins, especially with large specimens, so the surgeon should indicate which margins are of concern, preferably with identifying sutures. Margins adjacent to bone should be specified, because additional surgery may be performed if a carcinoma involves the soft tissue attached to bone (e.g., marginal mandibulectomy for a carcinoma that involves the soft tissue adjacent to the mandible).[4,8] Few laboratories have the capacity to evaluate all the margins on large specimens, so it is reasonable to first evaluate margins that are of concern to the surgeon, and then, after sectioning the specimen, to evaluate any other margin that is of concern to the pathologist.

The margins on small excisions can be evaluated in their entirety, using different color inks to identify different margins – similar to that described for skin specimens in Chapter 3, p. 27). Wedge resections of the lip should be evaluated by sampling the two peripheral margins with parallel sections (see Fig. 3.2, p. 27).

There are two methods of evaluating margins on large resection specimens: sections may be taken parallel to the margin or perpendicular to the margin. There is no evidence-based literature to support one approach over the other,[3] but each has its advantages. A reasonable approach is to customize the sampling based on the surgeon's concerns and the gross findings. For example, we recommend taking parallel sections when the carcinoma appears to be >5 mm from the margin, and perpendicular sections when the carcinoma is <5 mm from the margin (Fig. 4.1). When perpendicular sections are taken, at least three sections should be taken from the area of concern; these can all be placed in one or two FS blocks if the sample includes only the peripheral portion of the carcinoma. Similarly, more than one piece of tissue can be placed in the FS block when using the parallel sampling technique, if each is marked with a unique color (Fig. 4.1). When reporting the distance of a carcinoma from the margin, it

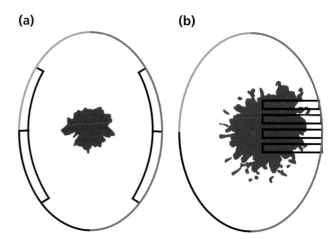

Fig. 4.1. (a) Excision specimen with the carcinoma well away from the surgical margins. Sections taken parallel to the closest margins are an efficient way to evaluate the surgical margins, and multiple pieces of tissue can be embedded in the FS block/s if the margins are color coded. (b) When the carcinoma is close to one margin, sections should be made perpendicular to that margin; multiple pieces of tissue can be embedded in the same FS block if the samples include only the peripheral zone of the carcinoma.

is worth remembering that the pathologist's measurement may differ significantly from the surgeon's estimate of tumor clearance, a difference that can be explained by shrinkage of the specimen after surgical removal.

In some cases, the surgeon will request margin evaluation on the main specimen and also submit biopsies from the resection bed. This situation requires close co-ordination with the surgeon to avoid any misunderstanding of what represents the true surgical margin.

Large keratotic lesions

When large keratotic lesions (e.g., verrucous carcinoma and papillary squamous carcinoma) are submitted for evaluation of margins, the specimen should be inked, sectioned and examined for gross evidence of invasion. If invasion is not visible with the naked eye, the peripheral margins of the specimen should be evaluated in areas of concern. The precise nature of the keratotic lesion may have to be deferred to permanent sections as these lesions may be difficult to classify on FS.

Tonsillectomy specimens

Carcinomas of the oropharynx are usually managed with an incisional biopsy for diagnosis, followed by radiation/chemoradiation, but suspected carcinomas of the tonsil are handled by tonsillectomy if the tonsil can be removed in its entirety. After inking the base of the tonsil, the specimen should be cut serially, and the most suspicious area should be submitted for FS. Confirmation of a carcinoma will allow the surgeon to curtail the search for a primary carcinoma elsewhere. If a carcinoma is not identified in the single section submitted for FS, the diagnosis should be deferred to permanent sections. We do not prepare more than one FS block because some well differentiated tonsillar carcinomas are difficult to recognize on FS, and there is no reason to compromise definitive interpretation by introducing freezing artifact in multiple blocks of tissue.

Thickness of frozen sections for margins

When the specimen contains a generous amount of submucosal fat, or if the tissue shows submucosal edema, frozen sections should be cut at 7–8 μm or even at 10–12 μm if necessary. Thicker sections are more likely to show the entire face of the tissue in the FS block, and tissue folds are less common. Some cytologic features, such as dyskeratosis, may become more evident in thicker sections and help in evaluating lesions such as mucosal dysplasia.

Reporting positive margins

When reporting the results of margins on a resected specimen, the location of the positive margin should be reported as accurately as possible; differential inking helps in this regard.[9,10] The pathologist should also report the length of the margin involved (in mm) and the tissue layer involved (mucosa vs submucosa vs skeletal muscle) as this will influence the extent and depth of re-excisions. One other point about reporting margins: the pathologist should be certain that the labeling of margins, such as anterior, posterior, medial and lateral, have the same meaning for the surgeon and pathologist. If the specimen is complex, these labels can be supplemented by the use of anatomic landmarks as this will ensure accurate reporting, especially if there is a positive margin.

SPECIFIC CLINICO-PATHOLOGIC ISSUES

Relevant pathologic characteristics of squamous cell carcinoma

Several characteristics of SCC are used to determine the extent of local excision, as well as the need for node dissection in patients who have clinically negative lymph nodes.[11,12] Some of these features can be assessed on clinical examination (e.g., size), others from the initial biopsy specimen (e.g.,

Table 4.1. Histologic features of squamous carcinoma that should be reported to surgeon

Histologic features	Comment
Size	Maximum surface dimension, especially in post-radiation cases where the carcinoma may have a wider surface dimension than can be appreciated clinically.
Tumor type	For example, distinguishing verrucous carcinoma from hybrid squamous carcinoma.
Grade	Well, moderately, and poorly differentiated.
Tumor thickness	As measured from the surface.
Invasion of skeletal muscle	
Angiolymphatic invasion	
Perineural invasion	More significant when large nerves are involved
Pattern of growth	Pushing margins, infiltrative, highly infiltrative
Associated carcinoma in situ	Relevant if extensive, and if it involves or approaches surgical margins.

grade), while still others may be identified for the first time during FS evaluation of surgical margins (Table 4.1). These features vary in their significance: some prompt the surgeon to perform a wider resection, while others will make the surgeon consider lymph node dissection (Fig. 4.2).[11,12]

It seems obvious that carcinomas with multiple poor prognostic factors will be more difficult to excise with adequate margins, and are more likely to require lymph node dissection. Some of these histologic features, including pattern of growth, appear to have relevance even for early stage carcinomas.

Impact of surgical margins in squamous cell carcinoma

The status of surgical margins is an important predictor of local recurrence, with recurrence rates of 25%–45% with negative margins and up to 80% with positive margins.[2,4,11–15] Overall survival may also be impacted by margin status, although the data are not conclusive. Even patients with negative surgical margins are at risk for developing local recurrence, presumably due to false negative interpretation of the margins,[17,20,21] discontinuous spread, and the field effect of SCC (Fig. 4.3).[2,16,17] It has also been reported that the outcome is more favorable when clear margins are achieved with the first excision compared to clear margins achieved after multiple re-excisions.[11,18,19] but this is hardly surprising because cases in the latter category are more likely to have poor prognostic features *ab initio*.

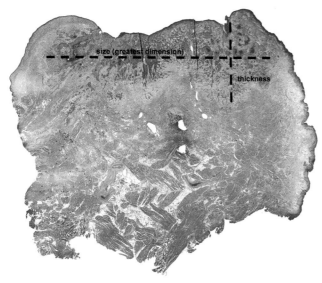

Fig. 4.2. Invasive squamous carcinoma with an infiltrative pattern. This histologic section illustrates three of the features that should be noted during intraoperative evaluation: size, tumor thickness, and invasion of skeletal muscle. Other features that should be reported to the surgeon include pattern of growth, tumor grade, lymphovascular invasion, and extent of any accompanying dysplasia.

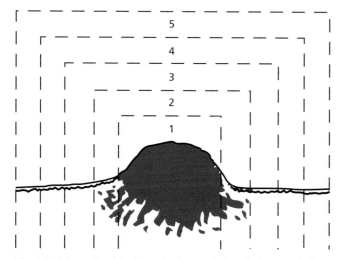

Fig. 4.3. Schematic of the biologic characteristics of a hypothetical squamous cell carcinoma. This schema provides one explanation why recurrences occur after seemingly complete excision. Zone 1: Clinically visible and palpable carcinoma. Zone 2: Extent of invasive carcinoma and mucosal dysplasia on histologic examination. Zone 3: Extent of "field effect" using immunohistochemical markers such as p. 53. Zone 4: Histologically normal mucosa with molecular abnormalities (e.g., loss of heterozygosity on chromosomes 3p and 9p). Zone 5: Normal mucosa.

Verrucous carcinoma

Clinical issues

Verrucous squamous cell carcinoma (VSCC) is a locally aggressive, non-metastasizing variant of SCC that occurs

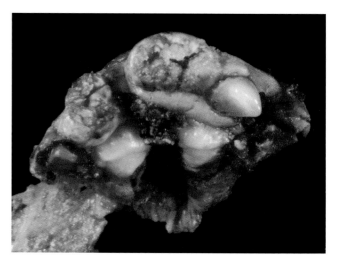

Fig. 4.4. Gross image of verrucous carcinoma of the anterior mandible. The exophytic, cauliflower-like lesion has displaced the remaining tooth to the right.

most commonly in the oral cavity and larynx, and presents as a white, warty, exophytic mass (Fig. 4.4).[22,25] While 5-year survival is reported as 86% in the National Cancer Database,[25] it is probably much higher, as the cases in this report were not subjected to central review and may have included hybrid carcinomas.

The clinical features are distinctive when the lesion is large. An incisional biopsy is performed to confirm the diagnosis, but the problem with VSCC is that the initial office biopsy is often interpreted as a benign keratosis, requiring repeat biopsy under anesthesia. The surgeon is usually certain that the lesion is a verrucous carcinoma and not a benign keratosis, but prefers to have a definite diagnosis before proceeding with resection.

Pathologic issues

Clinicopathologic correlation is essential in the diagnosis of VSCC. The pathologist should view the lesion in situ and encourage the surgeon to obtain a biopsy that is deep enough to include the base of the lesion to allow evaluation of the deep aspect of the lesion. The diagnosis can be made with confidence when the clinical aspects are combined with the histologic findings (Fig. 4.5).[24]

There are two main issues with regard to the IOD of VSCC. First, VSCC has to be distinguished from benign verrucous lesions, such as papillary keratosis and verruca vulgaris, a distinction that usually does not create a management problem because these lesions are small and easily excised in most locations. Proliferative verrucous leukoplakia is a rare disorder that has to be distinguished from conventional verrucous carcinoma; the main clues to the diagnosis

(a)

(b)

(c)

(d)

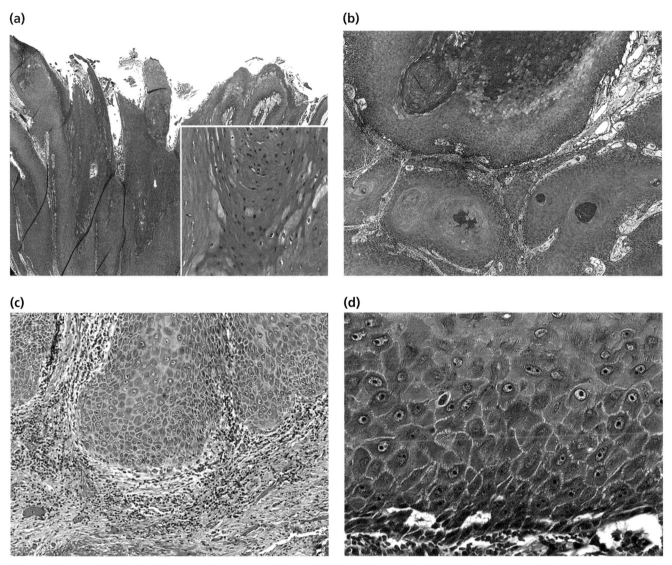

Fig. 4.5. Characteristic histologic features of verrucous carcinoma. (a) The surface consists of spire-like projections with a thick layer of keratin; parakeratosis is prominent between the spires (inset). (b) The rete pegs are characteristically bulbous. (c) A lymphoplasmacytic infiltrate is commonly present in the lamina propria. (d) Minimal cytologic atypia.

are that these patients have multiple lesions that show a range of histologic changes that include simple hyperplasia, verrucous hyperplasia, VSCC and conventional SCC.[26,27]

The second, and more important issue, is the distinction of VSCC from hybrid carcinomas (mixed verrucous carcinoma/conventional squamous carcinoma (Fig. 4.6); approximately 25% of cases in the oral cavity and 10% of laryngeal lesions diagnosed as verrucous carcinoma on clinical grounds are in fact hybrid carcinomas, a distinction that is important because the presence of conventional SCC may prompt lymph node dissection. The finding of conventional SCC on the initial biopsy submitted for FS should be reported to the surgeon because this may affect the extent of local surgical resection, but the relative

volume of conventional SCC in the lesion will be taken into account before deciding on regional lymph node dissection, a decision that will have to be deferred until permanent sections are examined.

It is not possible to evaluate all the peripheral surgical margins on large verrucous carcinomas, and the surgeon will have to accept that the margins will be evaluated selectively, based mainly on areas that the surgeon finds of concern. Occasionally, the periphery of a verrucous carcinoma shows what is descriptively termed verrucous hyperplasia (Fig. 4.7), but there is increasing evidence that verrucous hyperplasia in this setting is a precursor of verrucous carcinoma and should be excised completely, if feasible.

(a)   **(b)**

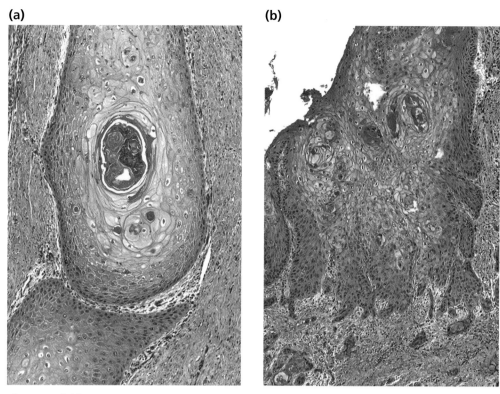

Fig. 4.6. Hybrid verrucous squamous carcinoma and conventional squamous carcinoma. (a) Verrucous carcinoma with blunt, pushing margins, and composed of bland cells. (b) Conventional SCC in the same lesion, with an infiltrative pattern of growth and cytologic atypia.

Basaloid squamous cell carcinoma

Clinical issues

Basaloid SCC, a rare variant of SCC that occurs mainly in the oropharynx and hypopharynx,[28–31] has a striking predilection for men (8:1), and when it occurs in the oropharynx, has a strong association with HPV infection.[32] Generally, basaloid SCC is more aggressive than conventional SCC, and up to 40% of patients have distant metastases at the time of presentation, but HPV-associated lesions in the oropharynx may have a more favorable prognosis.[28–32] Because of their location and advanced stage, many basaloid SCCs, are treated with chemoradiation.

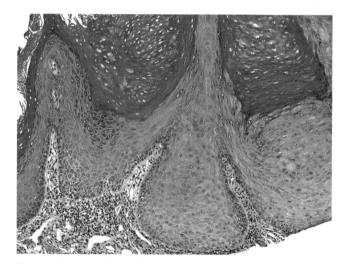

Fig. 4.7. Verrucous hyperplasia at the periphery of a verrucous carcinoma. This lesion is considered a precursor of verrucous carcinoma, and should be excised if feasible.

Pathologic issues

The usual specimen is an incisional biopsy for diagnosis and specimen adequacy. A touch preparation may be helpful for cytologic detail, but a FS should be performed to determine specimen adequacy. On FS, basaloid SCC may be difficult to distinguish from other cellular tumors with a high N/C ratio, but there is no reason to make a specific diagnosis intraoperatively. The occasional tumor that is resected will be submitted for evaluation of surgical margins.

Clues to the FS diagnosis of basaloid SCC include a lobular growth pattern with peripheral palisading, comedonecrosis, abrupt keratinization, pseudoglandular spaces and myxoid or hyaline stroma (Fig. 4.8). The differential diagnosis includes the solid variant of adenoid cystic carcinoma (Fig. 4.9) and small cell neuroendocrine carcinoma (Fig. 4.10).

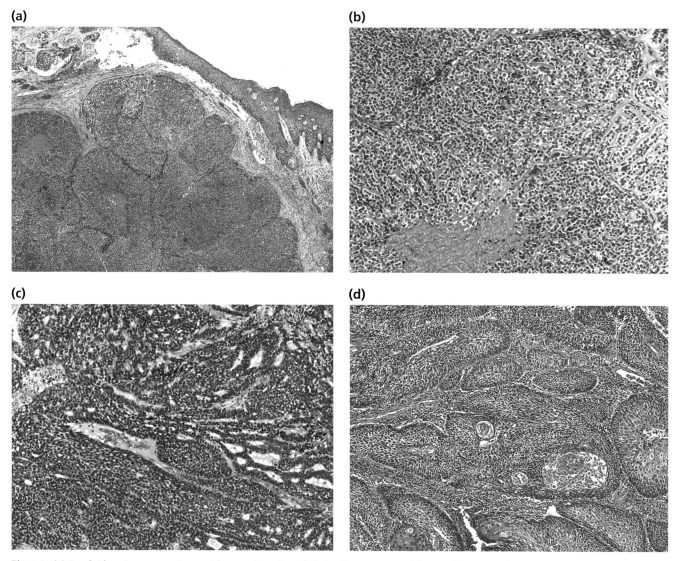

Fig. 4.8. (a) Basaloid squamous carcinoma. The neoplasm has a lobulated appearance with comedonecrosis. (b) The stroma may show hyalinization, mimicking a salivary gland neoplasm. (c) Pseudoglandular spaces may be present, and the cells at the periphery of the lobules are often palisaded. (d) Abrupt keratinization is typical of the basaloid variant of SCC.

Spindle cell squamous carcinoma

Clinical issues

Spindle cell SCC (sarcomatoid carcinoma, carcinosarcoma), a rare variant of SCC with mesenchymal differentiation, occurs most frequently in the larynx, followed by the oral cavity.

The clinical presentation is usually that of a polypoid mass (Fig. 4.11), although it may also present as an infiltrative mass in the oral cavity. Lymph node metastases at the time of presentation are more common in oral tumors. The prognosis is not significantly worse than conventional SCC when controlled for stage and other parameters.[24,33,34]

Pathologic issues

Spindle cell SCC ranges from a bland spindle cell lesion resembling reactive fibrosis, to a malignant neoplasm resembling pleomorphic spindle cell sarcoma. Conventional SCC is present in 50%–80% of cases but may be focal, and absent in the sample taken for FS. Heterologous elements are present in up to 15% of cases, mostly neoplastic bone or cartilage (Fig. 4.12).

The differential diagnosis includes reactive fibrosis, inflammatory myofibroblastic tumor, myoepithelial carcinoma, sarcoma, and spindle cell melanoma. The distinction between spindle cell SCC and other frank malignancies is of no immediate consequence and can be deferred to permanent

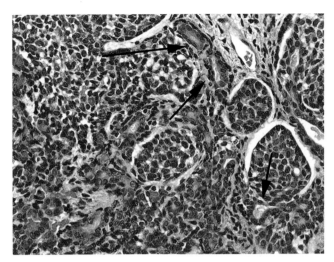

Fig. 4.9. Solid variant of adenoid cystic carcinoma, a neoplasm that may be difficult to distinguish from basaloid SCC on FS. The ductal structures are a clue to the diagnosis (arrows).

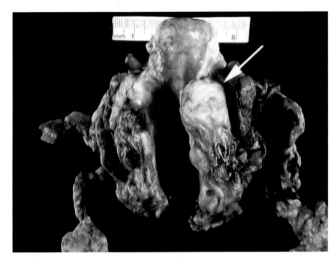

Fig. 4.11. Polypoid spindle cell squamous carcinoma in the hypopharynx of a laryngectomy specimen.

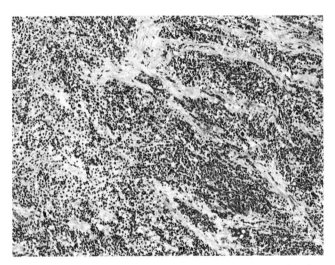

Fig. 4.10. Small cell neuroendocrine carcinoma may be mistaken for basaloid SCC on FS, but this neoplasm lacks a lobulated pattern of growth, punctuate necrosis and abrupt keratinization.

sections. The most important task at the time of IOD is to determine if the lesion has been adequately sampled when the FS shows a bland spindle cell lesion, because reactive fibrosis may be superimposed on the neoplasm if it is ulcerated. If necessary, the pathologist should encourage the surgeon to obtain a true incisional biopsy from a non-ulcerated area, and not a shave biopsy from an ulcerated area. The presence of high grade dysplasia in the non-ulcerated mucosa is a useful clue to the diagnosis.

Nasopharyngeal carcinoma

Clinical issues

Nasopharyngeal carcinoma is uncommon in the United States, but the incidence is at least twentyfold higher in

endemic regions of Southeast Asia, where it is associated with Epstein-Barr virus infection in almost 100% of cases. This carcinoma, which usually arises in the fossa of Rosenmuller, presents most often with a nodal metastasis and an occult primary. The initial diagnosis is made either by FNA of an enlarged lymph node or by incisional biopsy of the primary carcinoma. Nasopharyngeal carcinoma is treated with radiation or chemoradiation, so IOD is limited to confirming the presence of diagnostic tissue in the incisional biopsy specimen.

Pathologic issues

Nasopharyngeal carcinomas range from keratinizing to large cell non-keratinizing, to the prototypic lymphoepithelioma.[35] The diagnosis can be made with confidence when squamous differentiation is identified on FS, but the undifferentiated forms may be difficult to distinguish from large cell lymphoma, dendritic cell sarcoma and melanoma (Fig. 4.13). The main purpose of IOD is to ensure that the biopsy contains sufficient neoplastic tissue for diagnosis. A touch imprint should be made, but a portion of the specimen should be submitted for FS diagnosis because FS is more reliable for determining specimen adequacy.

Dysplasia and carcinoma in situ at the surgical margins

Clinical issues

Invasive SCC may be accompanied by mucosal dysplasia, usually appearing as leukoplakia or erythroplakia on clinical examination, but the lesion may be identified

(a)

(b)

(c)

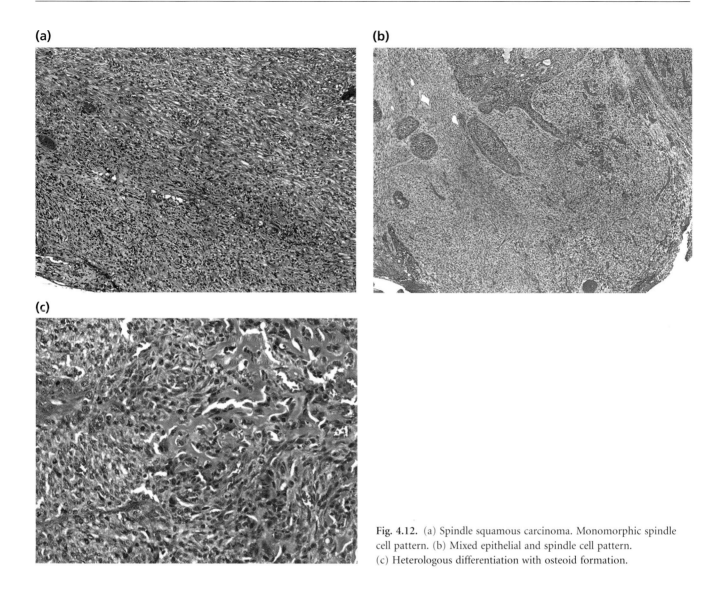

Fig. 4.12. (a) Spindle squamous carcinoma. Monomorphic spindle cell pattern. (b) Mixed epithelial and spindle cell pattern. (c) Heterologous differentiation with osteoid formation.

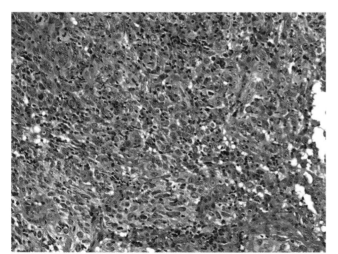

Fig. 4.13. Nasopharyngeal carcinoma, lymphoepithelial type. The carcinoma has a sheet-like growth pattern with an infiltrate of lymphocytes and plasma cells. At the time of FS, the differential diagnosis included large cell lymphoma and melanoma.

for the first time when margins are evaluated at the time of definitive resection. Since dysplasia is a precursor of invasive carcinoma, an attempt will be made to completely excise the lesion if feasible.[2,4,16,41] Some surgeons will expect the pathologist to grade the dysplasia because this may determine the extent of further resection.

Pathologic issues

There are two issues with regard to dysplasia. First, there should be clear communication between pathologist and surgeon about the surgeon's expectations with regard to grading the dysplasia, and how the grade of dysplasia will influence immediate surgical management. This point is made because there is inter-observer variation in the grading of dysplasia, and considerable variation in the diagnosis of mild dysplasia (Fig. 4.14). The second issue relates to the difficulty in

(a)　　　　　　　　　　**(b)**

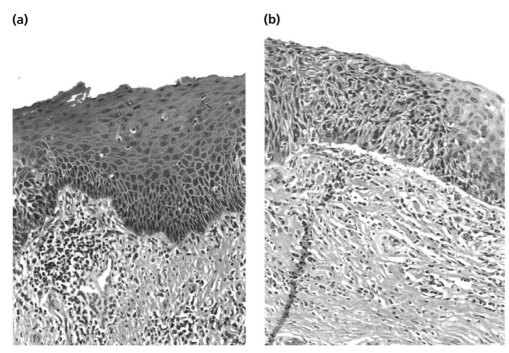

Fig. 4.14. Mucosa adjacent to an invasive squamous carcinoma. Some observers may interpret lesion
(a) as mild dysplasia, but this diagnosis is fraught with problems because of poor reproducibility; the diagnosis
of mild dysplasia should be made with caution because it may lead to unnecessary surgical resection. There
is a high level of inter-observer reproducibility for the diagnosis of high grade dysplasia, an example of which
is shown in (b).

distinguishing radiation-induced atypia from high grade
dysplasia, a distinction that can be challenging. Knowing
if the patient has received radiation therapy to this site is
crucial, but in addition, mitoses, especially atypical
mitoses, will favor high grade dysplasia (Fig. 4.14). In
addition, dysplasia tends to be sharply demarcated from
adjacent uninvolved mucosa, whereas radiation atypia
shows a gradual transition. If the diagnosis of dysplasia
is in doubt, it is prudent to report the changes as "surgical
margins involved by atypia of uncertain significance"
instead of committing to a diagnosis of dysplasia, thus
avoiding unnecessary surgery.

Evaluation of bone margins

Clinical issues
Carcinoma of the oral cavity may invade the mandible,
either because the carcinoma is advanced or because it has
arisen from mucosa close to the bone. CT scan and MRI are
sensitive for detecting bone invasion, but there are false
positives and false negatives. When there is good evidence
of bone invasion, the surgeon may ask for evaluation of
the bony surgical margin. When an invasive carcinoma is
close to a bone such as the mandible, the surgeon may be
interested in the distance of the carcinoma from the soft

tissue margin, because close proximity to the mandible
may prompt marginal resection of the mandible.*

Pathologic issues
It is difficult to evaluate mandibular bony margins accurately because most laboratories are unable to section bone
specimens for IOD.[36] When invasion of the medullary
cavity is suspected, cancellous bone from the surgical
margin can be scraped out with the tip of a blade and this
material can be used for touch preparations and FS. It
should be recognized however, that the accuracy rate for
evaluating bony margins is low, and the surgeon may have
to rely on imaging data to guide the extent of resection.

Evaluation of nerve margins

Clinical issues
Patients with invasion of large nerves may have symptoms related to that nerve (e.g., facial nerve palsy) or

---

* In segmental resection, a segment of the full thickness of the
mandible is removed, and this is done when there is evidence of
bone invasion, or a strong suspicion of bone invasion. Marginal
resection involves removal of the superior portion of the
mandibular bone, and is performed when the carcinoma
involves the soft tissue immediately adjacent to the bone.

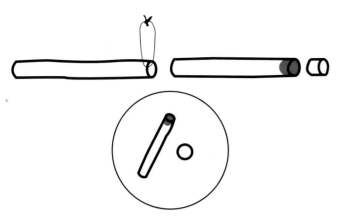

Fig. 4.15. Segment of nerve with a suture marking the margin of interest to the surgeon. A 3 mm long piece of nerve should be removed from the margin and embedded on end. The newly created margin should be inked, and this remaining portion of nerve should be embedded longitudinally. Multiple levels should be prepared routinely.

they may be asymptomatic and nerve involvement is suspected during surgery if the nerve is expanded and edematous. MRI can detect nerve invasion, but only when the nerve is grossly abnormal. Nerve invasion is a poor prognostic factor, and when radical resections are performed, any involved segment of nerve will be included in the surgical resection, and the surgeon will be interested in the status of the nerve margin before reconstruction of the nerve.[37,38,40]

Pathologic issues
When a short segment of unoriented nerve is submitted for IOD, the nerve should be cut in cross-section, and the entire specimen should be embedded for FS. Multiple levels should be prepared routinely because nerve invasion may have a skip pattern of growth. When a longer segment of nerve is submitted for FS evaluation, a single cross-section should be taken from the end identified as the surgical margin; the newly created surgical margin should be inked and the remainder of the nerve should be embedded longitudinally (Fig. 4.15). Multiple levels should be prepared routinely. This approach will evaluate if carcinoma is present anywhere in the nerve segment as well as the relationship of the carcinoma to the surgical margin.

Radiation atypia in resected specimens

Clinical issues
Squamous cell carcinomas of the UADT are frequently treated with chemoradiation, either as primary treatment or as adjuvant therapy. Tissues subjected to chemoradiation are encountered for IOD either as an incisional

biopsy to evaluate the response to treatment, or when surgical resection is performed as a salvage procedure for local recurrence.

Pathologic issues
If residual carcinoma is present, it may be more pleomorphic than the pre-treatment tumor, a point that is of little consequence if the pathologist is aware of the clinical history. What is more important is radiation atypia in benign tissue because this may be mistaken for a malignancy, a pitfall that can be avoided by familiarity with the clinical history, and by paying attention to subtleties that distinguish radiation atypia from recurrent carcinoma[42] (Fig. 4.16). The correct interpretation of radiation atypia is particularly important when it is present at the surgical margins.

Benign lesions that may be mistaken for dysplasia or invasive carcinoma

Pseudoepitheliomatous hyperplasia may occur in association with a variety of inflammatory and non-epithelial neoplasms, including deep fungal infections, granular cell tumor and T-cell lymphoma, but its relevance in the intraoperative setting is when it is present at the surgical margin in patients who have had previous surgery for SCC. One quick way to resolve the question of carcinoma versus pseudoepitheliomatous hyperplasia is to compare the FS findings with the patient's original malignancy; the issue is readily resolved if the original biopsy shows a high grade carcinoma. If there is no information about the original biopsy, clues to the diagnosis of pseudoepitheliomatous hyperplasia include the lack of cytologic atypia and limited extension of the proliferating epithelium into the underlying lamina propria.[43]

Necrotizing sialometaplasia, which may occur after radiation treatment, may be mistaken for SCC or muco-epidermoid carcinoma, a point that is significant if it is present at the margin of resection. The lobular outline and lack of significant cytologic atypia are the main clues to the diagnosis (Fig. 4.17).[44]

Normal structures that may be mistaken for squamous cell carcinoma

Odontogenic rests, either the epithelial remnants of Malassez and Serres in the gingiva[45] may be mistaken for SCC on FS (Fig. 4.18). Their proximity to tooth-bearing areas of the oral cavity and bland cytologic features are clues to the

(a) **(b)**

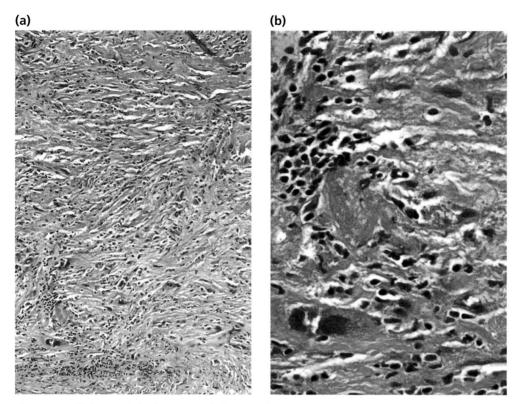

Fig. 4.16. Radiation atypia in the stroma of a laryngeal biopsy. (a) Atypical stromal cells that raise concern about spindle cell carcinoma. The atypical cells have moderate quantities of slightly basophilic cytoplasm, and (b) the nuclei have a smudged appearance, features that support radiation atypia. Familiarity with the appearance of the pre-treatment carcinoma is helpful in this situation.

(a) **(b)**

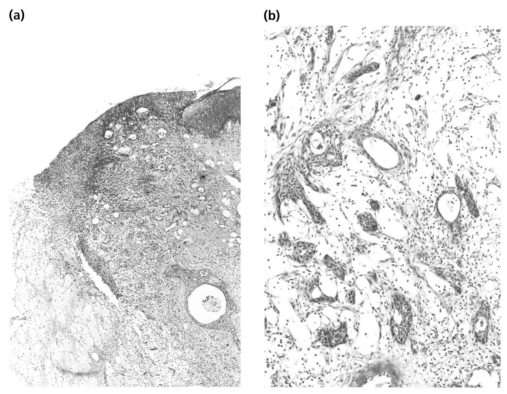

Fig. 4.17. Palatal biopsy with necrotizing sialometaplasia. (a) This low magnification view shows mucosal ulceration and extravasation of mucus (lower left). (b) Minor salivary gland ducts undergo squamous metaplasia, a finding that should not be misinterpreted as invasive carcinoma. The loose stroma argues against squamous carcinoma.

(a)

(b)

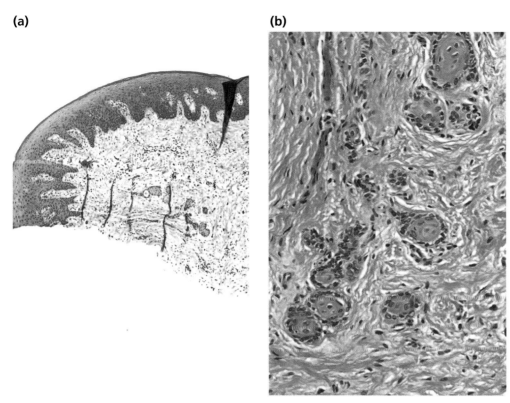

Fig. 4.18. Benign odontogenic rests with bland cytologic features. These rests may pose a problem when they are at a margin of a resection. Odontogenic rests should always be considered when the specimen is from the gingiva.

correct diagnosis. Comparison of the FS findings with the patient's original carcinoma may quickly settle the issue – one more reason to be familiar with the histologic features of the patient's known malignancy.

The Juxtaoral Organ of Cheivitz, located in the bucco-temporal space, consists of epithelium that is intimately associated with loose neurovascular tissue.[46] This normal structure should not be mistaken for SCC with perineural invasion. The anatomic location, nested appearance, and the lack of keratinization, atypia and desmoplasia should lead to the correct interpretation.

Cystic metastatic squamous cell carcinoma in cervical lymph nodes

Clinical issues

Up to 5% of cervical lymph node metastases from SCC are cystic, the majority taking their origin as occult primary carcinomas in Waldeyer's ring. The cystic change may be extensive enough to mimic a benign cyst clinically, an impression that is compounded by a negative FNA. A cystic metastasis is most often mistaken for a branchial cleft cyst, although other cystic lesions also enter the differential

diagnosis.[47–54] An open biopsy will be performed when there is a suspicion that the lesion may be malignant.

Pathologic issues

The specimen submitted may be an incisional biopsy, or an excision of the entire mass. If the specimen is an excision, it should be inked, since primary salivary gland tumors may occasionally occur in this location, making margin evaluation relevant. Metastatic SCC with cystic change usually takes the form of a multiloculated cyst with solid and pseudo-papillary areas (Fig. 4.19). The lesion may be mistaken for a branchial cyst if the FS sample shows lymphoid tissue with cysts lined by a thin layer of relatively bland epithelium. This error can be avoided by careful gross examination, sampling of the solid areas, and a high level of suspicion based on the clinical history.

Sentinel lymph node biopsy in squamous cell carcinoma

Clinical issues

The status of regional lymph nodes has a major influence on the management of SCC of the UADT. Sentinel lymph

(a)

(b)

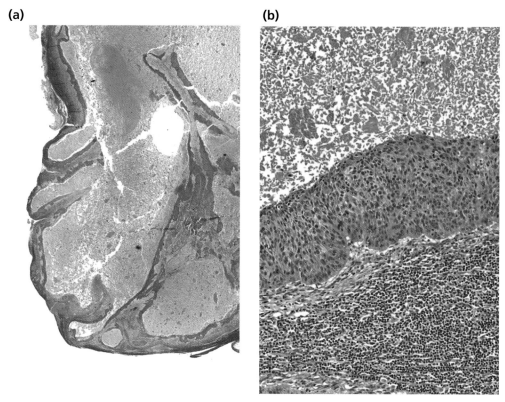

Fig. 4.19. Cystic metastatic squamous carcinoma in a cervical lymph node. (a) The architectural complexity and papillations should suggest a neoplasm and argue against a branchial cleft cyst. (b) The epithelial cells are sufficiently atypical to warrant a diagnosis of squamous carcinoma.

node biopsy has begun to gain traction as an alternative to elective neck dissection in patients with cT1/T2,N0,M0 disease, because this test can identify the approximately 25% of patients who have occult nodal metastases, allowing the surgeon to offer node dissection to these patients, and sparing the remaining patients from unnecessary surgery.[55–57] Currently, sentinel lymph node biopsy is not standard practice for evaluating malignancies of the UADT, but is likely to gain popularity as its benefits are validated.

Pathologic issues

The issues regarding intraoperative examination of sentinel nodes are discussed in detail in the Chapters 13 and 16, pp. 201 and 258. In summary, we feel that the goal of intraoperative examination is to detect larger nodal metastases, and that cytologic examination is sufficient in most cases. If the cytologic examination is negative, the sentinel node should be processed routinely, and examined with multiple levels and immunohistochemical stains to detect micrometastases. Failure to detect nodal metastases intraoperatively does mean a second operation for completion

lymphadenectomy, but for the present, we do not recommend exhaustive intraoperative evaluation of sentinel nodes with multiple frozen sections.

REFERENCES

1. Woolgar JA, Triantafyllou A. A histopathological appraisal of surgical margins in oral and oropharyngeal cancer resection specimens. *Oral Oncol* 2005; **41**(10): 1034–1043.
2. Bradley PJ, MacLennan K, Brakenhoff RH, *et al.* Status of primary tumour surgical margins in squamous head and neck cancer: prognostic implications. *Curr Opin Otolaryngol Head Neck Surg* 2007; **15**(2): 74–81.
3. Black C, Marotti J, Zarovnaya E, *et al.* Critical evaluation of frozen section margins in head and neck cancer resections. *Cancer* 2006; **107**(12): 2792–2800.
4. Batsakis JG. Surgical excision margins: a pathologist's perspective. *Adv Anat Pathol* 1999; **6**(3): 140–148.
5. Kerawala CJ, Ong TK. Relocating the site of frozen sections–is there room for improvement? *Head Neck* 2001; **23**(3): 230–232.
6. Ambrosch P, Brinck U, Fischer G, *et al.* [Special aspects of histopathologic diagnosis in laser microsurgery of cancers of the upper aerodigestive tract]. *Laryngorhinootologie* 1994; **73**(2): 78–83.
7. Cooley ML, Hoffman HT, Robinson RA. Discrepancies in frozen section mucosal margin tissue in laryngeal squamous cell carcinoma. *Head Neck* 2002; **24**(3): 262–267.

8. Cheng A, Cox D, Schmidt BL. Oral squamous cell carcinoma margin discrepancy after resection and pathologic processing. *J Oral Maxillofac Surg* 2008; **66**(3): 523–529.

9. Gnepp DR, Barnes L, Crissman J, *et al.* Recommendations for the reporting of larynx specimens containing laryngeal neoplasms. *Am J Clin Pathol* 1998; **110**(2): 137–139.

10. Zarbo RJ, Barnes L, Crissman JD, *et al.* Recommendations for the reporting of specimens containing oral cavity and oropharynx neoplasms. Association of Directors of Anatomic and Surgical Pathology. *Hum Pathol* 2000; **31**(10): 1191–1193.

11. Brandwein-Gensler M, Teixeira MS, Lewis CM, *et al.* Oral squamous cell carcinoma: histologic risk assessment, but not margin status, is strongly predictive of local disease-free and overall survival. *Am J Surg Pathol* 2005; **29**(2): 167–178.

12. Spiro RH, Guillamondegui O, Jr., Paulino AF, *et al.* Pattern of invasion and margin assessment in patients with oral tongue cancer. *Head Neck* 1999; **21**(5): 408–413.

13. Jones AS, Bin Hanafi Z, Nadapalan V, *et al.* Do positive resection margins after ablative surgery for head and neck cancer adversely affect prognosis? A study of 352 patients with recurrent carcinoma following radiotherapy treated by salvage surgery. *Br J Cancer* 1996; **74**(1): 128–132.

14. Haque R, Contreras R, McNicoll MP, *et al.* Surgical margins and survival after head and neck cancer surgery. *BMC Ear Nose Throat Disord* 2006; **6**: 2.

15. Cook JA, Jones AS, Phillips DE, *et al.* Implications of tumour in resection margins following surgical treatment of squamous cell carcinoma of the head and neck. *Clin Otolaryngol Allied Sci* 1993; **18**(1): 37–41.

16. Looser KG, Shah JP, Strong EW. The significance of "positive" margins in surgically resected epidermoid carcinomas. *Head Neck Surg* 1978; **1**(2): 107–111.

17. Ord RA, Aisner S. Accuracy of frozen sections in assessing margins in oral cancer resection. *J Oral Maxillofac Surg* 1997; **55**(7): 663–669; discussion 669–671.

18. Scholl P, Byers RM, Batsakis JG, *et al.* Microscopic cut-through of cancer in the surgical treatment of squamous carcinoma of the tongue. Prognostic and therapeutic implications. *Am J Surg* 1986; **152**(4): 354–360.

19. Jackel MC, Ambrosch P, Martin A, *et al.* Impact of re-resection for inadequate margins on the prognosis of upper aerodigestive tract cancer treated by laser microsurgery. *Laryngoscope* 2007; **117**(2): 350–356.

20. DiNardo LJ, Lin J, Karageorge LS, *et al.* Accuracy, utility, and cost of frozen section margins in head and neck cancer surgery. *Laryngoscope* 2000; **110**(10 Pt 1): 1773–1776.

21. Ribeiro NF, Godden DR, Wilson GE, *et al.* Do frozen sections help achieve adequate surgical margins in the resection of oral carcinoma? *Int J Oral Maxillofac Surg* 2003; **32**(2): 152–158.

22. Ackerman LV. Verrucous carcinoma of the oral cavity. *Surgery* 1948; **23**(4): 670–678.

23. Medina JE, Dichtel W, Luna MA. Verrucous-squamous carcinomas of the oral cavity. A clinicopathologic study of 104 cases. *Arch Otolaryngol* 1984; **110**(7): 437–440.

24. Barnes EL. *Surgical Pathology of the Head and Neck.* 3rd edn. Informa Healthcare; 2009, pp. 123–124.

25. Koch BB, Trask DK, Hoffman HT, *et al.* National survey of head and neck verrucous carcinoma: patterns of presentation, care, and outcome. *Cancer* 2001; **92**(1): 110–120.

26. Suarez P, Batsakis JG, el-Naggar AK. Leukoplakia: still a gallimaufry or is progress being made?--A review. *Adv Anat Pathol* 1998; **5**(3): 137–155.

27. Batsakis JG, Suarez P, el-Naggar AK. Proliferative verrucous leukoplakia and its related lesions. *Oral Oncol* 1999; **35**(4): 354–359.

28. Luna MA, el Naggar A, Parichatikanond P, *et al.* Basaloid squamous carcinoma of the upper aerodigestive tract. Clinicopathologic and DNA flow cytometric analysis. *Cancer* 1990; **66**(3): 537–542.

29. Banks ER, Frierson HF, Jr., Mills SE, *et al.* Basaloid squamous cell carcinoma of the head and neck. A clinicopathologic and immunohistochemical study of 40 cases. *Am J Surg Pathol* 1992; **16**(10): 939–946.

30. Winzenburg SM, Niehans GA, George E, *et al.* Basaloid squamous carcinoma: a clinical comparison of two histologic types with poorly differentiated squamous cell carcinoma. *Otolaryngol Head Neck Surg* 1998; **119**(5): 471–475.

31. Soriano E, Righini C, Faure C, *et al.* [Course and prognosis of basaloid squamous cell carcinoma: case-control study of 49 patients]. *Ann Otolaryngol Chir Cervicofac* 2005; **122**(4): 173–180.

32. Begum S, Westra WH. Basaloid squamous cell carcinoma of the head and neck is a mixed variant that can be further resolved by HPV status. *Am J Surg Pathol* 2008; **32**(7): 1044–1050.

33. Lewis JE, Olsen KD, Sebo TJ. Spindle cell carcinoma of the larynx: review of 26 cases including DNA content and immunohistochemistry. *Hum Pathol* 1997; **28**(6): 664–673.

34. Thompson LD, Wieneke JA, Miettinen M, *et al.* Spindle cell (sarcomatoid) carcinomas of the larynx: a clinicopathologic study of 187 cases. *Am J Surg Pathol* 2002; **26**(2): 153–170.

35. Chan JKC, Bray F, McCarron P, *et al.* Nasopharyngeal carcinoma. In Barnes L, Eveson JW, Reichart P, Sidransky D, eds. *Pathology and Genetics of Head and Neck Tumors.* Lyons: IARC; 2005, pp. 85–97.

36. Oxford LE, Ducic Y. Intraoperative evaluation of cortical bony margins with frozen-section analysis. *Otolaryngol Head Neck Surg* 2006; **134**(1): 138–141.

37. Carter RL, Pittam MR, Tanner NS. Pain and dysphagia in patients with squamous carcinomas of the head and neck: the role of perineural spread. *J Roy Soc Med* 1982; **75**(8): 598–606.

38. Wax MK, Kaylie DM. Does a positive neural margin affect outcome in facial nerve grafting? *Head Neck* 2007; **29**(6): 546–549.

39. Spiro JD, Spiro RH. Cancer of the parotid gland: role of 7th nerve preservation. *World J Surg* 2003; **27**(7): 863–867.

40. Vural E, Fan CY, Spring P, *et al.* Evaluation of the inferior and superior laryngeal nerve stumps for perineural spread in laryngeal cancer. *Otolaryngol Head Neck Surg* 2007; **137**(6): 889–892.

41. Slootweg PJ, Hordijk GJ, Schade Y, *et al.* Treatment failure and margin status in head and neck cancer. A critical view on the potential value of molecular pathology. *Oral Oncol* 2002; **38**(5): 500–503.

42. Kwong DL, Nicholls J, Wei WI, *et al.* Correlation of endoscopic and histologic findings before and after treatment for nasopharyngeal carcinoma. *Head Neck* 2001; **23**(1): 34–41.

43. Zarovnaya E, Black C. Distinguishing pseudoepitheliomatous hyperplasia from squamous cell carcinoma in mucosal biopsy specimens from the head and neck. *Arch Pathol Lab Med* 2005; **129**(8): 1032–1036.

44. Brannon RB, Fowler CB, Hartman KS. Necrotizing sialometaplasia. A clinicopathologic study of sixty-nine cases and review of the literature. *Oral Surg Oral Med Oral Pathol* 1991; **72**(3): 317–325.

45. Rincon JC, Young WG, Bartold PM. The epithelial cell rests of Malassez – a role in periodontal regeneration? *J Periodontal Res* 2006; **41**(4): 245–252.

46. Pantanowitz L, Balogh K. Significance of the juxtaoral organ (of Chievitz). *Head Neck* 2003; **25**(5): 400–405; discussion 400.

47. Devaney KO, Rinaldo A, Ferlito A, *et al.* Squamous carcinoma arising in a branchial cleft cyst: have you ever treated one? Will you? *J Laryngol Otol* 2008; **122**(6): 547–550.

48. Gourin CG, Johnson JT. Incidence of unsuspected metastases in lateral cervical cysts. *Laryngoscope* 2000; **110**(10 Pt 1): 1637–1641.

49. Schmalbach CE, Miller FR. Occult primary head and neck carcinoma. *Curr Oncol Rep* 2007; **9**(2): 139–146.

50. Goldenberg D, Sciubba J, Koch WM. Cystic metastasis from head and neck squamous cell cancer: a distinct disease variant? *Head Neck* 2006; **28**(7): 633–638.

51. McCoy KL, Yim JH, Zuckerbraun BS, *et al.* Cystic parathyroid lesions: functional and nonfunctional parathyroid cysts. *Arch Surg* 2009; **144**(1): 52–56; discussion 56.

52. Firat P, Ersoz C, Uguz A, *et al.* Cystic lesions of the head and neck: cytohistological correlation in 63 cases. *Cytopathology* 2007; **18**(3): 184–190.

53. Miseikyte-Kaubriene E, Trakymas M, Ulys A. Cystic lymph node metastasis in papillary thyroid carcinoma. *Medicina (Kaunas)* 2008; **44**(6): 455–459.

54. Goldenberg D, Begum S, Westra WH, *et al.* Cystic lymph node metastasis in patients with head and neck cancer: An HPV-associated phenomenon. *Head Neck* 2008; **30**(7): 898–903.

55. Devaney KO, Rinaldo A, Rodrigo JP, *et al.* Sentinel node biopsy and head and neck tumors where do we stand today? *Head Neck* 2006; **28**(12): 1122–1131.

56. Paleri V, Rees G, Arullendran P, *et al.* Sentinel node biopsy in squamous cell cancer of the oral cavity and oral pharynx: a diagnostic meta-analysis. *Head Neck* 2005; **27**(9): 739–747.

57. Bilde A, von Buchwald C, Therkildsen M, *et al.* Need for intensive histopathologic analysis to determine sentinel node metastases when using sentinel node biopsy in oral cancer. *Laryngoscope* 2008; **118**(3): 408–414.

5 LUNG

Charles M. Lombard and Linda W. Martin

INTRODUCTION

The pathologist's role in the intraoperative management of lung lesions has continued to evolve because of technical advances in the diagnosis and treatment of pulmonary diseases. In some situations, the pathologist's role has diminished because sensitive imaging techniques such as high resolution CT (HRCT) scans and PET scan have reduced the need for biopsy in some types of interstitial lung disease. In other situations, the pathologist has a role, but the role has changed; for example, percutaneous needle biopsy has replaced wedge biopsy as the principal method of making an initial diagnosis on mass lesions, and while wedge biopsies are still submitted for intraoperative diagnosis, the purpose is for evaluation of surgical margins.

The screening of high risk populations for lung cancer – which is still quite controversial[1] – as well as increased use of diagnostic imaging, has resulted in the detection of increasing numbers of small peripheral carcinomas that are amenable to limited surgical resection, often employing minimally invasive surgical techniques.

The non-surgical treatment of lung cancer and other pulmonary diseases has also evolved. Molecular based treatments are likely to find more applications, and the use of targeted therapies may call for further refinements in the classification of pulmonary carcinomas using immuno-histochemical and other techniques such as micro-array gene expression analysis as we move towards "personalized medicine." Fresh frozen tumor tissue may be required for these newer tests, and the procurement of tissue for this purpose may require the pathologist's participation.

MASS LESIONS OF THE LUNG

Indications for intraoperative diagnosis (IOD)

1. To render a diagnosis on a mass lesion when less invasive procedures have failed to provide a diagnosis.
2. To assist with planned staging of patients with a primary pulmonary malignancy, e.g., evaluation of mediastinal lymph nodes when immediate resection is planned.
3. To re-stage patients intraoperatively prior to resection because there are unexpected findings at the time of surgery (e.g., a small pleural metastasis outside of the operative field that was not detected by imaging, or the discovery of an additional pulmonary nodule in a non-tumor bearing lobe).
4. Evaluation of surgical margins in resected malignancies. This includes evaluation of parenchymal surgical margins in limited (wedge) resections, and evaluation of bronchial or vascular margins in lobectomy and pneumonectomy specimens.
5. To confirm that a localized lesion is present in a limited resection specimen when the lesion does not form a distinct mass (e.g., small peripheral carcinomas that present as ground glass opacities on HRCT scans).
6. To procure tissue for ancillary studies such as microbiological culture, chemosensitivity assays and micro-array analysis.
7. To assess mediastinal lymph nodes following induction chemotherapy and radiation, to confirm resolution of metastases prior to definitive resection in stage III NSCLC.

Intraoperative Consultation in Surgical Pathology, ed. Mahendra Ranchod. Published by Cambridge University Press.
© Cambridge University Press 2010.

Information needed before and during intraoperative consultation (IOC)

- The clinical history should be checked, especially for a history of prior malignancy, and treatment with preoperative chemotherapy or radiation. This can be done by checking the hospital information system and surgical pathology files, but when necessary, the information should be solicited directly from the surgeon.
- The pathology files should be checked for prior biopsies of the target lesion. The prior material should be reviewed whenever possible because this may help to interpret intraoperative findings if they are challenging.
- The pathologist should be aware of the surgeon's operative plan, and recognize that the surgeon's original plan may change during the procedure if there are unexpected findings. There is therefore, no substitute for direct communication with the surgeon.

SPECIFIC CLINICOPATHOLOGIC ISSUES

Handling wedge biopsy and wedge resection specimens for a solitary nodule

Clinical issues

The differential diagnosis of a solitary pulmonary nodule is quite extensive and includes inflammatory, infectious, and neoplastic lesions. The number of cases presenting for initial diagnosis has decreased significantly with improvements in radiographically directed biopsies and with the advent of real-time electromagnetic navigation bronchoscopy. Nevertheless, the pathologist will still encounter solitary pulmonary nodules for IOD for the following reasons: (a) The lesion may be small and in a location not readily accessible to percutaneous needle biopsy; (b) fine needle aspiration biopsy (FNA) and needle core biopsy were attempted but abandoned because of complications such as a large pneumothorax or bleeding; and (c) the needle biopsy yielded non-diagnostic benign cells but the radiographic and clinical findings remain suspicious for malignancy.

When the surgeon submits a wedge biopsy, it is important to know if the biopsy is for diagnosis or if it is an attempt at limited resection of a previously diagnosed small peripheral lung carcinoma. An increasing number of small peripheral lung lesions are being detected with screening HRCT scans and at least some of these are candidates for limited resection. The risk for local recurrence is three times greater when a wedge resection is performed compared to lobectomy,[2] but there are mitigating factors that favor limited resection. Patients with limited lung reserve may not tolerate lobectomy, and patients with significant cardiac disease, moderate to severe pulmonary hypertension, and poor performance status are at higher risk and may be offered a wedge resection instead of lobectomy. Limited resection may have the same outcome as lobectomy for small peripheral lesions (<2 cm) but this is still under investigation.

Pathologic issues

INITIAL SPECIMEN HANDLING

The specimen should be handled in a sterile fashion so that cultures can be obtained if the lesion is inflammatory/infectious. We recommend the following approach for potentially infectious lesions. The specimen should be placed on a sterile surface such as a telfa pad and handled under sterile conditions. After palpation, an initial section should be made perpendicular to the staple line, into but not through the lesion. Additional cuts are made if required and a sample should be taken for culture. The stapled margin of the specimen should then be grasped with a forceps and the staples should be removed with small, sharp scissors, conserving as much lung tissue as possible. The surgical margin is inked, and if the lesion is a neoplasm, a 2–3 mm thick section of tissue should be taken parallel to the margin for FS.

PROCURING TISSUE FOR CULTURES

A sample of the lesion should be taken for culture if there is any likelihood of an infectious process. Deciding which cultures are appropriate depends on the clinical information and the pathologic findings. If the cytoscrape shows typical granulomatous inflammation, cultures for Mycobacteria and fungi are usually sufficient, and there is usually no reason to submit tissue for aerobic and anaerobic bacterial cultures. When neutrophilic inflammation is present, we recommend aerobic and anaerobic bacterial cultures as well as cultures for Mycobacteria and fungi; cultures for acid fast organisms and fungi are usually redundant but it is prudent to be all encompassing just in case intraoperative evaluation failed to sample the granulomatous component of the lesion. Comprehensive cultures should be performed in immunocompromised patients – regardless of the nature of the inflammation – because of their muted reaction to infections. Cultures are often pre-ordered, and if it becomes apparent later that some or all of the cultures are not necessary, the orders should be cancelled after obtaining the surgeon's approval.

CYTOLOGIC PREPARATIONS

A scrape cytologic preparation should be the initial test on all solitary lesions, especially if the gross features suggest a granulomatous inflammatory process. Cytologic preparations will identify the majority of carcinomas with sufficient specificity to allow the surgeon to proceed with definitive surgical treatment, but more important, identifying the lesion as granulomatous inflammation will obviate the need for FS and all the consequences of freezing a potentially infectious lesion. Our preference is to prepare a fixed smear and an air-dried smear for H&E and Diff-Quik stains respectively

FROZEN SECTIONS

A FS should be performed if the cytologic findings are non-diagnostic or equivocal. There are two main reasons why carcinomas yield unsatisfactory cytologic preparations: First, carcinomas with marked desmoplasia tend to yield paucicellular smears and these may lack diagnostic features. Second, the cytologic preparation is cellular, but the neoplastic cells are bland and lack sufficient atypia to make a diagnosis of carcinoma; a FS is needed to evaluate the architectural features of the lesion.

Primary versus metastatic carcinoma in a wedge biopsy

It is sometimes difficult to distinguish primary lung carcinoma from metastatic carcinoma, but both gross and microscopic features may provide clues to the correct diagnosis. When a neoplasm is adjacent to the pleura, puckering of the overlying pleura favors a primary carcinoma; however, the converse is not as true as a number of subpleural primary malignancies do not involve the pleura and, like metastases, produce a dome-shaped subpleural nodule covered by a smooth pleural surface. The presence of an in situ component favors primary carcinoma, but this may not be present in the tissue sampled for FS. The periphery of a carcinoma may also provide clues because extensive lymphatic and/or vascular invasion favor a

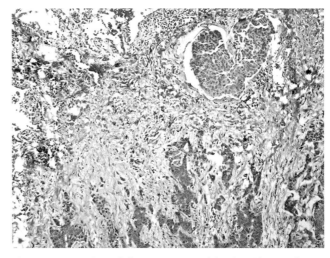

Fig. 5.1. Metastatic medullary carcinoma of the thyroid. Note the presence of lymphatic space involvement at the periphery of the tumor. The patient has a prior history of medullary carcinoma of the thyroid and the tumor is calcitonin positive. (Hematoxylin and eosin)

metastasis (Fig. 5.1). A metastasis should also be considered if the neoplasm has an unusual histologic appearance but keep in mind that primary lung carcinomas can assume a variety of appearances, some of which closely resemble metastases from other anatomic sites (Table 5.1).

A rapid Thyroid Transcription Factor 1 (TTF-1) stain has been described for intraoperative use, and it has been argued that this may help to determine if an adenocarcinoma is primary. However, 25% of non-mucinous bronchioloalveolar carcinomas and as many as 80% of mucinous bronchioloalveolar carcinomas are negative for TTF-1, and this, together with the lack of availability of this test in most laboratories, makes this stain of limited value at this time.

It is an axiom that a solitary lesion is more likely to be a primary malignancy and that multiple lesions favor metastases. However, this is not invariable as about 10% of metastases are solitary and occasional primary lung tumors present with multiple nodules (Table 5.2). Epithelioid hemangioendothelioma is an example of a primary pulmonary neoplasm that frequently presents with multiple lesions – although this neoplasm is treacherous for other reasons as well. It assumes a variety of patterns and may be mistaken for hyalinizing granulomatous inflammation, hamartomatous proliferations as well as other lesions. The intra-alveolar growth of hyalinized chondroid matrix, bland cells with large intracytoplasmic vacuoles, and intravascular growth are clues to the diagnosis (Fig. 5.2).

Table 5.1. Primary pulmonary malignancies that may be mistaken for metastases[23,36]

Metastases that are mimicked	Primary pulmonary carcinomas that may be mistaken for metastases
Clear cell renal cell carcinoma	Clear cell squamous cell carcinoma
	Clear cell adenocarcinoma
	Clear cell tumor
Metastatic endometrial carcinoma	Monophasic pulmonary blastoma
	Primary endometrioid-like adenocarcinoma
Metastatic colloid carcinoma	Primary colloid carcinoma
Metastatic squamous cell carcinoma	Primary squamous cell carcinoma
Metastatic lymphoepithelial carcinoma	Primary lymphoepithelial carcinoma
Metastatic adenocarcinoma with bronchioloalveolar growth pattern	Bronchioloalveolar carcinoma
Metastatic papillary carcinoma	Primary papillary/micropapillary carcinoma
Metastatic signet ring carcinoma	Primary signet ring adenocarcinoma
Metastatic hepatocellular carcinoma	Pulmonary hepatoid adenocarcinoma
Metastatic neuroendocrine carcinoma	Primary neuroendocrine carcinoma
Metastatic sarcoma	Primary pulmonary sarcoma
	Primary spindle cell carcinoma
	Primary carcinoma with metaplastic stroma
Metastatic GIST	Pulmonary solitary fibrous tumor
Germ cell tumor	Pulmonary choriocarcinoma
	Pulmonary carcinoma with choriocarcinomatous differentiation

Table 5.2. Primary lung tumors with multiple nodules

Epithelioid hemangioendothelioma

Sclerosing hemangioma

Bronchioloalveolar carcinoma

Lymphoma

Post-transplant lymphoproliferative disorder

Plasma cell granuloma (inflammatory myofibroblastic tumor)

Blastoma

Carcinoid

Chondroma (Carney Triad)

Hamartomas

examination; in other cases the surgeon may elect to stop at a wedge resection regardless of the final diagnosis. In an otherwise healthy patient, lobectomy carries a mortality rate of 1.5%–4.5%[3] and lesser resections on the order of 1% or less;[4] most surgeons consider this a significant difference and are hesitant to go on to lobectomy with questionable indications.

Classification of non-small cell carcinomas

A reasonable effort should be made to distinguish squamous carcinoma, adenocarcinoma and large cell undifferentiated carcinoma at the time of IOD, but the distinction does not influence surgical management – as long as the patient has no prior history of malignancy, and there is no reason to address the issue of primary versus metastatic carcinoma. Precise classification can be deferred to permanent sections.

With regard to adenocarcinomas, however, an attempt should be made to distinguish between bronchioloalveolar carcinoma (BAC) and invasive adenocarcinoma, as the former is an in situ carcinoma suited to limited resection, whereas invasive adenocarcinomas are best treated by lobectomy. The 2004 WHO classification of lung tumors defines BAC as lacking stromal, vascular and pleural invasion; as defined, BAC accounts for less than 3% of all lung carcinomas although it accounts for up to 16% of carcinomas detected by screening.[5]

Limited resection of pulmonary neoplasms

Clinical issues

Small, peripherally located lung carcinomas are candidates for limited (wedge) resection. These lesions may be difficult to localize at the time of video-assisted thoracoscopic

When a solitary pulmonary malignancy is encountered in a patient with a history of prior malignancy, and the distinction between primary and metastasis cannot be made with certainty, it is best to report this uncertainty to the surgeon. Ideally, a pre-operative biopsy would have been obtained and compared with the prior malignancy, but when this is not possible, the surgeon should decide ahead of time what she will do if the nature of the malignancy cannot be determined intraoperatively. In some cases a thoracoscopic wedge resection can be followed with completion lobectomy within a few days if primary NSCLC is confirmed on final pathologic

(a)
(b)

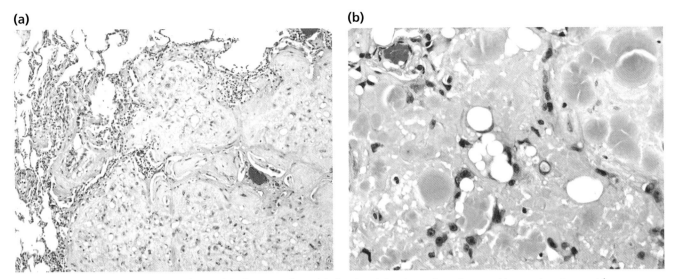

Fig. 5.2. Epithelioid hemangioendothelioma. (a) The tumor has a lobulated peripheral margin and a myxoid appearing stroma at low power. (b) The vacuolated cells are characteristic of epithelioid hemangioendothelioma.

surgery because of the limited tactile qualities of this procedure, but hookwire localization, radio-guided surgery with 99mTc albumin microsphere injection near the nodule;[6] and CT or three-dimensional bronchoscopy guided methylene blue labeling help the surgeon locate these lesions.[7]

Limited (wedge) resection is appropriate for resecting benign neoplasms, metastases, typical carcinoid tumors,[8] and small, pure bronchioloalveolar carcinomas (BAC). The criteria for limited resection of BAC-like tumors are:[9] a peripheral lesion ≤2 cm in maximum dimension; CT scan with ground glass appearance without alteration of the vascular pattern and without pleural indentations; FS shows BAC without evidence of invasion (Noguchi types A/B);* absence of pneumonic mucinous tumor; and the neoplasm can be excised with a 1 cm margin of normal tissue.

Pathologic issues
The margins should be evaluated initially by gross examination but even if the margins appear to be clear, we recommend evaluation by FS because bronchioloalveolar carcinomas may extend beyond the grossly visible lesion. Alternatively, touch preparations can be made from the stapled edges of the wedge resection as described by Sawabata,[10] but the accuracy of this method has not been established and is currently under study.

---

* Noguchi type A: Limited BAC without fibrosis. Noguchi type B: Limited BAC with fibrous collapse but without invasion.

Benign lesions that mimic bronchioloalveolar carcinoma (BAC)

Scar-associated reactive changes
Pulmonary scars may evoke atypical proliferation of pulmonary epithelium. Three main features distinguish scar-associated atypical epithelial proliferations from BAC: (a) an admixture of cell types, including ciliated, mucinous and/or squamous cells; (b) an absence of invasion; and (c) the inflammatory and fibrotic changes constitute the major component of the lesion (Fig. 5.3).

Apical cap lesions
Apical cap lesions occasionally present as radiographic mass lesions. They develop as a result of ischemic collapse of the subpleural tissues and are typically triangular in shape. The core of the lesion is composed predominantly of acellular fibrous and elastic tissue. The epithelial cells around the scar usually show some degree of hyperplasia but the degree of atypia is less than that seen in carcinoma (Fig. 5.4). The presence of ciliated columnar cells is another clue to the diagnosis.

Atypical adenomatous hyperplasia
Atypical adenomatous hyperplasia accompanies BAC in as many as 35% of cases.[11] This lesion is difficult to distinguish from BAC when it shows atypia (Fig. 5.5). Unfortunately, there are no reliable criteria for separating these two

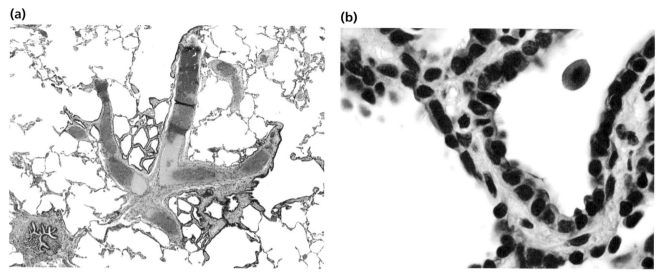

Fig. 5.3. Scar associated atypical epithelial proliferation. (a) There are small scars with areas of bronchioloalveolar proliferation which appear bronchiolocentric. (b) At high magnification admixed ciliated cells are noted.

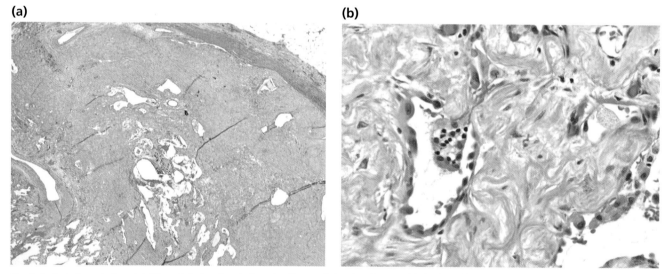

Fig. 5.4. Apical cap lesion. (a) There is ischemic subpleural collapse of alveolar tissues with hyaline change. (b) Atypical alveolar lining cells are identified in the areas of the apical cap lesion. The degree of atypia is generally less than that seen in bronchioloalveolar cell carcinoma.

entities and the distinction is rather arbitrary. Atypical adenomatous hyperplasia, which is defined as measuring <5 mm in size and is clinically and radiographically silent, is a problem when encountered at the margin of a wedge resection specimen performed for BAC. The degree of cytologic atypia at the periphery of the lesion should be compared to the target carcinoma and if it is significant, it is prudent to interpret it as BAC and not atypical adenomatous hyperplasia.

Papillary adenoma

Papillary adenoma, a benign neoplasm of type II pneumocytes, is rare. In contrast to BAC, it is well circumscribed and typically compresses the adjacent normal lung (Fig. 5.6). The alveolar walls are preserved, and the lesion is composed of a uniform population of cells that resemble activated type II pneumocytes. The neoplastic cells do not show significant atypia; the presence of marked cytologic atypia excludes this diagnosis.

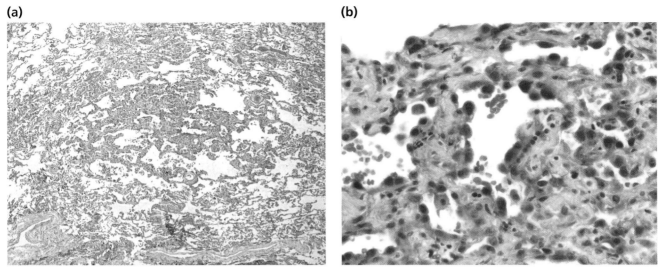

Fig. 5.5. Atypical adenomatous hyperplasia. (a) A 2.1-mm area of atypical adenomatous hyperplasia is present and appears well demarcated from surrounding normal alveolar tissues. (b) Atypical adenomatous hyperplasia may show variable degrees of atypia; however, the <5 mm size distinction has arbitrarily been defined to separate atypical adenomatous hyperplasia from small bronchioloalveolar cell carcinomas.

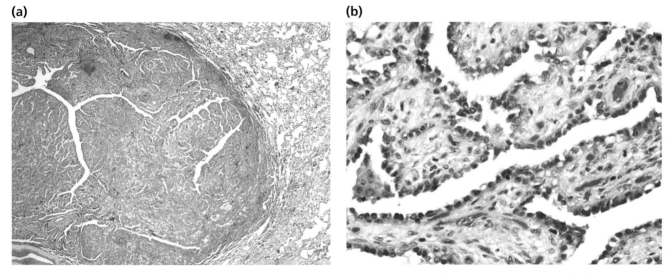

Fig. 5.6. Papillary adenoma of type II pneumocytes. (a) The tumor is well-circumscribed and there is compressed normal alveolar tissues at the periphery of this nodule. (b) The alveolar lining cells show a uniform population of bland appearing cells resembling activated type II pneumocytes.

Carcinomas that may be confused for bronchioloalveolar carcinoma

Papillary adenocarcinoma

Papillary and micropapillary adenocarcinomas of the lung have a destructive and invasive growth pattern. The spaces in the neoplasm lack the uniform spaces of alveoli and the neoplasm evokes a fibrous reaction, a feature that is usually absent in BAC (Fig. 5.7).

Invasive adenocarcinoma

The distinction between pure BAC and adenocarcinoma with a mixed pattern is usually straightforward when multiple sections are available for histologic examination, but the distinction is often more challenging on FS because of limited sampling. There are two subtypes of bronchioloalveolar cell carcinoma: The mucinous subtype, which is characteristically composed of multifocal proliferations of

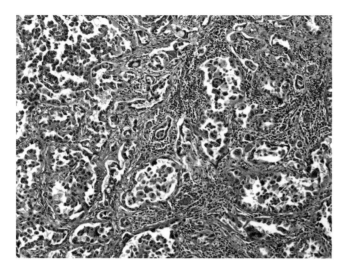

Fig. 5.7. Invasive papillary adenocarcinomas of the lung. This tumor shows a destructive growth pattern unlike that seen in bronchioloalveolar carcinoma.

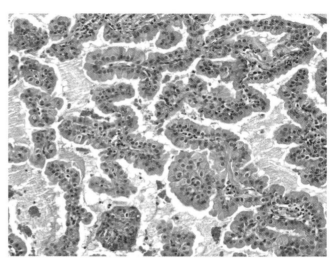

Fig. 5.9. Non-mucinous bronchioloalveolar cell carcinoma. Neoplastic cells line the normal alveolar spaces. By definition, there is no stromal invasion.

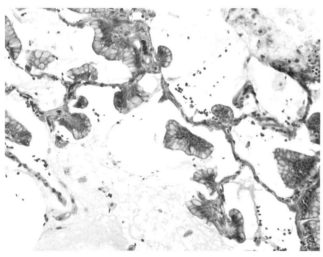

Fig. 5.8. Mucinous bronchioloalveolar carcinoma. Cytologically bland columnar mucinous epithelium appears to colonize preexistent alveolar spaces. Mucus and neoplastic cells are found free floating within the areas of mucinous consolidation of the lung.

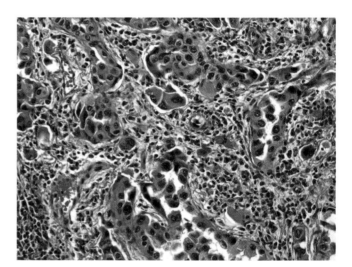

Fig. 5.10. Area of stromal invasion in a mixed adenocarcinoma. When stromal invasion characterized by irregular and single cell infiltration of the pulmonary interstitium by neoplastic cells is identified in a predominantly bronchioloalveolar cell carcinoma, the tumor is classified as an adenocarcinoma, mixed subtype with predominant bronchioloalveolar growth pattern.

columnar mucinous epithelial cells, grows along alveolar septae, shows prominent desquamation into alveoli and spreads into adjacent alveoli in pools of mucin (Fig. 5.8). In contrast, the non-mucinous subtype, which is composed of cuboidal cells with variable degrees of cytologic atypia, has an alveolar growth pattern, with or without areas of papillary tufting. Both subtypes may show variable alveolar fibrosis and inflammation but there is no stromal invasion (Fig. 5.9).

The key feature that differentiates mixed adenocarcinoma with a predominant BAC growth pattern, from pure BAC is the presence of invasion. Tissue for FS should be taken from the center of the grossly visible lesion as this area is more likely to show stromal invasion. Stromal invasion is characterized by irregular nests and single neoplastic cells infiltrating fibrous tissue (Fig. 5.10). It is uncommon to identify lymphatic and vascular space involvement but this would certainly constitute evidence of invasion. Some cases of BAC show restructuring of alveolar tissue, making it difficult to determine if invasion is present, but intraluminal alveolar histiocytes favor in-situ carcinoma.

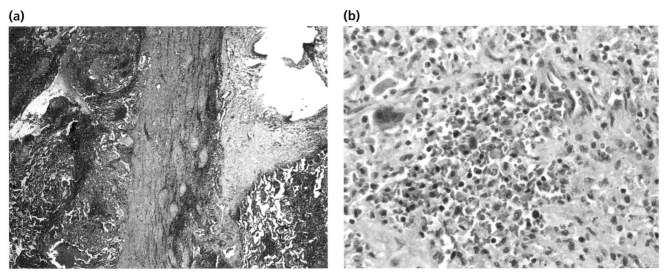

(a) **(b)**

Fig. 5.11. Needle biopsy tract in pulmonary parenchymal tissue. (a) A linear biopsy tract is identified at low power. (b) An entrapped neoplastic cell can be identified in the needle biopsy tract. The needle biopsy tract has a granulation tissue-like appearance with hemorrhage and hemosiderin laden macrophages.

Prior needle biopsy may produce artifactual changes that mimic invasive adenocarcinoma. Single and clusters of neoplastic cells may be entrapped in fibrous tissue but the needle tract can be recognized by the fibromyxoid nature of the stroma, as well as hemorrhage and hemosiderin laden macrophages arranged in a linear pattern (Fig. 5.11).

If the pathologist is unable to distinguish between BAC and a mixed lesion, limited resection is still appropriate for lesions <2 cm, Noguchi types A or B.[12] If the Noguchi type can not be determined with certainty, it is reasonable to go ahead with limited resection and return for completion lobectomy if invasive adenocarcinoma is identified on permanent sections.

Staging of lung carcinoma

Clinical issues

Accurate staging of pulmonary carcinoma is essential for proper management of the patient (Table 5.3). For non-small carcinomas, the principal question is whether the neoplasm is resectable or not, and this decision can only be made after thorough staging. Non-small cell carcinomas are considered potentially resectable when metastases to distant sites have been excluded. There is no consensus for resectability with regional disease, but bulky disease is sometimes resected after a suitable response to chemoradiation. Initial staging, which includes contrast enhanced CT scans, PET-CT scans[13,14] and ultrasound directed transbronchial needle aspiration biopsy of lymph nodes[15,16] direct the surgeon's attention to areas of concern, but mediastinoscopic examination with biopsies

remains the gold standard for evaluating the status of mediastinal lymph nodes. Sentinel lymph node biopsy evoked some interest when it was recognized that up to 30% of sentinel lymph nodes are in the mediastinum, by-passing lobar and hilar lymph nodes,[17] but its value is limited since most surgeons routinely perform mediastinal node dissection for all stages of resectable lung cancer.

There are two management scenarios with mediastinoscopic biopsies sent for IOD. First, the surgeon plans to proceed with definitive surgery (e.g., lobectomy) under the same anesthetic if the lymph node biopsies are interpreted as negative, and second, the surgeon does not plan to proceed with definitive surgery but submits biopsies for FS because a positive result will allow immediate termination of the surgical procedure.

Pathologic issues

When a lymph node biopsy shows a grossly visible metastasis, it is sufficient to confirm the diagnosis with a cytoscrape or touch preparation. If there is no grossly visible metastasis, a cytoscrape preparation should be made, and the entire specimen should then be submitted for FS. We suggest at least two levels routinely because metastases may be focal. The pathologist should be alert to the following pitfalls when evaluating FSs of mediastinal lymph nodes:

- Crush artifact can make it difficult to distinguish crushed small neoplastic cells from crushed lymphocytes on FS. Cytoscrape preparations will allow this

Table 5.3. Proposed AJCC/UICC 7th edition TNM classification of lung cancer[18]

Stage I A	T1a,b	N0	M0
Stage I B	T2a	N0	M0
Stage II A	T1a,b	N1	M0
	T2a	N1	M0
	T2b	N0	M0
Stage II B	T2b	N1	M0
	T3	N0	M0
Stage III A	T1, T2	N2	M0
	T3	N1, N2	M0
	T4	N2	M0
Stage III B	T4	N2	M0
	Any T	N3	M0
Stage IV	Any T	Any N	M1a,b

UICC/AJCC 6th edition T/M Descriptors	Revised 7th edition T/M
T1 ≤2 cm)	T1a
T1 (>2–3 cm)	T1b
T2 (3–5 cm)	T2a
T2 (5–7 cm)	T2b
T2 (>7 cm)	T3
T2/T3 invasion criteria[a]	T2/T3
T4 (same lobe nodules)	T3
T4 extension criteria[b]	T4
M1 (ipsilateral lung nodules)	T4
T4 malignant pleural effusion	M1a
M1 (contralateral lung nodules)	M1a
M1 distant	M1b

[a] T3 invasion criteria: (1) a tumor of any size directly invading chest wall, diaphragm, mediastinal pleura, parietal pericardium. (2) Tumor in the main bronchus less than 2 cm removed from the carina but without involvement of the carina. (3) Tumor associated with atelectasis/obstructive pneumonia of the entire lung.
[b] T4 extension criteria: (1) tumor of any size that invades the mediastinum, heart, great vessels, trachea, esophagus, vertebral body, or carina.

distinction to be made with greater confidence, which explains why we recommend making cytologic preparations routinely.

▪ Cautery induced artifacts cause the same challenges as crush artifact.
▪ The surgeon may inadvertently biopsy the thymus gland, and if atrophic thymus is not considered in the differential diagnosis, thymic epithelium may be misconstrued as metastatic carcinoma.

Evaluation of lobectomy and pneumonectomy specimens

Clinical issues

Because lobectomy and pneumonectomy are performed after a proven diagnosis of malignancy, the purpose of IOD is to evaluate the proximal bronchial margin of resection and not confirm the presence of malignancy. In general, the surgeon will send lobectomy and pneumonectomy specimens for intraoperative evaluation regardless of the proximity of the carcinoma to the proximal bronchial margin, and leave the pathologist to decide on how the specimen should be evaluated.

Sleeve resections are performed for tumors involving a mainstem bronchus that would otherwise require a pneumonectomy for complete resection. A "sleeve" of mainstem bronchus is resected and the remaining lobe(s) are re-attached to the remaining mainstem bronchus or even the lateral tracheal wall. Morbidity and mortality rates are lower, and long term survival from cancer is similar to lobectomy. For this approach to be successful, all bronchial margins must be negative and all nodal and parenchymal disease must be completely resected.

Pathologic issues

For lobectomy and pneumonectomy specimens, gross examination is reliable for evaluating the proximal bronchial margin if the carcinoma is >2–3 cm away from the margin, and in our opinion, gross examination will suffice for small carcinomas confined to the periphery of the lung. It has been proposed that a FS should be performed on the proximal bronchial margin when the carcinoma is within 2 cm of the margin;[19] we agree with this proposal, but in addition, recommend FS evaluation of the bronchial margin for any carcinoma >3 cm in maximum dimension – regardless of its distance from the margin. We take this approach because of the risk of a false-negative diagnosis; it is simple enough to perform a FS on the margin and avoid the risk of subjecting the patient to a second surgical procedure to achieve clear margins.

When the proximal bronchial margin is sampled, a 3 mm thick circumferential section should be taken parallel to the margin. If the bronchus is >1.5 cm in diameter, we cut the specimen in half and embed the two pieces of bronchial tissue parallel to one another because this results in fewer folds. The low serum content of cartilage predisposes the tissue to wash off the slide during staining, a frustration that can be minimized by using lysine-coated slides or charged slides, but if this fails, the alcohol- fixed slide should be air-dried for 1 minute, and then stained with minimal agitation. If tissue adherence remains a problem, the slide should be air dried and stained with a few drops of toluidine blue or some other metachromatic stain.

When the bronchial margin is involved by carcinoma, a distinction should be made between (a) in situ carcinoma; (b) invasive carcinoma involving the mucosa; (c) invasive carcinoma involving the peribronchial tissues; and (d) lymphatic/vascular invasion.[20–22] Direct invasion of the bronchial wall and peribronchial tissues in stages I and II disease will prompt the surgeon to remove additional bronchial tissue if the margin is reported as positive intraoperatively. Some surgeons will re-operate if there is a false-negative FS interpretation of the margin, so it is important to examine the bronchial margin with care. In contrast, a positive peribronchial margin in patients with stage III carcinoma does not appear to change the prognosis and additional surgery is not performed; systemic chemotherapy and radiation to the bronchial stump are usually undertaken in this situation.[22]

The significance of in situ carcinoma at the bronchial margin is not altogether clear. Because in situ carcinoma may regress after surgery, the surgeon may not remove additional tissue but follow the patient and treat the lesion with endoscopic ablation if necessary. In contrast, vascular and lymphatic space invasion at the bronchial margin usually implies non-resectable disease, but if lymphatic/vascular invasion is accompanied by direct stromal invasion in a patient with otherwise low stage disease (stages I and II), many surgeons will attempt further resection to obtain clear margins.

Neuroendocrine neoplasms

Clinical issues

This group of tumors includes typical carcinoid tumor, atypical carcinoid tumor, large cell neuroendocrine carcinoma, and small cell carcinoma. Eighty percent of typical carcinoid tumors are centrally located[23] and they are readily amenable to transbronchial biopsy. Peripheral lesions are usually diagnosed by radiographically directed needle biopsy or electromagnetic navigation bronchoscopic biopsy. Occasionally, the diagnosis is first made intraoperatively. Typical carcinoid tumors have a low incidence of spread to hilar lymph nodes (about 5%), and are treated either by lobectomy or wedge resection.

Atypical carcinoid tumors are more aggressive than typical carcinoid tumors.[24] About 60% are peripheral and 40% of patients present with stage II or more advanced disease. Resectable tumors are treated by lobectomy. Large cell neuroendocrine carcinoma, a highly aggressive form of carcinoma, usually occurs in the peripheral and mid zones of the lung. In general, these tumors are staged and treated in the same manner as conventional NSCLC, even though they have a poorer prognosis stage for stage.[25] Adjuvant therapy is recommended and some authors have used small cell lung cancer regimens (cisplatin + etoposide) rather than NSCLC protocols, but the optimal approach remains unclear.

Small cell carcinoma of the lung is usually treated with combination radiation and chemotherapy. At presentation, two-thirds of the patients have clinical evidence of distant metastases and most of the remaining patients have regional lymph node involvement. For these reasons, staging of small cell carcinoma of the lung is clinical rather than pathologic. An abbreviated clinical staging system divides these patients into two categories: limited disease (LD) or extensive disease (ED). Limited disease includes tumors confined to one hemithorax with regional lymph node metastases and an ipsilateral pleural effusion (regardless of cytologic findings). Extensive disease refers to extrathoracic metastasis. Rare patients with limited disease, such as a small peripheral nodule without apparent metastases, are staged as for non-small cell carcinoma and are treated by surgical resection, but adjuvant chemotherapy is recommended even for stage IA disease.

Pathologic issues

Most of the diagnostic issues concerning endocrine cell neoplasms are resolved pre-operatively, but two diagnostic problems may present for the first time during IOD.

The distinction between typical and atypical carcinoid tumor is usually straightforward but it is sometimes challenging. Typical carcinoid tumors have a variety of microscopic appearances, including trabecular, insular, glandular, rosette, papillary, spindle cell, oncocytic, and pigmented,[23] and they are distinguished from atypical carcinoid tumors by their low mitotic rate (<2/10 hpf) and the absence of necrosis.[26] Although most typical carcinoid tumors are composed of cells with uniform nuclei, occasional cases show marked cytologic pleomorphism (Fig. 5.12), so nuclear pleomorphism should not be the sole criterion for making a diagnosis of atypical carcinoid tumor. In addition, surface ulceration and necrosis due to prior

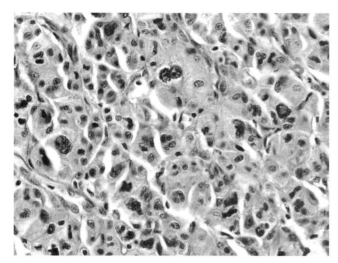

Fig. 5.12. Typical carcinoid tumor with pleomorphic cells. Significant nuclear pleomorphism may be identified in typical carcinoid tumors; however, this feature does not separate typical carcinoid from atypical carcinoid tumors. These tumors are separated by mitotic rate (<2 per 10 hpf in typical carcinoid) and by the presence or absence of tumor necrosis.

transbronchial or needle biopsy should not be confused for true tumor necrosis.

The distinction between atypical carcinoid, large cell neuroendocrine carcinoma, and large cell undifferentiated carcinoma can be difficult. Fortunately, this distinction is not critical at the time of IOD as all three neoplasms are treated with lobectomy if the tumor is resectable. The distinction between atypical carcinoid tumor and large cell neuroendocrine carcinoma is one of degree; both neoplasms retain their neuroendocrine characteristics, including organoid, rosette and trabecular patterns, and both neoplasms may have necrosis. The main distinction is that large cell neuroendocrine carcinomas are more pleomorphic and have higher mitotic counts (>10/HPF compared to 2–10/HPF in atypical carcinoid tumors) (Fig. 5.13).

Resection of metastatic malignancies

Clinical issues

Most pulmonary metastases occur in the setting of widespread metastatic disease; only 15%–25% of these patients have metastases confined to the lungs,[27] and a minority of these patients are candidates for surgical resection. The criteria for resection are as follows: (a) The primary malignancy has been successfully eradicated, or if detected synchronously, both the primary and the pulmonary metastasis are resectable; (b) the metastases are confined to the lung; (c) if a pleural or pericardial effusion is

present, the fluid should be negative for malignancy; (d) complete resection of the pulmonary metastasis/metastases is possible; (e) the patient is able to tolerate the surgical procedure; and (f) there is no alternative therapy equal or superior to surgery.

A wide variety of pulmonary metastases are treated surgically, and these include colorectal carcinoma, squamous cell carcinoma of head and neck origin, melanoma, osteosarcoma, soft tissue and uterine sarcomas, renal cell carcinoma, breast carcinoma, and germ cell tumors. In contrast to primary lung carcinoma, wedge resection of the metastasis with clear margins is sufficient because this preserves lung tissue in the event that further resections become necessary.

Pathologic issues

The wedge resection specimen should be evaluated as described for peripheral bronchioloalveolar carcinoma (see pp. 61 and 62).

DIFFUSE LUNG DISEASE AND LOCALIZED INFILTRATES

Indications for intraoperative diagnosis

1. To ensure that diagnostic tissue has been obtained in patients with infiltrative or diffuse pulmonary disease.
2. To provide information that will guide immediate postoperative management in an acutely ill patient with pulmonary infiltrative disease.
3. To identify a previously undiagnosed malignancy that will allow the surgeon to proceed with definitive resection if the neoplasm is resectable.

Information needed before and during intraoperative consultation (IOC)

The pathologist should be pro-active when handling open biopsies for interstitial lung disease because incorrect handling of the specimen may compromise patient care and cause a great deal of frustration for the surgeon and pulmonologist. The following guidelines should be followed before handling the specimen:

It is essential to have a good clinical history. If the surgeon is not familiar with the details of the clinical history, it is worthwhile discussing the case with the referring physician (pulmonologist, infectious disease specialist,

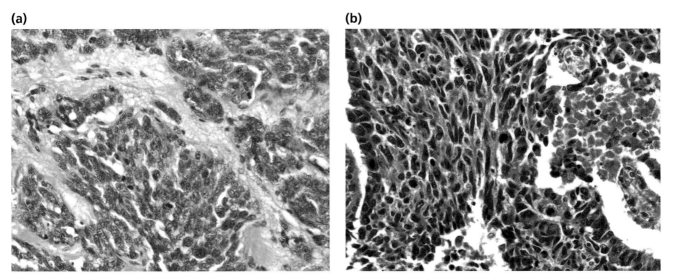

Fig. 5.13. Atypical carcinoid tumor versus large cell neuroendocrine carcinoma. (a) Atypical carcinoid tumor with nests of neoplastic cells showing mitotic activity up to 10 mitoses per high power field. (b) Large cell neuroendocrine carcinoma with increased cellular pleomorphism and increased mitotic activity (>10 per high power field).

rheumatologist, etc.) as this will help to frame a meaningful differential diagnosis, as well as ensure that all the appropriate ancillary tests are ordered.

The case should be discussed with the surgeon, and ideally, the images should be reviewed with the surgeon to ascertain which areas will be targeted for biopsy. In cases of chronic interstitial lung disease, the chances of rendering a specific diagnosis are greatly improved if biopsies are obtained from two different sites. One additional reason for discussing the case with the surgeon is to determine who will be responsible for procuring material for culture and other ancillary studies. We prefer the surgeon to select tissue samples for microbiologic studies because this minimizes the risk of contamination. For other studies such as tissue culture, chemosensitivity assay and micro-array analysis, a fresh specimen should be submitted to the laboratory in a sterile container with a request for the pathologist to triage the specimen.

If the surgeon requests a FS, the pathologist should enquire about the reason for the test and how this will influence immediate patient management; this is especially relevant if the specimen is small.

Clinical issues
Patients with diffuse lung disease and localized infiltrates usually have inflammatory/infectious lung disease but neoplastic processes such as lymphoma, lymphangitic carcinoma and bronchioloalveolar carcinoma can produce pulmonary infiltrates that mimic acute or chronic inflammatory disease. A carefully taken clinical history frequently provides clues to the diagnosis if the following questions are asked: What is the tempo of the disease (acute versus subacute versus chronic)? Does the patient have a history of underlying disease (collagen-vascular, autoimmune, neoplastic, other)? What is the medication history? Has the patient had treatment or bronchoscopic evaluation prior to the surgical biopsy? Have cultures been attempted and what are the results? Are there any other pertinent laboratory data such as CBC, blood chemistries and serologies? Radiologic findings are often helpful since the distribution of the disease (localized, multi-focal, diffuse), the character of the abnormality (interstitial, alveolar, nodular, or mixed) and the pattern (bronchiolocentric, peripheral, central, paraseptal) will often narrow the differential diagnosis.

The surgeon will usually discuss her biopsy strategy with the pulmonologist and/or radiologist prior to surgery to obtain agreement about areas that are likely to have the highest diagnostic yield. There are two axioms that guide surgeons about the selection of biopsy sites: (a) the tips of the lingula and right middle lobe are avoided because they often show non-specific changes; and (b) the biopsies should not be limited to the most abnormal areas because these may show advanced disease and lack specific diagnostic changes.

The optimal number of specimens procured depends on the clinical situation. A single biopsy specimen is usually sufficient when the patient has diffuse, acute pulmonary disease with uniform involvement of the lung. Similarly, sampling is limited to the abnormal area when the disease is localized. In contrast, when there is diffuse disease with heterogeneity to the character of the infiltrates, biopsies should be taken from more than one lobe because different lobes may show different histologic patterns.[28] Furthermore, in chronic interstitial lung disease, biopsies from two different sites should be obtained, preferably from the upper and lower lobes,[29] and a third biopsy should be considered if the radiologic images show heterogeneity of the infiltrates. It is also helpful if transitional areas between grossly abnormal and relatively normal lung are sampled.

Surgeons and pathologists may differ on what constitutes an adequate biopsy, but an experienced surgeon should be able to procure thoracoscopic biopsies that are at least 3 cm wide and 3 cm deep. Sometimes, a significant amount of tissue is lost during removal of the staples and obtaining samples of this size will ensure an adequate specimen.

Pathologic issues

FAMILIARITY WITH THE SURGEON'S OPERATIVE PLAN

Ideally, the pathologist should be familiar with the surgeon's operative plan and know why an IOC is needed, but if there was no opportunity for pre-operative discussion, it is prudent to discuss the case with the surgeon before handling the specimen. The following questions should be asked: If the lesion is neoplastic, how much surgery do you plan to undertake? Is the only purpose of IOD to determine if diagnostic tissue has been obtained? If the patient has acute respiratory failure, is the purpose of IOD to help with immediate post-biopsy treatment? Is there a need for special tissue handling, such as cultures, analysis for inorganic dusts, examination for immune deposits and tissue microarray analysis?

INFLATING THE SPECIMEN

Because compression of pulmonary parenchyma may be mistaken for interstitial fibrosis, techniques have been described for inflating fresh lung biopsies before cutting the specimen. The injection of normal saline through the pleural surface is the simplest, but an alternative method is to inject dilute OCT into the lung, using a ratio of 2 parts OCT to 3 parts saline. In a third method, the Yoshida technique, the specimen is inflated using negative pressure created in a 25 ml^3 syringe partially filled with saline. After removing the staples, the specimen is placed in the

syringe, the syringe is capped, and negative pressure is created by a few rapid movements of the plunger. The negative pressure expands the lung parenchyma, drawing the saline into the air spaces.

DETERMINING SPECIMEN ADEQUACY

Lung biopsy specimens are often submitted for IOD to determine specimen adequacy. This question can only be answered if the pathologist is familiar with the clinical and radiographic facts of the case. The following points should be considered before deciding on the adequacy of a biopsy:

- Was medical treatment given prior to biopsy? This is relevant because immunosuppressive therapy, such as steroids, may dramatically decrease the number of inflammatory cells in the biopsy, removing an important clue to the correct diagnosis. A related issue in immunocompromised patients, and one that is easily overlooked, is the way an infection may mask the patient's underlying pulmonary disease. It is good policy therefore, to consider the possibility of more than one pathologic process in immunocompromised patients.
- The presence of abnormal lung tissue on FS does not necessarily mean that the sample is adequate and representative of the patient's disease. The FS findings should be correlated with the clinical findings because failure to do so may lead to the wrong conclusions. Three examples will illustrate this point: (i) The biopsy is not representative if it shows mild non-specific or chronic changes but the patient has acute respiratory failure (Table 5.4). (ii) A patient with known chronic lung disease, who now has an accelerated clinical course or superimposed acute disease, should have histologic changes that reflect the acute process. (iii) If a patient with diffuse pulmonary infiltrates has a necrotic nodule on FS, lung tissue away from the nodule should also be sampled because non-specific inflammatory changes often occur around necrotic nodules, regardless of their etiology (Fig. 5.14).

PROCURING TISSUE FOR CULTURE

If the surgeon has not obtained tissue for culture, the initial handling of the specimen should be under sterile conditions. A portion of the specimen should be saved in a sterile container until completion of the FS, at which time

Table 5.4. Causes of acute respiratory failure

Diffuse alveolar damage/acute interstitial pneumonia

Wegener's granulomatosis

Diffuse alveolar hemorrhage

Malignant lymphoma

Embolism

    Clot

    Foreign material

    Tumor

    Fat

Radiation pneumonitis

Drugs/Toxic exposure

Allergic/Hypersensitivity pneumonitis

Acute eosinophilic pneumonia

Infection

    Pneumocystis carinii

    Viral pneumonia

    Mycoplasma pneumonia

    Legionella pneumonia

    Miliary granulomatous disease

    Other

Acute or chronic disease

Miscellaneous

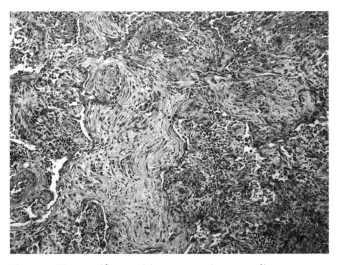

Fig. 5.14. Non-specific organizing pneumonia surrounding squamous cell carcinoma. The histologic appearance is identical to the changes seen in idiopathic cryptogenic organizing pneumonia (bronchiolitis obliterans with organizing pneumonia).

the FS findings can dictate whether cultures are needed. Unless the FS shows a neoplastic process, tissue should be submitted for culture even if the inflammatory changes are minor, a point that is certainly true of immunocompromised hosts.

Pleural based lesions

Clinical issues

Clinical history often provides clues to the diagnosis of pleural lesions. The pathologist should ask the following questions. Is there a history of a prior malignancy? Is the pleural disease unilateral or bilateral? Is the disease limited to the pleura or is there parenchymal involvement as well? Does the patient have a known pleural infection or inflammatory/autoimmune disease? Is there a history of exposure to asbestos?

Frozen sections of the pleura are usually requested to confirm the presence of diagnostic tissue in patients suspected of having granulomatous inflammation or non-resectable neoplastic disease. In patients scheduled for lobectomy, unexpected pleural lesions will be biopsied for FS diagnosis because positive biopsies will render the tumor unsuitable for surgical resection. A minority of patients with malignant mesothelioma are treated with extrapleural pneumonectomy or pleurectomy/decortication, but only after strict criteria are met.[30,31]

Pathologic issues

Pleural biopsies submitted for FS evaluation in patients with lung carcinoma should be interpreted with caution because reactive mesothelial lesions may show significant atypia and mitotic activity; invasion of the pleural connective tissue or pulmonary parenchyma are the only reliable criteria for making the distinction between a reactive mesothelial lesion and carcinoma. If the lesion is solitary and non-invasive, the surgeon should be given license to proceed with surgical resection, but if there are multiple lesions, the surgeon should be asked to biopsy more than one lesion because the additional tissue may help to determine if the lesion is benign or malignant (Fig. 5.15).

When the differential diagnosis is between epithelioid malignant mesothelioma and metastatic lung carcinoma, the purpose of the FS is to confirm that adequate diagnostic tissue has been procured for permanent sections and ancillary studies. The surgeon should be encouraged to obtain multiple biopsies from different sites, and the diagnosis should be deferred to permanent sections as immunohistochemical studies are required to make a definite diagnosis.

Spindle cell proliferations of the pleura include sarcomatoid mesothelioma, desmoplastic mesothelioma, spindle cell carcinoma, leiomyosarcoma, synovial sarcoma, melanoma and solitary fibrous tumor of the pleura.

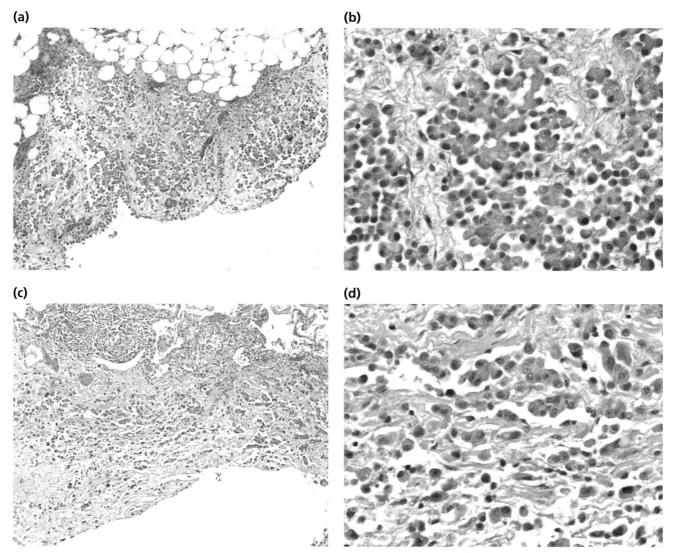

Fig. 5.15. Atypical mesothelial hyperplasia versus well differentiated epithelioid malignant mesothelioma. (a) Atypical mesothelial hyperplasia involving parietal pleural tissues. (b) The atypical mesothelial cells are admixed with fibrin, but no tissue invasion is identified. (c) Well-differentiated epithelioid malignant mesothelioma involving visceral pleura. (d) The malignant epithelioid mesothelioma is infiltrating collagenous tissues.

Desmoplastic malignant mesothelioma can appear deceptively bland and mimic fibrotic pleura or areas of organizing fibrinous pleuritis (Fig. 5.16).[32] Infiltration into surrounding structures such as the chest wall, mediastinum or lung is the best evidence of malignancy and the surgeon should be encouraged to obtain biopsies from areas of invasive disease. If invasion cannot be demonstrated on FS, additional tissue should be requested because obvious cytologic atypia may be present elsewhere in the lesion. Other findings that support the diagnosis of sarcomatoid mesothelioma include the lack of transition from reactive fibrinous pleuritis to hyalin fibrosis, a storiform pattern and patchy areas of infarct-like necrosis.

Accuracy of intraoperative diagnosis

The accuracy of intraoperative diagnosis depends on the question being asked.[33–35] For mass lesions (benign versus malignant) the accuracy is high, with 97% concordance between FS and permanent sections. A false-positive diagnosis of malignancy occurs in <1% of cases and false-negative diagnoses are rendered in <2% of cases. The accuracy for evaluation of bronchial margins is reported to be as high as 98%, and the accuracy of FS diagnosis on mediastinoscopic biopsies of lymph nodes is reported to be as high as 98%.

The accuracy of FS diagnosis for undefined infiltrative processes (infectious versus non-infectious, inflammatory

(a) (b)

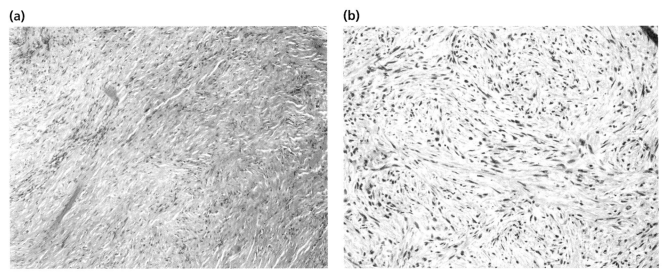

Fig. 5.16. Desmoplastic malignant mesothelioma. (a) Hypocellular area of desmoplastic malignant mesothelioma mimicking fibrotic pleura. A definitive diagnosis is not possible in these areas, but should prompt further evaluation. (b) Storiform area of malignant desmoplastic mesothelioma found in additional tissues taken from the same case.

versus neoplastic) is lower, with concordance rates of 85%–90%. These errors occur because of problems related to tissue sampling, technical problems, interpretive errors and failure to be conversant with the clinical and imaging findings.

REFERENCES

1. Midthun DE, Swensen SJ, Hartman TE *et al.* Lung cancer screening results: easily misunderstood. *Mayo Clin Proc* 2007; **82**: 14–15.

2. Ginsberg RJ, Rubinstein L. The comparison of limited resection to lobectomy for T1N0 non-small cell lung cancer. *LCSG 821. Chest* 1994; **106**: 318S–319S.

3. Ponn RB. Complications of pulmonary resection. In *General Thoracic Surgery*, Shields TW, LoCicero J, Ponn RB *et al.* eds. Philadelphia: Lippincott Williams & Wilkins; 2005: pp. 554–586.

4. Wada H, Nakamura T, Nakamoto K *et al.* Thirty-day operative mortality for thoracotomy in lung cancer. *J Thorac Cardiovasc Surg* 1998; **115**: 70–73.

5. Flieder DB. Screen-detected adenocarcinoma of the lung. Practical points for surgical pathologists. *Am J Clin Pathol* 2003; **119** Suppl: S39–S57.

6. Gonfiotti A, Davini F, Vaggelli L *et al.* Thoracoscopic localization techniques for patients with solitary pulmonary nodule: hookwire versus radio-guided surgery. *Eur J Cardio-Thoracic Surg* 2007; **32**: 843–847.

7. Seymour CW, Krimsky WS, Sager J *et al.* Transbronchial needle injection: a systematic review of a new diagnostic and therapeutic paradigm. *Respiration* 2006; **73**: 78–89.

8. Ferguson MK, Landreneau RJ, Hazelrigg SR *et al.* Long-term outcome after resection for bronchial carcinoid tumors. *Eur J Cardio-Thoracic Surg* 2000; **18**: 156–161.

9. Arenberg D. Bronchioloalveolar lung cancer: ACCP evidence-based clinical practice guidelines (2nd ed). *Chest* 2007; **132**: 306S–313S.

10. Sawabata N, Matsumura A, Ohota M *et al.* Cytologically malignant margins of wedge resected stage I non-small cell lung cancer. *Ann Thorac Surg* 2002; **74**: 1953–1957.

11. Garfield DH, Cadranel JL, Wislez M *et al.* The bronchioloalveolar carcinoma and peripheral adenocarcinoma spectrum of diseases. *J Thorac Oncol* 2006; **1**: 344–359.

12. Rusch VW, Tsuchiya R, Tsuboi M *et al.* Surgery for bronchioloalveolar carcinoma and "very early" adenocarcinoma: an evolving standard of care? *J Thorac Oncol* 2006; **1**: S27-S31.

13. Silvestri GA, Gould MK, Margolis ML *et al.* Noninvasive staging of non-small cell lung cancer: ACCP evidenced-based clinical practice guidelines (2nd ed). *Chest* 2007; **132**: 178S–201.

14. Erasmus JJ, MacApinlac HA, Swisher SG. Positron emission tomography imaging in nonsmall-cell lung cancer. *Cancer* 2007; **110**: 2155–2168.

15. Detterbeck FC, Jantz MA, Wallace M *et al.* Invasive mediastinal staging of lung cancer: ACCP evidence-based clinical practice guidelines (2nd edition). *Chest* 2007; **132**: 202S–220S.

16. Martin LW. Invasive mediastinal staging for non-small-cell lung cancer. *Gastrointestinal Endoscopy* 2008; **67**: 199–201.

17. Liptay MJ, Grondin SC, Fry WA *et al.* Intraoperative sentinel lymph node mapping in non-small-cell lung cancer improves detection of micrometastases. *J Clin Oncol* 2002; **20**: 1984–1988.

18. Goldstraw P, Crowley J, Chansky K *et al.* The IASLC Lung Cancer Staging Project: proposals for the revision of the TNM stage groupings in the forthcoming (seventh) edition of the TNM Classification of malignant tumours. *J Thorac Oncol* 2007; **2**: 706–714.

19. Kara M, Sak SD, Orhan D *et al.* Changing patterns of lung cancer; (3/4 in.) 1.9 cm; still a safe length for bronchial resection margin? *Lung Cancer* 2000; **30**: 161–168.

20. Kutlu CA, Urer N, Olgac G. Carcinoma in situ from the view of complete resection. *Lung Cancer* 2004; **46**: 383–385.

21. Thunnissen FB, den Bakker MA. Implications of frozen section analyses from bronchial resection margins in NSCLC. *Histopathology* 2005; **47**: 638–640.

22. Wind J, Smit EJ, Senan S *et al.* Residual disease at the bronchial stump after curative resection for lung cancer. *Eur J Cardiothorac Surg* 2007; **32**: 29–34.

23. Colby TV, Koss MN, Travis WD. Tumors of the lower respiratory tract. In *AFIP Atlas of Tumor Pathology.* Washington, DC: Armed Forces Institute of Pathology, 1995.

24. Beasley MB, Thunnissen FB, Brambilla E *et al.* Pulmonary atypical carcinoid: predictors of survival in 106 cases. *Hum Pathol* 2000; **31**: 1255–1265.

25. Iyoda A, Hiroshima K, Nakatani Y *et al.* Pulmonary large cell neuroendocrine carcinoma: its place in the spectrum of pulmonary carcinoma. *Ann Thorac Surg* 2007; **84**: 702–707.

26. Travis WD, Rush W, Flieder DB *et al.* Survival analysis of 200 pulmonary neuroendocrine tumors with clarification of criteria for atypical carcinoid and its separation from typical carcinoid. *Am J Surg Pathol* 1998; **22**: 934–944.

27. Greelish JP, Friedberg JS. Secondary pulmonary malignancy. *Surg Clin North Am* 2000; **80**: 633–657.

28. Flaherty KR, Travis WD, Colby TV *et al.* Histopathologic variability in usual and nonspecific interstitial pneumonias. *Am J Respir Crit Care Med* 2001; **164**: 1722–1727.

29. Riley DJ, Costanzo EJ. Surgical biopsy: its appropriateness in diagnosing interstitial lung disease. *Curr Opin Pulm Med* 2006; **12**: 331–336.

30. Rice DC, Erasmus JJ, Stevens CW *et al.* Extended surgical staging for potentially resectable malignant pleural mesothelioma. *Ann Thorac Surg* 2005; **80**: 1988–1992.

31. Rice DC, Stevens CW, Correa AM *et al.* Outcomes after extrapleural pneumonectomy and intensity-modulated radiation therapy for malignant pleural mesothelioma. *Ann Thorac Surg* 2007; **84**: 1685–1692.

32. Colby TV. Malignancies in the lung and pleura mimicking benign processes. *Semin Diagn Pathol* 1995; **12**: 30–44.

33. Gephardt GN, Rice TW. Utility of frozen-section evaluation of lymph nodes in the staging of bronchogenic carcinoma at mediastinoscopy and thoracotomy. *J Thorac Cardiovasc Surg* 1990; **100**: 853–859.

34. Oneson RH, Minke JA, Silverberg SG. Intraoperative pathologic consultation. An audit of 1,000 recent consecutive cases. *Am J Surg Pathol* 1989; **13**: 237–243.

35. Sawady J, Berner JJ, Siegler EE. Accuracy of and reasons for frozen sections: a correlative, retrospective study. *Hum Pathol* 1988; **19**: 1019–1023.

36. Moran CA. Pulmonary adenocarcinoma: the expanding spectrum of histologic variants. *Arch Pathol Lab Med* 2006; **130**: 958–962.

37. Tsuta K, Ishii G, Nitadori J *et al.* Comparison of the immunophenotypes of signet-ring cell carcinoma, solid adenocarcinoma with mucin production, and mucinous bronchioloalveolar carcinoma of the lung characterized by the presence of cytoplasmic mucin. *J Pathol* 2006; **209**: 78–87.

38. Motoi N, Szoke J, Riely GJ *et al.* Lung adenocarcinoma: modification of the 2004 WHO mixed subtype to include the major histologic subtype suggests correlations between papillary and micropapillary adenocarcinoma subtypes, EGFR mutations and gene expression analysis. *Am J Surg Pathol* 2008; **32**: 810–827.

39. Noguchi M, Morikawa A, Kawasaki M *et al.* Small adenocarcinoma of the lung. Histologic characteristics and prognosis. *Cancer* 1995; **75**: 2844–2852.

6 MEDIASTINUM

Saul Suster, César A. Moran, and David C. Rice

INTRODUCTION

The pathologist's role in the management of mediastinal lesions can be challenging because the mediastinum contains a multitude of structures and organs, all of which can be the site of pathologic processes. The mediastinum is also a frequent site of metastases from other locations, adding to the complexity of diseases that should be considered during intraoperative diagnosis (IOD).

GENERAL CLINICAL ISSUES

Most patients with mediastinal tumors present with non-specific symptoms related to the chest, but a minority present with superior vena caval obstruction or with a paraneoplastic syndrome, such as myasthenia gravis or Cushing's syndrome. In selected situations, laboratory tests can provide useful diagnostic information, as with tumor markers in malignant germ cell tumors, and chemical abnormalities in paraneoplastic syndromes.

A standard chest X-ray is usually the first imaging test performed to evaluate the patient, and when this is found to be abnormal, it is followed with CT scans, PET-CT scans and MRI. Imaging studies are important for narrowing the differential diagnosis because the majority of mediastinal tumors occur in predictable anatomic compartments (Fig. 6.1). Imaging may also provide other clues to the diagnosis; for example, a mediastinal mass accompanied by multiple enlarged lymph nodes favors a lymphoproliferative disorder, while a tooth in an anterior mediastinal mass would be diagnostic of a teratomatous component in the tumor. Imaging may also help to determine if the neoplasm is benign or malignant, as well as its resectability.

A tissue or cytologic diagnosis is almost always required before treatment is instituted, and this is obtained either by fine needle aspiration biopsy (FNA), needle core biopsy, incisional biopsy or by surgical resection. The method that is chosen depends on the preliminary clinical diagnosis, tumor resectability and accessibility to minimally invasive techniques. For example, complete surgical excision would be the first approach to a mass thought to be a non-invasive thymoma, but needle core biopsy or a limited incisional biopsy would be the technique of choice for a large infiltrative neoplasm of the anterior mediastinum suspected to be Hodgkin's lymphoma.

Metastatic carcinoma, which is the most common malignancy to involve the mediastinum, is discussed in detail in the chapter on Lung (see p. 67).

INDICATIONS FOR INTRAOPERATIVE CONSULTATION

1. To evaluate an incisional biopsy or an excised mass found incidentally during the course of open chest surgery for other reasons, such as coronary artery bypass surgery.
2. To determine if an incisional biopsy of a non-resectable mediastinal mass contains sufficient diagnostic tissue.
3. To evaluate an incisional biopsy of a mediastinal mass to determine if the lesion is benign or malignant, in situations where the IOD will dictate whether the surgeon will proceed with immediate surgical resection.
4. To render a diagnosis and evaluate the surgical margins of a resected primary malignancy of the mediastinum.
5. To evaluate biopsies of post-treatment mass lesions to determine if the lesion is recurrent neoplasm or post-treatment fibrosis.

Intraoperative Consultation in Surgical Pathology, ed. Mahendra Ranchod. Published by Cambridge University Press.
© Cambridge University Press 2010.

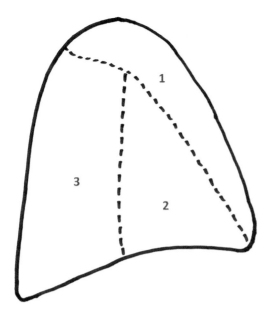

Fig. 6.1. Mediastinal compartments: (1) anterior superior mediastinum: thymoma, thymic cysts, thymic carcinoma, malignant lymphoma, germ cell tumors, spindle cell sarcomas, solitary fibrous tumor, ectopic thyroid/parathyroid; (2) middle mediastinum: malignant lymphoma, Hodgkin's disease, pericardial cyst, bronchogenic cyst; (3) posterior mediastinum: neurogenic tumors, gastroenteric cyst, sarcomas.

INFORMATION NEEDED BEFORE AND DURING SURGERY

The pathologist should not depend on the information provided on the pathology requisition form because this is often inadequate. Before handling the specimen, the patient's age and gender should be checked, and the pathologist should be familiar with the patient's past history, including previous neoplastic and non-neoplastic diseases and treatments. A clinical history of superior vena cava syndrome or paraneoplastic syndrome provides useful clues. Review of images is essential because precise location within the mediastinum often narrows the differential diagnosis, and in addition, CT scans and MRI provide information about the character of the mass, including the likelihood of malignancy. The pathologist should also be aware of the surgeon's operative plan, and in particular, whether surgical resection is dependent on the FS diagnosis. It is sometimes helpful to be familiar with the surgical findings because these may be different from what was anticipated; for this reason, it pays to visit the operating room in selected situations to receive an update of the surgical findings.

We cannot over-emphasize the importance of clinico-pathologic correlation. Many of the misdiagnoses on FS can be avoided if the FS findings are correlated with clinical and imaging data.

GENERAL PATHOLOGIC ISSUES

When the only purpose of the surgical procedure is to obtain diagnostic tissue, the pathologist has to ensure that sufficient tissue has been procured for routine histopathologic evaluation as well as for all ancillary studies. Because most incisional biopsies are obtained by minimally invasive surgical procedures, and not an open thoracotomy, tissue samples are small, sometimes making it difficult to decide if sufficient tissue has been obtained. Two precautions should be taken before declaring the specimen adequate:

- Crush artifact is liable to occur when a biopsy forceps is used to obtain tissue, a problem that is exaggerated when the tissue is fragile. Malignant lymphomas and small cell malignancies are particularly susceptible to crush artifact, especially if sclerosis is present in the stroma of the neoplasm. This problem can be mitigated by asking the surgeon for multiple biopsies and larger samples, and by alerting the surgeon to interpretive problems associated with crush artifact.
- Secondary changes are treacherous because they may be mistaken for the primary disease. For example, granulomatous inflammation is a common host reaction to a variety of neoplasms, and should not be taken as the principal disease if the patient has a large anterior mediastinal mass; if the FS shows only granulomatous inflammation, it should be assumed that there is an underlying neoplasm that has not been sampled. Similarly, cystic change in the thymus gland is a common secondary reaction to malignancies that involve the thymus, so a diagnosis of thymic cyst should only be made if that diagnosis is compatible with the clinical and imaging findings.

A resected mass should be inked regardless of the preoperative diagnosis, because inking will allow more reliable evaluation of the surgical margins if the mass harbors an unsuspected malignancy. When thymoma is suspected, we recommend inking with two colors, with a different color to identify the more critical deep surgical

Table 6.1. Pitfalls in the diagnosis of mediastinal lesions

Exclusive or predominant finding on FS	Underlying neoplasm that should be considered
Granulomatous inflammation	Hodgkin's lymphoma with secondary granulomatous inflammation
Seminoma with secondary granulomatous inflammation
Multiple benign thymic cysts	Hodgkin's lymphoma involving thymus
Seminoma involving thymus
Sclerosing process resembling sclerosing mediastinitis	Sclerosing large cell lymphoma
Sclerosing Hodgkin's lymphoma
Sclerosing seminoma
Lymphocytic-rich infiltrate	Lymphocyte-rich thymoma
Lymphoma

Table 6.2. Comparison of histologic classifications of thymic epithelial neoplasms

WHO Classification	"Traditional" (Mayo Clinic) Classification	Suster & Moran Classification
Type A	Spindle cell thymoma	Thymoma
Type AB	Lymphocyte-rich spindle cell thymoma	"
Type B1	Lymphocyte-rich thymoma	"
Type B2	Mixed lymphoepithelial thymoma	"
Type B3	Epithelial-rich thymoma	Atypical thymoma
Type C (thymic carcinoma)	Thymic carcinoma	Thymic carcinoma

margin. If other tissues, such as pleura, lung, pericardium, or great vessels are attached to the mass, these surfaces should be inked selectively if it will help to identify positive margins with greater specificity. The surgeon should be consulted when the orientation of the specimen is unclear.[2,3]

When a lymphoproliferative lesion is encountered, cytologic preparations should be made, and fresh tissue should be sampled for flow cytometry, and for molecular and cytogenetic studies – when appropriate. When sarcoma enters the differential diagnosis, a portion of fresh tissue should be sampled for cytogenetic studies, and a piece of tissue should be frozen for molecular assay, in the event that those studies become necessary. When an unusual neoplasm is encountered, a sample of the specimen should also be placed in gluteraldehyde for possible electron microscopic examination.

One of the problems with evaluating small biopsies of mediastinal masses is that malignant neoplasms may masquerade as benign processes, and the malignancy may be overlooked if the FS slides are examined in isolation; the most common of these are listed in Table 6.1.

SPECIFIC CLINICO-PATHOLOGIC ISSUES

Thymomas

Clinical issues
Most thymomas are detected incidentally on chest X-ray and only about 5% of patients present with myasthenia gravis. FNA and needle core biopsies are not performed

when a diagnosis of thymoma is favored on clinical grounds, as almost all thymomas are resected even if imaging studies show limited invasion into adjacent structures. At the time of surgical exploration, non-invasive thymomas are completely resected without prior incisional biopsy. The specimen will be submitted for IOD, with the expectation that the diagnosis of thymoma will be confirmed. Any histologic type of thymoma may be locally invasive without showing cytologic atypia, and when invasion is identified at surgery, an incisional biopsy will be submitted for IOD to confirm that the neoplasm is indeed thymoma and not some other malignancy. When the diagnosis is confirmed, the surgeon will excise the thymoma with an attempt to obtain clear surgical margins. If a histologically bland thymoma or thymic carcinoma is extensively invasive and not amenable to surgical resection, the surgical procedure may be limited to an incisional biopsy to obtain diagnostic tissue.

Pathologic issues
Thymomas range from very well-differentiated tumors that closely recapitulate the architecture of the normal thymus, to poorly differentiated tumors that no longer resemble the normal organ.[4] The terminology and classification of thymic neoplasms remain controversial;[5-7] the World Health Organization (WHO) classification is the most widely used,[8] but its validity has been challenged because of its complexity and difficulties in reproducibility (Table 6.2).[5,9-11] Fortunately, for purposes of IOD, the pathologist's role is limited to confirming the diagnosis of thymoma, and distinguishing it from thymic carcinoma.

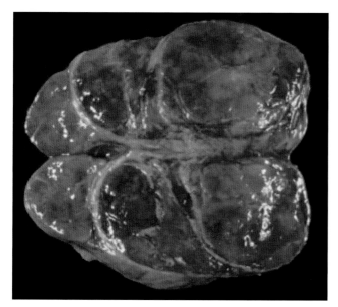

Fig. 6.2. Thymoma. Cut section of the gross specimen shows a well-encapsulated mass with fibrous bands dividing the tumor into lobules.

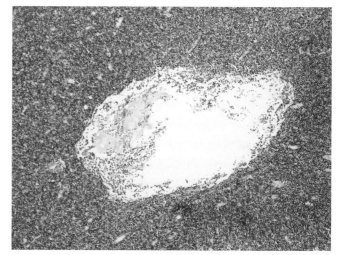

Fig. 6.4. Lymphocyte-rich thymoma with dilated perivascular space.

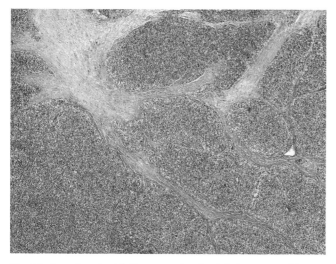

Fig. 6.3. Lymphocyte-rich thymoma showing lobules separated by broad bands of fibrous tissue.

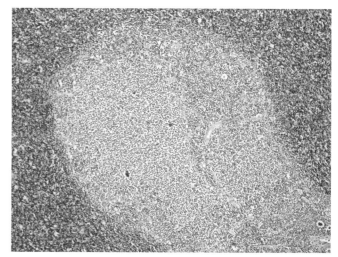

Fig. 6.5. Lymphocyte-rich thymoma with area of "medullary differentiation." Notice the relative paucity of small lymphocytes.

However, each of the histologic types of thymoma presents their own challenges on FS examination.

A common problem with *lymphocyte-rich thymomas* is that they may be mistaken for lymphoma. The distinction is of importance because mediastinal lymphomas are treated by chemotherapy and/or radiation therapy, whereas thymomas are treated by surgical resection. Features that support the diagnosis of thymoma are: (a) a firm encapsulated mass, with or without a grossly lobulated appearance due to fibrosis (Fig. 6.2); (b) a lobular pattern on scanning magnification, produced by lobules of cellular tissue separated by broad bands of fibrous tissue (Fig. 6.3); and (c) the presence of organotypical features of thymic differentiation such as dilated perivascular spaces and areas of "medullary differentiation" (Figs. 6.4 and 6.5). Features that support lymphoblastic lymphoma are: (a) a mass that is poorly defined and invasive as described by the surgeon; (b) a high mitotic count and necrosis, and (c) infiltration of atypical lymphocytes into mediastinal fat or adjacent structures (Fig. 6.6). Cytologic preparations are helpful, but are not always conclusive in making the distinction between lymphocyte-rich thymoma and lymphoma,[12] so that the diagnosis may have to be deferred to permanent sections. In this situation, the procedure would be limited to an incisional biopsy. It is obvious that the clinical, imaging and surgical findings should be taken into account to

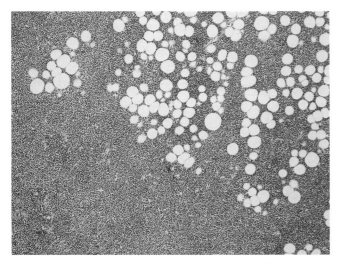

Fig. 6.6. Lymphoblastic lymphoma showing extensive infiltration but with preservation of the mediastinal fat.

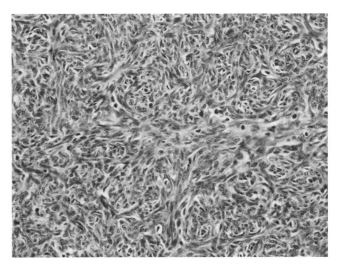

Fig. 6.7. Spindle cell thymoma with prominent storiform pattern resembling a "fibrohistiocytic" tumor.

Table 6.3. Differential diagnosis of lymphocyte-rich lesions of the mediastinum

Lymphocyte-rich thymoma

Lymphoblastic lymphoma

Diffuse large cell lymphoma with sclerosis

Hodgkin's lymphoma

Castleman's disease

Thymic hyperplasia

Table 6.4. Differential diagnosis of spindle cell neoplasms of the mediastinum

Spindle cell thymoma

Spindle cell thymic carcinoma

Solitary fibrous tumor

Schwannoma and neurofibroma

Spindle cell sarcoma

Spindle cell metastatic malignancies

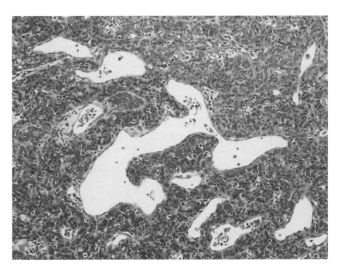

Fig. 6.8. Spindle cell thymoma with prominent staghorn pattern of vessels resembling "hemangiopericytoma."

reach a diagnosis in challenging cases, because these may provide helpful supportive data for one or other diagnosis.

Lymphocyte-rich thymomas should be also distinguished from other lymphocyte-rich lesions (Table 6.3).

Spindle cell thymomas may be difficult to separate from benign and malignant mesenchymal tumors, such as solitary fibrous tumor, schwannoma, synovial sarcoma and other types of spindle cell neoplasms (Table 6.4). The most common situation is distinguishing benign spindle cell thymoma from solitary fibrous tumor. These neoplasms have a great deal of morphologic overlap and it may not be possible to make the distinction on FS; fortunately, both are treated by complete excision and a diagnosis of "benign spindle cell neoplasm" is good enough for immediate surgical management.[6] Spindle cell thymoma may mimic sarcoma when it has a prominent storiform pattern, hemangiopericytoma-like areas, rosette-like structures and stromal hyalinization, and sometimes thymomas have a biphasic pattern that may be mistaken for carcinosarcoma (Figs. 6.7, 6.8, and 6.9).[13] Features that help to distinguish spindle cell thymoma from spindle cell sarcoma are the absence of nuclear atypia and the near absence of mitotic activity. The presence of marked nuclear pleomorphism, mitotic activity, and necrosis should suggest spindle cell sarcoma or spindle cell carcinoma of the

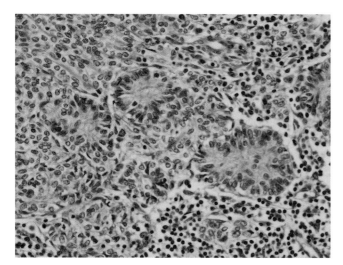

Fig. 6.9. Spindle cell thymoma with focal pseudo-rosette formation simulating a neuroendocrine neoplasm.

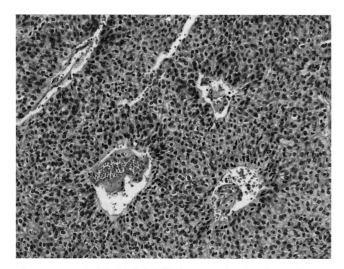

Fig. 6.10. Atypical (epithelial-rich) thymoma showing sheets of epithelioid cells with a few small perivascular spaces.

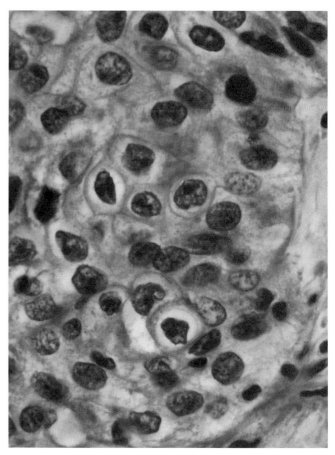

Fig. 6.11. Higher magnification of atypical thymoma showing epithelioid cells with large, hyperchromatic nuclei, abundant cytoplasm and sharply delineated cell membranes imparting them with a "squamoid" appearance.

thymus rather than a spindle cell thymoma, and the surgeon should be alerted to the potential aggressive nature of the neoplasm. Spindle cell thymoma has a tendency to undergo secondary cystic change, and when this is pronounced, the tumor can be mistaken for a benign thymic cyst; this distinction is not critical intraoperatively as both lesions are treated by complete surgical resection; the issue can be resolved with thorough sampling on permanent sections.

Thymomas rich in epithelial cells (WHO type B3, atypical thymoma) have to be distinguished from metastases to the anterior mediastinum, especially from pulmonary carcinoma. The neoplastic cells in atypical thymoma are often large, with abundant cytoplasm, and have enlarged hyperchromatic nuclei, prominent nucleoli and show

occasional mitoses.[5,14] Foci of squamous differentiation may be present, mimicking squamous carcinoma. The most helpful clue to the diagnosis of epithelial thymoma is the sheet-like growth of the neoplastic cells, compared to the islands or small clusters of infiltrative tumor cells seen in metastatic carcinoma (Figs. 6.10 and 6.11). In addition, the stroma in atypical thymomas often shows prominent dilated perivascular spaces containing lymphocytes, a clue to the thymic nature of the neoplasm.[13]

Thymic carcinomas resemble carcinomas that occur in other organs. A variety of histologic types have been described and these are listed in Table 6.5.[8,14] The most commonly encountered type in Western countries is the poorly differentiated, non-keratinizing (lymphoepithelioma-like) squamous cell carcinoma of the thymus (Fig. 6.12). The diagnosis of carcinoma is readily made intraoperatively, but its thymic origin may not be so obvious; the diagnosis can be made more confidently at a later date, after a metastasis has been excluded.[15] Most thymic

Table 6.5. Histologic types of thymic carcinoma

Histologic types of thymic carcinoma

Well and moderately-differentiated squamous cell carcinoma

Poorly-differentiated, non-keratinizing squamous cell carcinoma (lymphoepithelioma-like carcinoma)

Mucoepidermoid carcinoma

Basaloid carcinoma

Clear cell carcinoma

Spindle cell carcinoma

Mucinous and non-mucinous adenocarcinoma

Papillary carcinoma

Desmoplastic carcinoma

Anaplastic carcinoma

Carcinosarcoma

Neuroendocrine carcinoma

Other rare types

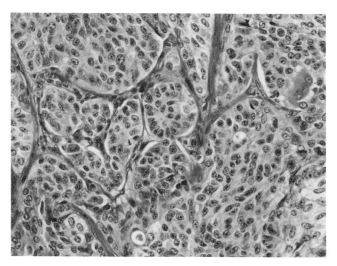

Fig. 6.13. Well-differentiated neuroendocrine carcinoma of the thymus (thymic carcinoid) showing nests of monotonous tumor cells separated by thin fibrovascular septa.

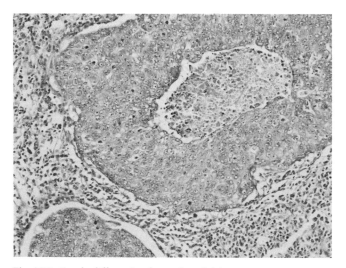

Fig. 6.12. Poorly differentiated, non-keratinizing (lymphoepithelioma-like) squamous cell carcinoma of the thymus showing islands of primitive tumor cells with central comedo-like areas of necrosis surrounded by a dense lymphoid infiltrate.

carcinomas are not resectable, so the purpose of IOD is to render a diagnosis, distinguish the carcinoma from other types of mediastinal malignancies, and ensure that an adequate sample is available for permanent sections and ancillary studies. A portion of fresh tumor tissue should be set aside for cytogenetic studies to determine if the tumor belongs to a particularly aggressive group of thoracic midline malignancies that are characterized by a specific 15;19 translocation.[16–18] Features that favor metastatic carcinoma to the mediastinum include associated mediastinal nodal metastases, abundant plasma cells in the stroma,

a history of prior carcinoma, and a histologic pattern that is similar to the prior tumor.

Mucoepidermoid and basaloid carcinoma of the thymus commonly undergo prominent cystic change, sometimes obscuring the neoplastic nature of the lesion.[19,20] Thorough sampling of the residual solid areas will reveal the diagnosis.

Neuroendocrine carcinomas of the thymus

Neuroendocrine carcinomas resemble their counterparts in other organs, but they are more aggressive, grade for grade.[21] They are classified as well-differentiated (conventional carcinoid tumor), moderately differentiated (atypical carcinoid), and poorly differentiated neuroendocrine carcinoma (small cell and large cell neuroendocrine carcinoma).[22]

Well-differentiated neuroendocrine carcinomas are circumscribed and composed of uniform, bland neoplastic endocrine cells that are arranged in nests, islands, trabeculae or ribbons with low mitotic activity (1–3/10 hpf) (Fig. 6.13). Punctate, comedo-like areas of necrosis with dystrophic calcification are often present (Fig. 6.14), a feature that is helpful for diagnosis. Moderately differentiated neuroendocrine carcinomas are usually poorly circumscribed with infiltrative margins. Histologically, these neoplasms retain an endocrine pattern of growth but may also show diffuse, sheet-like areas.[22] The neoplastic cells are usually enlarged with large, hyperchromatic nuclei, prominent nucleoli and frequent mitotic figures (4–9/10 hpf). Tumor necrosis is much more prominent than in the well-differentiated variants, and can often be

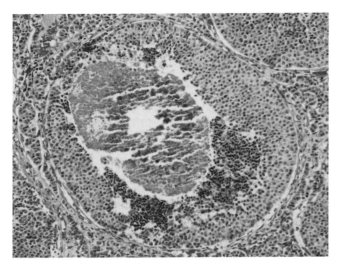

Fig. 6.14. Moderately differentiated neuroendocrine carcinoma of the thymus (atypical carcinoid) showing large ball of cells with central, comedo-like area of necrosis and dystrophic calcification.

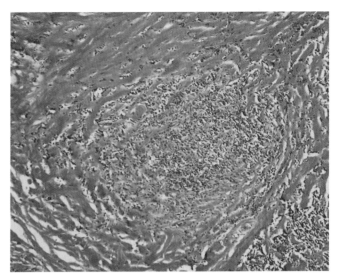

Fig. 6.15. Hodgkin lymphoma with extensive stromal fibrosis. A sparse lymphoid infiltrate without the characteristic Reed–Sternberg cells may be all that is present.

confluent and geographic. Vascular invasion and infiltration of adjacent structures is often seen.

Small cell neuroendocrine carcinomas and high grade, large cell neuroendocrine carcinomas are similar to their pulmonary counterparts. Small cell neuroendocrine carcinoma has to be distinguished from lymphoblastic lymphoma; the cells in both neoplasms have a high N/C ratio, show many mitotic figures and display the Azzopardi phenomenon (encrustation of vessel walls by DNA material). Infiltration of fat by single neoplastic cells favors lymphoblastic lymphoma, as do convoluted nuclei and cytoplasmic fragments (blue blobs on air dried, Romanowski stained cytologic preparations). The distinction may not be possible at times, but this is of little consequence because the purpose of the surgical procedure – for both neoplasms – is to obtain diagnostic tissue. The distinction of small cell neuroendocrine carcinoma from metastatic small cell carcinoma of pulmonary origin will depend on the sites involved.[19]

Lymphomas

Clinical issues

Both Hodgkin's lymphoma and non-Hodgkin's lymphomas can present as primary tumors of the mediastinum. Most occur in the anterior mediastinum, but they may occur in the middle or posterior mediastinal compartments as well.[23] When lymphoma is suspected, needle core biopsy will be attempted if the mass is accessible, but if this is not possible, tissue is obtained through a limited

thoracotomy incision or by thoracoscopy. The purpose of the surgical procedure is to obtain sufficient tissue for conventional and ancillary tests. The surgeon will depend on the pathologist to order the appropriate tests, including flow cytometry, cytogenetics and molecular tests.

Pathologic issues

Hodgkin's lymphoma is the most common lymphoma to involve the mediastinum. Most patients with mediastinal Hodgkin's lymphoma also have involved cervical lymph nodes, and the diagnosis is established by biopsy of a cervical lymph node. Occasionally however, the disease is limited to the anterior mediastinum and thoracoscopic biopsies or exploratory thoracotomy has to be performed to establish the diagnosis.[1] Nodular sclerosing Hodgkin's disease is the most common subtype. The diagnosis of Hodgkin's disease is usually straightforward but a number of problems may be encountered intraoperatively:

- When Hodgkin's lymphoma involves the thymus gland, it induces cystic change, mimicking benign cystic disease of the thymus (see Fig. 1.1, p. 7). If the clinical and imaging findings are those of a malignant neoplasm, the pathologist should insist that the surgeon obtain additional biopsies, and these should be submitted for FS until a diagnosis of malignancy is established.
- The biopsy may show extensive sclerosis and lack diagnostic neoplastic cells (Fig. 6.15). The sclerosis

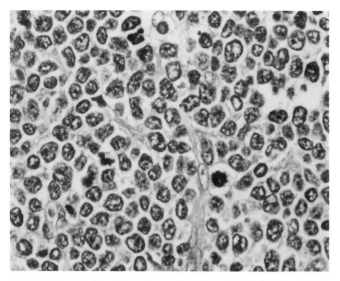

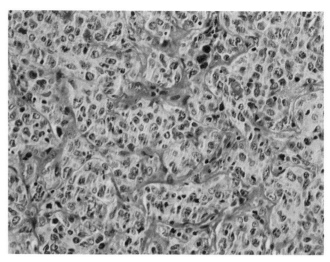

Fig. 6.16. Lymphoblastic lymphoma showing primitive lymphoid cells with convoluted nuclei, scattered chromatin with inconspicuous nucleoli, and numerous mitotic figures.

Fig. 6.17. Diffuse large cell lymphoma of the mediastinum with sclerosis. The compartmentalizing effects of the fine fibrous bands in the stroma may create a resemblance to an epithelial malignant neoplasm.

may be a secondary reaction to a deeper-lying Hodgkin's lymphoma or it may be an extensively sclerotic Hodgkin's lymphoma with near obliteration of neoplastic cells. Regardless of the origin of the fibrosis, the biopsy should be considered abnormal but nondiagnostic, and the surgeon should be asked to submit more tissue.

▪ The artifacts of freezing tissue for FS may compromise subsequent interpretation on permanent sections. If an incisional biopsy is large enough, the specimen should be bisected and one half should be saved for permanent sections. On the other hand, if the entire specimen has to be submitted for FS because of its small size, the pathologist should request additional tissue for permanent sections from the same site as the diagnostic biopsy.

Lymphoblastic lymphoma occurs most frequently in children and adolescents, although it may occur in adults as well. Patients usually present with a rapidly enlarging mediastinal mass, with airway obstruction, pleural effusion and superior vena cava syndrome, requiring urgent attention.[24] The neoplastic lymphoid cells have convoluted or non-convoluted nuclei, with finely dispersed chromatin and inconspicuous nucleoli (Fig. 6.16). Two characteristic features on FS are crush artifact and numerous "tingible-body" macrophages, imparting a "starry-sky" appearance. The Azzopardi phenomenon may also be present. The main differential diagnosis is lymphocyte-rich thymoma and small cell neuroendocrine carcinoma; patient age,

clinical presentation and imaging findings will usually favor one of these diagnoses over the other. The distinction between lymphoblastic lymphoma and small cell carcinoma can be deferred to permanent sections if necessary, but every attempt should be made to recognize lymphocyte-rich thymoma, because unlike the other two neoplasms, thymomas will be surgically resected.

Diffuse Large B-cell Lymphoma with sclerosis, a true primary thymic B-cell lymphoma,[23] usually occurs in adult women, and often presents with bulky disease and the superior vena cava syndrome. Histologically, the neoplasm shows compartmentalization of neoplastic cells by dense fibrous tissue, sometimes mimicking an epithelial malignancy (Fig. 6.17); the presence of entrapped thymic epithelium adds to the risk of misinterpreting the lesion as carcinoma. The diffuse sclerosis makes the specimen susceptible to crush artifact, so precautions should be taken to obtain sufficient non-traumatized tissue.

Germ cell tumors of the mediastinum

Clinical issues

Germ cell tumors of the mediastinum account for approximately 10–20% of all mediastinal masses and cysts.[1] All types of germ cell tumors occur in the mediastinum and, of these, teratomas are the most common, followed by seminoma.[25–27] The vast majority of germ cell tumors occur in the anterior mediastinum, but they have been described in the posterior mediastinum as well. Symptoms

Table 6.6. Histologic classification of germ cell tumors of the mediastinum

Teratomatous lesions	Non-teratomatous lesions
Mature teratoma	Seminoma
Immature teratoma	Yolk sac tumor
Teratoma with additional malignant components	Choriocarcinoma
■ Type I: Teratoma + non-teratomatous germ cell tumor (i.e., seminoma, yolk sac tumor, embryonal carcinoma, etc)	
■ Type II: Teratoma + epithelial malignancy (i.e., adenocarcinoma, squamous cell carcinoma)	
■ Type III: Teratoma + sarcoma (i.e., rhabdomyosarcoma, leiomyosarcoma, liposarcoma, etc)	
■ Type IV: Teratoma + more than one of the above	
	Embryonal carcinoma
	Combined non-teratomatous tumors (mixtures of the above)

are related mainly to compression of adjacent structures, although a significant number of cases are discovered incidentally on routine chest X-ray. Germ cell tumors affect young adults and show a striking predilection for men; non-teratomatous germ cell neoplasms are extremely rare in females. Elevated serum levels of embryonic hormones such as alpha-fetoprotein, placental-like alkaline phosphatase, and human beta-chorionic gonadotrophin provide strong evidence for a germ cell neoplasm.

Needle core biopsy is usually performed on an anterior mediastinal mass suspected to be malignant germ cell tumor. If the needle biopsy is non-diagnostic, an incisional biopsy will be performed, either by thoracoscopy or through a limited thoracotomy. Thoracotomy, with the intent of tumor resection, is undertaken for resectable germ cell tumors, and this includes clinically benign teratomas, resectable immature teratomas and occasionally, an encapsulated seminoma. Non-seminomatous malignant germ cell tumors, which are usually locally advanced, are subjected to biopsy only, and resected only if there is residual tumor after chemotherapy.

Pathologic issues
The classification of mediastinal germ cell tumors is listed in Table 6.6.[25]

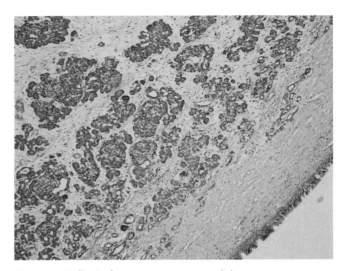

Fig. 6.18. Mediastinal mature teratoma containing mature pancreatic tissue.

Teratomas. Mature teratomas are more frequent than immature teratomas. One peculiar aspect of mediastinal teratomas is the frequency of mature pancreatic tissue, which on rare occasions, may be the seat of acute pancreatitis (Fig. 6.18). The majority of mature teratomas are cystic, and this feature, together with a tooth on chest X-ray, will clinch the diagnosis. Rupture of a mature teratoma will result in an inflammatory reaction that the surgeon may interpret as suspicious of an invasive malignancy. Biopsy of this area will show a florid granulomatous inflammatory reaction that may be mistaken for primary granulomatous inflammation if this is viewed out of context.

Immature teratomas are predominantly solid on gross examination, and have the same histologic appearance as immature teratomas in other locations. A variety of other malignant germ cell tumors, as well as carcinomas and sarcomas, may arise within mature and immature teratomas; these are more likely to be infiltrative and will prompt the surgeon to perform an incisional biopsy before attempting surgical resection.

Seminoma is the second most common type of germ cell tumor of the mediastinum.[24] Most cases are diagnosed by percutaneous needle core biopsy, but when this fails, an incisional biopsy is performed. There are four challenges to recognizing mediastinal seminoma on small biopsies:

■ The neoplasm may be obscured by a florid granulomatous reaction, a finding that could mislead the pathologist into believing that the disease is an inflammatory process (Fig. 6.19).

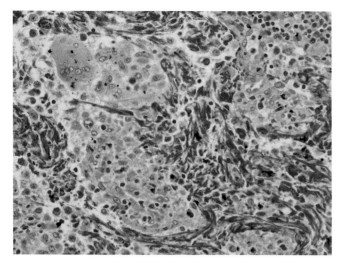

Fig. 6.19. Mediastinal seminoma with prominent granulomatous reaction. Notice the crushed and distorted seminoma tumor cells scattered in-between the granulomas.

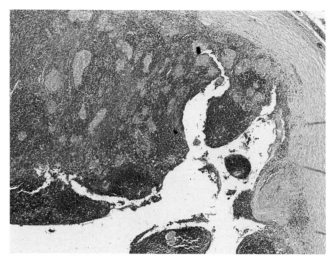

Fig. 6.21. Mediastinal seminoma with extensive secondary cystic changes. The neoplastic elements may be very subtle and only identified focally under higher magnification.

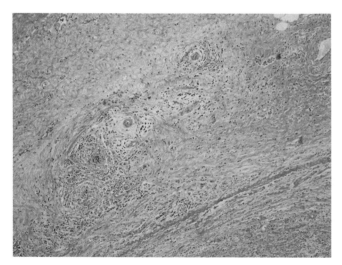

Fig. 6.20. Mediastinal seminoma with extensive stromal sclerosis. The neoplastic elements may be largely obscured by the fibrosing process, simulating sclerosing mediastinitis.

- Occasionally, seminomas evoke marked sclerosis, and this may obscure the neoplastic cells (Fig. 6.20).[28]
- Seminomas that involve the thymus evoke the development of cysts lined by thymic epithelium, mimicking a benign multilocular thymic cyst (Fig. 6.21).[29]
- The cells of seminoma are fragile and susceptible to crush artifact, sometimes making it difficult to identify the nature of the neoplasm.

Yolk sac tumor, embryonal carcinoma and choriocarcinoma only rarely occur in the pure form, but are more often seen in combination with other germ cell tumor

components.[27,31] Because these neoplasms have characteristics of malignancy on imaging, the diagnosis is usually made by percutaneous needle core biopsy, but if this fails, or if the diagnosis of malignant germ cell tumor has not been considered, the patient will have an incisional biopsy with a request for FS diagnosis. If the pathologist has not been primed to the possibility of a malignant germ cell tumor, the FS could easily be misinterpreted as anaplastic carcinoma. Rarely, yolk sac tumors undergo extensive cystic change, another feature that would direct the pathologist away from considering a malignant germ cell tumor.[30] These misdiagnoses are not important since the purpose of IOD is to ensure that sufficient neoplastic tissue is obtained for detailed evaluation on permanent sections.

Mesenchymal tumors

Clinical issues

Mesenchymal neoplasms present as a mass without specific clinical or imaging features, and they are approached in the same way as other mediastinal tumors; benign tumors are excised, and needle core biopsy or incisional biopsy are performed on non-resectable malignancies. Biopsies for FS will be submitted for evaluation of surgical margins in cases that are locally infiltrative or malignant because complete excision offers the best chance of cure. If a specific diagnosis or "good enough diagnosis" cannot be made, the surgeon will limit the surgical procedure to a diagnostic incisional biopsy, and resect the mass at a later date – if clinically indicated.

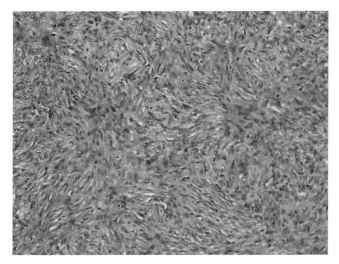

Fig. 6.22. Solitary fibrous tumor with prominent storiform pattern simulating a fibrohistiocytic neoplasm.

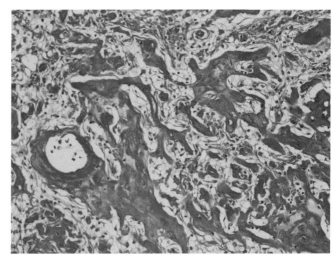

Fig. 6.24. Solitary fibrous tumor with extensive stromal sclerosis.

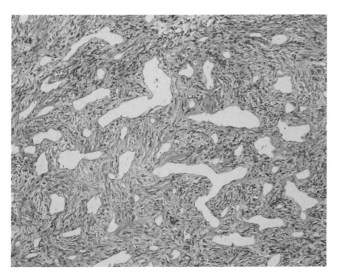

Fig. 6.23. Solitary fibrous tumor with prominent hemangiopericytoma-like vascular pattern.

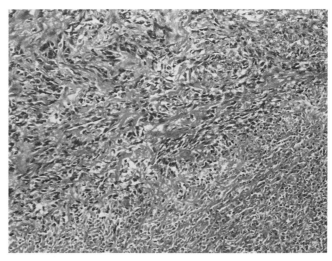

Fig. 6.25. Malignant solitary fibrous tumor showing increased cellularity, nuclear pleomorphism, and tumor necrosis (bottom).

Pathologic issues

Solitary Fibrous Tumor (SFT) is the most common mesenchymal tumor of the mediastinum. The majority occur in the anterior mediastinum, although they may also occur in the middle and posterior compartments. Solitary fibrous tumors of the mediastinum tend to be more aggressive than their counterparts in other anatomic locations, perhaps because they tend to be large and are often locally invasive at the time of diagnosis.[33] The histologic heterogeneity of SFT may make it difficult to distinguish this neoplasm on FS from other spindle cell tumors such as spindle cell thymoma and low grade sarcomas (Figs. 6.22–6.24).[34] Approximately 10% of SFTs will show histologic features of malignancy, including increased cellularity, marked nuclear pleomorphism, high mitotic activity and areas of necrosis (Fig. 6.25). A FS diagnosis of "spindle cell sarcoma" may be as specific as the pathologist can be; surgical management will depend on the resectability of the mass.

Synovial sarcoma of the mediastinum has been recognized with increasing frequency in recent years.[35] Most occur in the anterior mediastinum, and they are usually bulky and infiltrative at the time of diagnosis. If a diagnosis has not been made on needle biopsy, an incisional biopsy will be performed and submitted for FS. The tumor is easily recognized on frozen section as a malignant spindle cell neoplasm but it may be more difficult to make a specific diagnosis (Fig. 6.26). Synovial sarcoma will be

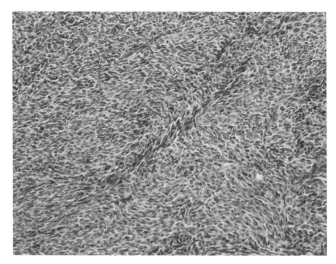

Fig. 6.26. Synovial sarcoma of the mediastinum showing monotonous atypical spindle cell population with focal herringbone pattern.

resected if this is possible. A sample of fresh tumor tissue should be set aside for cytogenetic studies whenever synovial sarcoma is suspected because 75%–80% of cases show the distinctive X;18 chromosomal translocation that is associated with this neoplasm. In the absence of adequate tissue for cytogenetic studies, identification of the specific fusion transcript for the X;18 translocation can be accomplished by PCR, FISH and other techniques. The differential diagnosis includes malignant solitary fibrous tumor and a malignant peripheral nerve sheath tumor.

Neural neoplasms are the most common tumors in the posterior mediastinum. They range from benign neural neoplasms (schwannoma, neurofibroma, ganglioneuroma, ganglioneurofibroma) to malignant (malignant peripheral nerve sheath tumor, neuroblastoma and ganglioneuroblastoma).[1] A fairly accurate pre-operative diagnosis can usually be made with a combination of clinical history, imaging studies, and needle core biopsy.[1,32] A needle core biopsy is usually performed, but often the diagnosis is not specific enough to plan treatment, leading to an open biopsy for diagnostic tissue. For example, a cellular schwannoma may not be readily distinguished from a low-grade malignant peripheral nerve sheath tumor on limited sampling and an open biopsy or resection may be required for definitive diagnosis. The pathologist's main charge is to make certain that sufficient tissue is obtained for ancillary studies.

Miscellaneous mesenchymal neoplasms

A large variety of other benign and malignant mesenchymal neoplasms occur in the mediastinum, all rare.[36–39]

Miscellaneous benign lesions

A variety of benign conditions occur in the mediastinum that may be confused pre-operatively for a malignant tumor, including infectious and inflammatory conditions (granulomatous inflammation, myofibroblastic inflammatory pseudotumor), hamartomatous lesions (thymolipoma, Castleman's disease), thymic cysts (congenital cysts, acquired multilocular thymic cysts), and thymic hyperplasia (lymphoid follicular hyperplasia and "true" thymic hyperplasia). It may not be easy to distinguish these lesions from some types of neoplasms, so the diagnosis may have to be deferred to permanent sections. It is advisable to take fresh samples for appropriate ancillary studies if sufficient material is available. When granulomatous inflammation is present, tissue should be collected for appropriate cultures.

Idiopathic sclerosing mediastinitis is another condition where it may not be possible to render a definitive diagnosis on FS.[40] Although commonly regarded as a sequel to a fungal infection, granulomas and/or organisms are absent in more than 50% of cases. The incisional biopsy will show diffuse sclerosis with scattered inflammatory cells, and the fibrosing process may be infiltrative, entraping nerve trunks and vessels. Although the process is non-neoplastic, it can be fatal when there is compromise of vital structures. Idiopathic sclerosing mediastinitis is a diagnosis of exclusion since many neoplastic conditions, such as Hodgkin's lymphoma, thymoma, thymic carcinoma and seminoma can evoke extensive sclerosis and hyalinization, masking the underlying neoplasm (Table 6.1).

Castleman's disease has the potential for being mistaken for lymphoma. Identification of the "lollipop" sign (longitudinal section of a small vessel traversing a lymphoid follicle) is a clue to the diagnosis (Fig. 6.27) but it may not be possible to make a specific diagnosis intraoperatively. Tissue samples should be procured for flow cytometry and molecular studies.

Multilocular thymic cyst is a reactive condition seen most often in adults. Radiographically, it presents as a multilocular cystic mass in the anterior mediastinum. The lesion is characterized by dilated cystic structures filled with clear to hemorrhagic fluid whose walls are lined by cuboidal, squamous or columnar epithelium.[41] The walls of the cysts usually show fibrosis, hemorrhage, acute and chronic inflammation, cholesterol granulomas and hyperplastic lymphoid follicles (Fig. 6.28). A reliable diagnosis cannot always be established on FS because identical

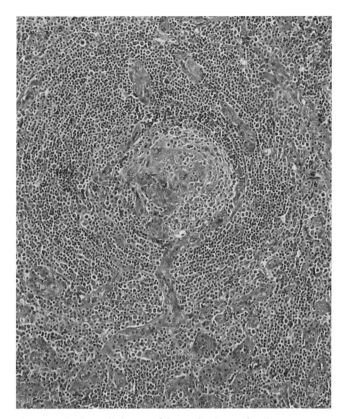

Fig. 6.27. Castleman's disease of the mediastinum showing characteristic onion-skin layering of lymphocytes around germinal center, with small blood vessel traversing the follicle (so-called "lollypop sign").

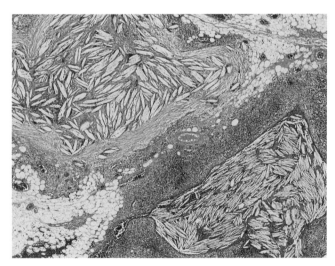

Fig. 6.28. Acquired multilocular thymic cyst showing cyst wall with severe chronic inflammation, fibrosis, and lined by a single cell layer of small cuboidal to squamoid epithelium. Notice the adjacent cholesterol-cleft granuloma.

changes can occur as a secondary reaction to a variety of neoplasms of the mediastinum, including thymoma, thymic carcinoma, Hodgkin's lymphoma, seminoma and yolk sac tumor.

REFERENCES

1. Suster S, Moran CA. The mediastinum. In *Modern Pathology*, Weidner N, Cote R, Suster S, Weiss L, (eds), Philadelphia: W.B. Saunders Co, 2003, pp. 439–504.
2. Marchevsky AM, Hammond EA, Moran CA, Suster S. Protocol for the examination of specimens from patients with thymic epithelial tumors located in any area of the mediastinum. *Arch Pathol Lab Med* 2003; **127**: 1298–1303.
3. Suster S. Diagnosis of thymoma. *J Clin Pathol* 2006; **59**: 1238–1244.
4. Suster S, Moran CA. Thymoma, atypical thymoma and thymic carcinoma. A novel conceptual approach to the classification of neoplasms of thymic epithelium. *Am J Clin Pathol* 1999; **111**: 826–833.
5. Suster S, Moran CA. Problem areas and inconsistencies in the WHO classification of thymoma. *Semin Diagn Pathol* 2005; **22**: 198–212.
6. Suster S, Moran CA. Thymoma classification: current status and future trends. *Am J Clin Pathol* 2006; **125**: 542–554.
7. Suster S, Moran CA. Classification of thymoma: the WHO and beyond. *Hematol Oncol Clin NA* 2008; **22**: 381–392.
8. Travis WD, Brambilla E, Muller-Hermelink HK *et al. Pathology and genetic of tumors of the lung, pleura, thymus and heart.* In *World Health Organization Classification of Tumors*, Lyon, IARC Press, 2004.
9. Rieker RJ, Hoegel J, Morresi-Hauf A *et al.* Histologic classification of thymic epithelial tumors: comparison of established classification schemes. *Int J Cancer* 2002; **98**: 900–906.
10. Marchevsky A, Gupta R, McKenna RJ *et al.* Evidence-based pathology and the pathologic evaluation of thymomas: The World Health Organization classification can be simplified into only 3 categories other than thymic carcinoma. *Cancer* 2008; **112**: 2780–2788.
11. Verghese ET, den Bakker MA, Campbell A *et al.* Interobserver variation in the classification of thymic tumors – a multicentre study using the WHO classification system. *Histopathology* 2008; **53**: 218–223.
12. Wakely PE, Jr. Cytopathology of thymic epithelial neoplasms. *Semin Diagn Pathol* 2005; **22**: 213–222.
13. Suster S, Moran CA. Primary thymic epithelial neoplasms. Spectrum of differentiation and histologic features. *Semin Diagn Pathol* 1999; **16**: 2–17.
14. Suster S. Thymic carcinoma: update of current diagnostic criteria and histologic types. *Semin Diagn Pathol* 2005; **22**: 198–212.
15. Moran CA, Suster S. Thymic carcinoma: current concepts and histologic features. *Hematol Oncol Clin NA* 2008; **22**: 393–407.
16. Kubonishi I, Takehara N, Iwata J *et al.* Novel t(15;19)(q15;p13) chromosome abnormality in a thymic carcinoma. *Cancer Res* 1991; **51**: 3327–3328.
17. Lee ACW, Kwong Y-I, Fu KH *et al.* Disseminated mediastinal carcinoma with chromosomal translocation (15;19). A distinctive clinicopathologic syndrome. *Cancer* 1993; **72**: 2273–2276.
18. Vargas SO, French CA, Faul PN *et al.* Upper respiratory tract carcinoma with chromosomal translocation 15;19. Evidence for a distinct disease entity of young patients with a rapidly fatal course. *Cancer* 2001; **92**: 1195–1203.
19. Suster S, Rosai J. Thymic carcinoma. Clinicopathologic study of 60 cases. *Cancer* 1991; **67**: 1025–1032.
20. Moran CA, Suster S. Mucoepidermoid carcinomas of the thymus. Clinicopathologic study of six cases. *Am J Surg Pathol* 1995; **19**: 826–834.

21. Suster S, Moran CA. Neuroendocrine neoplasms of the mediastinum. *Am J Clin Pathol* 2001; **115** (S1): 17–27.

22. Moran CA, Suster S. Neuroendocrine carcinomas of the thymus (thymic carcinoid). Clinicopathologic study of 80 cases with a proposal for histologic grading and clinical staging. *Am J Clin Pathol* 2000; **114**: 760–766.

23. Suster S. Primary diffuse large cell lymphomas of the mediastinum. *Semin Diagn Pathol* 1999; **16**: 51–64.

24. Jaffe ES, Berard CW. Lymphoblastic lymphoma: a term rekindled with new precision. *Ann Int Med* 1978; **89**: 415–417.

25. Moran CA, Suster S. Primary germ cell tumors of the mediastinum. I. Analysis of 322 cases with special emphasis on teratomatous lesions and a new proposal for histopathologic classification and clinical staging. *Cancer* 1997; **80**: 681–690.

26. Moran CA, Suster S, Przygodzki RM *et al.* Primary germ cell tumors of the mediastinum. II. Mediastinal seminomas: a clinicopathologic and immunohistochemical study of 120 cases. *Cancer* 1997; **80**: 691–698.

27. Moran CA, Suster S, Koss MN. Primary germ cell tumors of the mediastinum. III. Primary yolk sac tumor, embryonal carcinoma, and combined non-teratomatous germ cell tumors: a clinicopathological and immunohistochemical study of 64 cases. *Cancer* 1997; **80**: 699–707.

28. Suster S, Moran CA. Malignant thymic neoplasms that may mimic benign conditions. *Semin Diagn Pathol* 1995; **12**: 98–104.

29. Moran CA, Suster S. Mediastinal seminomas with prominent cystic changes. A clinicopathologic study of 10 cases. *Am J Surg Pathol* 1995; **19**: 1047–1053.

30. Moran CA, Suster S. Mediastinal yolk sac tumors associated with prominent multilocular cystic changes of thymic epithelium: a clinicopathological and immunohistochemical study of five cases. *Mod Pathol* 1997; **10**: 800–803.

31. Moran CA, Suster S. Primary mediastinal choriocarcinomas. A clinicopathologic and immunohistochemical study of 8 cases. *Am J Surg Pathol* 1997; **21**: 1007–1012.

32. Suster S, Moran CA, Koss MN. Epithelioid hemangioendothelioma of the anterior mediastinum. Clinicopathologic, immunohistochemical and ultrastructural study of 12 cases. *Am J Surg Pathol* 1994; **18**: 871–881.

33. Witkin GB, Rosai J. Solitary fibrous tumor of the mediastinum. A report of 14 cases. *Am J Surg Pathol* 1989; **13**: 547–557.

34. Moran CA, Suster S, Koss MN. The spectrum of histologic growth patterns in benign and malignant fibrous tumors of the pleura. *Semin Diagn Pathol* 1992; **9**: 169–180.

35. Suster S, Moran CA. Primary synovial sarcomas of the mediastinum. A clinicopathological, immunohistochemical and ultrastructural study of 15 cases. *Am J Surg Pathol* 2005; **29**: 569–578.

36. Suster S, Moran CA, Koss MN. Primary rhabdomyosarcomas of the anterior mediastinum. Report of 4 cases unassociated with germ cell, teratomatous or thymic carcinomatous components. *Hum Pathol* 1994; **25**: 349–356.

37. Moran CA, Suster S, Perino G *et al.* Malignant smooth muscle neoplasms presenting as mediastinal soft tissue masses: Clinicopathologic study of 10 cases. *Cancer* 1994; **74**: 2251–2260.

38. Suster S, Moran CA. Chordomas of the mediastinum. Clinicopathologic, immunohistochemical and ultrastructural examination of 6 cases presenting as posterior mediastinal masses. *Hum Pathol* 1995; **26**: 1354–1362.

39. Suster S, Moran CA. Malignant cartilaginous tumors of the mediastinum: clinicopathologic study of 6 cases presenting as extraskeletal soft tissue masses. *Hum Pathol* 1997; **28**: 588–594.

40. Flieder DB, Suster S, Moran CA. Idiopathic fibroinflammatory (fibrosing/sclerosing) lesions of the mediastinum: a study of 30 cases with emphasis on histologic heterogeneity. *Mod Pathol* 1999; **12**: 257–264.

41. Suster S, Rosai J. Multilocular thymic cysts: an acquired reactive process. Study of 18 cases. *Am J Surg Pathol* 1991; **15**: 388–398.

7 SALIVARY GLANDS

Mahendra Ranchod, John K.C. Chan, and David W. Eisele

Tumors of the salivary glands are treated primarily by surgical resection. The surgeon often has a good sense for whether the lesion is benign or malignant based on clinical and imaging findings. Often, this is supplemented with a cytologic diagnosis from fine needle aspiration biopsy (FNA) for neoplasms of the parotid and submandibular glands, or an incisional biopsy diagnosis on minor salivary gland lesions.

INDICATIONS FOR INTRAOPERATIVE DIAGNOSIS

1. To render an initial diagnosis on a mass in the parotid or submandibular gland.
2. To determine the adequacy of an incisional biopsy specimen for lesions arising in a minor salivary gland, e.g., biopsy of a lesion in the palate.
3. To evaluate the surgical margins in resections of salivary gland tumors.
4. To evaluate a cervical lymph node biopsy in situations where a diagnosis of metastatic carcinoma would prompt cervical lymph node dissection.
5. To procure tissue for ancillary studies.

GENERAL CLINICAL ISSUES

Salivary gland neoplasms usually present as an asymptomatic mass. The distinction between benign and malignant neoplasm cannot always be made on clinical examination. Pain and a history of rapid growth raise the possibility of malignancy, and fixation of the mass to surrounding tissues, nerve dysfunction (e.g., facial nerve palsy in association with an ipsilateral parotid mass), and associated lymphadenopathy are strong indicators of malignancy.

The frequency of neoplasms in different sites appears to be related to the mass of salivary gland tissue at risk. Approximately 80% of neoplasms arise in the parotid and submandibular glands, and more than 90% of parotid neoplasms arise in the superficial lobe. There is an inverse relationship between the frequency of malignancy and the size of the gland; >60% of minor salivary gland neoplasms are malignant compared to 20% in the parotid gland, a phenomenon for which there is no satisfactory explanation.

A FNA is usually performed for mass lesions in the submandibular region, partly to distinguish between a salivary gland lesion and an enlarged lymph node. Depending on size and location, FNA or an incisional biopsy is usually performed on a suspected minor salivary gland neoplasm because this helps to plan surgical resection as well as identify lesions that do not require surgical resection, such as necrotizing sialometaplasia and lymphomas. There is some disagreement about the value of FNA in the evaluation of mass lesions in the parotid area. Some surgeons argue that FNA is not needed for benign-appearing mass lesions that are limited to the superficial lobe because superficial lobectomy is both diagnostic and therapeutic; in addition, it is argued that FNA cannot always distinguish between benign neoplasms and low grade carcinomas. However, strong arguments can be made for performing FNA on all masses in the parotid area because: (a) FNA may identify the mass as a reactive lymph node and not salivary gland tissue, and thus avert an unnecessary superficial parotidectomy; (b) FNA facilitates discussion of treatment recommendations with the patient; and (c) FNA justifies evaluation with imaging studies such as CT, MRI and PET scans to determine the extent of local and regional disease; (d) FNA enables pre-operative consultation with other specialists such as radiation oncologists.

Intraoperative Consultation in Surgical Pathology, ed. Mahendra Ranchod. Published by Cambridge University Press.
© Cambridge University Press 2010.

Table 7.1. Managerial classification of salivary gland neoplasms

Category	Common neoplasms	Management
Benign recur infrequently and recurrences are innocuous	Warthin's tumor Basal cell adenoma Oncocytoma	Complete excision
Benign but high recurrence rate with incomplete excision; recurrences difficult to control	Pleomorphic adenoma	Complete excision with clear margins.
Low grade carcinoma	Low grade mucoepidermoid carcinoma Acinic cell carcinoma Polymorphous low grade adenocarcinoma Epithelial-myoepithelial carcinoma Basal cell adenocarcinoma Low grade adenocarcinoma ex pleomorphic adenoma	– Complete excision with clear margins. – Lymph node biopsy if node enlarged.
Histologically low grade but highly infiltrating	Adenoid cystic carcinoma	Wide excision with clear margins.
High grade carcinoma	High grade mucoepidermoid carcinoma High grade carcinoma ex pleomorphic adenoma Salivary duct carcinoma	– Complete excision with clear margins. – Radical resection if necessary. – Lymph node dissection for positive nodes. – Controversy about elective node dissection.

Surgical resection with adequate surgical margins is the treatment of choice for all resectable salivary gland neoplasms. Benign tumors of the parotid gland are treated by parotidectomy with an adequate surgical margin, and benign neoplasms of the submandibular gland are treated by complete resection of the gland. It is a well-known surgical axiom that benign neoplasms of the salivary glands should not be enucleated because pleomorphic adenomas in particular, have a high rate of local recurrence with incomplete removal.

Surgical resection with clear margins is the most effective treatment for salivary gland carcinomas. Resection of the facial nerve and removal of the deep lobe add complexity to the procedure and are performed only when necessary, i.e., when there is tumor involvement of the facial nerve or tumor invasion into deep lobe. Radical resections are performed for malignancies that extend into the extra-salivary gland tissue but are still resectable. Radical parotidectomy may include removal of the facial nerve, pre-auricular skin, auditory canal or temporal bone. Radical resection of the submandibular gland involves excision of the submandibular salivary gland, lingual or hypoglossal nerves, floor of mouth, digastric and mylohyoid muscles, and sometimes part of the mandible. Radical resection of malignancies in minor salivary gland locations are determined by the location of the neoplasm. It is sometimes difficult to obtain clear surgical margins on malignant neoplasms that appear resectable on clinical grounds, especially high grade carcinomas and highly infiltrative carcinomas such as adenoid cystic carcinoma. When clear microscopic surgical margins cannot be achieved, the grossly visible tumor is removed and adjuvant postoperative radiation therapy is delivered.

GENERAL PATHOLOGIC ISSUES

There are more than 40 named salivary gland neoplasms, but these can be distilled into four managerial groups (Table 7.1). This managerial classification is modeled on the classification of soft tissue neoplasms proposed by Kempson et al.[1] There are therefore two steps in the diagnosis of salivary gland neoplasms: first, making a specific morphologic diagnosis, and second, assigning the tumor to a managerial category. When a specific diagnosis cannot be reached intraoperatively, an attempt should be made to assign the tumor to a managerial category.

High-grade carcinomas of the salivary gland are readily recognized as malignant. The main issue is to distinguish between primary carcinoma and a metastasis from a cutaneous or other primary site. Metastases, especially to intra-parotid and peri-parotid lymph nodes, may be mistaken for a primary salivary gland malignancy, and it is prudent

(a)

(b)

(c)

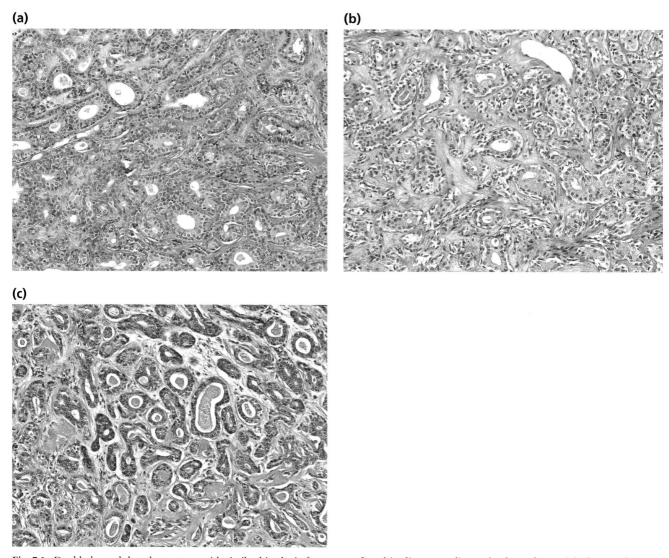

Fig. 7.1. Double-layered ductal structures with similar histologic features are found in disparate salivary gland neoplasms: (a) pleomorphic adenoma; (b) epithelial/myoepithelial carcinoma; and (c) adenoidcystic carcinoma.

therefore, to consider a metastasis when a salivary gland tumor is difficult to classify.

Low grade carcinomas may be difficult to distinguish from benign neoplasms for the following reasons:

- Low grade carcinomas show minimal to mild cytologic atypia and can be indistinguishable from benign neoplasms on cytologic grounds.
- Some adenomas and carcinomas have overlapping patterns. For example, pleomorphic adenoma (PA) characteristically contains ductal structures with a double layer of cells (epithelial and myopeithelial), but similar ductal structures are found in epithelial-

myoepithelial carcinoma and in the tubular component of adenoid cystic carcinoma (Fig. 7.1). Similarly, sheets of basaloid cells are present in basal cell adenoma, some cellular PAs and basal cell adenocarcinoma.

- A few neoplasms have characteristic histologic or cytologic features but these should be viewed in the context of the entire neoplasm. For example, a cribriform pattern is characteristic of adenoid cystic carcinoma but a focal cribriform pattern is occasionally seen in PA. Similarly, squamoid and mucus cells are typical of mucoepidermoid carcinoma but these cells are occasionally present in Warthin's tumors and pleomorphic adenomas.[2] These histologic features are of no clinical

(a)

(b)

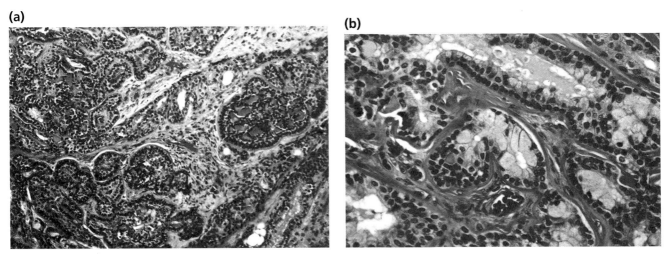

Fig. 7.2. (a) Microscopic cribriform foci, resembling adenoidcystic carcinoma were present in this PA of the parotid gland. (b) Focal squamoid and mucus cells, typical of the cells found in MEC, were found in this PA of the parotid gland. These incidental microscopic findings are of no clinical significance.

Table 7.2. Anatomic location of selected salivary gland neoplasms

Tumors that occur predominantly or exclusively in major salivary glands	Tumors that occur predominantly or exclusively in minor salivary glands
— Warthin's tumor	— Canalicular adenoma
— Acinic cell carcinoma	— Polymorphous L.G. adenocarcinoma
— Basal cell adenoma/carcinoma	— Cystadenoma/cystadenocarcinoma
— Epithelial/myoepithelial CA	— Inverted papilloma
— Oncocytoma and oncocytic CA	— Intraductal papilloma
— Salivary duct carcinoma	— Sialadenoma papilliferum
— Lymphoepithelial carcinoma	

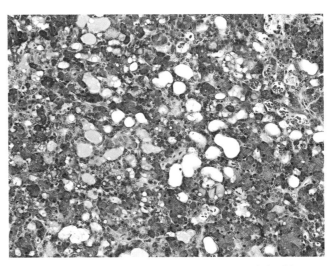

Fig. 7.3. Low-grade acinic cell carcinoma of the parotid gland in which the neoplastic cells have a close resemblance to normal acinar cells.

significance if they are microscopic in size and do not form an expansile mass (Fig. 7.2).

The following points are helpful for distinguishing between adenoma and low grade carcinoma:

▪ Certain neoplasms occur exclusively or predominantly in specific anatomic locations. For example, polymorphous low-grade adenocarcinoma occurs de novo in minor salivary gland locations, and it occurs in the parotid and submandibular glands only when it complicates a pre-existing PA. The diagnosis of primary polymorphous low grade carcinoma in the parotid gland should therefore, be made with caution; the neoplasm is more likely to be a cellular pleomorphic adenoma or hyalinized epithelial/myoepithelial carcinoma. Table 7.2 shows the distribution of selected neoplasms. This table does not necessarily distinguish between benign and low grade carcinoma but it emphasizes the point about distributional peculiarities.

▪ Certain cyto-histologic features are pathognomonic of carcinoma. A neoplasm composed entirely of acinic cells is a carcinoma no matter how bland the cytology (Fig. 7.3) as there is no benign counterpart to acinic cell carcinoma.

Table 7.3. Tumors with clear cell change in salivary gland locations

Primary malignant salivary gland neoplasms

    Epithelial-myoepithelial carcinoma

    Hyalinizing clear cell carcinoma

    Clear cell mucoepidermoid carcinoma

    Clear cell acinic cell carcinoma

    Clear cell oncocytic carcinoma

    Sebaceous carcinoma

    Myoepithelial carcinoma

Benign salivary gland neoplasms

    Clear cell oncocytoma

    Clear cell myoepithelioma

    Clear cell PA (rare)

Metastases

    Renal cell carcinoma

    Other clear cell malignancies

Clear cell odontogenic neoplasms (in the oral cavity)

- Benign neoplasms may show clear cell change, but the majority of salivary gland neoplasms with clear cytoplasm are low grade carcinomas (Table 7.3).
- Most carcinomas have infiltrative margins, and the appearance of the neoplasm at its interface with normal tissue is the single most helpful feature for distinguishing low grade carcinomas from adenomas (Fig. 7.4). Some low grade carcinomas, including acinic cell carcinoma and epithelial/myoepithelial carcinoma, have relatively smooth pushing margins but the majority have irregular pushing margins or a frankly infiltrative growth pattern. A chronic inflammatory infiltrate and a fibroblastic host reaction are also characteristic of carcinoma (Fig. 7.5).
- Perineural invasion is diagnostic of carcinoma, no matter how bland the neoplasm (Fig. 7.6). Perineural invasion is more readily identified at the periphery of the neoplasm, another reason for sampling the interface of tumor with normal tissue.

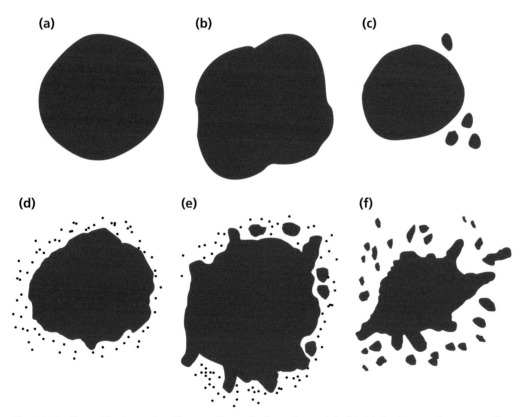

Fig. 7.4. Outlines of benign and malignant salivary gland neoplasms. (a), (b), (c) Benign neoplasms are well circumscribed/encapsulated and generally symmetrical. (b) Mixed tumors often have a lobulated outline. (c) The membranous variant of basal cell adenoma frequently has satellite lesions. (d) Carcinomas may have pushing margins, but (e), (f) most carcinomas have infiltrative margins. (f) Some carcinomas, such as adenoid cystic carcinoma, have highly infiltrative margins. A chronic inflammatory host reaction is often present at the periphery of carcinomas.

(a)

(b)

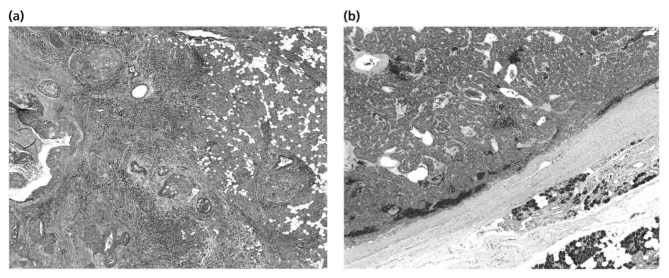

Fig. 7.5. (a) Well-differentiated mucoepidermoid carcinoma with an infiltrative margin and a chronic inflammatory host reaction. (b) Compare this with a benign neoplasm (basal cell adenoma) that is well circumscribed, encapsulated and lacks an inflammatory host reaction at the periphery.

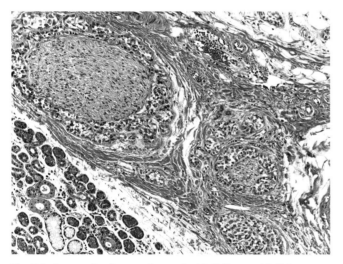

Fig. 7.6. Low-grade adenocarcinoma (epithelial/myoepithelial carcinoma) of the parotid gland with perineural invasion.

INFORMATION NEEDED BEFORE AND DURING INTRAOPERATIVE CONSULTATION (IOC)

The pathologist should be familiar with the clinical aspects of the disease including location of mass, size, if there are clinical signs of malignancy, and whether this is the initial surgical procedure or surgery for a recurrence. Prior FNA slides should be reviewed, and if these are not available, the pathologist should at least be familiar with the FNA report. As is true for all anatomic sites, it is helpful to know the surgeon's operative plan and to know what is at stake.

HANDLING SPECIMENS FOR INTRAOPERATIVE DIAGNOSIS

Inking the specimen is an essential first step because evaluation of the surgical margins has a critical bearing on management. The local recurrence rate is 20-fold higher with positive margins,[3] and post-operative radiation therapy may be recommended to the patient if the margins are positive. Failure to ink the margins would be a serious shortcoming if the status of the margins was in doubt because of this oversight.

The mass should be bisected after inking and additional sections should be made into the specimen if necessary. The cut surface should be carefully examined for undue softening and necrosis, and the periphery of the neoplasm should be examined for circumscription. The sample taken for FS should include the interface of tumor with normal tissue, and if part of the border of the neoplasm is poorly demarcated, that area should be selected for FS (Fig. 7.7).

Frozen section is superior to cytologic preparations for distinguishing low-grade carcinoma from adenoma because architectural features, such as infiltrative margins, can only be appreciated on tissue sections. However, it is our practice to supplement FSs with cytologic examination as the latter provides superior cytologic detail.

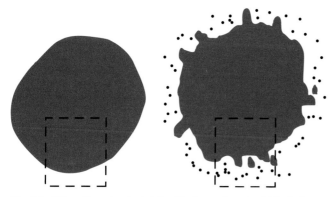

Fig. 7.7. When tissue is selected for FS, the section should include the interface of tumor with normal tissue. The appearance of the neoplasm at the interface is often the single most reliable way to distinguish between adenoma and low grade carcinoma.

The surgeon is unlikely to request IOC if a firm diagnosis of benign neoplasm such as PA or Warthin's tumor has been rendered on FNA. However, FS may be requested if there is no prior FNA, if there are untoward findings at the time of surgery, or if the surgeon wishes to confirm a FNA diagnosis of carcinoma before proceeding with a major resection. A FS should also be performed if there is a discrepancy between the gross appearance of the neoplasm and the FNA diagnosis, recognizing that there is a low and probably irreducible margin of error on FNA of salivary gland neoplasms; in the study by Seethala et al., false-negative and false-positive FNA diagnoses were rendered in 4% and 5% of cases, respectively,[4] and if a FS is performed, at least some of these FNA errors will be detected intraoperatively.

SPECIFIC CLINICO-PATHOLOGICAL ISSUES

Variants of pleomorphic adenoma (benign mixed tumor)

Clinical issues

It is a surgical dictum that benign salivary gland neoplasms should be excised with a margin of normal tissue. This is based on the high local recurrence rate of PAs following enucleation. Highly myxoid PAs are reputed to recur more frequently, probably because the capsule of myxoid PA is more easily disrupted during surgical removal. PAs are rarely enucleated in modern-day surgical practice, and when it occurs, it is because the surgeon has mistaken a low-lying PA in the tail of the parotid for an enlarged

cervical lymph node. It is prudent therefore, to consider a mass in the region of the parotid gland to be a salivary gland neoplasm until proven otherwise.

The vast majority of PAs arise in the superficial (lateral) lobe of the parotid gland. When large, the neoplasm often extends right up to the branches of the facial nerve and may splay or displace the branches of the nerve. When a PA is in close proximity to the facial nerve, the tumor is carefully dissected away from the branches of the facial nerve, and as a result, the deep margin is composed of a delicate fibrous capsule. PAs do not have infiltrative margins, so there is no reason to remove the deep lobe in this situation. Infrequently, PAs arise in the deep lobe and extend into the parapharyngeal space. Surgical removal of the neoplasm involves careful identification of the facial nerve branches, followed by removal of the deep lobe.

Recurrent PAs most often present as multiple tumor nodules in the residual parotid gland and/or peri-parotid soft tissue. Surgical resection usually involves removal of the residual parotid gland and wide excision of the peri-parotid soft tissue.

Pathologic issues

CLASSICAL AND CELLULAR PLEOMORPHIC ADENOMA

The majority of PAs are easily recognized because they are circumscribed, solid and at least partially myxoid on gross examination (Fig. 7.8). Microscopically, the combination of epithelial cells, myoepithelial cells and myxoid stroma makes the neoplasm recognizable at a glance. In contrast, cellular PAs have a non-distinctive fleshy cut surface, and the area sampled for FS may lack the characteristic myxochondroid differentiation. Cellular PAs have three main patterns: predominantly ductal, predominantly myoepithelial and predominantly basaloid. Cellular PA has to be distinguished from low grade carcinoma, and this can be done most reliably by including the interface of tumor with normal tissue in the FS sample. Well-circumscribed margins without a host reaction favor PA, whereas infiltrative margins, a host reaction and perineural invasion, if present, are characteristic of carcinoma. In challenging situations, a different area of the neoplasm should be sampled for FS, with the hope of finding a minor myxoid component, or blending between ductal structures and spindle myoepithelial cells, a feature that is very helpful for identifying the neoplasm as a PA. (Fig. 7.9). Rarely, the pathologist may not be able to distinguish between PA and low grade carcinoma, and in this situation, the diagnosis should be deferred to permanent sections.

(a)

(b)

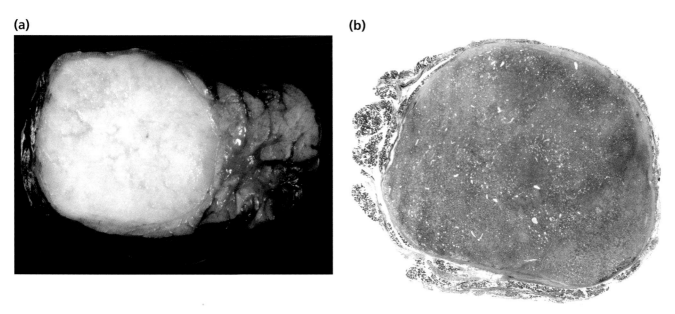

Fig. 7.8. (a) Most pleomorphic adenomas have a myxoid cut surface and are readily identified as PA. (b) Cellular PA can be challenging but the circumscription and lack of an inflammatory host reaction are clues to a benign diagnosis. Focal myxoid areas, and blending of epithelium with myoepithelium should be sought.

(a)

(b)

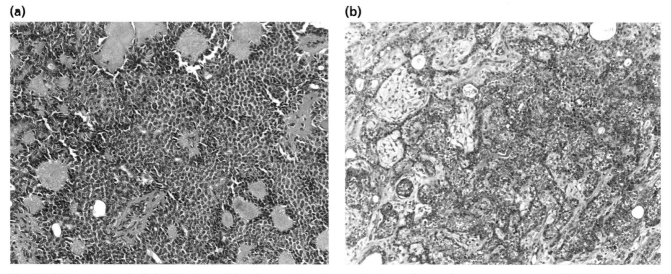

Fig. 7.9. (a) A minority of cellular PAs show mild nuclear atypia and scattered mitoses, features that may cause concern. (b) A blending between epithelial and spindle myoepithelial cells, best seen in the upper left, is characteristic of PA. Cellular PAs behave in a benign fashion, even when they show atypia and mitoses.

EVALUATION OF MARGINS

In the case of a superficial parotidectomy, the deep margin will be the primary margin of interest. The superficial surface of a parotidectomy is covered by fascia but the deep surface is composed of salivary gland tissue. There is no histologic barrier between the superficial and deep lobes; the plane between these lobes is demarcated by the branches of the facial nerve. If a PA is large and bulges from the deep aspect of the superficial lobe, the deep margin will be composed of a delicate layer of connective tissue (Fig. 7.10). After inking the specimen, a single section should be made into the specimen in the area where the mass is closest to the deep surface. The thin capsule will retract from the cut surface, making it difficult to include the capsule in the FS sample. It is disconcerting for the pathologist to evaluate the deep margin in this situation

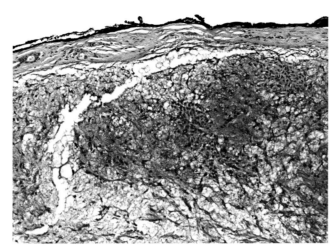

Fig. 7.10. Deep margin of a pleomorphic adenoma. The neoplasm was separated from the facial nerve by a thin layer of fibrous tissue. This is an adequate deep margin for PA.

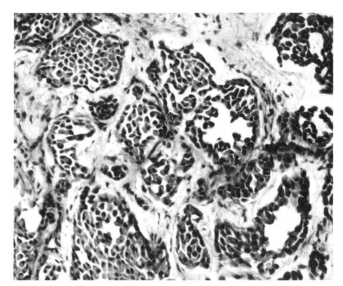

Fig. 7.11. Pleomorphic adenoma of the palate with plasmacytoid hyaline cells. These epithelioid myoepithelial cells are seen most often in PAs of the palate.

but the surgeon will not be surprised by the pathologist's findings. Discussion of the pathologic findings with the surgeon will quickly put the pathologist at ease because the surgeon will be fully aware of the paucity of tissue at the deep margin. The surgeon is unable to obtain a more generous margin because the next anatomic plane is formed by the facial nerve – and there is no reason to obtain a wider margin and compromise the facial nerve for resection of a benign neoplasm. It is appropriate to record the IOD as "pleomorphic adenoma; deep margin composed of thin layer of connective tissue. Findings discussed with Dr. . . . . . ."

Pleomorphic adenoma in minor salivary glands

Clinical issues
PAs account for about 50% of tumors that arise in minor salivary glands. The palate is the most common site but PAs can occur in other sites as well, such as the lip and buccal mucosa. For anatomic reasons, PAs located in the hard palate are non-mobile and cannot be distinguished from carcinomas by clinical examination alone. Small lesions may be excised in their entirety, whereas larger lesions will very likely be subjected to incisional biopsy, followed by definitive resection.

Pathologic issues
PAs in the palate tend to be less well circumscribed compared to major glands and they frequently have prominent

epithelioid myoepithelial (hyaline) cells that at first glance have a plasmacytoid appearance (Fig. 7.11). The main issue with resections of palatal PA is the correct interpretation of secondary changes following an incisional biopsy. Squamous metaplasia and fibrosis may occur after incisional biopsy, and these features, combined with the lack of circumscription, may suggest the diagnosis of MEC (Fig. 7.12). However, familiarity with the findings in the prior incisional biopsy should lead the pathologist to correctly interpret the squamous epithelium and fibrosis as reactive.

Carcinoma arising in pleomorphic adenoma

Clinical issues
Less than 5% of PAs are complicated by the development of a carcinoma (carcinoma ex-PA). Approximately 20% of patients who develop carcinoma ex PA have a history of one or more prior resections for recurrent PA, so a history of recurrent disease should alert the surgeon to the possibility of carcinoma. A malignancy will be suspected when there is rapid growth, fixation to adjacent tissues, nodal metastases or nerve palsy, but in a minority of patients, the carcinoma is discovered only after surgical resection of what is thought to be an uncomplicated PA.

Surgical treatment is based on the grade and stage of the malignancy. Complete resection is performed whenever possible, and if clinically appropriate, node dissection is performed for high grade carcinomas.

(a)

(b)

(c)

(d)

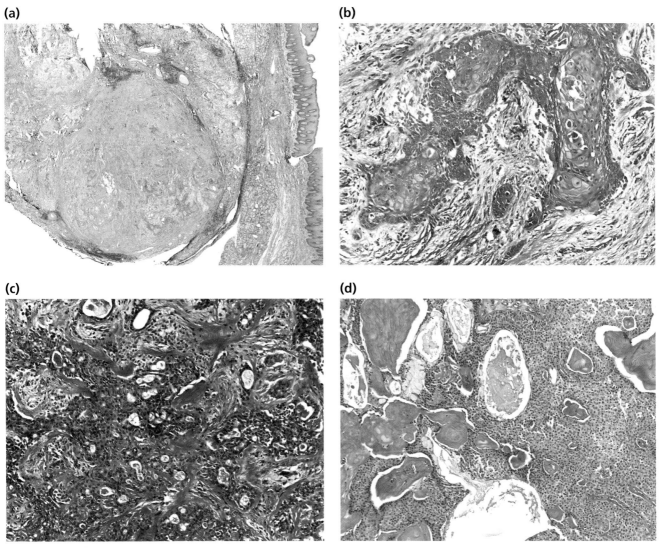

Fig. 7.12. (a) Pleomorphic adenoma of the palate with secondary changes due to prior incisional biopsy. (b) Much of the lesion shows nests of squamous cells embedded in loose connective tissue, but (c) residual areas of PA were also present. (b) The loose connective tissue stroma is characteristic of a reactive process; (d) mucoepidermoid carcinomas typically have dense, paucicellular fibrous stroma, as in this MEC of the palate.

Pathologic issues

The majority of carcinomas that arise in PA are poorly differentiated adenocarcinomas that have overgrown the underlying PA, with gross and histologic features of a malignant neoplasm. Sometimes however, the underlying PA is dominant and the carcinoma is identified only after thorough sampling.[5] About 20% are low grade adenocarcinomas, either adenocarcinoma N.O.S., myoepithelial carcinoma (Fig. 7.13) or polymorphous low grade adenocarcinoma.[6,7] It is curious that specific salivary gland carcinomas, such as MEC and adenoid cystic carcinoma, rarely arise from PAs.

When a carcinoma ex-PA is confined to the salivary gland, an attempt should be made to determine if the malignancy is confined to the PA or if it has invaded beyond the capsule of the PA, because carcinomas limited to the PA have an extremely good prognosis, even if high grade (Fig. 7.14).[7] The extent of the invasive carcinoma may influence surgical resection, but it is often difficult to determine the extent of the invasive carcinoma relative to the underlying PA intraoperatively. The pathologist should, however, be prepared to address the surgeon's enquiry about this issue.

Even though carcinoma ex PA is infrequent, it should be considered whenever a large PA is encountered, if there is a history of recurrent disease, if the margins are poorly defined, if necrosis is present, or if there are large areas of hyalinization (Fig. 7.15).

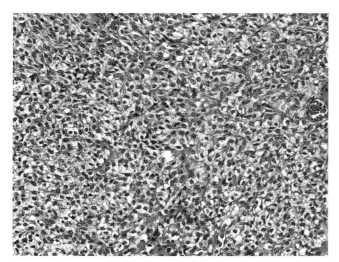

Fig. 7.13. Low grade clear-cell myoepithelial carcinoma arising in a pleomorphic adenoma. The diagnosis of carcinoma cannot be made on cytologic grounds, but was based on the infiltrative nature of the spindle cell component and its extension beyond the boundaries of the underlying PA.

Cystic lesions

Clinical issues

Extravasation mucocele is the most common cystic lesion of salivary gland origin. The majority are located in the lower lip and oral cavity. They are recognized clinically and treated without need for intraoperative evaluation. Ranula is an extravasation mucocele arising from the sublingual gland, and it is referred to as a plunging ranula when it presents as a mass in the suprahyoid area of the neck. The diagnosis is made clinically and the lesion is excised without need for IOD. Non-neoplastic cysts of major salivary glands are rare, lymphoepithelial cysts of the parotid gland being the most frequent. Benign and malignant neoplasms may undergo cystic change, and pathologic examination is required to make the correct diagnosis.

Pathologic issues

The diagnosis of extravasation mucocele should not be made in the parotid and submandibular glands because the lesion is more likely to be a cystic, low grade mucoepidermoid carcinoma. Benign neoplasms that undergo cystic change include Warthin's tumor, cystadenoma, sebaceous cystadenoma, and basal cell adenoma, while PAs only rarely undergo significant cystic change.

The most important issue about cystic lesions is to recognize that some low grade carcinomas undergo cystic change, and that occasionally the cystic change is

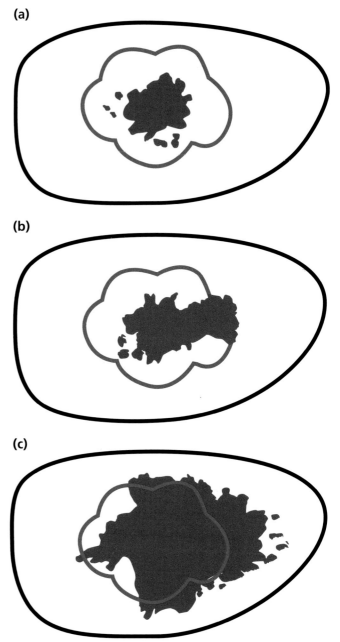

Fig. 7.14. When carcinoma complicates a PA, the relationship of the carcinoma to the underlying PA influences prognosis. (a) Carcinomas that are limited to the PA have an excellent prognosis and almost all patients are free of disease after complete surgical resection. (b), (c) When the carcinoma extends beyond the boundaries of the underlying PA, the prognosis depends on the volume of carcinoma beyond the confines of the PA.

extensive enough to be mistaken for a benign cyst (Fig. 7.16). MEC is the most treacherous, especially when macrocysts rupture and evoke a histiocytic and granulation tissue reaction that mimics an extravasation mucocele. If the specimen is a surgical resection, such as a superficial parotidectomy, the solid component should

(a) **(b)**

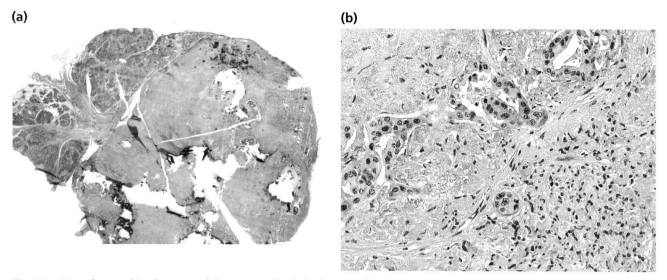

Fig. 7.15. (a) A pleomorphic adenoma with large areas of hyalinization as well as dystrophic calcification. Extensive hyalinization should prompt extensive sampling of the lesion because of the high association with malignancy. (b) Areas of poorly differentiated adenocarcinoma and small foci of residual PA were present in this neoplasm.

(a) **(b)**

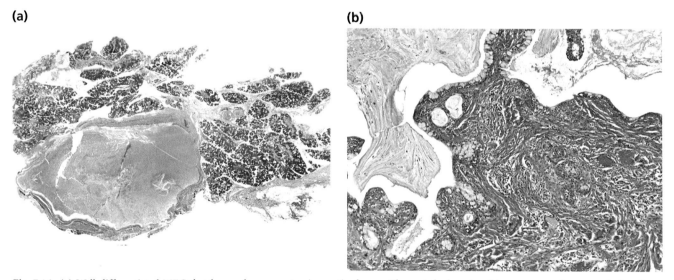

Fig. 7.16. (a) Well-differentiated MEC that has undergone extensive cystic change. The cysts had ruptured in areas to evoke a granulation tissue and histiocytic reaction resembling an extravasation mucocele. (b) Residual solid areas or thickened areas in the wall of the cyst/s should be sampled for FS as these are likely to show the typical intermediate and mucus cells of MEC.

be sampled and not the wall of a macrocyst. Incisional biopsies of cystic minor salivary gland neoplasms are more challenging because the biopsy may only include the mucocele-like macrocystic component. Clinico-pathologic correlation will usually help in suspecting a poorly sampled cystic neoplasm; extravasation mucoceles are small and occur primarily in the lip and buccal mucosa, whereas mucoepidermoid carcinomas tend to be larger

and occur in the palate as well as other minor salivary gland locations.

Acinic cell carcinoma usually forms microcysts (Fig. 7.17) but the neoplasm occasionally contains large cysts. One should be alert to the possibility of cystic acinic cell carcinoma if the cyst shows papillary structures projecting into the cavity, if the lining cells show small cytoplasmic vacuoles, or if small solid cell islands are found in the wall.[8]

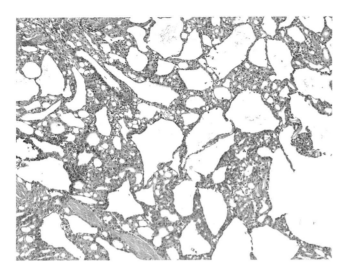

Fig. 7.17. Acinic cell carcinoma with microcysts.

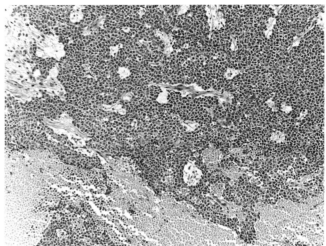

Fig. 7.18. Small cell carcinoma of the parotid gland. The cohesiveness, molding, nuclear features and the absence of cytoplasmic fragments should allow ready distinction from large cell lymphoma.

Lymphoid lesions

Clinical issues

Benign and malignant lymphoid lesions may present as a solitary mass in the parotid and submandibular glands. Depending on whether a pre-operative FNA was performed, the surgeon may approach the lesion as a salivary gland neoplasm of unknown type, or as a lymphoid lesion for which an open biopsy is required for definitive diagnosis. A superficial parotidectomy is usually performed for lesions involving the parotid gland, and the entire gland is removed for lesions of the submandibular salivary gland. The main goal of surgery is to obtain sufficient tissue for diagnosis. There is no role for extensive surgery in the management of lymphomas.

Pathologic issues

The purpose of IOD is to confirm that the lesion is a lymphoproliferative lesion, and to ensure that there is sufficient tissue for diagnosis. Large cell lymphoma, which is easily recognized as neoplastic on cytologic preparations (see Fig. 2.9, p. 22) should not be confused for small cell carcinoma (Fig. 7.18), a tumor that is treated with extensive surgical resection, a form of treatment that is inappropriate for lymphoma.

Small cell lymphomas (MALTomas) cannot be confidently distinguished from benign lymphoid lesions such as lymphoepithelial sialadenitis (LESA) in the parotid gland, and sclerosing sialadenitis (Kuttner tumor) in the submandibular gland (Fig. 7.19). A preliminary diagnosis of "lymphoproliferative lesion" should be made, with deferral to permanent sections.

Clear cell neoplasms

Clinical issues

Clear cell change occurs in a variety of primary salivary gland neoplasms, both benign and malignant. The differential diagnosis in all sites should include metastatic carcinoma, and clear cell odontogenic tumors should be included for lesions in the oral cavity. Treatment depends on the diagnosis.

Pathologic issues

Many salivary gland neoplasms show focal clear cell change that may go unnoticed or is simply observed as an interesting feature. Occasionally, however, clear cells are the dominant cell type in neoplasms such as MEC (Fig. 7.20) and acinic cell carcinoma, obscuring the underlying nature of the neoplasm. Clear cells are always the dominant cell type in hyalinizing clear cell carcinoma and epithelial-myoepithelial carcinoma (Fig. 7.20).[8–10] The majority of primary clear cell neoplasms are low-grade carcinomas (Table 7.3). A specific diagnosis may be difficult to make at the time of FS but the pathologist's main charge is to distinguish between benign and malignant, a distinction that is best done by examining the interface of the neoplasm with normal tissue.

A metastasis should always be considered when a clear cell neoplasm is encountered in major and minor salivary gland sites. Metastatic renal cell carcinoma, the most frequent metastasis composed of clear cells, should be suspected when the neoplasm has a prominent vascular pattern and intraglandular hemorrhage (see Fig. 11.18, p. 175).

Clear cell odontogenic neoplasms, both benign and malignant, should be included in the differential diagnosis

(a)

(b)

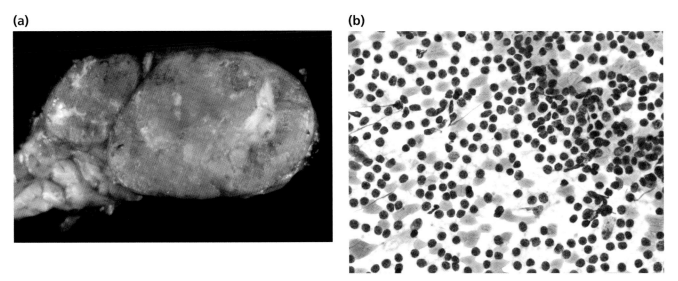

Fig. 7.19. Lymphoproliferative lesion of the submandibular salivary gland. (a) The gland was enlarged, firm and showed a loss of its normal lobulated appearance. (b) The cytoscrape preparation is dominated by small round lymphocytes. A diagnosis of small cell lymphoproliferative lesion is "good enough" for purposes of IOD. The lymphoid infiltrate was proven to be a marginal cell lymphoma on permanent sections.

(a)

(b)

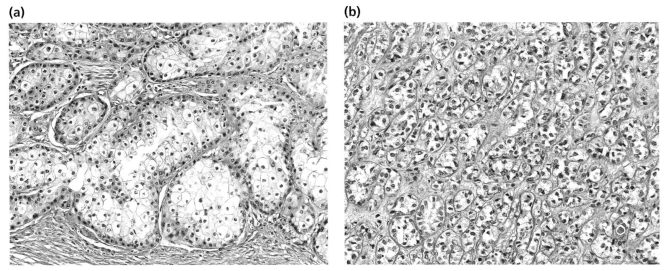

Fig. 7.20. (a) Clear cell variant of mucoepidermoid carcinoma. Other areas of the neoplasm showed conventional intermediate cells and mucus cells. (b) Clear cells may dominate parts of epithelial/myoepithelial carcinoma, but thorough sampling will usually reveal typical bilayered ductal structures with clear myoepithelial cells.

for lesions in the oral cavity.[9] The presence of a lytic lesion in the underlying maxillary or mandibular bone is an important clue to the diagnosis, again emphasizing the need for clinico-pathologic correlation.

Epithelial tumors with a heavy lymphoid component

Three groups of salivary gland neoplasms have a dense lymphoid component. A lymphoid component is integral to some benign salivary gland neoplasms such as Warthin's tumor, lymphadenoma, and sebaceous lymphadenoma (Fig. 7.21), and in this group of neoplasms, the lymphoid element is probably a secondary reactive phenomenon induced by the neoplastic epithelial cells. Infrequently, salivary gland neoplasms arise from ectopic intra-nodal salivary gland tissue, and in this situation, the heavy lymphoid component represents residual lymph node; the main issue is to recognize this as a primary neoplasm and not a metastasis.

(a)

(b)

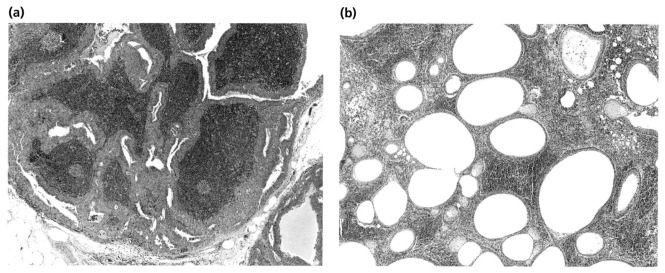

Fig. 7.21. (a) Classical Warthin's tumor and (b) sebaceous lymphadenoma. By definition, both neoplasms contain benign lymphoid cells.

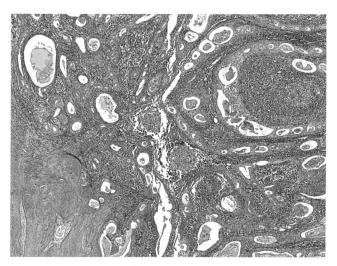

Fig. 7.22. Mucoepidermoid carcinoma of the parotid gland with a heavy lymphoid infiltrate. The lymphoid infiltrate is heavy enough to raise the possibility of metastatic carcinoma in a lymph node.

Low grade carcinomas frequently evoke a chronic inflammatory host reaction, and this is usually mild and concentrated in the periphery of the carcinoma. Occasionally, especially in acinic cell and mucoepidermoid carcinomas, the lymphoid infiltrate is heavy, includes lymphoid follicles, and is dense enough to mimic a lymph node with metastatic carcinoma (Fig. 7.22). Lymphoepithelial carcinoma and sebaceous lymphadenocarcinoma are other carcinomas that are accompanied by a heavy lymphoid infiltrate.

Oncocytic neoplasms

Warthin's tumor is the most frequent salivary gland neoplasm containing oncocytic cells and this neoplasm is easily distinguished from other tumors containing oncocytic cells. Oncocytoma forms a circumscribed or encapsulated nodule and is readily separated from the rare oncocytic carcinoma with its characteristic infiltrating pattern of growth. Oncocytoma with nodular oncocytic hyperplasia (nodular oncocytosis) should not be confused with oncocytic carcinoma; the satellite nodules of nodular oncocytic hyperplasia are circumscribed, cytologically bland and do not evoke a host reaction.[11] For some odd reason, nodular oncocytic hyperplasia is often composed of clear cells (Fig. 7.23).

There are two additional issues concerning neoplasms with oncocytes. First, MEC may occasionally have a prominent oncocytic component and be mistaken for a benign oncocytoma (Fig. 7.24). The characteristic squamoid and mucus cells of MEC are always present but may not be in the FS block. A FS taken from the margin of the neoplasm will very likely reveal the infiltrative character of the neoplasm, excluding a benign oncocytoma. The second issue is the distinction between benign oncocytoma and well-differentiated acinic cell carcinoma: both neoplasms have granular cytoplasm but the cytoplasmic characteristics are different; the granules of oncocytoma are eosinophilic and larger, whereas the granules of acinic cell carcinoma are amphophilic or basophilic, and smaller. Furthermore, the nuclei of oncocytes are centrally located in the cell, whereas the nuclei in acinic cell carcinoma are basal in location (Fig. 7.25).[11]

(a) **(b)**

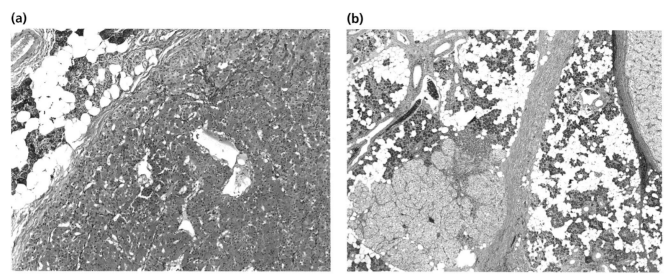

Fig. 7.23. An oncocytoma of the parotid gland. (a) The neoplasm is circumscribed and composed of uniform benign oncocytes. (b) Clear cell oncocytoma with oncocytosis. The edge of the main oncocytoma is in the upper right and one of the small clear cell oncocytic nodules is in the lower left. Nodular oncocytosis may raise concern about clear cell carcinoma because of the multiplicity of nodules. The absence of histologic and cytologic features of malignancy, the circumscription of all the nodules, and the absence of a host reaction are clues to the correct diagnosis.

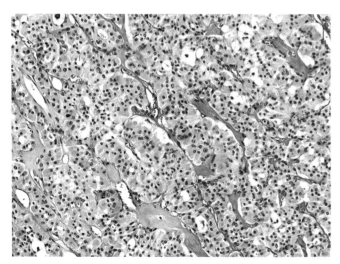

Fig. 7.24. Mucoepidermoid carcinoma with extensive oncocytic change.

Multiple neoplasms in major salivary glands

Clinical issues

Table 7.4 lists the neoplasms that most frequently present as multiple palpable masses, or are found to be multifocal on histologic examination.[12] Warthin's tumor is the most common neoplasm to present with bilateral parotid masses, with about 12% of patients having bilateral disease or multiple lesions in a single parotid gland. Clinical history may be helpful in narrowing the differential diagnosis.

The history of a previously resected PA naturally favors recurrent PA. Multiple salivary gland nodules accompanied by enlarged lymph nodes should suggest lymphoma, especially if the enlarged nodes are distant from the mass in the salivary gland. FNA can reliably distinguish between the common causes of multiple mass lesions and is a useful initial diagnostic test.

Pathologic issues

Multiple lesions that present as clinically palpable masses are usually subjected to FNA and so the pathologist is likely to have the benefit of a prior cytologic diagnosis at the time of IOD. When the resected specimen contains multiple lesions, the larger nodules should be examined grossly to determine if they are part of a single neoplasm or if they are different neoplasms. For example, recurrent PA may be complicated by carcinoma, and gross examination may identify something unusual about one or more of the nodules (Fig. 7.26). Cytoscrape preparations are useful for the evaluation of multiple nodules because they can quickly determine if there is significant cytologic variance between different nodules.

Membranous basal cell adenoma may have nonpalpable satellite lesions in addition to the palpable mass (Fig. 7.27). If one or more satellite lesions are included in the FS sample, they should not be misconstrued as evidence of infiltrating carcinoma. The following features support a benign diagnosis: the circumscribed

(a)
(b)

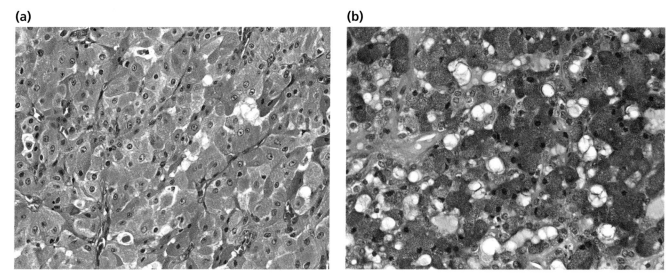

Fig. 7.25. Comparison of oncocytoma with well differentiated acinic cell carcinoma. (a) The cells of oncocytoma have centrally placed nuclei and granular, eosinophilic cytoplasm, whereas (b) the cells of acinic cell carcinoma have basally located nuclei and basophilic or amphophilic cytoplasm.

Table 7.4. Multiple tumor nodules in major salivary glands

Neoplasms that may present as multiple palpable masses
Warthin's tumor
Recurrent pleomorphic adenoma
Metastatic malignant neoplasms
Malignant lymphoma
Multiple unrelated primary neoplasms (rare)
Neoplasms that are found to be multifocal on pathologic examination
Membranous basal cell adenoma
Oncocytoma with nodular oncocytic hyperplasia

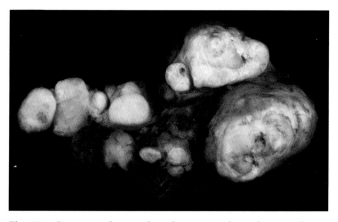

Fig. 7.26. Recurrent pleomorphic adenoma involving the parotid gland and peri-parotid soft tissue. The larger nodules have a variegated appearance, warranting cytologic or FS examination.

nature of the dominant lesion; the jig-saw shape of the smaller foci; the presence of perfectly normal salivary gland tissue between the lesions; the absence of a host reaction; the lack of cytologic atypia, and familiarity with this feature of the neoplasm.[13]

As stated above, oncocytoma may be accompanied by nodular oncocytic hyperplasia, the latter being microscopic in size and appearing as a surprise on FS.

Metastatic malignancies

Clinical issues

Metastatic malignancies can mimic a primary carcinoma clinically, and this can be a problem when the surgeon is not aware of the history of prior malignancy. About 80% of metastases are from some other head and neck location, and 20% are from infraclavicular sites. The most common metastases are of cutaneous origin, namely squamous carcinoma and melanoma, whereas the lung and kidney are the main extra-cutaneous primary sites. Depending on the clinical situation, management involves complete surgical resection of the primary tumor, parotidectomy, with or without a neck dissection, and adjuvant postoperative radiation therapy. Management of disease from infraclavicular sites usually includes systemic therapy with or without radiation therapy.

Pathologic issues

It is good policy to consider a metastasis whenever it is difficult to classify a salivary gland neoplasm. The problem, of course, is that salivary gland neoplasms have such diverse

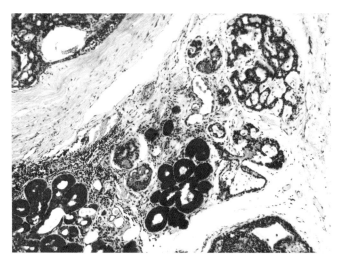

Fig. 7.27. Membranous basal cell adenoma with a satellite nodule on the right. The satellite nodules associated with membranous adenoma have a characteristic checker board appearance.

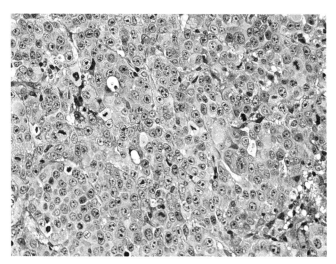

Fig. 7.28. Metastatic melanoma to the parotid gland and intra-parotid lymph nodes. This neoplasm contained pseudoglandular structures simulating high grade adenocarcinoma. Note the similarity to the high grade MEC illustrated in Fig. 7.29(b).

appearances that it is tempting to force an unusual tumor into some known category of primary neoplasm. Multiple tumor nodules, disproportionate involvement of lymph nodes and an unusual pattern are clues to the correct diagnosis.

Metastatic melanoma is a major challenge when it is amelanotic. The spindle cell pattern can simulate myo-epithelial carcinoma, and the epithelioid variant can be mistaken for poorly differentiated salivary gland carcinoma (Fig. 7.28). Intranuclear inclusions are a clue to the diagnosis and should prompt a search for melanin pigment. The problem with metastatic melanomas is compounded by long periods of latency so that the connection between a parotid mass and removal of a skin lesion many years earlier may have escaped everyone's attention.

Metastatic squamous carcinoma should be considered whenever a pure squamous malignancy is encountered because primary squamous cell carcinoma of the salivary gland is extremely rare. High grade MEC should enter the differential diagnosis even if mucus cells are inapparent at the time of IOD, but distinct squamous differentiation with keratinization favors a metastasis since mucoepidermoid carcinomas do not show squamous differentiation with keratinization (Fig. 7.29).[8,14]

Changes secondary to fine needle aspiration biopsy

Clinical issues
FNA is a safe and useful procedure for evaluating salivary gland tumors. Occasionally, the tumor undergoes extensive infarction after FNA and the infarction may cause pain and swelling. The granulation tissue that develops after infarction may sufficiently alter the characteristics of the neoplasm at the time of surgery to cause concern about malignancy.

Pathologic issues
In most cases, post-FNA infarction is focal and does not interfere with making the correct diagnosis. On the other hand, extensive infarction can be disconcerting on gross examination, as necrosis is usually considered a feature of malignancy. The issue is usually resolved when the history of FNA and the prior cytologic diagnosis are taken into account.

Metaplastic squamous and mucus cells may occur as part of the repair process after FNA, and when these changes occur in benign neoplasms such as Warthin's tumor and PA, they may suggest the diagnosis of muco-epidermoid carcinoma (Fig. 7.30). Errors can be avoided by viewing these focal changes in the context of the entire neoplasm, and by correlating the FS findings with the clinical and prior FNA findings.[15,16]

Frozen section evaluation of the facial nerve

Clinical issues
The facial nerve is intimately related to the parotid gland and arbitrarily divides the gland into superficial and deep lobes. Carcinomas arising in either the superficial lobe or deep lobe may compromise the facial nerve. A segment of the facial nerve will be resected if there is direct invasion

(a)

(b)

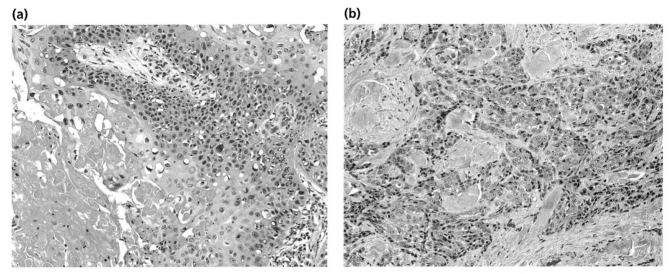

Fig. 7.29. Keratinization in a squamoid lesion should suggest metastatic squamous carcinoma, (a) as in this case of cutaneous squamous carcinoma metastatic to the parotid gland and peri-parotid lymph nodes. (b) High grade mucoepidermoid carcinomas are composed predominantly of intermediate cells, and while they may show focal squamous differentiation, keratinization is most unusual.

(a)

(b)

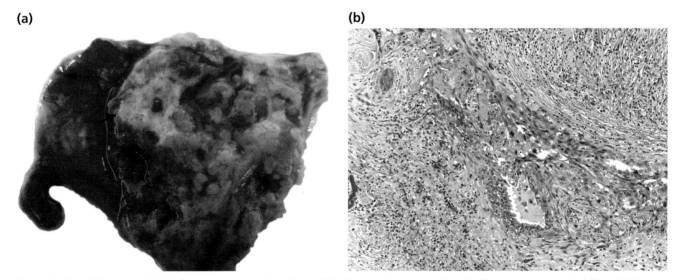

Fig. 7.30. Warthin's tumor with focal squamous metaplasia due to FNA. The neoplasm showed a pale fibrous area (arrow in [a]) and this area was included in the FS sample, confounding interpretation. (b) The focal nature of the squamous differentiation, the history of recent FNA, and the granulation tissue background are clues to the diagnosis of post-FNA changes.

of the nerve or if the nerve is firmly embedded within the substance of a carcinoma. Carcinomas vary in their propensity to invade the facial nerve, and while all carcinomas are capable of invading this nerve, adenoid cystic carcinoma has the greatest potential of all. Involvement of the facial nerve may be obvious at the time of surgery, but carcinomas may track along the nerve without producing grossly visible changes. This is the reason for obtaining FSs on the nerve stumps; after the segment of putative abnormal nerve has been resected, biopsies are taken from each end of the remaining nerve for FS evaluation before performing a nerve graft.

Pathologic issues

If a nerve biopsy is submitted, the entire specimen should be embedded for FS evaluation. The biopsy should be embedded on end, and because of the skip pattern of growth, at least three levels should be cut routinely. Additional levels should be prepared if necessary. Tissue should not be intentionally spared for permanent sections because the surgeon is interested in the status of the nerve during the surgical procedure, not the following day. If a longer segment of nerve is submitted, the specimen should be evaluated as described in Chapter 4, p. 52.

REFERENCES

1. Kempson RL, Fletcher CDM, Evans HL, Hendrickson MR, Sibley RK. *Tumors of Soft Tissues Atlas of Tumor Pathology Armed Forces Institute of Pathology* Washington DC, 2001.
2. Seifert G, Bull HG, Donath K. Histologic subclassification of the cystadenolymphoma of the parotid gland. *Virch Arch A Pat Anat and Histol* 1980; **388**: 13–38.
3. Healey WV, Perzin KH, Smith L. Mucoepidermoid carcinoma of salivary gland origin: clasification, clinico-pathologic correlation, and results of treatment. *Cancer* 1970; **26**: 368–388.
4. Seethala RR, LiVolsi VA, Baloch ZW. Relative accuracy of fine-needle aspiration and frozen section in the diagnosis of lesions of the parotid. *Head Neck* 2005; **27**: 217–223.
5. LiVolsi VA, Perzin KH. Malignant mixed tumors arising in salivary glands 1. Carcinomas arising in benign mixed tumors. A clinico-pathologic study. *Cancer* 1977; **39**: 2209–2230.
6. Savera AT, Sloman A, Huvos AG, et al. Mucoepidermoid carcinoma of the salivary glands: a clinicopathologic study of 25 patients. *Am J Surg Pathol* 2000; **24**: 761–774.
7. Tortoledo ME, Luna MA, Batsakis JG. Carcinoma ex pleomorphic adenoma and malignant mixed tumors. *Arch Otolaryngol* 1984; **110**: 172–176.
8. Cheuk W, Chan JKC. Salivary gland tumors. In *Diagnostic Histopathology of Tumors*, Fletcher CDM, ed. 3rd edn. Churchill Livingstone Elsevier, 2007; pp. 239–326.
9. Maiorano E, Altini M, Favia G. Clear cell tumors of the salivary glands, jaws, and oral mucosa. *Seminars Diagn Pathol* 1997; **14**: 203–212.
10. Milchgrub S, Gnepp DR, Vuitch F, Delgado R, Albores-Saavedra J. Hyalinizing clear cell carcinoma of salivary gland. *Am J Surg Pathol* 1994; **18**: 74–82.
11. Capone RB, Westra WH, Pilkington TM, Sciubba JJ, Koch WM, Cummings CW. Oncocytic neoplasms of the parotid gland: a 16-year institutional review. *Otolaryngol Head Neck Surg* 2002; **126**: 657–662.
12. Gnepp DR, Schroeder W, Heffner D. Synchronous tumors arising in a single major salivary gland. *Cancer* 1989; **63**: 1219–1224.
13. Batsakis JG, Brannon RB, Sciubba JJ. Monomorphic adenomas of major salivary glands: a histologic study of 96 tumors *Clin Otolaryngol.* 1981; **6**: 129–143.
14. Ellis GL, Auclair PL. *Tumors of the Salivary Glands Atlas of Tumor Pathology*. Washington DC, Armed Forces Institute of Pathology, 1996.
15. Li S, Baloch ZW, Tomaszewski JE, et al. Worrisome histologic alterations following fine needle aspiration of benign parotid lesions. *Arch Pathol Lab Med* 2000; **124**: 87–91.
16 Taxy JB. Necrotizing squamous/mucinous metaplasia in oncocytic salivary gland tumors. *Am J Clin Pathol* 1992; **97**: 40–45.

8   GASTROINTESTINAL TRACT

Steven D. Hart and Sarah M. Dry

INTRODUCTION

The types of gastrointestinal (GI) specimens sent for intraoperative diagnosis have changed in the past two decades because of technological advances in endoscopy, developments in imaging, improvements in medications, and advances in treatment modalities. Traditional endoscopy has expanded to include endoscopic ultrasound, new diagnostic techniques such as endoscopic-guided fine needle aspiration of mural lesions, and endoscopic mucosal resections. Capsule endoscopy now permits visualization of small bowel lesions in the outpatient setting, in contrast to prior push enteroscopy performed in the OR suite. Effective medical therapies for H. pylori-associated peptic ulcer disease have essentially eliminated vagotomy, pyloroplasty, and resection of benign ulcers, and positron emission technology (PET) scans permit sensitive detection and staging of malignancies. Non-surgical modalities, such as photodynamic therapy, are now being used to treat dysplasia arising in Barrett's esophagus, and endoscopists routinely tattoo the GI mucosa adjacent to clinically suspicious lesions to help the surgeon locate the target lesion. Collectively, these have resulted in more specific preoperative diagnoses, improved treatment planning, facilitated definitive surgery and in the process, reduced the need for intraoperative diagnosis (IOD). Nonetheless, the pathologist still has an important role to play in selected situations.

INDICATIONS FOR INTRAOPERATIVE DIAGNOSIS

1. To evaluate surgical margins. In the GI tract, gross examination is often sufficient but frozen section (FS) diagnosis has a role in certain situations, such as margin evaluation following neoadjuvant chemoradiation of malignant neoplasms.
2. To render a diagnosis that may change the scope of the surgical procedure. For example, finding adenocarcinoma in an ampullectomy for adenoma may change the resection from local excision to a pancreaticoduodenectomy.
3. To stage cancers in situations where loco-regional spread will lead to cancellation of the planned surgical resection.
4. To confirm adequacy of an incisional biopsy specimen and to allocate tissue for appropriate ancillary studies. This occurs infrequently as most tumors, including lymphoma, can be sampled either endoscopically or via imaging-guided biopsy.

GENERAL CLINICAL ISSUES

Gastroenterologists usually provide detailed diagnostic and staging information to surgeons prior to resection of GI tract malignancies. This includes mapping of malignant, dysplastic and normal mucosa, ultrasound evaluation of depth of invasion, and ultrasound evaluation of lymph node involvement. They also will tattoo the mucosa, either to mark the extent of the malignancy prior to neoadjuvant therapy or to identify a target lesion that may be difficult to locate at surgery, such as a subtotally removed malignant colonic polyp. In the GI tract, most resections include regional lymph nodes, unlike other organs, such as lung, where regional lymph node groups have to be removed separately for staging.

Intraoperative diagnosis may change the extent of surgical resection, and some of these changes are associated

Intraoperative Consultation in Surgical Pathology, ed. Mahendra Ranchod. Published by Cambridge University Press.
© Cambridge University Press 2010.

with significant patient morbidity; these include conversion from partial gastrectomy to total gastrectomy, conversion of an ampullectomy to a Whipple procedure, and conversion from a proximal rectal resection to an abdominoperineal resection.

GENERAL PATHOLOGIC ISSUES

The pathologist should be aware of pre-operative therapies given to the patient because these may significantly alter the pathologic appearance of the specimen.
Here are a few examples:

- New treatment modalities for Barrett's esophagus, such as photodynamic therapy, may cause mature squamous epithelium to grow over underlying dysplastic and non-dysplastic glandular mucosa, making gross examination unreliable for evaluating surgical margins.
- Neoadjuvant chemoradiation therapy can result in complete or near-complete regression of a mass lesion (Fig. 8.1). Mucosal ulceration is usually present, but often does not reflect the size of the original mass. Mucosal tattoos, if present, can guide the pathologist to the prior tumor site, but frozen section (FS) evaluation may be required to ensure clear margins.
- Neoadjuvant chemoradiation induces epithelial atypia in normal tissue and this may be misdiagnosed as dysplasia or carcinoma.
- Premalignant lesions at resection margins should be reported to the surgeon. For example, intestinal metaplasia at the proximal margin of an esophagectomy for adenocarcinoma arising in Barrett's esophagus, may prompt resection of additional esophageal tissue – depending on the clinical situation. Similarly, dysplasia at the margin of an ampullectomy for adenoma may prompt further local resection or conversion to a pancreaticoduodenectomy, depending on the clinical context. The pathologist should be aware of the surgical algorithm for the specific case because of the potential impact of the FS diagnosis; if there is any doubt about the nature of the lesion at the margin, and if the stakes are high, additional levels should be prepared and/or colleagues should be consulted for their opinion.
- Considerable caution should be exercised when evaluating the margins on poorly differentiated invasive carcinomas, especially signet ring cell carcinomas,

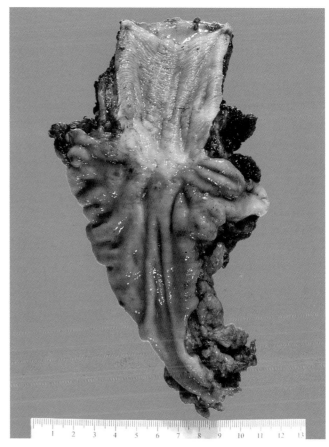

Fig. 8.1. Adenocarcinoma of the gastroesophageal junction. Neoadjuvant chemoradiation therapy led to almost complete regression of this carcinoma. A subtle area of thickening immediately proximal to the gastric folds represents the residual tumor.

because of their tendency to infiltrate widely without forming a grossly visible lesion. False negative interpretation of the margins can be avoided by thorough sampling of the surgical margins.
- Some neoplasms of the gastrointestinal tract are challenging for surgeons and pathologists, although our understanding of these neoplasms, especially mucinous neoplasms of the appendix, pseudomyxoma peritonei and gastrointestinal stromal tumors (GIST) has improved considerably in recent years.

INFORMATION NEEDED BEFORE AND DURING IOD

The pathologist should be familiar with the clinical aspects of the case as well as the results of prior biopsies. Knowing the type of neoplasm (e.g., squamous cell versus adenocarcinoma), degree of differentiation, specific anatomic location and prior margin status can make it easier to interpret the surgical margins in problematic situations. It is also necessary to know if the patient has received pre-operative radiation or chemotherapy because these therapies may significantly change the pathologic appearance of the neoplasm. It is also useful to be familiar with the surgeon's operative plan, especially if IOD will significantly change the nature of the surgical procedure.

SPECIFIC CLINICO-PATHOLOGIC ISSUES

Appendiceal neoplasms

Appendiceal neoplasms are uncommon, accounting for 1%–2% of all appendectomies and about 1% of all GI tract malignancies. The vast majority are endocrine (carcinoid) tumors and epithelial neoplasms; mesenchymal tumors and lymphomas occur only rarely. There are significant differences in the frequency with which different epithelial tumors occur in the appendix compared to the colon: hyperplastic polyps and tubular adenomas are infrequent, and are usually found incidentally during histologic examination of an appendix removed for acute appendicitis. Conventional colonic-type adenocarcinomas, including cytologically high grade mucinous carcinoma, are relatively uncommon and are treated in the same way as carcinomas arising in the cecum. In contrast, cytologically bland mucinous neoplasms, the most common epithelial tumors of the appendix, have unique clinical and pathologic characteristics.[1–8]

Low grade mucinous neoplasms of the appendix

Clinical issues

In this section of the chapter, mucinous neoplasm and mucinous carcinoma refer to cytologically bland mucinous neoplasms. These uncommon neoplasms have been the source of a great deal of confusion because they show an unusual pattern of spread, and were only recently accepted as the source of virtually all cases of pseudomyxoma peritonei. If the neoplasm is confined to the appendix, complete resection is curative, but when spread occurs beyond the appendix, with local (Fig. 8.2) or diffuse peritoneal dissemination, the prognosis is markedly poorer, with survival rates of 100% at 3 years, 86% at 5 years and only 45% at 10 years.[1,5]

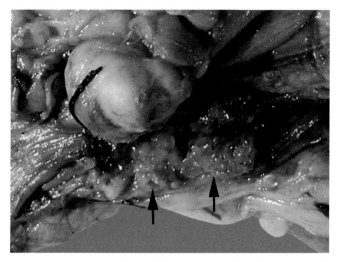

Fig. 8.2. Mucinous neoplasm of the appendix with subtle deposits of extra-appendiceal mucin (arrows) in peri-appendiceal adipose tissue.

Mucinous neoplasms present in four main ways and each is relevant to IOD.

1. A significant proportion of patients present with pain in the right lower quadrant of the abdomen. If a CT scan is performed, an enlarged and distended appendix* may be identified. These are best approached by an open surgical procedure, and not laparoscopy, because of precautions that are necessary to avoid rupture of the lesion and spillage of neoplastic cells into the peritoneal cavity. If there is no other disease in the abdomen at the time of exploratory laparotomy, the surgeon will perform a right hemicolectomy, given the high probability that the lesion will be neoplastic.[9,10] When a right hemicolectomy is performed, the margins of resection will be clear, and if IOD is requested, gross examination is all that is necessary (Fig. 8.3).

2. Infrequently, a mucinous neoplasm is complicated by acute appendicitis, and the neoplastic nature of the process is only discovered at the time of laparoscopic surgery. The surgeon is likely to convert the surgical procedure to an open laparotomy for reasons described in (1) above.

---

* Mucocele refers to an enlarged, dilated appendix, the lumen of which is filled with mucin. The term does not provide any information about the pathologic nature of the lesion and should be used as a generic descriptive term. The majority of mucoceles are mucinous neoplasms. Rarely, mucoceles have an inflammatory origin, with obstruction of the lumen and stasis of mucin.

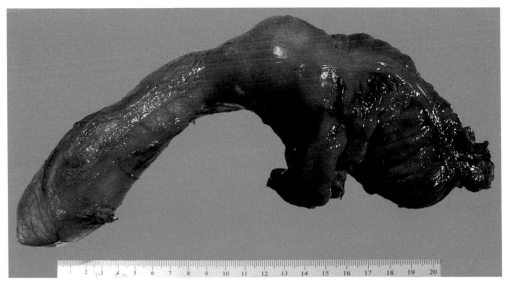

Fig. 8.3. Ileocolectomy specimen with enlarged and distended appendix (left) containing a low-grade mucinous neoplasm. No extra-appendiceal mucin was present.

3. The patient has vague abdominal symptoms, a mass or abdominal distension, and is found to have pseudomyxoma peritonei at the time of laparotomy. The appendix may be grossly abnormal, enlarged, and distended, or it may have a normal or near-normal diameter, presumably because it had ruptured and released its lumenal mucin. The surgeon should remove the appendix regardless of its gross appearance as it is almost certainly the source for the pseudomyxoma peritonei. Right hemicolectomy may not offer a survival advantage over appendectomy because of the advanced peritoneal disease, and simple appendectomy is adequate.[6,11,12]

The surgeon should remove the bulk of the intra-abdominal mucin for three reasons: (a) it is part of the treatment (coupled with intraperitoneal chemotherapy); (b) to relieve symptoms of distension; and (c) to allow thorough histologic examination on permanent sections because even scanty epithelial cells in the mucin are associated with a high risk of intra-abdominal recurrence. In addition, in a minority of cases, there is discordance in the appearance of the neoplastic cells in the appendix and the extra-appendiceal mucin; the extra-appendiceal mucin deposits contain cells with high grade cytologic atypia, a finding that is associated with more aggressive behavior.[1,5,6,11,13,14]

4. The patient has ovarian masses, usually bilateral, and is explored with a provisional diagnosis of primary ovarian carcinoma. The presence of pseudomyxoma peritonei is strong evidence of a primary appendiceal mucinous neoplasm, and should prompt an appendectomy, regardless of the gross appearance of the appendix.[15] In the absence of pseudomyxoma peritonei, there is a risk that the appendiceal primary may be overlooked, and the ovarian neoplasms interpreted as primary mucinous neoplasms. It is worth repeating the pathologic dictum that the appendix (and other gastrointestinal sites) should be examined whenever handling an unusual mucinous neoplasm of the ovary.

Pathologic issues

When handling mucinous neoplasms of the appendix, the pathologist should be familiar with the findings at surgery, a task that is easily accomplished by a visit to the operating room.

By definition, the lining epithelium of mucinous neoplasms is low-grade, either flat, undulating, serrated or villiform (Fig. 8.4)[1,5]. In some cases, clear foci of penetration into or through the wall are seen and this invasion is frequently accompanied by mural fibrosis and atrophy of the lymphoid tissue (Fig. 8.4). It is important to document extra-appendiceal mucin or appendiceal rupture when it is present, a finding that can be subtle but is of clinical significance (Fig. 8.2).

Appendiceal mucinous neoplasms should be handled as follows.

■ If the surgeon has performed an appendectomy for an enlarged, distended appendix -instead of the

(a)

(b)

(c)

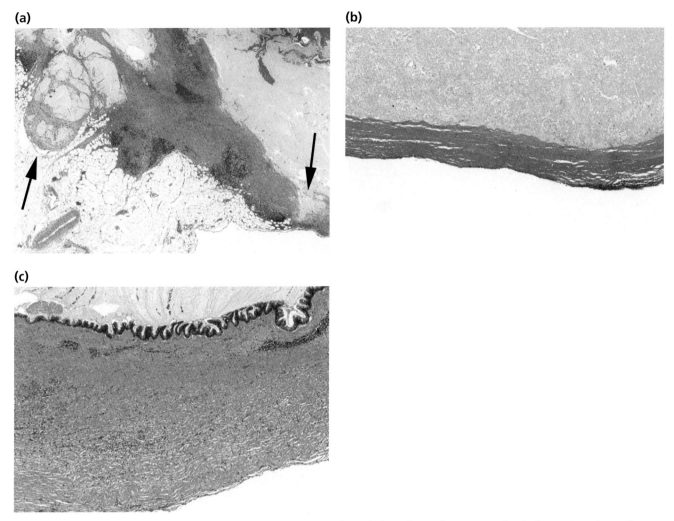

Fig. 8.4. (a) Low-grade mucinous neoplasm showing direct penetration through the wall into the periappendiceal adipose tissue (arrows). This is the same tumor as shown in Fig. 8.2. Invasive low-grade mucinous neoplasms of the appendix showing mural fibrosis with effacement of the submucosa and muscularis propria. Note the marked atrophy of lymphoid tissue. (b) Most of this tumor lacked an identifiable epithelial lining, but (c) some areas showed residual lining epithelium with a villiform pattern and low-grade cytomorphology.

recommended right hemicolectomy – and there is no other intra-abdominal disease, the main goal of IOD is to evaluate the proximal margin of the appendix. A single section should be taken parallel to the proximal margin for FS evaluation. If an invasive mucinous neoplasm is present at the margin, the surgeon will very likely proceed with a right hemi-colectomy; on the other hand, if the proximal margin is free of invasive neoplasm, the surgeon should be informed that the appendiceal lesion is very likely a mucinous neoplasm, and that the final diagnosis will be made on permanent sections. There is no reason to perform frozen sections on the remainder of the appendix; invasion of the appendiceal wall may be present, but this is often focal,

requiring examination of the entire appendix, and may not affect immediate surgical management.

■ If the surgeon performs a right hemicolectomy for a presumed mucinous neoplasm and there are no other intra-abdominal lesions, gross examination is adequate because the surgical margins will be clear. There is no reason to perform FSs on the appendix.

■ In the two situations listed above, the appendix should be fixed overnight, inked on the external surface (to distinguish true serosal implants of mucinous material from contaminants caused by sectioning) and submitted in its entirety for histologic examination. The fresh appendix should not be sectioned serially because this may complicate the distinction between true

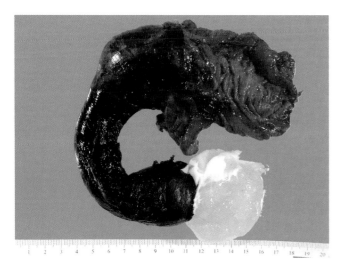

Fig. 8.5. Low grade mucinous neoplasm of the appendix to show the importance of inking the external surface before cutting into the specimen. A small incision was made into the lesion, resulting in extrusion of abundant mucinous material through the defect. Unless the appendix is inked prior to sectioning, mucinous contamination of the serosal surface may be incorrectly interpreted as clinically-significant extra-appendiceal mucin.

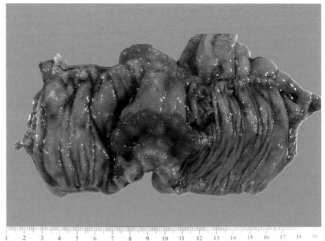

Fig. 8.6. Adenocarcinoma of the colon. Gross examination is usually sufficient for confirming that the margins are clear of carcinoma.

serosal implants and artifactual extravasation due to sectioning (Fig. 8.5). Even limited extra-appendiceal mucin has an adverse effect on long term survival; this is not an issue that should be resolved intraoperatively, but it is mentioned here because the evaluation of minimal extra-appendiceal mucin calls for proper handling of the fresh specimen, a responsibility that lies with the pathologist on FS duty.

▪ If the appendix is submitted for IOD in a patient with pseudomyxoma peritonei, there is no reason to perform a FS if the appendix is grossly abnormal. However, if the appendix is near normal (disregarding mucinous material on the serosal surface), one or two FS should be performed to determine if a mucinous neoplasm is present. If the appendix is histologically normal, the surgeon should be encouraged to examine other organs as the source for the pseudomyxoma peritonei.

▪ When a patient has pseudomyxoma peritonei, the surgeon will very likely send a sample of the peritoneal mucinous material for IOD. It is reasonable to perform a FS on the specimen to confirm the presence of epithelial cells. From a practical point of view, the surgical findings are what matter, and FS of the mucinous material usually adds little to guiding intraoperative management. If the FS of the peritoneal mucin fails to show epithelial cells, there is no reason to routinely

perform additional FSs, since the neoplastic epithelium in pseudomyxoma peritonei is variable in distribution, and multiple sections may be required to demonstrate the cellular component.

▪ If the patient has unilateral or bilateral mucinous neoplasms of the ovary, with or without pseudomyxoma peritonei, it is reasonable to perform a FS on the appendix because the presence of a mucinous neoplasm will stop the surgeon from staging the patient for a gynecologic malignancy.

Colorectal carcinoma

Colectomies for colon carcinoma are among the most common specimens received in the surgical pathology laboratory, but the role of IOD is limited since most cases are diagnosed and staged prior to surgical resection, and the surgeon has sufficient clinical information to perform the appropriate procedure with adequate margins. Sometimes, however, colectomy specimens are submitted for confirmation that the margins are clear, and gross examination is sufficient in almost all cases (Fig. 8.6).

There are a number of situations where intraoperative evaluation is justified.

▪ When a colectomy is performed after subtotal endoscopic removal of a polypoid lesion containing carcinoma, the surgeon may wish to confirm that the polypectomy site has been included in the resection; IOD may be requested even if a tattoo is present.

- Occasionally, a colectomy is performed to remove a carcinoma as well as one or more residual biopsy proven adenomatous polyps. If the surgeon is unable to palpate these polyps, the specimen will be sent for IOD to confirm that the polyps are present in the specimen. Gross examination is all that is needed but the pathologist should discuss the findings with the surgeon, and if necessary, show the open colectomy specimen to the surgeon to ensure that there is concordance between the pathologic findings and the surgeon's expectations.

- Patients who present with acute obstruction or colonic perforation usually undergo colonic resection without prior endoscopic examination. The specimen may be submitted for IOD if the surgeon suspects carcinoma, and especially if the diagnosis of carcinoma will alter the extent of colonic resection. A FS of the lesion will readily distinguish carcinoma from other lesions in the differential diagnosis, including lymphoma, endometriosis and inflammatory conditions such as diverticulitis and Crohn's disease.

- When a colectomy is performed to remove a sessile polyp that is too large to remove endoscopically, the surgeon may request a FS to rule out carcinoma. These lesions are difficult to evaluate intraoperatively because of the inability to examine the entire lesion, and the difficulty in obtaining well oriented sections. In most cases, the FS diagnosis of invasive carcinoma should not change the extent of surgical resection because the surgeon should perform a resection that is adequate to treat an occult invasive carcinoma.[16] If, however, the surgeon insists on a FS diagnosis, careful palpation is an important first step, and any unusually firm area should be sampled for FS. If the FS fails to demonstrate an invasive carcinoma, the surgeon should be told of the risk of a false-negative diagnosis.

- Rectal carcinomas that are pre-treated with chemoradiation usually undergo extensive regression, with the rectum containing either minimal residual carcinoma, or pools of mucin without residual neoplastic cells. The rectum in the area of the treated carcinoma will show mucosal ulceration without a grossly visible mass (Fig. 8.7). Gross examination may not be reliable for evaluating the distal margin, and if the surgeon is concerned, a request will be made for FS evaluation of this margin. The distal margin of the specimen should be inked, and sections should be taken perpendicular to the inked margin. Because the specimen will contract

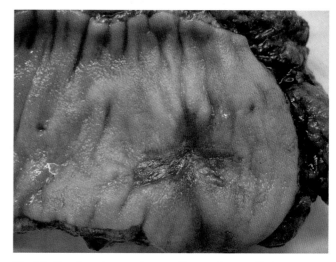

Fig. 8.7. Rectal carcinoma after neoadjuvant chemoradiation treatment. A superficial ulcer was present in the area of treated carcinoma, and histologically, all that remained was a 2 mm focus of residual invasive carcinoma.

after surgical removal, the surgeon's estimate of the length of normal tissue at the margin will be different from the pathologist's measurement of the margin of clearance.

Hirschprung's disease

See chapter on Pediatric pathology, p. 330.

Idiopathic chronic inflammatory bowel disease

Clinical issues

The treatment of idiopathic chronic inflammatory bowel disease (IBD) is primarily medical, but surgical intervention is occasionally required during the course of the disease. For ulcerative colitis (UC), colectomy is performed for dysplasia that cannot be managed endoscopically, for invasive carcinoma, and for severe intractable disease or fulminating colitis with toxic megacolon.[17]

In Crohn's disease, surgery is performed to treat strictures and obstructions, and less commonly, to treat carcinoma. When Crohn's disease of the small intestine causes obstruction, it is treated by conservative surgery: resection of ileocecal disease and stricturoplasty for segments of small bowel disease. The goal of surgical treatment is to preserve as much of the small bowel as possible in order to avoid complications of short gut syndrome. When colonic Crohn's disease leads to obstruction, it is treated with either segmental or total colectomy depending on the location and extent of disease.[17]

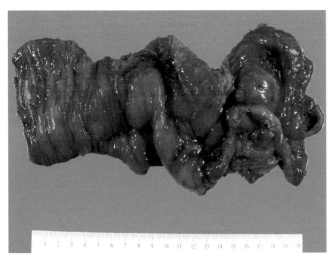

Fig. 8.8. Crohn's disease of the small intestine causing a stricture. Normal bowel mucosa is present at the proximal and distal margins by gross examination. There is no reason to perform frozen sections of the surgical margins if the margins appear to be clear by gross examination.

Pathologic issues

In resections for dysplasia arising in UC, the goal is to remove all the mucosa at risk. There is some debate about whether this should include anal mucosectomy, which may be of some benefit but may also lead to a worse functional outcome.[18] If a mucosectomy is included as part of the resection, the surgeon may request intraoperative examination of the rectal sleeve resection to ensure that the distal margin includes anal squamous mucosa.

If there is known carcinoma diagnosed by endoscopic biopsy in either UC or Crohn's disease, the specimen is treated as any other resection for carcinoma.

For segmental resections of intestine in known Crohn's disease uncomplicated by dysplasia or carcinoma, FS evaluation is not necessary (Fig. 8.8). The extent of resection is governed by the surgeon's evaluation of the diseased area, and microscopic disease at the surgical margins has no bearing on the likelihood of recurrence.[19] Small intestinal strictures due to Crohn's disease are treated by stricturoplasty, and the surgeon will very likely submit a biopsy for FS to exclude dysplasia and invasive carcinoma before completing the stricturoplasty.[16]

Occasionally, the first presentation of Crohn's disease will be intestinal obstruction. A segmental resection will be performed and the specimen will be sent to IOD to determine the cause of the obstruction. The differential diagnosis will include diverticulitis, carcinoma, lymphoma and endometriosis among others.[20]

Ischemic bowel disease

Clinical issues

The diagnosis of acute ischemia is made on clinical grounds. The nature of the disease and the extent of ischemia are obvious to the surgeon at the time of surgical resection. In contrast, the diagnosis of chronic ischemia is more difficult to establish pre-operatively, and when surgery is performed, the surgeon is likely to resect an area of intestinal stenosis and submit the specimen for IOD.

Pathologic issues

There is no need for IOD in acute ischemia. In chronic ischemia, the resected specimen will very likely be sent for IOD to determine the cause of the stenosis. The differential diagnosis includes Crohn's disease, lymphoma and carcinoma.

Esophagus and gastroesophageal junction

Surgical resection plays an important role in the management of carcinomas involving the esophagus and gastroesophageal junction, and the surgical approach and extent of resection are guided by the anatomic location of the carcinoma, its extent, histologic type, and whether there is associated dysplasia.

General clinical issues

The incidence of esophageal cancer continues to increase in the United States and this is attributed to an increased incidence of adenocarcinoma.[21] The diagnosis is usually established pre-operatively by endoscopic biopsy, and preoperative staging includes PET CT and endoscopic ultrasound (EUS). Endoscopic ultrasound can determine the depth of tumor invasion, evaluate para-esophageal lymph nodes and guide fine needle aspiration of para-esophageal lymph nodes for pathologic staging.[22–25] Laparoscopic staging has also been used but remains controversial.[26–28] Location of the carcinoma, pathologic type, stage, and the patient's general condition are taken into account when deciding on treatment, and after complete evaluation, <50% of patients are candidates for curative surgical resection.[29]

General pathologic issues

The usual specimen received in the laboratory is an esophagogastrectomy with a variable length of esophagus and approximately 5 cm of gastric wall.[30,31] The purpose of

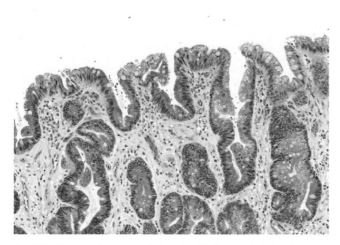

Fig. 8.9. Chemoradiotherapy-induced epithelial atypia in benign esophageal epithelium. The resection was for adenocarcinoma arising in Barrett's esophagus. Note the serrated appearance of the pits lined by pseudostratified cells. There is no significant pleomorphism, no atypical mitoses, and in many areas, the epithelium appears to mature as it reaches the surface.

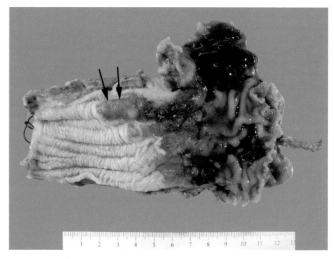

Fig. 8.10. Adenocarcinoma of the distal esophagus arising in association with Barrett's esophagus and dysplasia. Note the normal white, ribbed squamous epithelium of the esophagus is irregularly replaced by glistening, smooth columnar epithelium, which has a pink appearance in the fresh specimen (arrows).

IOD is to evaluate the proximal and distal margins of the resection; routine evaluation of the radial margin is not indicated since it is not feasible to remove additional tissue from this margin.

Both adenocarcinoma and squamous cell carcinoma may be multifocal,[32] so careful gross examination should be performed to look for lesions close to the surgical margins. We take a parallel section of the entire circumference of the proximal esophagus and submit this for FS evaluation; this is easily done as the tissue can usually fit into one or two FS blocks. Opinions vary in how to handle the distal margin; adenocarcinomas, and to a lesser extent, squamous cell carcinomas, show microscopic extension beyond the grossly visible lesion,[30] so there is a risk of obtaining false negative margins with inadequate sampling. We prefer to perform FS evaluation of the entire distal gastric margin if the carcinoma is within 5cm of the margin, but it is perfectly reasonable to limit the sampling to areas of the margin closest to the carcinoma.

The pathologist should be aware of prior neoadjuvant chemoradiotherapy as this can induce atypia in non-neoplastic tissue and be mistaken for malignancy, an issue that is relevant if the atypia is at a surgical margin (Fig. 8.9).[34] When there is marked regression of a carcinoma following adjuvant chemoradiation therapy, and the original boundaries of the carcinoma cannot be identified on gross examination, we perform complete enface FS evaluation of both margins (Fig. 8.1).

SQUAMOUS CELL CARCINOMA

Squamous cell carcinoma (SCC) is the most common esophageal malignancy worldwide, with especially high incidence rates in Iran, central China, South Africa and Brazil. This tumor is much less common in the United States, and occurs most frequently in males, with a much higher incidence in African-American males.[21] Resectable SCCs are usually pre-treated with chemoradiation, often with complete or near complete regression,[35] and when this occurs, gross examination is unreliable as a guide for evalauation of margins. Opinions vary about the minimum acceptable proximal margin in esophagogastrectomies for SCC; if the patient has not received neoadjuvant chemoradiation treatment, then a margin of 5 cm is ideal, but a margin of 2 cm is acceptable if the patient has received prior chemoradiation therapy.[33]

Squamous cell dysplasia is often found in association with invasive SCC,[21] and about 20% of superficially invasive (mucosal and submucosal) SCCs are multicentric, requiring careful gross and microscopic evaluation of the surgical margins.

ADENOCARCINOMAS

Adenocarcinomas most commonly arise in the distal esophagus of older white males in the background of Barrett's esophagus and dysplasia (Fig. 8.10). These may be treated by surgical resection alone, although neoadjuvant chemoradiation is used in some situations to facilitate surgical resection.[29] Adenocarcinoma often spreads in the submucosal plane, and this may be grossly invisible and subtle on microscopic examination, especially with poorly differentiated carcinomas.[40] Intestinal metaplasia (Barrett's esophagus) at the margin should be reported to the surgeon, since this might lead to further resection.

Recently, local endoscopic ablation techniques have successfully eradicated dysplastic and non-dysplastic Barrett's mucosa,[36] but there are no data about the response of residual Barrett's esophagus, with or without dysplasia, to post-operative endoscopic ablation. For the present, most surgeons prefer to surgically resect all the Barrett's mucosa, if technically feasible (Maish, personal communication).

Endoscopic mucosal resection (EMR) has recently emerged as an alternative to esophagogastrectomy in the treatment of early (TIS and T1)* adenocarcinoma arising in Barrett's esophagus.[37] One of the primary advantages of EMR is reduced morbidity, but positive margins are associated with tumor recurrence, and it has been proposed that FS be used to evaluate the surgical margins of these specimens.[38,39] At this time, EMR is limited to specialized medical centers.

Lymphomas of the gastrointestinal tract

See chapter on Lymph node, spleen and extranodal lymphomas (p. 262).

Adenomas and adenocarcinomas of the peri-ampullary region

Clinical issues

While adenomas may occur throughout the small bowel, they are most frequent in the ampulla and periampullary region. Most are sporadic, but some are associated with familial adenomatous polyposis, in which case, the adenomas are usually multiple.[41] Approximately 25% of all periamullary adenomas harbor an invasive carcinoma.[42] Most patients initially have endoscopic biopsies and other staging procedures, such as endoscopic ultrasound. The sensitivity of pre-operative endoscopic biopsy for diagnosing adenocarcinoma is generally around 75%–80%,[42–46] although some studies report higher rates.[47–48]

Treatment consists of resection with negative margins, but there is no consensus about the optimal resection technique.[42,43,46] Local resection options include endoscopic resection and ampullectomy, while wide resection is achieved by pancreaticoduodenectomy (PD) or Whipple's procedure. Endoscopic resection is least invasive but technically challenging, and complete resection can be difficult to achieve, especially with large sessile lesions.[45,49] Pancreaticoduodenectomy offers the best opportunity for cure, but is associated with significant morbidity and mortality.[46] Recurrence rates for locally resected sporadic adenomas vary from zero to 25%,[42,43,46,48,50] and the recurrence rates are equally variable (0–75%) in patients with familial adenomatous polyposis.[48,50] Local recurrences have been reported in both sporadic and polyposis-associated adenomas, even in patients with pathologically confirmed negative margins, and in the polyposis syndrome, it is difficult to determine if these are local recurrences or new lesions.[45,50]

If an adenocarcinoma is identified in an excised adenoma, the surgical procedure will very likely be converted from local excision to PD if the patient can tolerate a Whipple's procedure.[44,46,19] Known adenocarcinomas of the periampullary region are resected by PD, with the goal of achieving negative margins,[46,49] while patients with medical contraindications to PD may be treated with palliative local resection, with understandably poorer overall and disease free survival rates.[49,51]

Pathologic issues

Surgeons usually submit local resections of peri-ampullary adenomas for intraoperative evaluation.[44,46,50] The pathologist should exercise great caution when examining these specimens because of the risk of false negative and false positive diagnoses of carcinoma; a false positive diagnosis may result in an unnecessary PD, whereas a false negative diagnosis may require the patient to undergo a second major surgical procedure. The sensitivity of FS identification of carcinoma arising in an adenoma ranges from 25%–88%, with negative predictive values ranging from 38%–84%.[44–47,50]

The specimen should be palpated for an unduly firm area that may correspond to a focus of invasive carcinoma, and this should be sampled for FS. The main reason for false positive diagnosis is the over-interpretation dysplasia involving pancreatic and biliary ductal structures. The pancreatic and bile ducts have lobular aggregates of ductules in the ampulla,[52] and when these are involved by the dysplastic epithelium of an adenoma, the irregular branching nature of the ducts and the way they are embedded in dense fibromuscular tissue may be mistaken for invasive

---

* TIS = carcinoma in situ. T1 = carcinoma invading into the lamina propria or submucosa.

(a)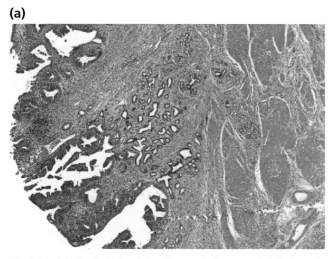

(b)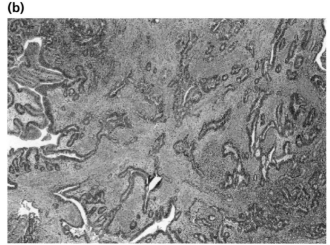

Fig. 8.11. (a) Dysplasia involving the terminal pancreatic/bile ducts in the sphincter of Oddi can mimic adenocarcinoma. The lobular architecture is a clue to the correct diagnosis. (b) Invasive adenocarcinoma of the ampulla. Note the more haphazard architectural pattern of invasive carcinoma.

carcinoma (Fig. 8.11). When faced with this problem, it is prudent to examine the lesion on low magnification, because this will bring about an appreciation for the underlying lobular architecture of these benign ductal/glandular structures.

Gastric carcinoma

Clinical issues

Gastric adenocarcinoma is the most common reason for surgical resection of the stomach. The diagnosis is made pre-operatively by endoscopic biopsy, except in the rare situation when endoscopic biopsies have failed to yield a firm diagnosis, requiring FS diagnosis on an incisional biopsy. Pre-operative staging with imaging (such as CT, PET-CT, percutaneous ultrasound for metastatic disease, and endoscopic ultrasound for depth of tumor invasion) is used to triage patients for surgical resection,[53] supplemented by laparoscopic staging in selected patients.[26]

When gastrectomy is performed with curative intent, an attempt will be made to obtain clear margins of 2–5 cm. On the other hand, when palliative gastrectomy is performed for high stage disease with complications such as obstruction, bleeding and perforation, the specimen may be submitted for IOD if the diagnosis of carcinoma has not been previously established; the purpose of IOD in this situation is to confirm the provisional clinical diagnosis, with less concern about the status of the surgical margins.

Pathologic issues

The pathologist should be familiar with the clinical aspects of the case and know if the intent of the gastrectomy is curative or palliative. Although pre-operative chemotherapy or chemoradiotherapy may be used as an adjuvant, surgery is the only potentially curative option and the goal is to obtain a resection with clear margins and adequate lymph node dissection.[54] There is an advantage in being familiar with the nature of the carcinoma when evaluating surgical margins, especially with signet ring cell carcinomas. The problems with signet ring cell carcinoma are:

- The gastric tissue at the margin may be grossly normal and yet harbor microscopic disease (Fig. 8.12);
- Skip foci of carcinoma may be present distant from the main tumor and these can be overlooked (Fig. 8.13);
- When the neoplastic cells are bland, they may be mistaken for prominent vessels and inflammatory cells (Fig. 8.14).

In the future, rapid immunohistochemistry may be available to aid in the evaluation of surgical margins in challenging situations.[55]

There are different opinions on how to evaluate the surgical margins in gastrectomy specimens. Because of the length of the gastric margins, microscopic evaluation of the entire margin by FS is time consuming and may not be necessary if the grossly visible tumor is well away from the margin; sections should be taken from the closest margins and embedded in one or more FS blocks. More extensive sampling is warranted when the carcinoma is close to the margins on gross examination, and for signet ring cell carcinomas; our preference is to evaluate the entire gastric margin with en face sections for signet ring cell carcinomas.

Endocrine tumors of the GI tract

Well-differentiated endocrine tumors occur throughout the GI tract and their behavior is determined by anatomic

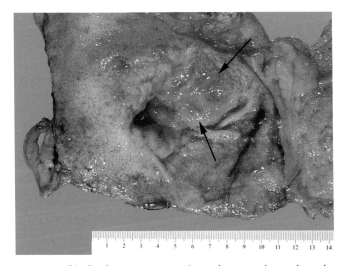

Fig. 8.12. This distal gastrectomy specimen shows an ulcerated poorly differentiated signet ring cell gastric carcinoma (arrows). Where the mucosa is not ulcerated, there is extensive subepithelial infiltration by tumor, extending for 1–2 cm beyond the boundary of the grossly visible mass.

location and size. Small neoplasms in the appendix and rectum are almost always confined to the primary site at the time of diagnosis, are readily resected, and behave in a benign fashion; however, large tumors in these same locations show much higher rates of lymph node metastases at presentation and can pursue a clinically aggressive course. In contrast, small bowel endocrine tumors, regardless of size, show a high propensity for nodal and distant metastases and thus tend to be clinically aggressive.

Gastric endocrine tumors comprise about 5% of all GI endocrine tumors and 1% of all gastric neoplasms. They are divided into Types 1, 2 and 3. About 70% are Type I and are associated with non-syndromic hypergastrinemia, usually in the setting of atrophic gastritis. These are usually small, typically limited to the mucosa, with only rare nodal (<5%) or distant (<2%) metastases. Small mucosal tumors (<1 cm) are indolent and are treated by endoscopic resection. Tumors that invade into the submucosa or deeper, or tumors that are large or multifocal may require partial gastrectomy. *Type 2* tumors (5%) arise in the setting of Zollinger-Ellison syndrome in patients with multiple endocrine neoplasia type I (MEN1). These neoplasms are 1–2 cm in size, often multiple, and most patients have synchronous or metachronous endocrine tumors in the duodenum or peripancreatic tissues, making it challenging for the surgeon to detect and remove all the neoplasms. Type 2 gastric endocrine tumors have an intermediate clinical course, with nodal and liver metastases in up to 30% and 20% of patients, respectively. Large gastric tumors are treated by gastrectomy, and small (<1 cm) gastric

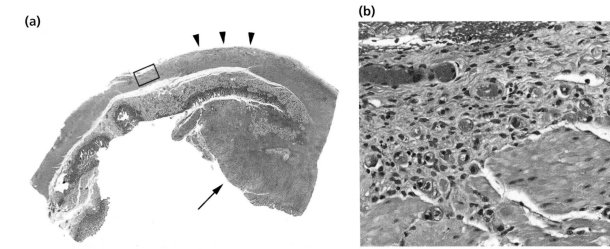

(a)

(b)

Fig. 8.13. Microscopic of tumor shown in Fig. 8.12. (a) On low power, the tumor mass is seen at the antral-pyloric junction (arrow), but tumor cells are seen to infiltrate for several centimeters into the duodenal muscularis propria and serosa (arrowheads). (b) On high power, malignant cells are readily identified in the area within the box. This invasion was not appreciated on gross examination.

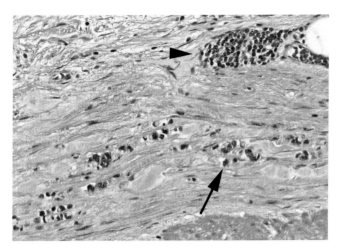

Fig. 8.14. Poorly differentiated gastric carcinoma usually shows a range of morphologies, including cells with identifiable cytoplasmic mucin with or without a signet ring morphology, as well as individual hyperchromatic cells (arrow). The latter may be mistaken for inflammatory cells, but they are usually larger and more pleomorphic than lymphocytes (arrowhead).

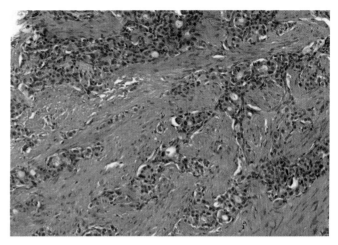

Fig. 8.15. Somatostatinoma, with a glandular pattern, invading through the duodenal muscularis propria. The uniform bland cytology and psammoma bodies are helpful clues to the diagnosis.

tumors via endoscopic resection. *Type 3 tumors* (20%) usually behave aggressively. They are sporadic and not associated with hypergastrinemia, Zollinger-Ellison syndrome or any of the multiple endocrine neoplasia syndromes. At the time of diagnosis, most are large (>2 cm), deeply invasive and up to 50% have nodal metastases. These patients may show an "atypical carcinoid syndrome" with cutaneous edema, patchy flushing, salivary gland swelling and brochospasm. Gastrectomy, the extent of which depends on the clinical situation, is recommended.[56]

Well-differentiated endocrine tumors of the stomach resemble typical carcinoid tumors, and the diagnosis is usually made on endoscopic biopsy. Resections are seldom sent for IOD except in patients with Zollinger–Ellison syndrome, when the surgeon is trying to locate and excise lesions in lymph nodes or peripancreatic soft tissues.

Duodenal endocrine tumors, which comprise about 3% of all GI tract endocrine tumors, are often associated with either neurofibromatosis Type 1 (NF1) or multiple endocrine neoplasia type 1 (MEN1). Most are located in the first and second portions of the duodenum, are multifocal, measure <1 cm, and are limited to the mucosa or submucosa. The majority (about 65%) are gastrin producing (G-cell) tumors and have nodal metastases in about 30% of cases. Somatostatin producing (D-cell) tumors are often associated with NF1, arise in the periampullary area, and are associated with pancreatic endocrine tumors.[56–58]

Duodenal endocrine tumors limited to the mucosa or submucosa can be treated by endoscopic resection. Tumors that are larger, have nodal metastases, or are associated with the Zollinger–Ellison syndrome are usually resected surgically, and pancreaticoduodenectomy may be required for selected peri-ampullary tumors, especially those that cause bile duct obstruction.[56] Most endocrine tumors of the duodenum have the typical histologic features of carcinoid tumor; but somatostatinomas have a cribriform pattern of growth and may be mistaken for adenocarcinoma; the presence of psammoma bodies and the absence of pleomorphism and are clues to the correct diagnosis (Fig. 8.15).

Gangliocytic paraganglioma presents as variably sized (1–10 cm) polypoid mass in the periampullary region. This neoplasm contains a mixture of epithelioid cells arranged in nests or clusters, ganglion cells, and spindle cells. Despite their large size, they tend to be encapsulated, and are only rarely associated with nodal metastases or local recurrence after excision.[59]

Endocrine neoplasms of the *jejunum and ileum* account for about 25% of all endocrine tumors of the GI tract and for about one-third of all tumors in this location. They are clinically aggressive, and the time of presentation, up to 80% of patients have nodal metastases, and up to 40% have liver metastases. The carcinoid syndrome, present in 20% of patients, occurs when there are liver metastases or when there is a large tumor burden in retroperitoneal lymph nodes.[56–58,60] The desmoplasia induced by the tumor causes a characteristic "kinking" of the involved segment of bowel (Fig. 8.16), and some neoplasms evoke marked

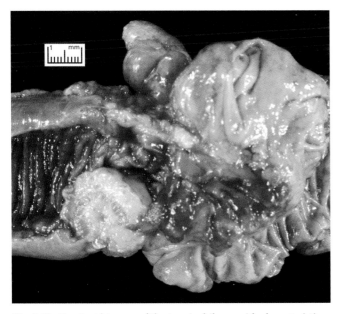

Fig. 8.16. Carcinoid tumor of the terminal ileum with characteristic "kinking" of the bowel wall.

mesenteric fibrosis and vascular changes, resulting in bowel obstruction or intestinal ischemia. Symptoms include abdominal pain, weight loss, nausea, vomiting, diarrhea and valvular heart disease, some of which are thought to be due to excessive tumor peptide production.[56,58]

A number of laboratory tests and imaging studies, including capsule endoscopy and double balloon enteroscopy, can be used to make the diagnosis pre-operatively,[60] but the diagnosis is often made for the first time during surgical exploration for symptoms of obstruction. Up to 20% of patients with small intestinal endocrine tumors will have synchronous or metachronous non-carcinoid tumors (both GI and non-GI primaries), so the surgeon should explore the abdomen for other neoplasms.[56,58]

The treatment of localized jejunal and ileal tumors consists of segmental bowel resection. Tumor that has spread into the mesentery or to the liver is resected, if clinically feasible, because of improved survival with aggressive surgical treatment.[56,58]

On gross examination, jejunal and ileal endocrine tumors are sclerotic, often with a kink in the bowel wall, and have a yellow cut surface (Fig. 8.16). Microscopically, the neoplasm usually has an insular pattern and is not likely to be confused for any other tumor. The presence of cytologic atypia and mitoses will not influence surgical management. If the neoplasm appears to be limited to the bowel wall, the surgeon will attempt to obtain a surgical margin of at least 2 cm on either side of the mass. If liver

lesions are discovered during surgery, a biopsy may be submitted for FS diagnosis before proceeding with hepatic resection.

Appendiceal endocrine tumors, which comprise 25% of all GI endocrine neoplasms, usually have a benign clinical course. Approximately 90% measure <1 cm and are usually first identified during pathologic examination of an appendix removed for acute appendicitis. Right hemicolectomy is recommended for tumors >2 cm, as up to 30% will have nodal metastases.[6,8–10,56,58] The appropriate surgical procedure for tumors 1–2 cm in size remains controversial; recommendations include simple appendectomy for tumors confined to the appendiceal wall with clear surgical margins, and right hemicolectomy for tumors that extend into the mesoappendix, involve the base of the appendix, or show extensive lymphovascular invasion.[6,56,58,61]

When the tumor forms a visible mass, the surgeon is likely to request IOD.[6,56] If margin evaluation is requested on an appendix that contains a small neoplasm (<2 cm), a complete en face section of the proximal margin should be submitted for FS evaluation. There is no reason to examine the surgical margins of a right hemicolectomy specimen, but if this is requested, gross examination is sufficient.

Goblet cell carcinoid, a histologic variant of carcinoid tumor, runs a more aggressive clinical course.[4] Unlike the typical carcinoid tumor, goblet cell carcinoids tend to be diffusely infiltrating, often involving the base of the appendix, requiring right hemicolectomy for optimal treatment.[6,56]

Colonic endocrine tumors comprise about 5% of all GI tract tumors, occur in older patients, and are located mainly in the right colon. Most behave aggressively with nodal metastases in about 80% of tumors >2 cm, and in about 20% of tumors <2 cm. Standard segmental resection or hemicolectomy is recommended.[58,61]

Rectal carcinoid tumors: Approximately15% of GI tract endocrine tumors occur in the rectum. Approximately 60% measure <1 cm, extend no deeper than the submucosa, and can be removed via endoscopic resection or transanal endoscopic microsurgery.[62] They usually pursue a benign clinical course, with nodal metastases occurring in <3% of cases. Rectal carcinoid tumors 1–2 cm in size show an increased rate of metastasis and require more aggressive resection. Tumors >2 cm have high rates of metastases (over 60%); tumors in the upper rectum are treated by anterior resection, while the treatment of tumors in the

(a)

(b)

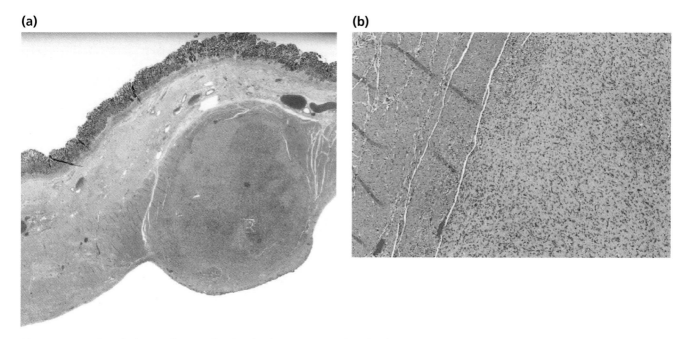

Fig. 8.17. Gastrointestinal stromal tumor showing the characteristic pushing border on microscopic examination. This pattern of growth allows the surgeon to perform complete excision with close but clear margins when there are anatomic constraints.

lower rectum is controversial because of the morbidity of abdominoperoneal resection.[56,61]

The diagnosis is made pre-operatively, so the purpose of IOD is to evaluate the margins of resection; a 2 cm margin is optimal, but the surgeon will settle for a lesser margin with local excisions of rectal tumors.

Gastrointestinal stromal tumors

Clinical issues

Gastrointestinal stromal tumors (GIST) are the most common mesenchymal tumor of the GI tract and occur most frequently in the stomach, followed by small intestine. Because these tumors are centered on the muscularis propria, pre-operative endoscopic biopsy is often non-diagnostic, and as a result, the surgeon will often approach the surgical procedure without a pathologic diagnosis, but with GIST as the favored diagnosis based on clinical and imaging findings.[63,64]

When a GIST is localized to the primary site, the goal of surgery is complete resection of the tumor with clear margins, taking care to avoid rupture of the neoplasm and the risk of peritoneal seeding. Small gastric neoplasms are successfully removed by laparoscopic resection.[63–65]

GISTs have pushing rather than infiltrative borders (Fig. 8.17), so that when necessary, complete resection

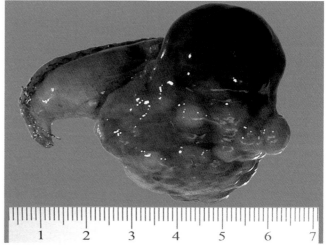

Fig. 8.18. Gastric stromal tumor removed by a typical wedge resection.

can be achieved with narrow margins (<1 cm); wide resection does not offer the patient any added benefits. Most gastric resections are achieved with a wedge resection (Fig. 8.18), and jejunal and ileal neoplasms are removed with a limited segmental resection. Because of anatomic factors, tumors of the esophagus, second part of the duodenum and low rectum may require more extensive surgery.[63–65]

The clinical significance of positive microscopic margins remains unclear, especially in those tumors that are considered malignant based on anatomic location, size and mitotic rate. While these patients are at higher risk for intra-abdominal recurrence, the impact on overall survival is less clear when the data are adjusted for the malignant potential of the primary tumor. There are no data to support re-operation in patients who have gross total tumor resection with positive microscopic margins; current recommendations are for these patients to be evaluated by a multidisciplinary team with expertise in treating GISTs.[63,65]

Patients with potentially malignant GISTs of the esophagus, duodenum and rectum may be managed differently if radical surgery will have significant functional consequences. Chemotherapy with imatinib (Gleevac) may be used as first-line neoadjuvant therapy in an effort to shrink the tumor and facilitate surgery.

Optimal treatment for patients with metastatic GIST remains the focus of investigation. If intra-abdominal metastases are suspected at the time of initial surgery, biopsy of a metastasis may be sent for IOD. Surgery alone is rarely effective in treating metastatic GIST, and there are on-going trials evaluating the efficacy of combining surgery with first and/or second generation tyrosine kinase inhibitors.[63,64,66]

Pathologic issues

If the diagnosis has not been previously established, the main goal of IOD is to determine if the neoplasm is a GIST. Gastrointestinal stromal tumors can be readily distinguished from carcinoma and lymphoma, but is sometimes more difficult to distinguish GIST from other mesenchymal neoplasms, such as scwannoma (stomach), mesenteric fibromatosis involving the small intestine, and metastatic mesenchymal tumors of uterine origin.

On occasion, anatomic location, size, and mitotic activity, will allow for a definite diagnosis of malignant GIST, but in most cases, the aggressive potential of the neoplasm will have to be deferred to permanent sections; this is of no immediate consequence as the surgical approach is the same.[63,64]

GISTs are typically well-circumscribed, with pushing margins (Figs. 8.17 and 8.18). If the surgeon requests evaluation of the surgical margins, sections should be taken perpendicular or parallel to the surgical margins, depending on the distance of the neoplasm from the surgical margin.[63,66] There are currently no data to show a difference in prognosis between immediate versus delayed re-excision of a microscopically positive margin;[64] if

a positive margin on FS will entail significant added complexity to the surgical procedure, it is reasonable to delay the final interpretation to permanent sections, and then decide on appropriate management based on the potential malignancy of the neoplasm.

ACKNOWLEDGEMENT

The authors would like to thank Drs. Mary Maish and Jonathan Sack, members of the UCLA Department of Surgery, for their helpful comments.

REFERENCES

1. Misdraji J, Yantiss RK, Graeme-Cook FM, Balis UJ, HYR. Appendiceal mucinous neoplasms; a clinicopathologic analysis of 107 Cases. *Am J Surgi Pathol* 2003; **2003**(27): 8.

2. Bucher P, Mathe Z, Demirag A, Morel P. Appendix tumors in the era of laparoscopic appendectomy. *Surg Endosc.* 2004; **18**(7): 1063–1066.

3. Gustafsson BI, Siddique L, Chan A, *et al.* Uncommon cancers of the small intestine, appendix and colon: an analysis of SEER 1973–2004 and current diagnosis and therapy. *Int J Oncol* 2008; **33**(6): 1121–1131.

4. McCusker ME, Cote TR, Clegg LX, Sobin LH. Primary malignant neoplasms of the appendix: a population-based study from the surveillance, epidemiology and end-results program, 1973–1998. *Cancer* 2002; **94**(12): 3307–3312.

5. Misdraji J, Young RH. Primary epithelial neoplasms and other epithelial lesions of the appendix (excluding carcinoid tumors). *Semin Diagn Pathol.* 2004; **21**: 120–133.

6. Murphy EM, Farquharson SM, Moran BJ. Management of an unexpected appendiceal neoplasm. *Br J Surg* 2006; **93**(7): 783–792.

7. Renshaw AA, Kish R, Gould EW. Sessile serrated adenoma is associated with acute appendicitis in patients 30 years or older. *Am J Clin Pathol* 2006; **126**(6): 875–877.

8. Tchana-Sato V, Detry O, Polus M, *et al.* Carcinoid tumor of the appendix: a consecutive series from 1237 appendectomies. *World J Gastroenterol* 2006; **12**(41): 1699–1701.

9. McGory ML, Zingmond DS, D Nanayakkara, Maggard MA, Ko CY. Malignancies of the appendix: beyond case series reports. *Dis Colon Rectum* 2005; **48**(12): 2264–2271.

10. Walters KC, Paton BL, Schmelzer TS, *et al.* Treatment of appendiceal adenocarcinoma in the United States: penetration and outcomes of current guidelines. *Am Surg* 2008; **74**(11): 1066–1068.

11. Gonzalez-Moreno S, Brun E, Sugarbaker PH. Lymph node metastases in epithelial malignancies of the appendix with peritoneal dissemination does not reduce survival in patients treated by cytoreductive surgery and perioperative intraperitoneal chemotherapy. *Ann Surg Oncol* 2005; **12**(1): 72–80.

12. Gonzalez-Moreno S, Sugarbaker PH. Right hemicolectomy does not confer a survival advantage in patients with mucinous carcinoma of the appendix and peritoneal seeding. *Br J Surg* 2004; **91**(3): 304–311.

13. Stewart JH, Shen P, Russell GB, *et al.* Appendiceal neoplasms with peritoneal dissemination: outcomes after cytoreductive surgery and intraperitoneal hyperthermic chemotherapy. *Ann Surg Oncol* 2006; **13**(5): 624–634.

14. Yantiss RK, Shia J, Klimstra DS, *et al.* Prognostic significance of localized extra-appendiceal mucin deposition in appendiceal mucinous neoplasms. *Am J Surg Pathol* 2009; **33**(2): 248–255.

15. Young RH. Pseudomyxoma peritonei and selected other aspects of the spread of appendiceal neoplasms. *Semin Diagn Pathol* 2004; **21**: 134–150.

16. Sack J. Personal communication: Resection of colonic neoplasms. 2009.

17. Hancock L, Windsor AC, Mortensen NJ. Inflammatory bowel disease: the view of the surgeon. *Colorectal Dis* 2006; **8** (Suppl 1): 10–14.

18. Chambers WM, McCMortensen NJ. Should ileal pouch-anal anastomosis include mucosectomy? *Colorectal Dis* 2007; **9**(5): 384–392.

19. Fazio VW, Marchetti F, Church M, *et al.* Effect of resection margins on the recurrence of Crohn's disease in the small bowel. A randomized controlled trial. *Ann Surg* 1996; **224**(4): 563–571; discussion 71–3.

20. Fry R, Mahmoud N, Maron D, Ross H, Rombeau J. Colon and small bowel. In Townsend CM, Beauchamp RD, Evers BM, Mattox KL, eds. *Sabiston Textbook of Surgery*, **18**th edn. Saunders Elsevier: Philadelphia, PA, 2008.

21. Glickman JN, Odze RD. Epithelial neoplasms of the esophagus. In Odze RD, Goldblum JR (eds). *Surgical Pathology of the GI Tract, Liver, Biliary Tree and Pancreas*, Saunders Elsevier: Philadelphia, 2009.

22. Anand D, Barroeta JE, Gupta PK, Kochman M, Baloch ZW. Endoscopic ultrasound guided fine needle aspiration of non-pancreatic lesions: an institutional experience. *J Clin Pathol* 2007; **60**(11): 1254–1262.

23. Bergman JJ. The endoscopic diagnosis and staging of oesophageal adenocarcinoma. *Best Pract Res Clin Gastroenterol* 2006; **20**(5): 843–866.

24. Peng HQ, Greenwald BD, Tavora FR, *et al.* Evaluation of performance of EUS-FNA in preoperative lymph node staging of cancers of esophagus, lung, and pancreas. *Diagn Cytopathol* 2008; **36**(5): 290–296.

25. Vazquez-Sequeiros E, Wiersema MJ. The role of endoscopic ultrasound in esophageal carcinoma. In *UpToDate*, Howell AD, ed. Vol. Waltham, MA: Wolters Kluwer, 2008.

26. Chang L, Stefanidis D, Richardson WS, Earle DB, Fanelli RD. The role of staging laparoscopy for intraabdominal cancers: an evidence-based review. *Surg Endosc* 2009; **23**: 2073–2077.

27. de Graaf GW, Ayantunde AA, Parsons SL, Duffy JP, Welch NT. The role of staging laparoscopy in oesophagogastric cancers. *Eur J Surg Oncol* 2007; **33**(8): 988–992.

28. Kaiser GM, Sotiropoulos GC, Fruhauf NR, *et al.* Value of staging laparoscopy for multimodal therapy planning in esophago-gastric cancer. *Int Surg* 2007; **92**(3): 128–132.

29. Maish M. Esophagus. In Townsend CM, Beauchamp RD, Evers BM, Mattox KL eds. *Sabiston Textbook of Surgery*, **18**th edn. Saunders Elsevier: Philadelphia, PA, 2008.

30. Casson AG, Darnton SJ, Subramanian S, Hiller L. What is the optimal distal resection margin for esophageal carcinoma? *Ann Thorac Surg* 2000; **69**(1): 205–209.

31. Law S, Arcilla C, Chu KM, Wong J. The significance of histologically infiltrated resection margin after esophagectomy for esophageal cancer. *Am J Surg* 1998; **176**(3): 286–290.

32. Altorki NK, Lee PC, Liss Y, *et al.* Multifocal neoplasia and nodal metastases in T1 esophageal carcinoma: implications for endoscopic treatment. *Ann Surg* 2008; **247**(3): 434–439.

33. Maish M. Personal communication: Resection of esophageal tumors. 2009.

34. Brien TP, Farraye FA, Odze RD. Gastric dysplasia-like epithelial atypia associated with chemoradiotherapy for esophageal cancer: a clinicopathologic and immunohistochemical study of 15 cases. *Mod Pathol* 2001; **14**(5): 389–396.

35. Forastiere A, Choi N, Gibson M. Radiation therapy, chemotherapy, and neoadjuvant approaches for localized cancers of the esophagus and GE junction. In Goldbery, R, Willett C, eds. Up To Date Waltham, MA, 2009.

36. Shaheen NJ, Sharma P, Overholt BF, *et al.* Radiofrequency ablation in Barrett's esophagus with dysplasia. *New England Journal of Medicine* 2009; **360**(22): 2277–2288.

37. Wright C, Saltzman J. Management of superficial esophageal cancer. In *UpToDate*, Tanabe K (ed). Waltham, MA: Wolters Kluwer, 2008.

38. Prasad GA, Buttar NS, Wongkeesong LM, *et al.* Significance of neoplastic involvement of margins obtained by endoscopic mucosal resection in Barrett's esophagus. *Am J Gastroenterol* 2007; **102**(11): 2380–2386.

39. Prasad GA, Wang KK, Lutzke LS, *et al.* Frozen section analysis of esophageal endoscopic mucosal resection specimens in the real-time management of Barrett's esophagus. *Clin Gastroenterol Hepatol* 2006; **4**(2): 173–178.

40. Nishimaki T, Tanaka O, Suzuki T, *et al.* Patterns of lymphatic spread in thoracic esophageal cancer. *Cancer* 1994 1; **74**(1): 4–11.

41. Yantiss RK, Antonioli DA. Polyps of the Small Intestine. In *Surgical Pathology of the GI Tract, Liver, Biliary Tract and Pancreas*, Odze RD, Goldblum JR, eds Philadelphia: Saunders Elsevier, 2009.

42. Treitschke F, Beger HG. Local resection of benign periampullary tumors. *Ann Oncol* 1999; **10**(Suppl 4): S212–S214.

43. Branum GD, Pappas TN, Meyers WC. The management of tumors of the ampulla of Vater by local resection. *Ann Surg* 1996; **224**(5): 621–627.

44. Clary BM, Tyler DS, Dematos P, Gottfried M, Pappas TN. Local ampullary resection with careful intraoperative frozen section evaluation for presumed benign ampullary neoplasms. *Surgery* 2000; **127**: 628–633.

45. Meneghetti AT, Safadi B, Stewart L, Way LW. Local resection of ampullary tumors. *J Gastrointest Surg* 2005; **9**: 1300–1306.

46. Roggin KK, J YJJ, R FC, *et al.* Limitations of ampullectoromy in the treatment of nonfamilial ampullary neoplasms. *Ann Surg Oncol* 2005; **12**(12): 971–980.

47. Grobmyer SR, Stasik CN, Draganov P, *et al.* Contemporary results with ampullectomy for 29 "benign" neoplasms of the ampulla. *J Am Coll Surg* 2008; **206**: 466–471.

48. Ouaissi M, Panis Y, Sielezneff I, *et al.* Long-term outcome after ampullectomy for ampullary lesions associated with familial adenomatous polyposis. *Dis Colon Rectum* 2005; **48**: 2192–2196.

49. Dittrick GW, Mallat DB, Lamont JP. Management of ampullary lesions. *Curr Treatm Options Gastroenterol* 2006; **9**: 371–376.

50. Dixon E, Jr CMV, Sahajpal A, *et al.* Transduodenal resection of peri-ampullary lesions. *World J Surg* 2005; **29**: 649–652.

51. DiGiorgio A, Alfieri S, Rotondi F, *et al.* Pancreatoduodenectomy for tumors of Vater's ampulla: report on 94 consecutive patients. *World J Surg* 2005; **29**: 513–518.

52. Klimstra DS. Pancreas. In Sternberg SS ed. *Histology for Pathologists* Lippincott-Raven: Philadephia, 1997.

53. Ly QP, Sasson AR. Modern surgical considerations for gastric cancer. *J Natl Compr Canc Netw* 2008; **6**(9): 885–894.

54. Van Cutsem E, Van de Velde C, Roth A, *et al.* Expert opinion on management of gastric and gastro-oesophageal junction adenocarcinoma on behalf of the European Organisation for Research and Treatment of Cancer (EORTC) – gastrointestinal cancer group. *Eur J Cancer* 2008; **44**(2): 182–194.

55. Monig SP, Luebke T, Soheili A, *et al.* Rapid immunohistochemical detection of tumor cells in gastric carcinoma. *Oncol Rep* 2006; **16**(5): 1143–1147.

56. Akerstrom G, Hellman P. Surgery on neuroendocrine tumours. *Best Pract Res Clin Endocrinol Metab* 2007; **21**(1): 87–109.

57. Graeme-Cook FM. Neuroendocrine tumors of the GI tract and appendix. In *Surgical Pathology of the GI Tract, Liver, Biliary Tract and Pancreas*, Odze RD, Goldblum JR eds. Philadelphia: Saunders Elsevier, 2009.

58. Sutton R, Doran HE, Williams EM, *et al.* Surgery for midgut carcinoid. *Endocr Relat Cancer* 2003; **10**(4): 469–481.

59. Noffsinger A. Epithelial neoplasms of the small intestine. In *Surgical Pathology of the GI Tract, Liver, Biliary Tract and Pancreas*, Odze RD, Goldblum JR eds. Philadelphia: Saunders Elsevier, 2009.

60. Bellutti M, Fry LC, Schmitt J, *et al.* Detection of neuroendocrine tumors of the small bowel by double balloon enteroscopy. *Dig Dis Sci* 2009; **54**(5): 1050–1058.

61. Roumeliotis A, Barkas K, Amygdalos G. Carcinoid: modern aspects on its therapy. *Tech Coloproctol* 2004; **8**(Suppl. 1): s164–s166.

62. Suzuki H, Furukawa K, Kan H, *et al.* The role of transanal endoscopic microsurgery for rectal tumors. *J Nippon Med Sch* 2005; **72**(5): 278–284.

63. Chaudhry UI, DeMatteo RP. Management of resectable gastrointestinal stromal tumor. *Hematol Oncol Clin North Am* 2009; **23**(1): 79–96.

64. Demetri GD, Benjamin RS, Blanke CD, *et al.* NCCN Task Force Report: management of patients with gastrointestinal stromal tumor (GIST) – update of the NCCN clinical practice guidelines. *J Natl Compr Canc Netw* 2007; **5**(Suppl. 2): S1–529.

65. Everett M, Gutman H. Surgical management of gastrointestinal stromal tumors: analysis of outcome with respect to surgical margins and technique. *J Surg Oncol* 2008; **98**(8): 588–593.

66. Blay JY, Bonvalot S, Casali P, *et al.* Consensus meeting for the management of gastrointestinal stromal tumors. Report of the GIST Consensus Conference of 20–21 March 2004, under the auspices of ESMO. *Ann Oncol* 2005; **16**(6): 566–578.

9 LIVER, GALLBLADDER, AND EXTRAHEPATIC BILIARY TRACT

Julia C. Iezzoni, Timothy M. Schmitt, and Reid B. Adams

INTRODUCTION

While intraoperative diagnosis (IOD) remains an important part of the surgical management of mass lesions of the liver, gallbladder, and extrahepatic biliary tract, its specific role has changed due to advances in multiple medical specialties.

Improvements in imaging techniques, including high-resolution ultrasound, multiphase contrast-enhanced computed tomography, and magnetic resonance, and nuclear scintigraphic modalities such as positron emission tomography, have greatly enhanced the pre-operative evaluation of hepatobiliary masses.[1,2] As a result, imaging studies alone often will: (a) differentiate between benign and malignant liver neoplasms; (b) detect and stage primary hepatobiliary malignancies; (c) detect metastatic disease; (d) determine the resectability of a neoplasm; and (e) provide reliable follow-up of treated hepatobiliary malignancies. When the radiographic features are not diagnostic, image guided fine needle aspiration (FNA) and needle core biopsies frequently provide a specific diagnosis in advance of possible surgical resection.

When surgical intervention is necessary, advances in operative techniques, instrumentation, anesthesia, and post-operative care have made surgical resection a safe and accepted modality for treating hepatobiliary neoplasia. Expanded knowledge of segmental hepatic anatomy, mainly from the field of liver transplantation, has dramatically reduced the morbidity and mortality of hepatic surgery. Further improvements in safety have been realized by techniques such as pre-operative portal vein embolization to induce pre-operative hypertrophy of the future liver remnant to minimize the risk of post-operative liver failure, inflow, and outflow vascular exclusion to minimize hemorrhage, low central venous pressure anesthesia to minimize blood loss, and ex-vivo resections with re-implantation for complex resections. As a result of these surgical and technological advances, laparoscopic resection of hepatic masses now is a routine approach at many medical centers. In addition, total hepatectomy with liver transplantation and live donor partial hepatectomy for transplantation are performed routinely in many specialized transplantation centers; this increasing use of liver transplantation has added new issues to be addressed at the time of frozen section (FS) diagnosis.

This chapter will focus on the role of IOD in the contemporary surgical management of hepatobiliary diseases in adults. The role of IOD in the management of neoplasms in infants and children is discussed in the chapter on pediatric pathology (Chapter 20, p. 329).

INFORMATION NEEDED BEFORE AND DURING INTRAOPERATIVE DIAGNOSIS

The pathologist should be familiar with the clinical aspects of the case to optimize the intra-operative evaluation of hepatobiliary specimens. This includes:

- Familiarity with patient demographics (age and gender), relevant clinical history (e.g., history of cirrhosis, oral contraceptive or androgenic steroid use in a patient with a hepatic mass), laboratory data including serum tumor markers (e.g., alpha-fetoprotein, carcinoembryonic antigen, and carbohydrate antigen 19–9), history of prior malignancy, and information about prior treatment of the mass, if applicable.
- Familiarity with the imaging characteristics of the lesion and the radiologist's interpretation.

Intraoperative Consultation in Surgical Pathology, ed. Mahendra Ranchod. Published by Cambridge University Press.
© Cambridge University Press 2010.

- Review of prior FNA or biopsy of the mass or a separate prior primary malignancy. Ideally, these slides should be available before the surgical procedure so they may be reviewed in advance, and compared to the intra-operative pathologic material, if necessary.
- Familiarity with surgeon's operative plan and awareness of how IOD will impact surgical management. It is prudent for the pathologist and surgeon to discuss the specific management issues of a case prior to surgery when a case is likely to be challenging.

LIVER

Indications for intraoperative diagnosis

Requests for IOD of the liver occur in a relatively limited number of clinical circumstances, as follows[3]:

1. To evaluate the surgical margins on partial hepatectomy specimens for primary or metastatic neoplasms
2. To diagnose a previously undetected liver nodule in a patient having non-hepatic surgery.
3. To make a diagnosis on additional hepatic nodule/s found unexpectedly in a patient scheduled for resection of a hepatic mass, especially when this diagnosis may influence the surgical procedure.
4. To provide an initial diagnosis on a hepatic mass in a patient scheduled for hepatic resection, in cases where it was not possible to make a pre-operative pathologic diagnosis; this is especially important if the diagnosis will influence the surgical procedure.
5. To evaluate the suitability of a potential donor liver for transplantation.

Specific clinico-pathologic issues

Evaluation of surgical margins in partial hepatectomy specimens

Since resection of a hepatic mass is almost always undertaken after the diagnosis has been established by imaging or on a pre-operative biopsy, the goal of IOD is usually limited to evaluation of surgical margins. Sometimes, however, partial hepatectomy specimens are not submitted for intraoperative evaluation, either because the margins are obviously clear on gross examination of the specimen, or resection of additional tissue is prohibited by anatomic or physiologic constraints. While the goal of surgical

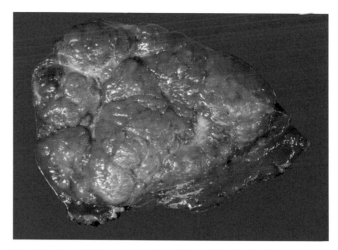

Fig. 9.1. In partial hepatectomies performed for benign lesions, as in this case of focal nodular hyperplasia, excision of uninvolved liver tissue is kept to a minimum, and gross examination is typically sufficient for evaluation of the surgical margins. (Photograph courtesy of William A. Kanner, MD)

resection of a mass is its complete excision, the following caveats apply:

PARTIAL HEPATECTOMY FOR BENIGN LESIONS

In partial hepatectomies performed for benign lesions, excision of uninvolved liver tissue is kept to a minimum, and it is acceptable for the mass to closely approximate the surgical margin.[4] Gross examination is sufficient to evaluate margins on cases of focal nodular hyperplasia and hepatic adenoma, and resections of hemangiomas may not be submitted for IOD because marginal excision* is adequate (Fig. 9.1). If a clear distinction between hepatic adenoma and well-differentiated hepatocellular carcinoma was not possible on pre-operative radiologic evaluation or the original biopsy material, we recommend that the mass be approached as a potential hepatocellular carcinoma with regard to evaluation of surgical margins (see below).

PARTIAL HEPATECTOMY FOR PRIMARY CARCINOMAS OF THE LIVER

The traditional approach to resecting primary carcinomas (i.e. hepatocellular carcinoma, intrahepatic cholangiocarcinoma) is to obtain a margin of benign liver tissue no less than 1 cm around the tumor.[4] However, especially in the resection of large tumors, surgical or clinical factors may dictate a margin of clearance that is <1 cm. Because long-term

* In a marginal excision, the plane of excision is along the "capsule" at the junction of the tumor and normal tissue, without regard to microscopic clearance.

131

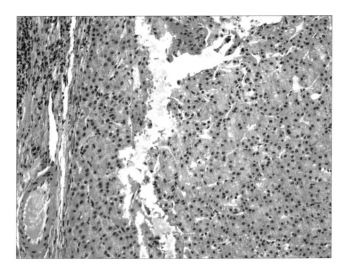

Fig. 9.2. In cases where it is difficult to distinguish between hepatic adenoma and well-differentiated hepatocellular carcinoma, as in this case, a margin of 0.5 cm should be obtained to insure adequate resection even for the more aggressive of these lesions. On permanent sections, this lesion was diagnosed as well-differentiated hepatocellular carcinoma.

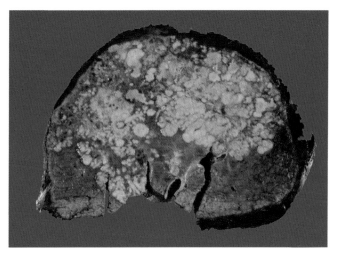

Fig. 9.3. Because hepatocellular carcinoma may be multifocal, the pathologist should carefully examine the partial hepatectomy specimen for previously undetected satellite tumor nodules near the surgical margin. (Photograph courtesy of Elizabeth B. Brunt, MD)

survival has been documented with close margins, the resection of a malignant neoplasm is generally considered adequate even if the tumor is <1 cm from the margin – provided that the margin is negative.[4] Because of the proclivity of hepatocellular carcinoma for intrahepatic spread, a minimal margin of 0.5 cm is recommended to avoid the possibility of micrometastases at the surgical margin, a phenomenon that would increase the risk of local recurrence.[5,6] This point is especially relevant in cases where it is difficult to distinguish between hepatic adenoma and well-differentiated hepatocellular carcinoma (Fig. 9.2). Also, because hepatocellular carcinoma may be multifocal, the pathologist should carefully examine the resection specimen for previously undetected satellite nodules of tumor near the margin (Fig. 9.3). Any suspicious nodules <0.5 cm from the margin should be submitted for IOD. In contrast to hepatocellular carcinoma, intrahepatic cholangiocarcinoma has a propensity to spread along bile ducts; a request for IOD may therefore, include evaluation of the bile duct margin in addition to the hepatic parenchymal margin.[7,8] For discussion of the FS evaluation of the bile duct margin, see p. 137.

PARTIAL HEPATECTOMY FOR METASTATIC COLON CARCINOMA

In partial hepatectomies for metastatic colon carcinoma, studies have shown that the extent of margin clearance – ranging from 0.1 cm to >1 cm – has no influence on the local recurrence rate or overall 5-year survival.[9,10] Only cases with positive surgical margins have a higher local recurrence rate and worse survival. As a result, the excision should be considered adequate even if the margins are close (<1.0 cm).

PARTIAL HEPATECTOMY IN PATIENTS WITH CIRRHOSIS

Many patients with cirrhosis are not suitable candidates for partial hepatectomy because of baseline hepatic dysfunction and the risk of post-operative liver failure due to the limited regenerative capacity of the cirrhotic liver. However, it has been demonstrated that partial hepatectomy for hepatocellular carcinoma can be performed safely in patients with well compensated cirrhosis, defined as a MELD* score <10.[11,12] As in non-cirrhotic patients, the distance of the carcinoma from the margin does not impact prognosis, provided that the margin is free of tumor.[13] The margin of benign tissue at the margin will be modest, because the surgeon will attempt to perform the resection with maximum conservation of non-neoplastic tissue.

HANDLING PARTIAL HEPATECTOMY SPECIMENS FOR EVALUATION OF SURGICAL MARGINS

The first step in the evaluation of the surgical margins in partial hepatectomy specimens is to examine the intact specimen for visible tumor at the margins. The surgical margins should be carefully inked, and the specimen should be "breadloafed" perpendicular to the surgical

---

* The model for end-stage liver disease (MELD) score is used to determine the severity of liver disease, and it is based on serum creatinine, total bilirubin, and INR (international normalized ratio).

(a)
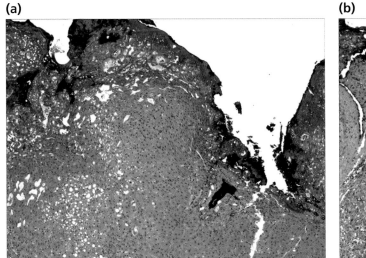

(b)
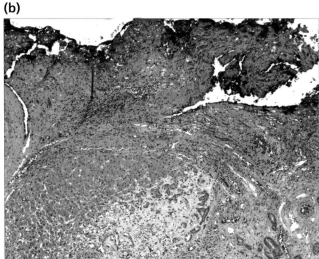

Fig. 9.4. (a) The surgical margin of a partial hepatectomy specimen is an irregular surface with crevices formed by parenchymal protrusions and depressions of variable size. (b) Ink can seep into these crevices making it difficult to determine the location of the true surgical margin, as in this case of intrahepatic cholangiocarcinoma.

margin, using a large knife to obtain full thickness sections of the specimen. The cut surfaces should be examined carefully, and the distance of the closest tumor nodule from the margin should be measured and recorded. If the tumor is close (<0.5 cm) to the margin, or if the status of the margin is in doubt, one or more sections should be taken perpendicular to the margin and submitted for FS evaluation. Sometimes, the surgeon will place a suture to mark an area along the margin that is of particular concern, and this area too, should be sampled for FS.

The appearance of the surgical margin will depend on the surgical technique used to perform the partial hepatectomy. The margin will be irregular when the resection is performed by blunt dissection/finger fracturing, whereas the surface will be smoother when an ultrasound dissector or water jet device is used. If, instead, radiofrequency ablation or bovie electrocautery is used, a zone of cauterized tissue will be present at the margin. Regardless of the resection technique, the surgical margins of a partial hepatectomy specimen will take the form of an irregular surface with crevices formed by parenchymal protrusions and depression of variable size (Fig. 9.4).[5] Awareness of the inherent irregularity of the surface of the margin is crucial when the tumor is close to the margin, because ink will seep into the crevices within the hepatic parenchyma, making it difficult to determine the location of the true surgical margin. In this circumstance, the limitations of the margin evaluation should be clearly communicated to the surgeon.

Intraoperative diagnosis of hepatic lesions

While a variety of mass lesions or nodules may require intraoperative diagnosis, the vast majority can be classified into two morphologic categories: lesions with ductal/glandular differentiation, and lesions with hepatocellular differentiation.

LESIONS WITH DUCTAL/GLANDULAR DIFFERENTIATION

Hepatic lesions with ductal/glandular differentiation include bile duct hamartoma, bile duct adenoma, and metastatic adenocarcinoma. Intrahepatic cholangiocarcinoma also falls into this category, but in the majority of cases, the clinical and imaging studies are characteristic of this neoplasm, allowing the surgeon to proceed with surgical resection without pre-operative or intraoperative histologic confirmation.[14] Accordingly, the usual question on IOD of lesions with ductal/glandular differentiation is to distinguish the benign entities (bile duct hamartoma and bile duct adenoma) from metastatic adenocarcinoma, a distinction that can be challenging on FS.[3,15]

Bile duct hamartoma (also known as von Meyenburg complex) presents as multiple small, whitish nodules scattered throughout the liver.[16] These nodules are composed of a disorderly collection of bile duct structures embedded in abundant fibrous stroma (Fig. 9.5). The duct structures, which are variably dilated and sometimes form microcysts, are lined by a single layer of cytologically bland, low cuboidal or flat epithelium. The lumen often contains bile, a useful diagnostic clue.

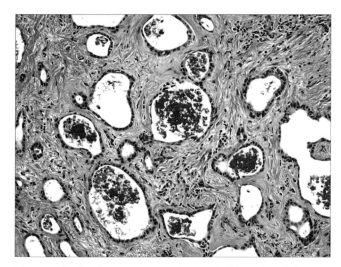

Fig. 9.5. Bile duct hamartomas are characterized by a disorderly collection of variably dilated bile duct structures embedded in abundant fibrous stroma and lined by a single layer of cytologically bland, low cuboidal or flat epithelium. The lumen often contains bile, a useful diagnostic clue.

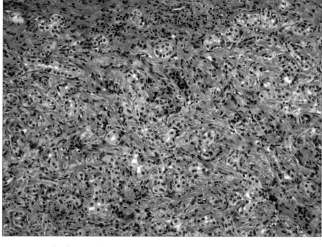

Fig. 9.6. Bile duct adenomas are composed of a well-circumscribed proliferation of small tubular structures with little or no lumen and lined by a single layer of cytologically bland cuboidal epithelium.

Bile duct adenoma is solitary in over 80% of the cases.[16] The lesion is usually <1 cm in diameter, subcapsular in location, and grossly appears as a well-circumscribed wedge-shaped white mass. Microscopically, it is composed of small tubular structures with little or no lumen and lined by a single layer of cytologically bland cuboidal epithelium (Fig. 9.6). Inflammation and/or fibrosis are often present. The clear cell variant of bile duct adenoma may be mistaken for metastatic renal cell carcinoma.[17]

These two benign lesions may be difficult to distinguish from well-differentiated metastatic adenocarcinoma that shows minimal cytologic atypia. The presence of mitotic activity, cellular atypia, and necrosis/apoptosis favors the diagnosis of metastatic adenocarcinoma.[3] This situation is particularly challenging when the patient is scheduled for a major resection for malignancy (e.g., pancreaticoduodenectomy for pancreatic carcinoma), because the resection would be abandoned if the liver biopsy is interpreted as metastatic carcinoma. If a definitive diagnosis cannot be made on FS, the surgeon should be encouraged to explore the rest of the abdomen for metastatic disease, because finding metastases elsewhere will resolve the dilemma.

LESIONS WITH HEPATOCELLULAR DIFFERENTIATION
Well-differentiated hepatocellular lesions include focal nodular hyperplasia (FNH), hepatic adenoma, a macroregenerative nodule of cirrhosis, and well-differentiated hepatocellular carcinoma. The clinical features (patient age, gender, history of oral contraceptive or androgenic steroid use, history of cirrhosis) and the radiographic findings often, but not always, allow differentiation between these entities. However, similar areas may be found in each of these lesions, making it difficult to offer a firm diagnosis, either intraoperatively or after routine processing.[18] Fortunately, in most situations, the intraoperative distinction between the benign entities (FNH and hepatic adenoma) and well-differentiated hepatocellular has limited impact on immediate surgical management, because complete excision with clear margins – a margin of at least 0.5 cm – is considered adequate treatment even for the most aggressive of these lesions, i.e., hepatocellular carcinoma. However, there is a caveat: there are clinical situations when FNH and hepatic adenoma may be managed differently; focal nodular hyperplasia is resected only if the lesion is large (>10 cm), subcapsular or symptomatic, whereas hepatic adenomas are resected regardless of size because of the risk of rupture and rarely, progression to malignancy.[19] When the pre-operative diagnosis is not clear, a needle core biopsy may be submitted for FS evaluation, with a request to distinguish between hepatic adenoma and FNH. If the biopsy sample shows the characteristic features of FNH (fibrous regions containing dystrophic arteries, ductular structures and a lymphocytic infiltrate, combined with nodules of hepatocytes), then the diagnosis of FNH can be made with confidence (Fig. 9.7).[19] However, if the biopsy is from the periphery of a FNH, containing hepatocytes only, or if the FNH is a variant with atypical histologic features (e.g., a paucity of

(a)
(b)

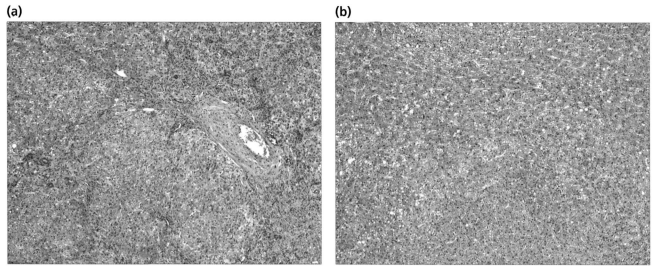

Fig. 9.7. Sampling effect in focal nodular hyperplasia (FNH). (a) If the tissue sample demonstrates the classic features (fibrous regions containing dystrophic arteries, ductular reaction, lymphocytic infiltrate, and nodules of hepatocytes), the diagnosis of FNH can be made. (b) However, if the biopsy is from the periphery of an FNH, thereby sampling predominantly the nodules of hepatocytes, the distinction between hepatic adenoma and FNH may be difficult.

ductal structures), it will be difficult to make the distinction between FNH and hepatic adenoma on limited sampling.[20] In this situation, additional biopsy samples should be requested for FS evaluation in an attempt to make this distinction.

Evaluation of the suitability of a donor liver for transplantation

Clinical issues

In the United States, approximately 6000 liver transplants are currently performed each year for a wide variety of clinical conditions.[21] The decision to use a potential donor liver for transplantation incorporates a variety of factors, many of which are unrelated to the organ itself; however, histologic evaluation of the liver for macrovesicular steatosis helps to exclude those organs associated with a high incidence of severe post-transplant dysfunction.[22,23] Because of the time constraints inherent in the transplant setting, the evaluation for macrovesicular steatosis is performed on a FS of a needle core or wedge biopsy of the donor liver. As such, the most common request for an IOD of a potential donor liver is to evaluate the extent of macrovesicular steatosis.

Pathologic issues

Extensive macrovesicular steatosis of the donor liver carries a significantly increased risk of poor post-transplant function of the allograft, and as a general rule, donor livers with greater than 40% to 50% macrovesicular steatosis are considered unsuitable for transplantation.[23–25] When determining the amount of fat in a potential donor liver, macrovesicular steatosis has to be distinguished from microvesicular steatosis. Microvesicular steatosis, which is common in potential allografts, is a reversible change due to the temporary ischemia inherent to the transplant procedure. While it is well established that macrovesicular steatosis affects allograft function, microvesicular steatosis of any degree, even severe, is not associated with a long-term worse prognosis.[26–28] Since macrovesicular steatosis can be identified readily on the H&E stain of a FS, and because it is relatively easy to misinterpret microvesicular steatosis as macrovesicular steatosis on histochemical stains for fat (such as Oil red O), the extent of macrovesicular steatosis should be assessed on a routine H&E stained FS, not on a fat stained tissue section (Fig. 9.8).[29] This approach helps to avoid the misintrepretation of microvesicular steatosis as macrovesicular steatosis, an error that could result in discarding a useful allograft.

In addition to macrovesicular steatosis, the FS donor liver biopsy should be evaluated for inflammation, fibrosis, necrosis, cholestasis, and bile duct changes. While there are no established criteria, the presence of these features may disqualify the organ as an allograft. Attempts are being made to develop a universal worksheet to standardize the FS evaluation and reporting of donor liver biopsies, but this is not yet available.[30]

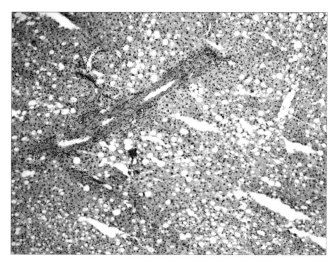

Fig. 9.8. The most common request for an IOD of a potential donor liver is for evaluation of the extent of macrovesicular steatosis. This frozen section of a wedge biopsy demonstrates approximately 30% macrovesicular steatosis.

GALLBLADDER

Clinical issues

Gallbladder cancer is rare, with an estimated rate of 6 to 15 cases per 1000 cholecystectomies. Carcinoma of the gallbladder is notorious for being asymptomatic in its early stages, and when symptoms occur, they are indistinguishable from chronic cholecystitis.[31] Sometimes, however, the clinical features and radiographic features suggest gallbladder carcinoma, and if the tumor appears resectable, a pre-operative biopsy is considered unnecessary.[31]

The surgical treatment of gallbladder carcinoma varies with the tumor stage.* Simple cholecystectomy is recommended for T1a tumors, while T1b, T2, and T3 tumors are treated by radical cholecystectomy, which involves resection of the liver surrounding the gallbladder fossa, and portal lymphadenectomy. Some surgeons advocate opening and inspecting all gallbladders in the operating room after laparoscopic and open cholecystectomy, and to submit the specimen for FS evaluation if the gross findings

are suspicious of gallbladder carcinoma.[32] This approach is valid in specialized medical centers with expertise in major resections of gallbladder malignancies, since a surgical team will be in place to proceed with immediate radical resection if a higher stage carcinoma is diagnosed on FS. However, in non-specialized medical centers, where a surgical team is not available to perform immediate radical surgery, we recommend that the gallbladder be submitted to the laboratory for routine gross and microscopic examination since an IOD of carcinoma will not impact immediate surgical management.

Pathologic issues

Poorly differentiated carcinomas are easily recognized on FS but well-differentiated carcinomas can be challenging. The following points should be kept in mind:

- Well-differentiated polypoid or exophytic carcinomas are difficult to diagnose on FS, but fortunately, many exophytic carcinomas are superficial (T1a), and simple cholecystectomy is the appropriate surgical treatment.
- In the early stages (either T1a or T1b), well differentiated, non-polypoid adenocarcinomas may be difficult to distinguish from dysplasia or reactive atypia in Rokitanski–Aschoff sinuses.
- The diagnosis of carcinoma on FS is more reliable when there is mural invasion, and when the carcinoma is at least stage T2 (Fig. 9.9).[3]
- As described above, the depth of tumor invasion into the gallbladder wall is a critical determinant of the surgical management for gallbladder carcinoma. The distinction on FS between T1 (either T1a or T1b) and T2 tumors however, is notoriously difficult,[33] and for this reason, if the depth of tumor invasion cannot be determined with certainty, this assessment should be deferred to permanent sections. This is particularly relevant when the surgical team is poised to perform radical surgery.
- Gallbladder carcinoma is often accompanied by dysplasia in the cystic duct, so FS evaluation of the cystic duct margin should be performed to ensure that it is free of high-grade dysplasia; if the margin is positive, additional cystic duct or even common bile duct resection may be necessary. For evaluation of bile duct margin, see below.

---

* Gallbladder carcinoma stage: T1a – tumor invades into lamina propria; T1b – tumor invades muscle layer; T2 – tumor invades into extramuscular connective tissue, but no extension beyond the serosa and no invasion into liver; T3 – tumor invades the liver (≤2 cm into liver) or penetrates the serosa and directly invades into an adjacent organ such as duodenum, colon, omentum, etc.

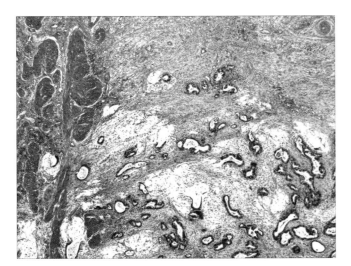

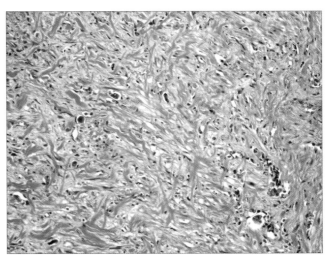

Fig. 9.9. The depth of tumor invasion in gallbladder carcinoma is notoriously difficult to determine on IOD. In this case, the tumor definitely invades through the muscular wall and into the extramuscular connective tissue (stage T2).

Fig. 9.10. Infiltrative cholangiocarcinomas characteristically have an associated desmoplastic response, with only sparse malignant cells scattered within the abundant fibrotic stroma. This feature may result in the tumor cells being overlooked on FS.

EXTRAHEPATIC BILIARY TRACT

Lesions of the proximal extrahepatic biliary tract

Clinical issues

Cholangiocarcinoma of the proximal biliary tract, so-called hilar cholangiocarcinoma or Klatskin tumor, is often unresectable at the time of diagnosis. In cases that are potentially resectable, histological confirmation of malignancy is not required prior to surgical exploration and excision if the clinical and radiographic features support the diagnosis.[14] Segmental bile duct resection and biliary reconstruction are feasible with some tumors, but the majority of cases require partial hepatectomy because the proximal extent of the tumor often involves intrahepatic bile ducts. The pathologist may therefore, be asked to perform FSs to evaluate the intrahepatic bile duct (proximal) margin in addition to the extrahepatic bile duct (distal) margin.[34–36] If portal vein invasion by tumor is suspected, the portal vein margin also will require evaluation.

Pathologic issues

Evaluation of the intrahepatic and extrahepatic bile duct margins is challenging for three main reasons.

- Carcinomas with an infiltrative pattern of growth characteristically evoke an intense inflammatory and/or prominent desmoplastic reaction.[37] When the neoplastic cells are scanty, they may be obscured by the dense

inflammatory infiltrate or overlooked when present within abundant desmoplastic stroma (Fig. 9.10).

- Reactive atypia in benign peri-biliary glands may be mistaken for well differentiated invasive adenocarcinoma.[38] A lobular or circumscribed configuration on low power favors a benign process, whereas an infiltrative pattern of growth supports the diagnosis of malignancy (Fig. 9.11).

- Instrumentation and the placement of stents in the intrahepatic and extrahepatic bile ducts may produce reactive changes in the surface epithelium that are marked enough to mimic high-grade dysplasia.[34,38] Marked nuclear enlargement, nuclear irregularities, hyperchromasia, loss of polarity, mitotic figures, apoptotic cells, and intraluminal necrosis favor high-grade dysplasia over a reactive process (Fig. 9.12). Sometimes, however, there is significant morphologic overlap between reactive atypia and dysplasia, requiring deferral to permanent sections. This is a difficult situation because the IOD will determine whether or not to remove additional bile duct tissue. Close communication between surgeon and pathologist is imperative, so that a joint decision can be made about the best way to handle this dilemma.

Lesions of the distal extrahepatic biliary tract, ampulla, and periampullary region

The ampulla of Vater and surrounding periampullary region is a small, but anatomically complex site that includes the distal common bile duct, the main pancreatic

(a)

(b)

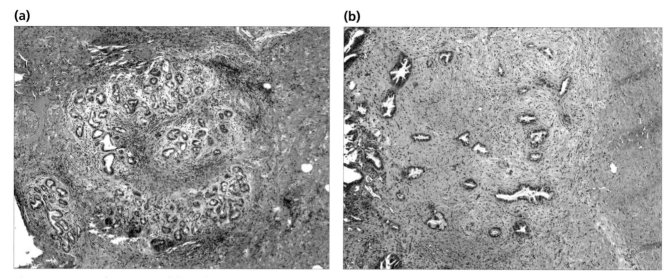

Fig. 9.11. Reactive changes in peribiliary glands in the wall of extrahepatic bile ducts can mimic invasive adenocarcinoma. A lobular or circumscribed configuration favors a benign process, whereas an infiltrative pattern of growth supports the diagnosis of malignancy. (a) Peribiliary glands with reactive atypia. (b) Invasive adenocarcinoma.

(a)

(b)

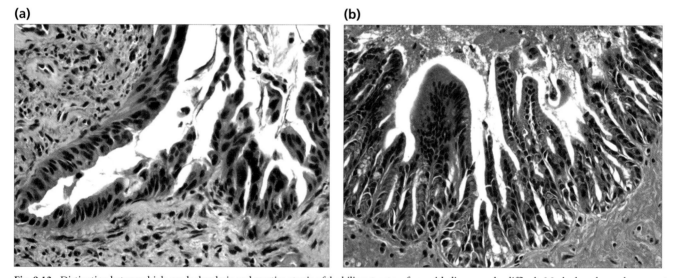

Fig. 9.12. Distinction between high-grade dysplasia and reactive atypia of the biliary tract surface epithelium may be difficult. Marked nuclear enlargement, hyperchromasia, loss of polarity, and mitotic figures favor high-grade dysplasia. (a) High-grade dysplasia. (b) Reactive atypia.

duct, the duodenum, pancreas, and the ampulla itself. This close proximity may make it difficult to determine the exact site of origin of tumors in this location until examination of the resection specimen.[39] One series of 443 resected carcinomas from this region demonstrated the following distribution: pancreas 63%, ampulla 16%, distal common bile duct 15%, and perivaterian duodenum 6%.[40] In patients with potentially resectable tumors, a tissue diagnosis is not required prior to surgery if the clinical and radiographic features are suspicious for malignancy.[39] The typical surgical procedure is a pancreaticoduodenectomy, and the bile duct margin and the

pancreatic neck margin are regularly submitted for FS. The handling of specimens from the bile duct and pancreatic margins is discussed in Chapter 10, p. 144).

REFERENCES

1. Ros PR, Mortele KJ. Hepatic imaging: an overview. *Clin Liver Dis* 2002; **6**: 1–16.
2. Choi BI, Lee JM. Neoplasms of the gallbladder and biliary tract. In *Textbook of Gastrointestinal Radiology*, Gore RM, Levine MS, (eds) 3rd edn, Saunders/Elsevier, 2008.
3. Lechago J. Frozen section examination of the liver, gallbladder and pancreas. *Arch Pathol Lab Med* 2005; **129**: 1610–1618.

4. Blumgart LH, Belghiti J. Liver resection for benign disease and for liver and biliary tumors. In *Surgery of the Liver, Biliary Tract, and Pancreas*, ed. LH Blumgart. Saunders/Elsevier, 4th edn, 2007.

5. Zimmerman A. Tumors of the liver – pathologic aspects. In *Surgery of the Liver, Biliary Tract, and Pancreas*, Blumgart LH, (ed.) 4th edn, Saunders/Elsevier, 2007.

6. Lai EC, Ng IO, You KT, *et al*. Hepatectomy for larger hepatocellular carcinomas: the optimal resection margin. *World J Surg* 1991; **15**: 141–145.

7. Uenishi T, Hirohashi K, Yamamoto T, *et al*. Clinicopathologic factors predicting outcome after resection of mass-forming intrahepatic cholangiocarcinoma. *Br J Surg* 2001; **88**: 969–974.

8. Hirohashi K, Uenishi T, Kube S, *et al*. Histologic bile duct invasion by a mass-forming intrahepatic cholangiocarcinoma. *J Hepatobiliary Pancreat Surg* 2002; **9**: 233–236.

9. Pawlik TM, Scoggins CR, Zorzi D, *et al*. Effect of surgical margin status on survival and site of recurrence after hepatic resection for colorectal metastases. *Ann Surg* 2005; **241**: 715.

10. Are C, Gonen M, Zazzali K, *et al*. The impact of margins on outcome after hepatic resection for colorectal metastasis. *Ann Surg* 2007; **246**: 295.

11. Llovet JM, Fuster J, Bruix J. Intention-to-treat analysis of surgical treatment for early hepatocellular carcinoma: resection versus transplantation. *Hepatology* 1999; **30**: 1434–1440.

12. Teh SH, Christein J, Donohue J, *et al*. Hepatic resection of hepatocellular carcinoma in patients with cirrhosis: model of end-stage liver disease (MELD) score predicts perioperative mortality. *J Gastrointest Surg* 2005; **9**. 1207–1215.

13. Ochiai T, Takayama T, Inoue K, *et al*. Hepatic resection with and without surgical margins for hepatocellular carcinoma in patients with impaired liver function. *Hepato-Gastroenterol* 1999; **46**: 1885–1889.

14. Jarnagin WR, D'Angelica M, Blumgart LH. Intrahepatic and extrahepatic biliary cancer. In *Surgery of the Liver, Biliary Tract, and Pancreas*, Blumgart LH. (ed.) 4th edn, Saunders/Elsevier, 2007.

15. Rakha E, Ramaiah S, McGregor A. Accuracy of frozen section in the diagnosis of liver mass lesions. *J Clin Pathol* 2006; **59**: 352–354.

16. Rosai J. Liver: Tumor and tumorlike conditions. In Rosai and Ackerman's *Surgical Pathology*, Rosai J. (ed.) 8th edn, Mosby, 2004.

17. Albores-Saavedra J, Hoang MP, Murakata LA, *et al*. Atypical bile duct adenoma, clear cell type. *Am J Surg Pathol* 2001; **25**: 956–960.

18. Snover D. Neoplasms and other mass lesions of the liver. In *Biopsy Diagnosis of Liver Disease*, Snover D. (ed). Williams and Wilkins, 1992.

19. Bioulac-Sage P, Balabaud C, Bedossa P, *et al*. Pathologic diagnosis of liver cell adenoma and focal nodular hyperplasia: Bordeaux update. *J Hepatol* 2007; **46**: 521–527.

20. Nguyen BN, Flejou JF, Terris B, *et al*. Focal nodular hyperplasia of the liver: a comprehensive pathologic study of 305 lesion and recognition of new histologic forms. *Am J Surg Pathol* 1999; **23**: 1441–1454.

21. cited; Available from: http://www.optn.org/.

22. Starzl TE, Miller CM, Broznick B, *et al*. An improved technique for multiple organ harvesting. *Surg Gynecol Obstet* 1987; **165**: 343–348.

23. Markin RS, Wisecarver JL, Radio SJ, *et al*. Frozen section evaluation of donor livers before transplantaion. *Transplantation* 1993; **56**: 1403–1409.

24. Selzner M, Clavien P-A. Fatty liver in liver transplantation and surgery. *Sem Liver Dis* 2001; **21**: 105–113.

25. Perez-Daga JA, Santoyo J, Suarez MA, *et al*. Influence of the degree of hepatic steatosis on graft function and postoperative complications of liver transplantation. *Transplant Proc* 2006; **38**: 2468–2470.

26. Crowley H, Lewis WD, Gordon F, *et al*. Steatosis in donor and transplant liver biopsies. *Hum Pathol* 2000; **31**: 1209–1213.

27. Zamboni F, Franchello A, David E, *et al*. Effect of macrovesicular and other donor and recipient characteristics on the outcome of liver transplantation. *Transplant* 2001; **15**: 53–57.

28. Fishbein TM, Fiel MI, Emre S, *et al*. Use of livers with microvesicular fat safely expands the donor pool. *Transplantation* 1997; **64**: 248–251.

29. Iezzoni JC. Diagnostic histochemistry in hepatic pathology. In *Diagnostic Histochemistry*. Wick MR. ed. Human Press/Oxford University Press, 2008.

30. Lo IJ, Lefkowitch JH, Feirt N, *et al*. Utility of liver allograft biopsy obtained at procurement. *Liver Transpl* 2008; **14**: 639–646.

31. D'angelica M, Jarnagin WR. Tumors of the gallbladder. In *Surgery of the Liver, Biliary Tract, and Pancreas*, Blumgart LH (ed.) 4th edn, Saunders/Elsevier, 2007.

32. Romano F, Franciosi C, Caprotti R, *et al*. Gallbladder carcinoma and laproscopic cholecystecomy: an emergent problem. *Minerva Chir* 2000; **55**: 817–822.

33. Yamaguchi K, Chijiiwa K, Saiki S, *et al*. Reliability of frozen section diagnosis of gallbladder tumor for detecting carcinoma and depth of its invasion. *J Surg Oncol* 1997; **65**: 132–136.

34. Endo I, House MG, Klimstra DS, *et al*. Clinical signficance of intraoperative bile duct margin assessment for hilar cholangiocarcinoma. *Ann Surg Oncol* 2008; **15**: 2104–2112.

35. Okazaki Y, Horimi T, Kotaka M, *et al*. Study of the intrahepatic surgical margin of hilar bile duct carcinoma. *Hepato-Gastroenterol* 2002; **49**: 625–627.

36. Wakai T, Shirai Y, Moroda T, *et al*. Impact of ductal resection margin status on long-term survival in patients undergoing resection for extrahepatic cholangiocarcinoma. *Cancer* 2005; **103**: 1210–1216.

37. Bosma A. Surgical pathology of cholangiocarcinoma of the liver hilus (Klatskin tumor). *Semin Liver Dis* 1990; **10**: 85–90.

38. Adsay NV, Klimstra DS. Tumors of the bile ducts – Pathologic aspects. In *Surgery of the Liver, Biliary Tract, and Pancreas*, Blumgart LH, (ed.) 4th edn, Saunders/Elsevier. 2007.

39. Nakakura EK, Yeo CJ. Periampullary and pancreatic cancer. In *Surgery of the Liver, Biliary Tract, and Pancreas*, Blumgart LH, (ed.) Saunders/Elsevier, 4th edn, 2007.

40. Yeo CJ, Cameron JL, Sohn TA, *et al*. Six hundred fifty consecutive pancreaticoduodenectomies in the 1990s: pathology, complications, and outcomes. *Ann Surg* 1997; **226**: 248–260.

10 PANCREAS

Ralph H. Hruban, Jon M. Davison, Richard D. Schulick, Karen M. Horton,
Elliot K. Fishman, and Syed Z. Ali

INTRODUCTION

Large numbers of surgeons are being trained with expertise in pancreatic surgery, the only effective therapy for neoplasms of the pancreas. As a result, surgical pathologists are encountering a growing number of pancreatic specimens. These frequently require intraoperative consultation, the results of which can have a dramatic impact on patient management. A rational approach to intraoperative consultation of pancreatic specimens is therefore a critical part of the armamentarium of all practicing surgical pathologists.[1]

The fundamental clinical questions that have to be addressed are:

- Is the lesion neoplastic or non-neoplastic? If the lesion is neoplastic, surgical resection is almost always the best treatment. In contrast, non-neoplastic lesions, such as pseudocysts are often managed medically or simply drained.
- If the lesion is neoplastic, what type of neoplasm is it? The answer to this question not only has profound prognostic significance, but also impacts the surgical management of the patient. For example, a patient may benefit from the surgical resection of a well-differentiated pancreatic endocrine neoplasm that has metastasized to the liver, but there is little, if any, clinical value in resecting an adenocarcinoma of the pancreas that has metastasized to distant sites.
- If the lesion has been resected, are the margins free of tumor? Curative resection requires clear margins, and it is obviously much easier to remove additional pancreatic tissue from an involved margin at the time of initial surgery, than to re-explore the patient at a later date. Accurate intraoperative interpretation of margins is therefore critical.

Because of the diversity of clinical situations that may be encountered during surgery, clear communication between the surgeon and surgical pathologist is essential for quality patient care.

INDICATIONS FOR INTRAOPERATIVE CONSULTATION

The indications for intraoperative consultations are natural extensions of the fundamental clinical questions that need to be addressed, and include:

1. To render a diagnosis that will determine the type of surgery.
2. To evaluate an extrapancreatic lesion, such as a liver nodule, to determine the resectability of a pancreatic neoplasm.
3. To determine the status of the surgical margins.

INFORMATION NEEDED BEFORE AND DURING INTRAOPERATIVE CONSULTATION

Clinical and radiological findings help to define the intraoperative issues that have to be addressed, and in some instances, they can significantly narrow the differential diagnosis for a lesion. The information needed for an efficient intraoperative consultation includes:

- The age and gender of the patient. For example, pancreatoblastoma should be considered in a child, solid-pseudopapillary neoplasm in a woman in her twenties, and pancreatic adenocarcinoma in an elderly patient,[1]

Intraoperative Consultation in Surgical Pathology, ed. Mahendra Ranchod. Published by Cambridge University Press.
© Cambridge University Press 2010.

Table 10.1. Cystic neoplasms of the pancreas

	Mucinous cystic neoplasm	Intraductal papillary mucinous neoplasm	Solid-pseudopapillary neoplasm	Serous cystic neoplasm
Gender (F:M)	20:1	1:1.5	10:1	7:3
Head/tail	Tail	Head	Tail = head	Tail = head
Relation to duct	None	Always	None	None
Central scar	None	None	None	Often, may be calcified
Cyst contents	Mucinous	Mucinous	Necrotic/Hemorrhagic	Serous
Epithelium	Mucinous	Mucinous	Poorly cohesive	Glycogen-rich
Stroma	Ovarian type	Non-specific	Delicate vessels	Non-specific

$^{+}$ Reprinted with permission of the American Registry of Pathology. From the Fourth Series Fascicle on Tumors of the Pancreas.[1]

- The results of imaging studies. In particular, which part(s) of the pancreas does the lesion involve, is the lesion solid or cystic, and does the lesion involve the larger pancreatic ducts? As shown in Table 10.1, the correct diagnosis of a cystic neoplasm of the pancreas can almost be established on clinical grounds alone.[1]
- The results of relevant laboratory tests, particularly cancer antigens (such as CA 19–9), serum IgG4 levels, and, if the patient is suspected of having an endocrine neoplasm, blood hormone levels (e.g., insulin). For example, significantly elevated serum IgG4 levels suggest the diagnosis of autoimmune/lymphoplasmacytic sclerosing pancreatitis.[2]
- The results of pre-operative biopsy or cytologic studies, and any history of extra-pancreatic neoplasms. For example, the presence of single prominent nucleoli in a neoplasm may suggest the diagnosis of an acinar cell carcinoma, but the same finding in a patient with a history of deeply invasive melanoma should also raise the possibility of melanoma metastatic to the pancreas.
- The patient's family history, particularly any family history of an inherited neoplasia syndrome. For example, patients with multiple endocrine neoplasia, type 1 (MEN1), often have multiple pancreatic endocrine microadenomas, a finding that can confuse the interpretation of a margin if one is not aware of the patient's syndrome.

It is unwise for a pathologist to undertake intraoperative consultation on a pancreatic specimen without being familiar with the clinical and imaging facts of the case. It is prudent to discuss the case with the surgeon before or during surgery, and to be familiar with the surgeon's operative plan.

ALGORITHMIC APPROACH

An algorithmic approach to the diagnosis of pancreatic lesions was presented by David Klimstra in the fourth edition of the *Fascicle on Tumors of the Pancreas*.[1] We find this approach extremely practical and worth repeating here (Fig. 10.1).

The first distinction to be made in this algorithm is between grossly solid and grossly cystic lesions (Fig. 10.2). If the lesion is solid, the relative contributions of stroma and epithelium to the mass should be evaluated, and lesions with few individual glands and abundant stroma should be distinguished from lesions with abundant epithelium and little stroma (Fig. 10.3). The major differential diagnosis for solid lesions composed of a few glands admixed with abundant stroma is between chronic pancreatitis and infiltrating adenocarcinoma of the pancreas, while acinar cell carcinoma, pancreatoblastoma, pancreatic endocrine neoplasm and the solid-pseudopapillary neoplasm should be considered if the lesion is solid and composed of abundant epithelium with little stroma.

The first step in evaluating grossly cystic lesions with an epithelial lining is to determine if the epithelium is serous (cuboidal with clear cytoplasm) or mucinous (Table 10.1). If the epithelium is serous, then the lesion is most likely a serous cystic neoplasm. If the epithelium contains large amounts of mucin, then the differential diagnosis should include the mucinous cystic neoplasm and an intraductal papillary mucinous neoplasm. Mucinous cystic neoplasms do not connect to the larger pancreatic ducts and they have a distinctive type of ovarian stroma, while intraductal papillary mucinous neoplasms arise within the larger ducts and lack a distinctive stroma.

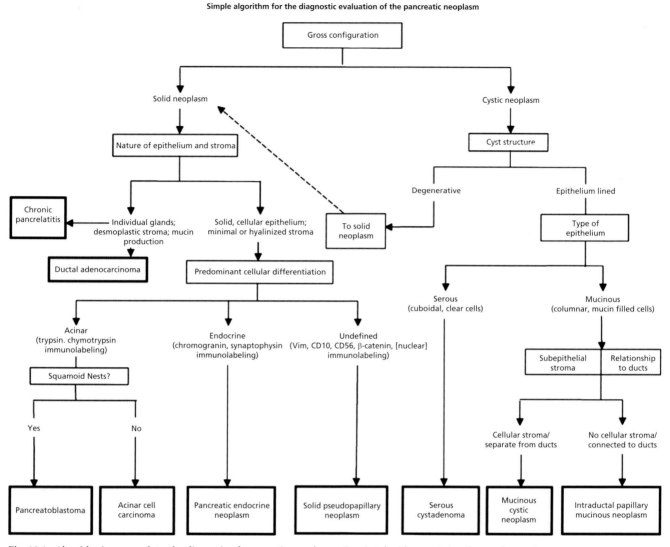

Fig. 10.1. Algorithmic approach to the diagnosis of pancreatic neoplasms. Reprinted with permission from reference 1.

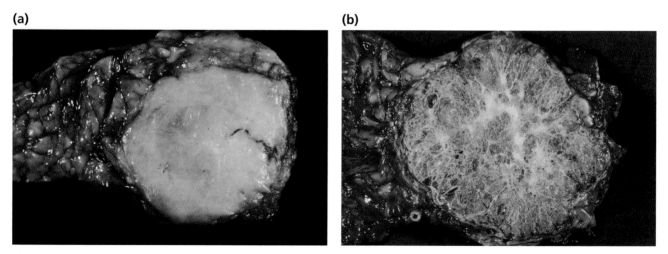

Fig. 10.2. Cross-sections of solid and cystic pancreatic neoplasms. (a) This solid neoplasm is a well-differentiated endocrine neoplasm. (b) This cystic lesion is a serous cystadenoma.

(a) **(b)**

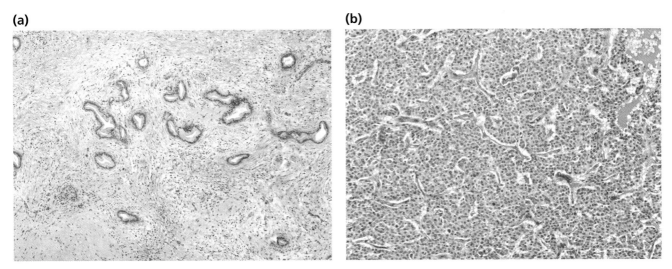

Fig. 10.3. (a) Histological sections of a sparsely cellular neoplasm with abundant stroma and (b) a cellular neoplasm with little stroma. The sparsely cellular neoplasm is an invasive ductal adenocarcinoma, the cellular neoplasm a well-differentiated pancreatic endocrine neoplasm.

While this simple algorithmic approach can be extremely helpful in narrowing down the differential diagnosis, a deeper understanding of the diagnostic criteria for each of the major entities in the pancreas is needed to arrive at a definitive diagnosis. In the following sections we provide brief overviews of the major diagnostic entities.

SPECIFIC CLINICO-PATHOLOGIC ISSUES

Pancreatic adenocarcinoma

Infiltrating adenocarcinoma of the pancreas, also known as "pancreatic cancer," is one of the deadliest of all of the solid malignancies.[3] Surgical resection is the best hope to prolong life, yet pancreatic surgery is technically complex and the interpretation of the pathology can be treacherous. It is not surprising therefore, that surgical resection of an adenocarcinoma of the pancreas requires close co-operation between surgeons and pathologists.

Clinical issues
The single most important clinical issue for a patient with a solid mass lesion in the pancreas is determining if the lesion is cancer or not. Clinically, chronic pancreatitis can mimic pancreatic cancer and yet the prognosis and treatment of patients with chronic pancreatitis differ dramatically from those of pancreatic cancer. The distinction between chronic pancreatitis and pancreatic cancer is particularly important in patients without a preoperative tissue or cytologic diagnosis. While many surgeons will

surgically resect pancreatic mass lesions without confirmatory tissue/cytologic diagnosis, the extent of the surgery will often depend on the underlying pathology.

After a diagnosis is established, the next step is to localize the lesion. Most pancreatic cancers arise in the head of the gland, and carcinomas that arise in the head of the gland, because they typically obstruct the bile duct and produce the clinically apparent sign of jaundice, are more often resectable than are carcinomas that arise in the body or tail of the gland. Carcinomas in the head of the gland are usually resected by a pancreatoduodenectomy, while those that arise in the tail by a distal pancreatectomy with splenectomy.

Once the neoplasm has been diagnosed and localized, the next step is to determine if the lesion is surgically resectable. Pancreatic cancers which locally invade a critical structure, such as the celiac artery, are deemed unresectable, as are cancers that have metastasized to distant organs not included in the resection. There is little benefit and significant operative morbidity associated with resecting adenocarcinomas of the pancreas that have metastasized to distant organs. By contrast, surgery is often performed if metastases to regional lymph nodes included in the standard resection are identified. Common sites of metastases include lymph nodes, the liver, lung, adrenal glands and peritoneal surfaces.[1] Modern imaging technologies, such as 64-slice CT scanning, detect most of these metastases preoperatively, but small metastases may only be identified or suspected at the time of abdominal exploration. Before embarking on resection of the pancreas, the surgeon will carefully explore the peritoneal cavity and submit biopsies of any suspect lesions for frozen section (FS) evaluation.

The presence of invasive carcinoma at a surgical margin is a significant negative prognostic indicator, and the surgeon will therefore request FS evaluation of surgical margins. As noted earlier, if invasive carcinoma extends to involve a margin, it is much easier to excise an additional portion of pancreatic parenchyma from the involved margin at the time of initial surgery than to subject the patient to a second surgical procedure. The main margins for a pancreatoduodenectomy are the uncinate margin (retroperitoneal margin), the pancreatic neck margin, the bile duct margin, and the proximal and distal bowel margins.

If a pancreatic carcinoma is found to be unresectable at the time of surgical exploration, a core biopsy or fine needle aspiration (FNA) biopsy will be submitted for intraoperative diagnosis (IOD) to confirm the diagnosis, and if the patient has obstructive jaundice, a palliative procedure – such as a cholejejunostomy – will be performed.

Pathologic issues
The major issues for the pathologist parallel the clinical issues.[4]

- Is the lesion cancer or chronic pancreatitis? Both chronic pancreatitis and pancreatic cancer can produce solid masses composed of a few glands admixed with abundant stroma. As listed in Table 10.2, features supporting the diagnosis of pancreatic cancer on FS include: haphazardly arranged glands, glands immediately adjacent to muscular vessels, vascular invasion, perineural invasion, incomplete lumina, luminal necrosis, and significant variation in nuclear area in a single gland (the "4 to 1 rule") (Fig. 10.4).[1,4–6] Cytologic features of malignancy on FNA include nuclear crowding and overlapping, nuclear contour irregularity, and irregular chromatin distribution. Additional "minor criteria" of malignancy on FNA include nuclear enlargement, single epithelial cells, necrosis, and mitoses.

- Has the carcinoma spread to the liver? Bile duct adenomas and bile duct hamartomas can both mimic metastases to the liver (Fig. 10.5). As listed in Table 10.3, the number of lesions, the size of the lesions, the shape and spacing of the glands, the nuclear morphology, the stroma and the presence or absence of bile and mucin are all useful diagnostic features. Even when the criteria listed in Table 10.3 are rigorously applied, it can sometimes be impossible to arrive at a definitive diagnosis

Table 10.2. Ductal adenocarcinoma versus chronic pancreatitis[+]

	Carcinoma	Pancreatitis
Arrangement of the glands	Haphazard	Lobular
Nuclear size	Varies >4:1 or more in a single gland	Uniform
Luminal necrosis	May be present	Absent
Incomplete glands	May be present	Absent
Perineural invasion	May be present	Absent
Vascular invasion	May be present	Absent
Glands immediately adjacent to muscular artery	May be present	Absent

[+] Reprinted with permission of the American Registry of Pathology. From the Fourth Series Fascicle on Tumors of the Pancreas.[1]

intraoperatively. In these instances clear communication between the pathologist and surgeon is critical. Our bias has been to give the patient the "benefit of the doubt" and to proceed with the resection unless a definitive diagnosis of metastatic carcinoma can be established intraoperatively.

- Has the carcinoma spread to other intra-abdominal sites, such as lymph nodes and peritoneum? Biopsies from these sites should be evaluated thoroughly because the IOD may determine if the surgeon will proceed with pancreatic resection. Cytologic preparations can aide in the diagnosis, especially if the biopsy contains a lot of fat, so remember to prepare the appropriate smears before the tissue is submitted for FS. After any cytologic preparations are made, the entire biopsy should be submitted for FS evaluation. Multiple levels of the FS block should be prepared routinely. Unless otherwise indicated, tissue should not be intentionally spared for permanent sections. If the patient has distant metastases, the goal is to detect them intraoperatively and not after the patient has been closed.

- Does the invasive carcinoma extend to a margin? In contrast with our bias to err on under calling distant metastases on intraoperative consultation, our bias has been to slightly "overcall" margins unless it means the patient will have a total pancreatectomy. We do this because it is much easier to resect additional pancreatic tissue at the time of surgery than it is to re-explore the patient. Intraoperatively, the most important margins for a pancreatoduodenectomy include:

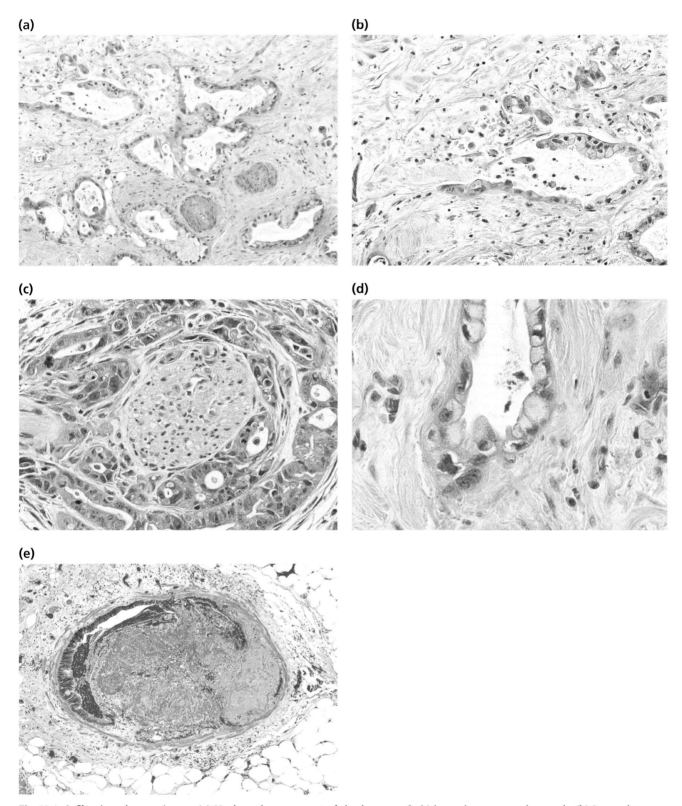

Fig. 10.4. Infiltrating adenocarcinoma. (a) Haphazard arrangement of glands, some of which are close to muscular vessels. (b) Incomplete lumina are a feature of invasive adenocarcinoma. (c) Perineural invasion. (d) The "4 to 1" rule with the area of one nucleus exceeding four times the area of other nuclei in the same gland. (e) Vascular invasion.

Table 10.3. Benign liver lesions versus metastatic ductal adenocarcinoma

	Bile Duct Hamartoma	Bile Duct Adenoma	Reactive Bile Ductular Proliferation	Metastatic Ductal Adenocarcinoma
Size	1–3 mm	1–20 mm	Variable	Variable
Number	May be multiple	Usually solitary	Variable	Usually solitary
Gland spacing	Regular	Regular	Variable; May be lobular	Irregular
Gland shape	Ectatic	Tubular/Acinar	Tubular/Acinar	Irregular
Luminal bile	Present	Absent	Absent	Absent
Nuclear morphology	Bland	Mildly atypical	Reactive features	Moderately to markedly atypical
Stroma	Hyalinized	Hyalinized/Inflamed	Variable	Desmoplastic
Cytoplasmic mucin	Absent	May be present	Absent	Often present

[+] Reprinted with permission of the American Registry of Pathology. From the Fourth Series Fascicle on Tumors of the Pancreas.[1]

(a) **(b)**

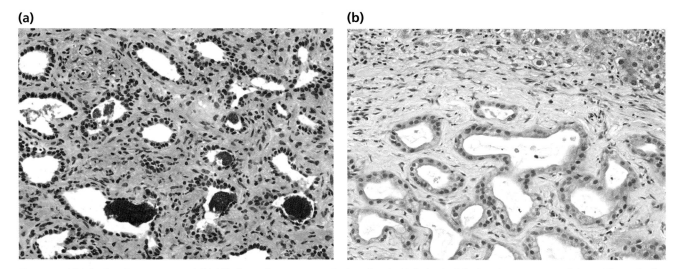

Fig. 10.5. (a) Bile duct hamartoma and (b) bile duct adenoma. Note the intraluminal bile in the bile duct hamartoma and the uniform glands without atypia in the adenoma.

■ *The pancreatic neck margin.* We like to take this as a 2–3 mm thick shave section parallel to the margin so that the entire margin surface can be evaluated in a single section. If the actual margin is severely cauterized, this section can be embedded such that the true margin is deep in the block and the non-cauterized, and therefore, evaluable parenchyma, is sectioned for frozen section evaluation. Deeper sections moving towards the true margin can always be taken if carcinoma is identified in these initial sections.

■ *The uncinate margin.* The surgeon may request intraoperative evaluation of this margin, but because this area of the pancreas abuts the mesenteric vessels, the surgeon is usually unable to remove more tissue if the margin is reported as positive. We typically take a section perpendicular to the margin, either

from the area designated by the surgeon or by feeling and looking for the point at which the lesion most closely approaches this margin. If this margin is not evaluated intraoperatively, it should certainly be evaluated during later, more comprehensive examination of the resected specimen.

■ *The bile duct margin.* The bile duct margin may be submitted separately by the surgeon, or it may be part of the resection specimen. This margin is best taken as a shave section parallel to the proximal margin.

■ *The proximal and distal bowel margins.* The distal bowel margin is usually so far from the neoplasm that there is little value in evaluating this margin intraoperatively. We do not routinely evaluate the proximal margin intraoperatively if it is grossly unremarkable and grossly clear of tumor. Nonetheless, we do have a

(a)   **(b)**

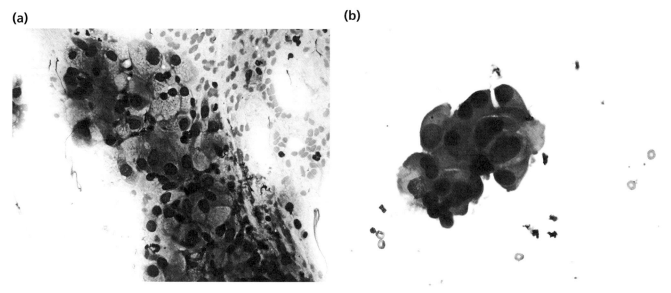

Fig. 10.6. Ductal adenocarcinoma. (a) A loosely cohesive group of ductal cells with prominent anisonucleosis, occasional macronucleoli and a disorganized architecture. (b) A small fragment of tumor cells with high N/C ratios and a prominent variation in nuclear size and shape. (Diff Quik stains)

very low threshold for freezing this margin, as it is one of the margins for which it is relatively easy for the surgeon to take additional tissue.

The major *intraoperative* margin for a distal pancreatectomy is the proximal pancreatic parenchymal margin.

When evaluating pancreatic tumors, cytologic preparations should be used in addition to frozen sections. As we will show throughout this chapter, a touch preparation made from the cut surface of a neoplasm can be invaluable in establishing the direction of differentiation of the neoplasm (Fig. 10.6).

Lymphoplasmacytic sclerosing pancreatitis

Lymphoplasmacytic sclerosing pancreatitis deserves special note because in some instances this entity cannot be clinically distinguished from invasive pancreatic cancer.[1]

Clinical issues

Most patients with lymphoplasmacytic sclerosing pancreatitis have elevated serum IgG4 levels, leading some to suggest that all patients with a provisional diagnosis of pancreatic cancer should have their serum IgG4 levels tested.[2] Lymphoplasmacytic sclerosing pancreatitis can produce a mass lesion, but it usually produces diffuse enlargement of the head of the gland on imaging.[7] Most

patients respond well to steroid therapy, but unfortunately, the diagnosis is not always made pre-operatively and the lesion is resected because it mimics a carcinoma.

Pathologic issues

The lesion is characterized by a duct-centric mixed inflammatory cell infiltrate and there is often an associated venulitis (Fig. 10.7).[1] At times there is a spindle cell proliferation similar to plasma cell granuloma of the lung. The fibrosis and inflammation can extend beyond the gland, mimicking a particularly aggressive pancreatic neoplasm. When performing frozen sections of the margins, a dense lymphoplasmacytic infiltrate at the pancreatic parenchymal and bile duct margins may suggest the diagnosis of lymphoplasmacytic sclerosing pancreatitis, but we usually reserve making a definitive diagnosis until the entire case has been reviewed on permanent sections, and the presence of an invasive cancer has been ruled out.

Acinar carcinoma

Acinar carcinomas are relatively rare, but they are important to recognize because of their distinct clinical features, pathology, and treatment.

Clinical issues

Fifteen percent of patients with an acinar carcinoma present with the syndrome of metastatic fat necrosis

(a)

(b)

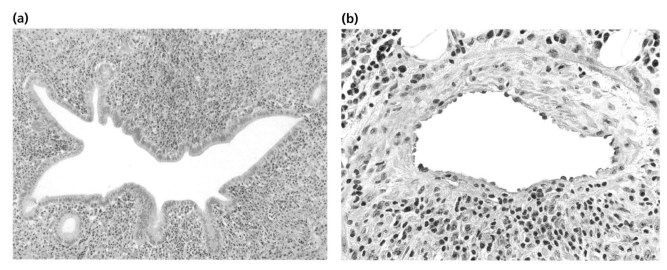

Fig. 10.7. Lymphoplasmacytic sclerosing pancreatitis. (a) Note the duct-centric inflammatory infiltrate and (b) the venulitis.

characterized by multiple foci of fat necrosis, blood eosinophilia, polyarthralgias, and elevated serum lipase levels.[1] This clinical syndrome can be a clue to the diagnosis, and portends a poor prognosis. The majority of acinar carcinomas however, do not have distinctive clinical features and present in the same way as conventional pancreatic ductal adenocarcinomas. Serum alpha-fetoprotein levels are often elevated in acinar carcinomas and this can be used to support the diagnosis as well as track response of the neoplasm to treatment.

The surgical approach is the same as for pancreatic ductal adenocarcinoma. The presence of intra-abdominal fat necrosis may mimic metastatic carcinoma and prompt biopsies for intraoperative consultation.

Pathologic issues

The neoplastic cells usually form small lumina, similar to non-neoplastic acini, with basally placed nuclei and granular apical cytoplasm.[8] Despite the name, acinar carcinomas often do not form well-developed acinar structures. In a significant fraction of cases the neoplastic cells form solid sheets of cells. Single prominent nucleoli are characteristic and are a clue to the diagnosis (Fig. 10.8). Cytologic examination with touch preparations can be very helpful in making the diagnosis (Fig. 10.9). "Naked" neoplastic nuclei (nuclei stripped of their cytoplasm) in touch preparations are a clue to the diagnosis; if the cytoplasm is intact, the neoplastic cells are surprisingly bland, polygonal, with a low nuclear to cytoplasmic ratio and uniform nuclei with single prominent nucleoli.

Because they both form solid cellular neoplasms, acinar cell carcinoma can be confused with the well-differentiated

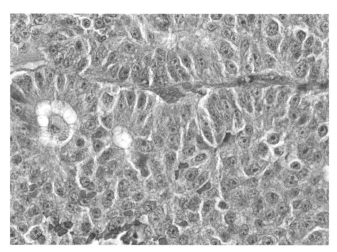

Fig. 10.8. Acinar cell carcinoma. Granular cytoplasm, polarization around small lumina, and single prominent nucleoli are clues to the diagnosis.

pancreatic endocrine neoplasms (islet cell tumor). This distinction can become an issue intraoperatively, because the surgeon may be more aggressive in resecting a metastatic well-differentiated pancreatic endocrine neoplasm. In these instances the nuclear features described above can be extremely helpful.

Peritoneal biopsies of fat necrosis may be submitted by the surgeon with a clinical diagnosis of metastatic carcinoma. Be on guard to not over-interpret the cellular phase of fat necrosis as carcinoma.

Pancreatic endocrine neoplasms

Well-differentiated pancreatic endocrine neoplasms, previously known as "islet cell tumors," are "functional," or "syndromic," when associated with clinical syndromes

(a)

(b)

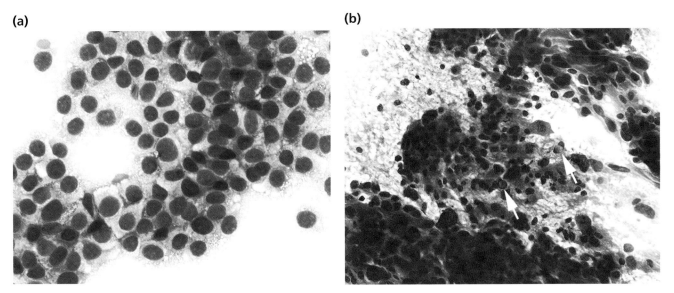

Fig. 10.9. Acinar carcinoma. (a) Loosely cohesive neoplastic cells with faintly basophilic and granular cytoplasm. The neoplastic cells have a fragile cytoplasm, which is easily stripped off resulting in occasional naked nuclei. (b) Pleomorphic tumor cells with marked variation in nuclear size and shape. The cells have a granular cytoplasm and nuclei show occasional well-formed pseudoinclusions (arrows). (Diff Quik and H&E stains)

caused by the production and release of endocrine hormones by the neoplasm, and "non-functional," or "non-syndromic." when they are not associated with a clinical syndrome.[1] The clinical syndrome, multiple endocrine neoplasia, type 1 (MEN1), is associated with multiple endocrine neoplasms of the pancreas, parathyroid glands, pituitary, and gastrointestinal tract.

Clinical issues

Three main questions have to be answered when a well-differentiated endocrine neoplasm is considered in the diagnosis: (a) Is the neoplasm functional or non-functional?; (b) is the tumor sporadic or associated with MEN 1 syndrome?; and (c) if the tumor is functional, which hormone is being produced? These questions are relevant because, for example, endocrine neoplasms are often multifocal in patients with MEN 1, and the surgeon may leave in a small (<0.5 cm) endocrine neoplasm at the margin of a resection for a larger tumor.

On CT these neoplasms typically appear as single well-defined solid neoplasms that enhance during the arterial phase, but some can be cystic, and others, particularly those in patients with MEN 1, can be multifocal. FNAs are often performed when a well-differentiated endocrine neoplasm is clinically suspected, because the diagnosis has such a significant impact on therapy. These neoplasms typically produce a cellular smear of uniform cells with monomorphic nuclei with fine, evenly dispersed nuclear chromatin (so-called "salt and pepper" chromatin), only inconspicuous nucleoli, infrequent mitoses and scant granular, basophilic to amphophilic cytoplasm.

The surgeon will identify and resect the neoplasm if the patient has a significant clinical syndrome caused by the tumor, but the identification of the neoplasm can be challenging if the tumor is small, and the resection difficult if the tumor is large. Patients with multiple endocrine neoplasia, type 1 (MEN1) can have multiple pancreatic endocrine neoplasms, and these neoplasms can range in size from microadenomas (<5 mm) to large unresectable masses. Imaging techniques are constantly improving, and as a result, larger numbers of small, non-functional endocrine neoplasms will be detected and resected. Some are so small that they cannot be palpated at the time of surgery, causing the surgeon to rely on intraoperative ultrasound examination for their detection.

In contrast to most other neoplasms of the pancreas, the resection of well-differentiated primary endocrine neoplasms that are metastatic to the liver benefits many patients. Some well-differentiated endocrine neoplasms, such as gastrinomas, may be extra-pancreatic in location. These neoplasms are often small and difficult to locate, and as a result, the surgeon may send multiple biopsies of extra-pancreatic lesions for intraoperative consultation in search of the tumor.

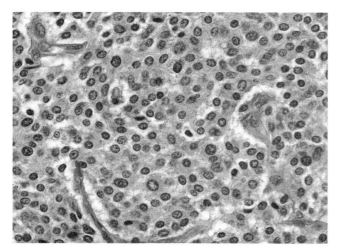

Fig. 10.10. Well-differentiated pancreatic endocrine neoplasm. This cellular neoplasm is composed of cells with uniform "salt and pepper" nuclei.

Pathologic issues

The distinction of functional from non-functional pancreatic endocrine neoplasms cannot be made on FS or on cytologic examination; this is a clinical distinction.

The specimen submitted for IOD is usually a biopsy, a partial pancreatectomy, or in rare cases a total pancreatectomy. As is true for ductal adenocarcinomas, surgery is often performed without a pre-operative FNA or biopsy diagnosis.

In a resected specimen, the gross appearance of the pancreatic endocrine neoplasm often provides a clue to the diagnosis (Fig, 10.2). They typically are well-demarcated and red-tan to yellow. Many are soft, but some can be firm. Cystic change can grossly mimic a cystic neoplasm of the pancreas.

The diagnosis can usually be suspected based on the low-power architectural features of these neoplasms such as nests, trabeculae, or sheets of cells (Figs. 10.3[b] and 10.10). The vast majority of pancreatic endocrine neoplasms are well-differentiated with uniform nuclei and a very low mitotic rate. Intraoperative cytologic preparations provide helpful confirmatory information, highlighting the uniformity of the nuclei and the characteristic "salt and pepper" chromatin pattern (Fig. 10.11). Well-differentiated pancreatic endocrine neoplasms often have a plasmacytoid appearance in touch preparations.

The surgical margins on a solitary endocrine neoplasm are usually easy to interpret because the microscopic findings mirror the gross findings. However, patients with MEN 1 have multiple endocrine cell neoplasms, many of them microadenomas. When a microadenoma is identified close to or at the surgical margin on FS, the size of the adenoma should be reported to the surgeon because microadenomas <5 mm may not justify additional pancreatic resection. The extent of surgical resection will be guided by other factors, to ensure that the surgical resection is not more burdensome to the patient than the neoplasm.

Pancreatoblastoma

Pancreatoblastomas are distinctive neoplasms with acinar differentiation and squamoid nests.[9] They can also have mesenchymal and ductal differentiation. They occur predominantly, but not exclusively, in children.

Clinical issues

The mean age at diagnosis is 10 years, and pancreatoblastoma should top the differential diagnosis for a pancreatic mass in a child.[1] This neoplasm is more common in Asians than in Caucasians, and they are associated with the Beckwith–Weidemann syndrome. In general, pancreatoblastomas are similar in behavior to acinar cell carcinoma and they are treated in the same way. Alpha-fetoprotein levels can be elevated, and when they are elevated, alpha-fetoprotein levels can help track response of the neoplasm to treatment.

Pathologic issues

Pancreatoblastomas have a low power appearance of lobules separated by fibrous bands. At high magnification at least two components are present- cells with acinar differentiation and squamoid nests (Fig. 10.12). Because they are so distinctive, the squamoid nests are a reliable clue to the diagnosis. Pancreatoblastoma may show other lines of differentiation as well, including ductal, mesenchymal and endocrine differentiation.

Solid-pseudopapillary neoplasm

Solid-pseudopapillary neoplasms of the pancreas are distinctive neoplasms that predominantly affect women in their twenties and thirties.[1] These neoplasms can be solid, but cystic degeneration can be very prominent, giving most cases a solid and cystic appearance.

Clinical issues

Solid-pseudopapillary neoplasm should top the differential diagnosis of a solid and cystic pancreatic mass in a young woman. The mean age at diagnosis is 28 years, and 90% are female. Computerized tomography typically reveals a

(a)

(b)

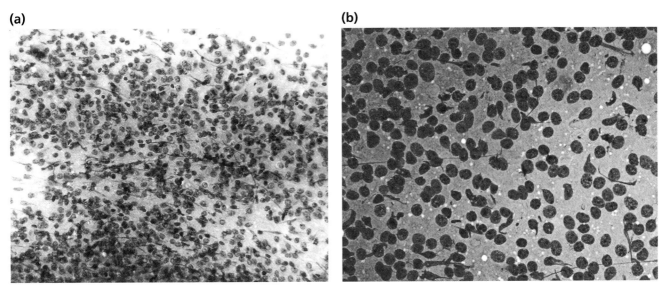

Fig. 10.11. Well-differentiated pancreatic endocrine neoplasm (a) Hypercellular smears with discohesive population of uniform "lymphocyte-like" cells. The cells lack prominent nucleoli and have a faintly granular chromatin pattern. (b) Higher magnification reveals cellular monotony with a predominant population of naked round to oval nuclei. ((a) H&E stain and (b), Diff Quik stain)

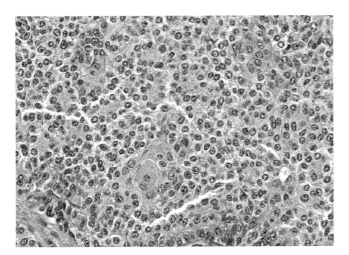

Fig. 10.12. Pancreatoblastoma. Squamoid nests emerge from a background of cells with acinar differentiation. Note the single prominent nucleoli in the cells with acinar differentiation.

well-circumscribed neoplasm with both solid and cystic components (Fig. 10.13). Most patients are cured by surgical resection, but a significant fraction (~10%) recurs and/or metastasizes, and they are considered malignant. As is true for well-differentiated endocrine neoplasms, some patients do well following the surgical resection of liver metastases. Although low-grade, the solid-pseudopapillary neoplasm is malignant, and solid-pseudo-papillary neoplasms can metastasize to the liver. When this happens, surgical resection of the metastasis may benefit the patient.

Pathologic issues

Clues to the diagnosis include uniform nuclei with nuclear grooves, foam cells, intracytoplasmic eosinophilic hyaline globules, and pseudopapillae formed around delicate vessels (Fig. 10.14). The poorly cohesive nature of the neoplastic cells is another strong clue to the diagnosis. The main differential diagnosis is from well-differentiated pancreatic endocrine neoplasm, which can mimic a solid-pseudopapillary neoplasm both clinically and pathologically. Touch preparations can be very helpful, highlighting the delicate vasculature, nuclear grooves, hyaline globules, and the poorly cohesive properties of the neoplastic cells (Fig. 10.15).

The vast majority of solid-pseudopapillary neoplasms are relatively well defined and readily excised with clear margins. FS is often used to evaluate surgical margins. These sections are usually relatively easy to evaluate because the neoplasm is quite distinctive.

Cystic neoplasms

As shown in Table 10.1, one can often arrive at the diagnosis of a cystic neoplasm from clinical findings alone.[1] Features such as the patient's gender and age, the location of the neoplasm in the pancreas, the presence or absence of connectivity of the cysts to native pancreatic ducts, and the quality of the cyst contents, can all help narrow the differential diagnosis substantially. For example, mucinous cystic neoplasm tops the list of differential diagnoses for

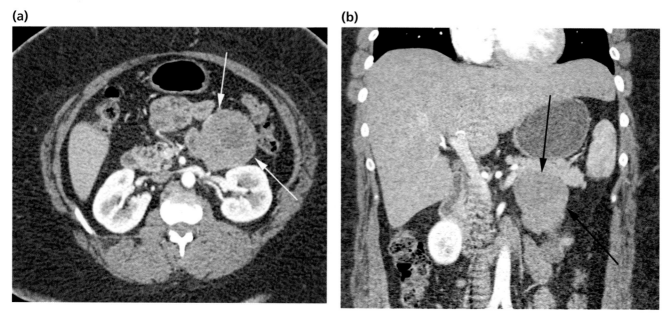

Fig. 10.13. Solid-pseudopapillary neoplasm. (a) Axial and (b) coronal CT scans revealing a large solid mass (arrows) with focal cystic degeneration in the tail of the pancreas.

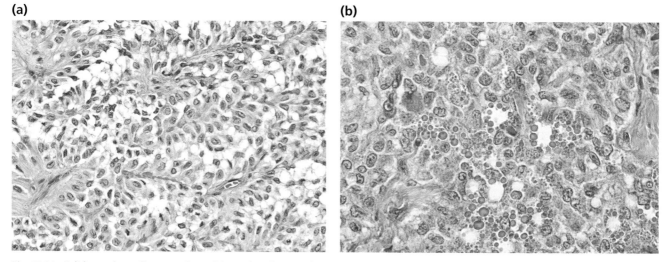

Fig. 10.14. Solid-pseudopapillary neoplasm. (a) Poorly cohesive cells surround delicate blood vessels. (b) Eosinophilic globules are a clue to the diagnosis of a solid-pseudopapillary neoplasm.

a mucin-producing cystic mass in the tail of the pancreas in a 45-year-old woman, particularly if the cysts do not communicate with the larger pancreatic ducts.

Serous cystic neoplasms

Serous cystic neoplasms are important to recognize because they are the least aggressive of all of the neoplasms of the pancreas. Only a small fraction of these distinctive neoplasms are locally aggressive, and metastases are extraordinarily rare.[10]

Clinical issues

The vast majority of serous cystic neoplasms of the pancreas are non-syndromic, and only a small minority is associated with the von Hippel Lindau syndrome. Patients with von Hippel–Lindau syndrome have other abdominal neoplasms including microadenomas of the pancreas. Computerized tomography typically reveals a well-defined mass with innumerable small cysts and a central, often calcified, stellate scar (Fig. 10.16). The pancreas may be more diffusely involved in patients with the von Hippel–Lindau syndrome.

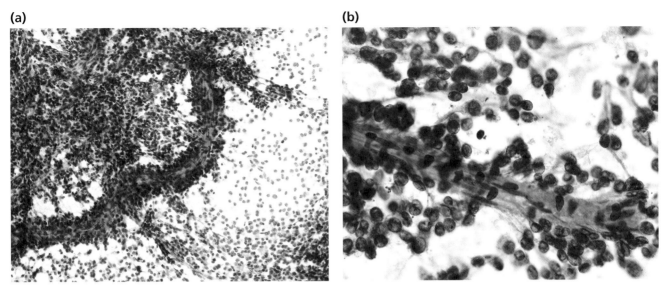

(a)

(b)

Fig. 10.15. Solid-pseudopapillary neoplasm. (a) Hypercellular smear with numerous fragments of branching, "cord-like" cells. Numerous small single cells are present in the background. (b) Uniform, round to oval nuclei with scant to barely perceptible cytoplasm in intimate association with capillary endothelial cells. The cellular monomorphism, round to oval nuclear shapes and lack of prominent nucleoli often raises the possibility of a well differentiated pancreatic endocrine neoplasm in these cases. (Papanicolaou stains)

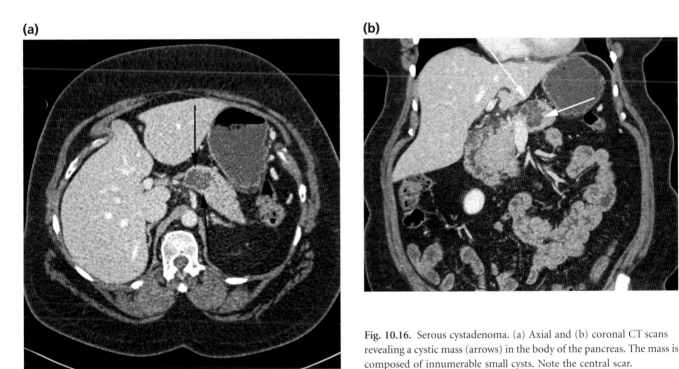

(a)

(b)

Fig. 10.16. Serous cystadenoma. (a) Axial and (b) coronal CT scans revealing a cystic mass (arrows) in the body of the pancreas. The mass is composed of innumerable small cysts. Note the central scar.

Pathologic issues

While most serous cystic neoplasms form small cysts, macrocystic and solid variants also exist.[1] The nature of the cyst fluid can help make the diagnosis. Note the color and viscosity of the cyst fluid when the lesion is first sectioned. Watery straw-colored fluid is characteristic of a serous cystic neoplasm, in contrast to the thick, tenacious, cloudy fluid of a mucin-producing neoplasm. The gross appearance can be virtually diagnostic (Fig. 10.2[b]). A well-demarcated neoplasm composed of innumerable small (1–3 mm) cysts with a central stellate scar is classic.

Microscopically, the small cysts are lined by cuboidal epithelium with clear cytoplasm and round uniform nuclei (Fig. 10.17). On touch preparations the cells have

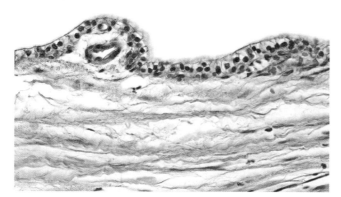

Fig. 10.17. Serous cystadenoma. The cysts are lined by a layer of uniform cuboidal cells with clear cytoplasm.

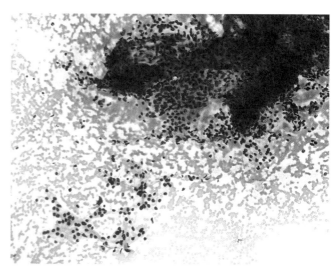

Fig. 10.18. Serous cystadenoma. Small bland-looking epithelial cells in a non-mucinous background. The cells have uniform round nuclei and fragile clear/wispy cytoplasm. (Diff Quik stain)

uniform round nuclei and fragile clear/wispy cytoplasm (Fig. 10.18). Since these neoplasms are almost always benign, surgical margins are not as critical as they are for most of the other neoplasms of the pancreas. Certainly, most surgeons will attempt to completely remove the lesion without compromising the patient's health.

Mucinous cystic neoplasm

Mucinous cystic neoplasms are distinctive tumors that occur predominantly in the tail of the pancreas in middle-aged women.[11] Up to a third harbor an invasive carcinoma. In contrast to intraductal papillary mucinous neoplasms, mucinous cystic neoplasms are almost always unifocal.

Clinical issues
The patient's age, gender and the location of the neoplasm can suggest the diagnosis. The female to male ratio is 20 to 1, the mean age at diagnosis is between 40 and 50 years, and most arise in the tail of the pancreas.[1] Patients with non-invasive mucinous cystic neoplasms are 5 to 10 years younger than are patients with mucinous cystic neoplasms with an associated invasive carcinoma.

Individual cysts are usually large enough to be visualized by computerized tomography, and they do not communicate with the larger pancreatic ducts (Fig. 10.19).

Pre-operative FNA can demonstrate the mucinous epithelium, but the characteristic stroma is usually not seen. Incisional biopsy of the lesion should never be performed as it may greatly underestimate the malignant potential of the neoplasm and, at the same time, risks seeding of the abdomen. Patients with a completely resected non-invasive

mucinous cystic neoplasm are usually cured. The presence or absence of an invasive carcinoma is the best prognosticator, but invasion cannot be excluded unless the neoplasm is completely resected and thoroughly, if not completely, evaluated histologically.

The criteria for surgical resection of an invasive carcinoma arising in association with a mucinous cystic neoplasm are generally the same as for conventional pancreatic ductal adenocarcinoma.

Pathologic issues
The specimen usually received is the definitive resection specimen. The surgeon expects confirmation of the diagnosis of mucinous neoplasm, would like to know if there is invasive carcinoma, and is interested in the status of the surgical margins. Keep in mind that the columnar lining cells may be desquamated and the FS may be misinterpreted as a pseudocyst unless the characteristic "ovarian-type" of stroma is appreciated.

The contents of the cysts can help establish the correct diagnosis. Thick sticky mucoid material should suggest either a mucinous cystic neoplasm or an intraductal papillary mucinous neoplasm. The cysts do not communicate with the larger pancreatic ducts, and the relationship between the cysts and the pancreatic duct system is best evaluated by first placing a probe in the main pancreatic duct and then bivalving the specimen along the probe.

The cysts are lined by tall columnar mucin-producing epithelium with varying degrees of architectural and cytologic dysplasia (Fig. 10.20). The mucinous epithelium may be

(a)

(b)

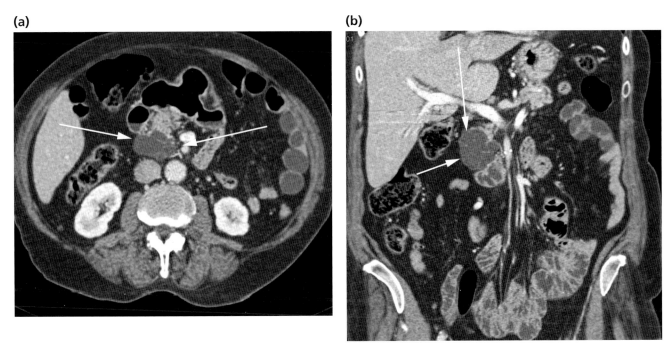

Fig. 10.19. Mucinous cystic neoplasm. (a) Axial and (b) coronal CT scans revealing a cystic mass (arrows) in the head of the pancreas. The cysts are larger and have thicker walls than the cysts in serous cystic neoplasms.

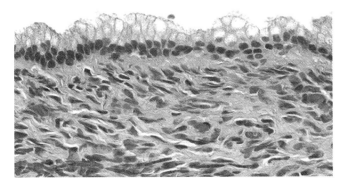

Fig. 10.20. Mucinous cystic neoplasm with low grade dysplasia. Tall columnar mucin-containing cells line the cysts. Note the ovarian-type stroma.

denuded, in which case the characteristic ovarian-type stroma in the cyst wall should suggest the diagnosis (Fig. 10.20). Touch preparations will reveal glandular mucinous epithelium with pale/clear cytoplasm (Fig. 10.21). The ovarian stroma is usually not appreciated in touch preparations.

Mucinous cystic neoplasms should be examined carefully for invasion. Gross clues to invasion include the presence of mural and solid nodules. These areas should be sampled first when selecting a piece of tumor for frozen

section diagnosis. While the demonstration of tissue invasion may not alter the surgical procedure, it will help guide sampling for permanent sections. If partial sampling of the tumor at the time of FS does not show invasive carcinoma, the surgeon should be made aware that invasive carcinoma may be found later after extensive sampling.

Intraductal papillary mucinous neoplasm

These distinctive neoplasms are characterized by prominent intraductal growth and abundant extracellular mucin production.[1] One-third of the cases harbor an associated invasive carcinoma. In contrast to mucinous cystic neoplasms, intraductal papillary mucinous neoplasms can be multifocal.

Clinical issues

In contrast to mucinous cystic neoplasms, intraductal papillary mucinous neoplasms affect men more frequently than women (male to female ratio 3:2), and they involve the head of the gland more often than the tail.[1] The diagnosis is often suggested preoperatively based on the identification of mucin oozing from the ampulla of Vater on endoscopy, cytologic sampling at the time of ERCP, or the demonstration of a markedly dilated pancreatic duct on computerized tomography (Fig. 10.22).[12] About 30% of

(a) **(b)**

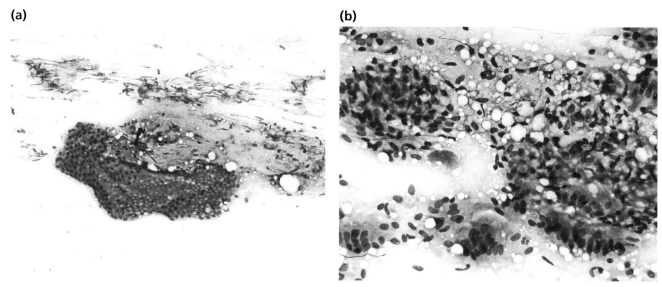

Fig. 10.21. Mucinous cystic neoplasm with low grade dysplasia. (a) A large tissue fragment of glandular mucinous epithelium with pale/clear cytoplasm and minimal nuclear crowding or atypia. (b) Higher magnification illustrates mildly atypical glandular epithelium with focally stratified oval nuclei and background mucin. (Diff Quik stains)

(a) **(b)**

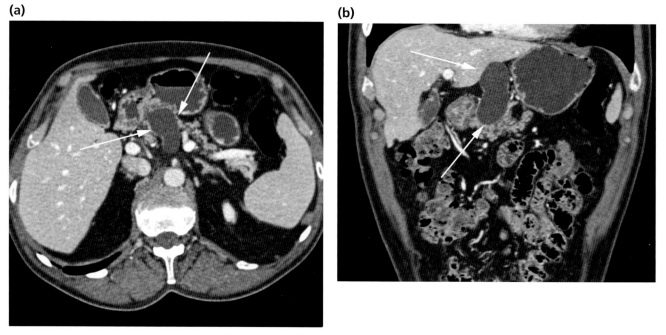

Fig. 10.22. Intraductal papillary mucinous neoplasm. (a) Axial and (b) coronal CT scans revealing a cystic mass (arrows) in the head of the pancreas. In contrast to mucinous cystic neoplasms, intraductal papillary mucinous neoplasms communicate with one of the larger pancreatic ducts.

IPMNs have an associated invasive ductal adenocarcinoma, a finding that is more common in IPMN of the main duct compared to branch duct IPMN. CT scans are used to determine if an invasive carcinoma is likely to be associated with the IPMN, and this test has a sensitivity of about 85%. The surgeon is therefore, usually well informed about the possibility of invasive carcinoma, and will approach cases with invasive carcinoma in the same way as cases of conventional invasive ductal adenocarcinoma. Minimally invasive carcinomas may not be detected pre-operatively, but this does not change the surgical approach to the disease.

Small intraductal papillary mucinous neoplasms are common and some may be followed clinically with periodic CT scans. There is international agreement that intraductal papillary mucinous neoplasms greater than 3 cm, associated with dilatation of the main pancreatic duct, or with a mural nodule should be resected if possible.[13] Non-invasive intraductal papillary mucinous neoplasms can be multifocal, and some involve the entire length of the gland. In these instances the surgeon has to balance the benefit of resecting a given lesion with the potential morbidity of the procedure.

As is true for mucinous cystic neoplasms, the presence or absence of an invasive carcinoma is the best indicator of prognosis. The surgical management of an invasive carcinoma

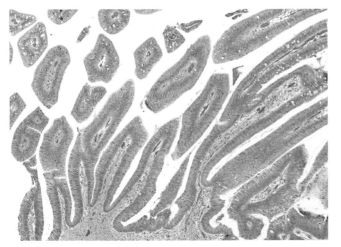

Fig. 10.23. Intraductal papillary mucinous neoplasm with moderate dysplasia. Note the long finger-like papillae, the columnar mucin-producing epithelium, and the absence of a distinctive stroma.

arising in association with an intraductal papillary mucinous neoplasm is generally the same as the management of a conventional pancreatic ductal adenocarcinoma.

Surgical resection is undertaken with a confident working diagnosis of IPMN, but the specimen will be submitted for IOD to determine if there is a grossly visible invasive carcinoma, and if the surgical margins are clear.

Pathologic issues

As is true for almost all cystic neoplasms of the pancreas, the nature of the cyst contents can help narrow the differential diagnosis. Thick sticky mucoid material should suggest either a mucinous cystic neoplasm or an intraductal papillary mucinous neoplasm.

By definition, the cysts in papillary intraductal mucinous neoplasm communicate with the larger pancreatic ducts. As noted earlier, this relationship is best evaluated by first placing a probe in the main pancreatic duct and then bivalving the specimen along the probe.

The larger pancreatic ducts are lined by tall columnar mucin-producing epithelium with varying degrees of architectural and cytologic dysplasia (Fig. 10.23). In contrast to mucinous cystic neoplasm, the intraductal papillary mucinous neoplasm does not have a distinctive stroma. Touch preparations usually contain fragments of mucinous glandular epithelium with papillary-like branching (Fig. 10.24).

The diagnosis is usually suspected pre-operatively based on endoscopic and imaging findings, so intraoperative consultation is used to evaluate the margins of

(a)

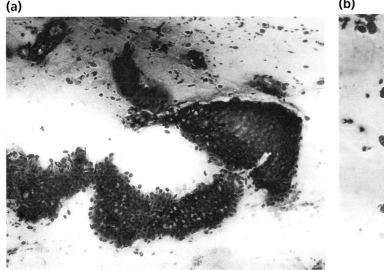

(b)

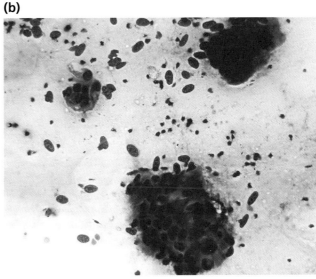

Fig. 10.24. Intraductal papillary mucinous neoplasm. (a) A large fragment of mucinous glandular epithelium with a vague papillary-like branching. Background shows abundant mucin. (b) Higher magnification depicts significant atypia with nuclear enlargement, crowding and overlap. Few discohesive bare nuclei are seen in the background. Follow-up showed IPMN with focal high grade dysplasia. (Diff Quik stains)

resection, as well as to determine if there is a grossly visible invasive carcinoma. It can be particularly difficult to distinguish between focal involvement of the margin by an intraductal papillary mucinous neoplasm and pancreatic intraepithelial neoplasia; long finger-like papillae and abundant intraluminal mucin favor the diagnosis of an intraductal papillary mucinous neoplasia but the distinction between these two lesions is less important than determining the grade of dysplasia in the lesion.

The full face of the surgical margin should be selected for FS. In the Mayo Clinic series, about 20% of cases required additional resection because of a positive margin. If an intraductal lesion is present at a margin, it is important to communicate to the surgeon, both the degree of dysplasia and the size of the lesion. Small papillary mucin-producing lesions (<1 cm) without significant dysplasia are common in the pancreas, particularly in pancreata with an intraductal papillary mucinous neoplasm. These lesions should not be overcalled, particularly in elderly patients, because they are less likely to harm the patient than overly aggressive surgery.

After the margins have been sampled, we like to bivalve the specimen along a probe placed in the main pancreatic duct. This is a great way to determine if the neoplasm is a branch-duct or a main-duct type of IPMN and it can help localize any invasive component. If clinically indicated, any areas worrisome for invasion can be submitted for FS evaluation.

REFERENCES

1. Hruban RH, Pitman MB, Klimstra DS. *Tumors of the Pancreas. Atlas of Tumor Pathology.* Fourth Series, *Fascicle 6* ed. Washington, DC: American Registry of Pathology and Armed Forces Institute of Pathology, 2007.

2. Hamano H, Kawa S, Horiuchi A, *et al.* High serum IgG4 concentrations in patients with sclerosing pancreatitis. *N Engl J Med* 2001; **344**: 732–738.

3. American Cancer Society. *Cancer Facts & Figures 2007.* Cancer, 1–52. 2007. New York, New York, American Cancer Society.

4. Cioc AM, Ellison EC, Proca DM, Lucas JG, Frankel WL. Frozen section diagnosis of pancreatic lesions. *Arch Pathol Lab Med* 2002; **126**: 1169–1173.

5. Sharma S, Green KB. The pancreatic duct and its arteriovenous relationship: an underutilized aid in the diagnosis and distinction of pancreatic adenocarcinoma from pancreatic intraepithelial neoplasia. A study of 126 pancreatectomy specimens. *Am J Surg Pathol* 2004; **28**: 613–620.

6. Hyland C, Kheir SM, Kashlan MB. Frozen section diagnosis of pancreatic carcinoma: a prospective study of 64 biopsies. *Am J Surg Pathol* 1981; **5**: 179–191.

7. Kawamoto S, Siegelman SS, Hruban RH, Fishman EK. Lymphoplasmacytic sclerosing pancreatitis with obstructive jaundice: CT and pathology features. *Am J Roentgenol* 2004; **183**: 915–921.

8. Klimstra DS, Heffess CS, Oertel JE, Rosai J. Acinar cell carcinoma of the pancreas. A clinicopathologic study of 28 cases. *Am J Surg Pathol* 1992; **16**: 815–837.

9. Klimstra DS, Wenig BM, Adair CF, Heffess CS. Pancreatoblastoma. A clinicopathologic study and review of the literature. *Am J Surg Pathol* 1995; **19**: 1371–1389.

10. Galanis C, Zamani A, Cameron JL, *et al.* Resected serous cystic neoplasms of the pancreas: a review of 158 patients with recommendations for treatment. *J Gastrointest Surg* 2007; **11**: 820–826.

11. Wilentz RE, Albores-Saavedra J, Hruban RH. Mucinous cystic neoplasms of the pancreas. *Semin Diagn Pathol* 2000; **17**: 31–42.

12. Kawamoto S, Lawler LP, Horton KM, *et al.* MDCT of intraductal papillary mucinous neoplasm of the pancreas: evaluation of features predictive of invasive carcinoma. *Am J Roentgenol* 2006; **186**: 687–695.

13. Tanaka M, Chari S, Adsay NV, *et al.* International consensus guidelines for management of intraductal papillary mucinous neoplasms and mucinous cystic neoplasms of the pancreas. *Pancreatology* 2006; **6**: 32.

11 THYROID GLAND

Mahendra Ranchod, John K.C. Chan, and Electron Kebebew

The pathologist's role in the intraoperative management of thyroid lesions has changed in recent years, and this is due to four main factors:

Fine Needle Aspiration Biopsy (FNA) is now used routinely to evaluate thyroid nodules and as a result, a diagnosis or a differential diagnosis is available in the majority of cases at the time of surgery.

Ultrasonography (U/S) plays an increasing role in the evaluation of nodular goiters and is used in the following situations: (a) To determine the number of nodules in the thyroid gland when only a single nodule is palpable, to ascertain if the nodule is solid or cystic, and to determine if there are imaging characteristics of malignancy. (b) To evaluate cervical lymph nodes in patients with a confirmed diagnosis of thyroid carcinoma. In one report,[1] U/S led to the detection of abnormalities in non-palpable lateral compartment lymph nodes in nearly 15% of cases, leading to a change in surgical management. The detection of nodal disease is even higher in patients who have neck surgery for recurrent thyroid carcinoma. (c) To direct FNA of non-palpable nodules. (d) With the availability of portable U/S units, palpable nodules are now being aspirated with ultrasound guidance, resulting in improved diagnostic yields.

The use of *Frozen Section* (FS) in the intraoperative evaluation of a solitary thyroid nodule has come into question because of the low accuracy rate, and it has been argued that gross examination is all that is necessary intraoperatively.

The majority of thyroid surgeons advocate *total thyroidectomy* for the treatment of clinically significant thyroid carcinomas. This has reduced the stakes for distinguishing between different types of thyroid carcinoma intraoperatively as almost all resectable carcinomas are now treated by total thyroidectomy.

GENERAL CLINICAL ISSUES

Thyroid nodules are common. Approximately 4% of adults in the US have a palpable thyroid nodule but only 5% of palpable nodules are malignant. The main reason for evaluating asymptomatic thyroid nodules is to identify nodules that are malignant so that these patients may be treated in a timely fashion. In the past, only palpable lesions came to clinical attention, but now, increasing numbers of non-palpable nodules are identified during imaging for other head and neck diseases, and many of these lesions – especially nodules >1 cm – are subjected to U/S FNA.[2] There is heightened concern about a solitary thyroid nodule because of the increased risk of malignancy, but the majority of solitary nodules are benign; malignancies also occur in the setting of multinodular goiter but this is uncommon in the United States.[3]

The causes of a solitary thyroid nodule are listed in Table 11.1. Occasionally, a nodule develops in patients with diffuse thyroid disease such as Graves' disease and Hashimoto's disease; these patients are managed in the same way as a solitary nodule without diffuse disease. In one series, 38% of nodules that occurred in Graves' disease were malignant.[4] In contrast, the majority of nodules that occur in Hashimoto's disease are nodular areas of chronic thyroiditis or benign follicular/Hurthle cell nodules.[5]

A nodule is suspicious of malignancy if the patient has any one of the following: cervical adenopathy, distant metastases, a thyroid mass that is fixed to adjacent soft tissue, or local obstructive symptoms such as a hoarseness, dysphagia, and stridor. However, 80%–90% of patients with a thyroid malignancy have a nodule that cannot be distinguished from a benign nodule on clinical grounds. In addition, patients with a thyroid nodule and a family history of thyroid cancer or a history of radiation exposure

Intraoperative Consultation in Surgical Pathology, ed. Mahendra Ranchod. Published by Cambridge University Press.
© Cambridge University Press 2010.

Table 11.1. Causes of a solitary thyroid nodule (in approximate order of frequency)

Dominant adenomatous nodule in a multinodular goiter

Solitary adenomatous (hyperplastic) nodule

Follicular adenoma

Hurthle cell adenoma

Papillary carcinoma

Minimally invasive follicular carcinoma

Minimally invasive Hurthle cell carcinoma

Hyalinizing trabecular neoplasms

Medullary carcinoma

Lymphoma

Metastasis

(e.g. Chernobyl) have a significantly increased risk of malignancy.

FNA is usually the first diagnostic test employed to evaluate a thyroid nodule because it is cost-effective, safe, and provides a rapid and accurate diagnosis. In the hands of experienced practitioners, approximately 65% of thyroid nodules are interpreted as benign, 10% malignant, 12%–15% indeterminate, 7%–8% suspicious, and 5%–8% unsatisfactory.[6] The percentage of "unsatisfactory" FNA specimens however, varies by institution and exceeds 15% in many series. It is clear that intraoperative consultation (IOC) has a role to play in cases where the FNA was interpreted as "suspicious" or "unsatisfactory," but there is no consensus for the role of intraoperative diagnosis (IOD) in cases where a firm diagnosis of a benign nodule or carcinoma has been rendered. This lack of consensus is partly related to the level of confidence the surgeon has in the pathologist's FNA diagnosis. While FNA is highly accurate in the hands of experts, there are inter-observer differences in interpretation. Baloch *et al.* report a significant reversal of FNA diagnoses in 10% of cases reviewed at their institution,[7] a situation that warrants review of FNA slides prior to surgery or for IOC on selected resected specimens.

INDICATIONS FOR INTRAOPERATIVE CONSULTATION

1. Evaluation of a lobectomy specimen in a patient who has a multinodular goiter with suspicious nodules. The presence of a carcinoma could lead to total thyroidectomy.

2. Evaluation of a solitary nodule in a patient whose FNA diagnosis is "follicular neoplasm" or "Hurthle cell neoplasm."

3. Evaluation of a lobectomy specimen when the FNA is suspicious, but not diagnostic, of papillary carcinoma, and the surgeon requests confirmation of the diagnosis before proceeding with total thyroidectomy.

4. Evaluation of an incisional biopsy of a thyroid mass suggestive of lymphoma on FNA, or when the FNA is inconclusive in suspected anaplastic carcinoma. The purpose of IOD is to confirm that the specimen contains diagnostic material.

5. Evaluation of an enlarged cervical lymph node in a patient who has thyroid carcinoma, when a diagnosis of metastatic carcinoma will lead to lymph node dissection.

INFORMATION NEEDED BEFORE AND DURING SURGERY

It is often possible to handle a thyroid specimen with the information available on the pathology requisition form, but there are advantages to being familiar with the clinical history, imaging findings, FNA results and the surgeon's operative plan.

HANDLING SPECIMENS INTRAOPERATIVELY

Lobectomy specimens

The most common thyroid specimen is a lobectomy or lobectomy/isthmusectomy. The specimen should be inked, even if a diagnosis of benign was rendered on FNA, because the final diagnosis may reveal a malignancy, and inking the specimen will allow the surgical margins to be evaluated with more confidence. If there are multiple nodules on palpation, one or when necessary, more than one section should be made into the specimen to permit gross evaluation of all the nodules, or at least the larger nodules. If a solitary nodule is present, a single section should be made in the coronal plane of the lobectomy specimen, bisecting the nodule. Further evaluation will depend on the gross findings.

If the specimen contains multiple, circumscribed, colloid-rich nodules characteristic of a multinodular goiter

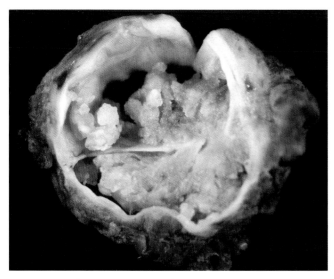

Fig. 11.1. Papillary carcinoma that has undergone marked cystic change, mimicking a benign nodule. The residual nodule in the wall of the cyst has a papillomatous appearance and it is this area that should be sampled intraoperatively.

(MNG), the diagnosis of MNG can be made by gross examination alone. There is no reason to perform frozen sections on a typical MNG.

If a solitary cystic lesion is present, the lesion is likely to be an adenomatous nodule or adenoma with cystic change but a minority of cystic lesions are cystic papillary carcinomas (Fig. 11.1).[8] A cytoscrape preparation should be made of the residual solid component if there is any concern about papillary carcinoma, and this should be supplemented with a FS if necessary.

If a solitary, encapsulated colloid-poor nodule is present, the differential diagnosis includes follicular adenoma, minimally invasive follicular carcinoma, encapsulated papillary carcinoma (about 10% of papillary carcinomas are encapsulated), a hyalinizing trabecular neoplasm and the rare encapsulated medullary carcinoma. The lesion is likely to be Hurthle cell adenoma or minimally invasive Hurthle cell carcinoma if the cut surface of the nodule is brown.

There is controversy on how best to evaluate a solitary encapsulated nodule with a prior FNA diagnosis of "follicular neoplasm." In the past, attempts were made to distinguish between follicular adenoma and minimally invasive follicular carcinoma by FS, but there is growing evidence that this distinction should be left to permanent sections. In the only randomized prospective study of FSs on solitary encapsulated nodules, Udelsman et al. have demonstrated that the yield is low enough to question the value of this test.[9] These authors recommend gross examination of the lobectomy specimen and deferral of the

diagnosis to permanent sections if a solitary encapsulated nodule is present. Not all surgeons will accept this approach, so we recommend the following compromise: (a) a single section is made through the equator of the nodule (Fig. 11.2); (b) a cytoscrape preparation is made of the cut surface of the nodule; and (c) if the cytologic findings are not clearly benign or malignant, a single section is taken parallel to the first cut (this sample includes part of the nodule, the capsule and normal thyroid tissue) and subjected to FS. There are three reasons for this approach. (i) Disparities can occur between FNA and final diagnosis,[10–11] and intraoperative evaluation provides another opportunity to make the correct diagnosis. (ii) Occasionally, the single section may spuriously include an area of capsular/vascular invasion and allow the pathologist to suggest the diagnosis of minimally invasive follicular carcinoma. (iii) It may re-assure the surgeon that every attempt has been made to arrive at a definitive diagnosis, even though it should be understood that intraoperative evaluation is not a sensitive test for detecting the follicular variant of PTC and minimally invasive follicular carcinoma, two common reasons for false-negative diagnoses.

A solid, firm pale lesion with poorly demarcated margins is characteristic of papillary carcinoma and medullary carcinoma. The diagnosis of medullary carcinoma is usually made pre-operatively but this neoplasm may occasionally be encountered for the first time during intraoperative consultation. The distinction between papillary and medullary carcinoma can usually be made with ease on microscopic examination.

Necrosis is rare in well-differentiated carcinomas and its presence should suggest a poorly differentiated or undifferentiated component to the carcinoma, or a metastasis. Tumor necrosis should be distinguished from infarction, a phenomenon that occurs most often in Hurthle cell neoplasms that have been subjected to FNA.

If soft tissue, either fibrofatty tissue or muscle, is adherent to the specimen, the underlying tumor is likely to be malignant. The sample taken for FS should include the soft tissue because the surgeon is likely to be interested in the status of the soft tissue margin.

Subtotal and total thyroidectomy specimens

Subtotal and total thyroidectomy are performed for a known malignancy as well as Graves' disease, MNG and infrequently, Hashimoto's disease. There is no reason for IOD in uncomplicated cases of Graves' disease and

(a)

(b)

(c)

(d)

(e)

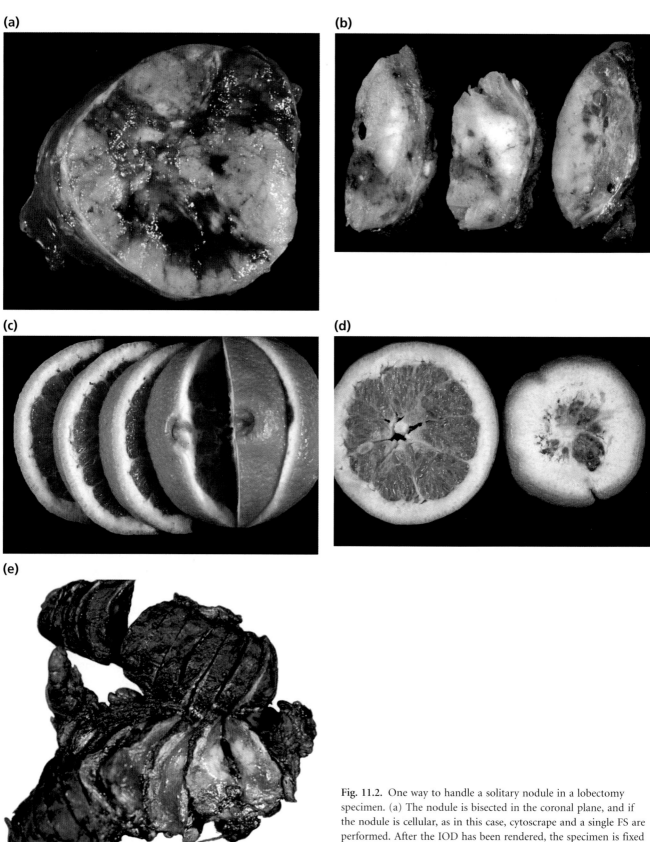

Fig. 11.2. One way to handle a solitary nodule in a lobectomy specimen. (a) The nodule is bisected in the coronal plane, and if the nodule is cellular, as in this case, cytoscrape and a single FS are performed. After the IOD has been rendered, the specimen is fixed overnight, and each half is cut radially. (b) Radial sections of a solitary nodule, showing the nodule, capsule, and the rim of normal thyroid tissue. (c) Radial sections ensure that sections are cut perpendicular to the capsule, in contrast to (d) where tangential sections of the capsule may occur at the polar aspects of the nodule with parallel sections. (e) This is not the way to cut a solitary nodule of the thyroid.

Hashimoto's disease but if a nodule is present, IOD of the nodule is appropriate, and the specimen should be handled as a thyroid specimen containing a potential malignancy. Subtotal thyroidectomy differs from total thyroidectomy in that a nubbin of thyroid tissue (1 gram or less) is left in the area where the recurrent laryngeal nerves penetrate the crico-thyroid membrane. This is an acceptable procedure for benign and malignant disease when the surgeon wishes to avoid any compromise of the recurrent laryngeal nerves. Subtotal and total thyroidectomy specimens for a suspected or known malignancy should always be inked.

SPECIFIC CLINICAL AND PATHOLOGIC ISSUES

Multinodular goiter

Clinical issues

Multinodular goiter (MNG) is the most common cause of goiter. Surgery is performed if there is rapid enlargement of a nodule, lack of response to thyroxin suppression, pressure symptoms on the trachea, suspicion of malignancy and for esthetic reasons. The frequency of carcinoma in MNGs is higher in iodine-deficient areas of the world and these are usually follicular thyroid cancers. The frequency of carcinoma in MNGs in the US is reported to be as high as 5%,[12] and this risk is said to be higher when there are 2–3 nodules and lower when there are >3 nodules.[3] In our experience, however, clinically significant papillary and follicular carcinomas in MNG are much less frequent and occur in <1% of all patients with MNG. Dyshormonogenetic goiter should be considered when a MNG occurs in a young patient or if the patient is hypothyroid. The reasons for surgery in dyshormonogenetic goiter are the same as for other MNGs.

A MNG may be treated by either a lobectomy/isthmusectomy or subtotal or total thyroidectomy, depending on the distribution and size of the nodules. The specimen is not always sent for IOD because most of these patients would have had a benign diagnosis on prior FNA of the dominant or suspicious nodule. An intraoperative diagnosis of malignancy will usually lead to total or near total thyroidectomy.

Pathologic issues

Gross examination is usually all that is necessary to evaluate a MNG. A confident diagnosis of multiple benign adenomatous nodules can be made if the nodules are

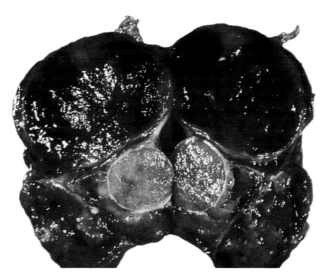

Fig. 11.3. Multinodular goiter with one nodule that is pale and encapsulated. Most pale, encapsulated nodules in MNG are benign nodules with a predominantly microfollicular pattern. Whether a pale, encapsulated nodule is a microfollicular adenomatous nodule or a true adenoma is a moot point as the management is the same. A colloid-poor nodule in a MNG should be thoroughly sampled to rule out malignancy.

circumscribed but poorly encapsulated, with a colloid-rich cut surface. Hemorrhage, fibrosis, and calcification may be present in one or more nodules but should not cause concern in the appropriate context. Occasionally, one of the nodules in a MNG is different; it may be encapsulated with a pale cut surface reflecting its increased cellularity (Fig. 11.3). This nodule should be approached as described for a solitary nodule above (p. 161).

The nodules in a dyshormonogenetic goiter are more cellular and do not have the colloid-rich appearance of the usual MNG. The gross findings may be puzzling in the absence of the clinical history and this may prompt the pathologist to perform a FS. Unlike other MNGs, these nodules are cellular, often microfollicular, and the follicular epithelial cells may show nuclear pleomorphism (Fig. 11.4).

In the US, papillary carcinoma is the most common malignancy in MNGs. Most papillary carcinomas are occult and identified only on permanent sections. If a papillary carcinoma is identified during intraoperative examination, it should be handled as discussed below (see below).

Papillary carcinoma

Clinical issues

Papillary thyroid carcinoma (PTC) constitutes approximately 80% of thyroid malignancies. Eighty-five percent

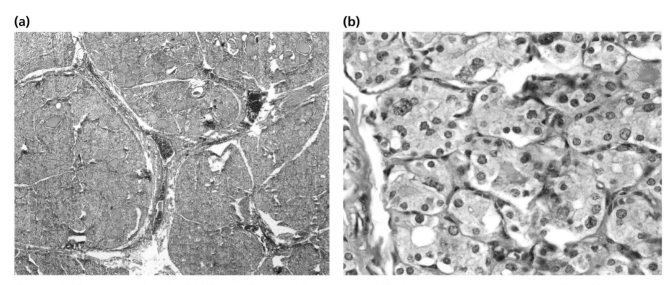

Fig. 11.4. Dyshormonogenetic goiter. (a) The hyperplastic nodules have a microfollicular pattern that may cause concern if the history is not known. (b) The follicular epithelial cells often show nuclear enlargement and pleomorphism somewhat reminiscent of papillary carcinoma.

of PTCs present as a solitary nodule, 7%–10% present as a thyroid nodule accompanied by cervical adenopathy, 1%–2% present as a nodal metastasis accompanied by an occult primary, and an occasional patient will present with distant metastases at the time of presentation. Rarely, PTC presents with a diffusely enlarged gland and elevated thyroid antibodies simulating Hashimoto's disease. In recent years, incidental non-palpable PTCs have been detected more frequently as a result of the widespread use of imaging techniques to evaluate unrelated diseases of the head and neck.

While there are still proponents for treating low-risk PTC by lobectomy, most thyroid surgeons prefer to treat all clinically significant PTCs by total thyroidectomy. The rationale for this approach is as follows. (a) PTC is frequently multifocal with involvement of both lobes. (b) The frequency of local recurrence is lower after total thyroidectomy. (c) If ^{131}I has to be administered post-operatively, it is more effective after total thyroidectomy. (d) In experienced hands, total thyroidectomy does not carry any increased surgical risk. (e) For purposes of clinical follow up, serum thyroglobulin is a more sensitive marker of recurrent/persistent disease if there is no remnant thyroid tissue. Lobectomy may however, be appropriate in certain clinical situations, given that conventional PTC is an indolent malignancy, and that loco-regional recurrences can be treated effectively by surgical and non-surgical modalities.

With FNA, a firm diagnosis of PTC can be made in 70%–90% of cases. With a firm diagnosis in hand, many surgeons will proceed with total thyroidectomy and not request intraoperative confirmation of the diagnosis. A FNA diagnosis of "suspicious of PTC" is made in about 10% of cases, and in this situation, the surgeon is likely to submit a lobectomy specimen for IOD, and proceed with total thyroidectomy if the diagnosis of PTC is confirmed. Invasion of PTC into the peri-thyroid soft tissue increases the risk of local and distant recurrences, and an attempt will be made to remove all grossly visible disease because the long-term outcome is significantly worse when there is residual macroscopic disease.[13] This explains why the surgeon is likely to request FS evaluation of the soft tissue margin.

Cervical lymph node metastases are present in about 40% of cases of conventional PTC[14] and most of these are not clinically apparent. Although nodal metastases do not affect long-term survival, they are associated with more frequent loco-regional recurrences. As a result, pre-operative U/S is used to evaluate cervical lymph nodes. The lymph nodes in the central compartment are usually the first to be involved, and this has led to the recommendation for central compartment neck dissection in certain situations. A lymph node biopsy will be performed on any lymph node in the lateral neck that is suspicious by U/S, and a positive diagnosis will result in ipsilateral neck dissection.[15] Functional compartmental en-bloc dissection is favored over selective node dissection ("berry picking"). There is rarely a need for radical neck dissection in the initial treatment of PTC.

(a)

(b)

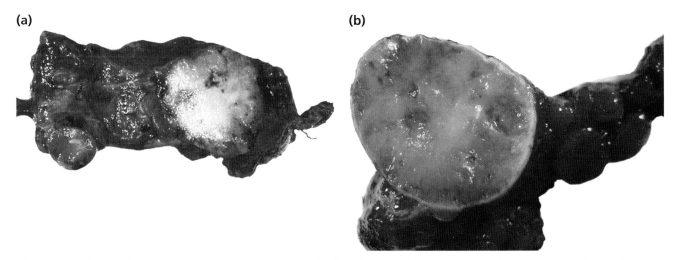

Fig. 11.5. (a) Most papillary carcinomas (PTC) are solid, firm, and pale with poorly defined margins. (b) A minority of papillary carcinomas are circumscribed, at least partially encapsulated, and not distinguishable from a benign thyroid nodule on gross examination. The specimen in image (b) also contains multiple benign adenomatous nodules.

Pathologic issues

There is no reason for intraoperative evaluation of the thyroidectomy specimen if a firm diagnosis of PTC was made on prior FNA. On the other hand, the surgeon is likely to request an IOD if the FNA was interpreted as "suspicious" or if the cytologic specimen was inadequate. The diagnosis of PTC may be more challenging intraoperatively because one of the primary features – nuclear clearing, an artifact of fixation – is absent in cytology preparations and FSs. The diagnosis is even more challenging when papillary structures and psammoma bodies are absent, a ready explanation for the frequent failure to recognize the follicular variant of papillary carcinoma intraoperatively.

CONVENTIONAL PAPILLARY CARCINOMA

Most papillary carcinomas are easily distinguished from benign nodules on gross examination because the neoplasm forms a poorly defined, firm, pale mass that sometimes has a gritty consistency on sectioning (Fig. 11.5). If there is a request for IOD, a cytologic preparation may be all that is needed to confirm the diagnosis. However, a FS should be performed if the cytologic preparation is not diagnostic, because the FS may show architectural features such as papillary structures and a trabecular pattern (Fig. 11.6) that are not apparent in cytologic preparations.

There are many variants of PTC and these are listed in Table 11.2.

PAPILLARY MICROCARCINOMA

Papillary microcarcinoma refers to papillary carcinomas that are <1 cm in maximum dimension. This definition

is somewhat arbitrary but serves to identify a group of PTCs that have a more favorable outcome. These lesions are true carcinomas; in the series by Hay et al.,[16] nodal metastases were present in 32% of patients, a frequency that approaches that seen in larger PTCs. Approximately 6% of patients with papillary microcarcinoma have loco-regional recurrences and this correlates with multifocal disease in the thyroid gland and nodal metastases at the time of initial diagnosis. Occult papillary microcarcinomas (i.e., carcinomas that present with a metastasis and have a clinically occult primary tumor) are treated by total thyroidectomy and appropriate lymph node dissection.[17] The treatment of latent papillary microcarcinoma (i.e., a microcarcinoma found incidentally during routine histologic examination of lobectomy and subtotal thyroidectomy specimens for benign disease) is not in the purview of intraoperative management, but as an aside, these neoplasms are usually minute and can be managed by observation alone. However, completion thyroidectomy may be considered if they are multicentric and if any one of the tumors is >5 mm in size. The 2004 WHO classification, which divides microcarcinomas into "occult" and "latent," does not take into account microcarcinomas that are detected during imaging studies of the neck for unrelated clinical diseases. Management of these carcinomas will depend on the size of the primary neoplasm, U/S status of cervical lymph nodes, patient's age and other clinical factors.

FOLLICULAR VARIANT OF PTC (FVPTC)

FVPTC is the most troublesome of the variants of PTC and accounts for most of the false negative intraoperative

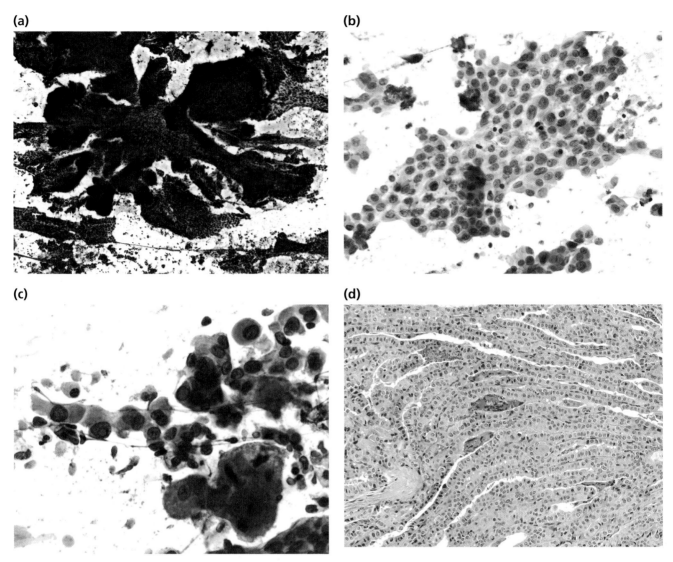

Fig. 11.6. (a) Cytologic findings in PTC. Occasionally, papillary structures are visible on a cytoscrape preparation. (b) Nuclear clearing is absent in cytologic preparations but nuclear enlargement, mild nuclear pleomorphism and abundant nuclear grooves should prompt a search for other primary features (c) such as metaplastic cells and intranuclear incusions. (d) When other architectural features of papillary carcinoma are absent on the FS slide, elongated follicles are a clue to the diagnosis of PTC, and are often associated with aborted papillary structures.

diagnoses of PTC. The reasons are clear: this variant lacks papillary structures and psammoma bodies, and because nuclear clearing is absent in FSs and cytoscrape preparations, the diagnosis is based on fewer cytologic features. Intraoperatively, FVPTC should be recognized when a lesion has the sclerotic and infiltrative pattern of PTC, since benign lesions do not have this architectural pattern (Fig. 11.7). The problem, however, is recognizing the encapsulated, non-sclerotic subtype of FVPTC. In the series by Jain et al.,[18] 60% of FVPTCs were interpreted as "follicular neoplasms" on FNA, so the pathologist on FS duty does not benefit from the correct FNA diagnosis in the majority of cases. This is an argument in support of limited FS and cytologic examination of encapsulated follicular neoplasms as it gives the pathologist a second opportunity to make the correct diagnosis. There is one other explanation for the under-recognition of FVPTC intraoperatively: its over-diagnosis on permanent sections. Since there is significant inter-observer variation in the diagnosis of FVPTC by expert thyroid pathologists,[19,20] it is possible that follicular adenomas with some degree of nuclear clearing are incorrectly interpreted as FVPTC, accounting for the disproportionate number of encapsulated FVPTCs. We should heed John Chan's appeal to use strict criteria for the diagnosis of encapsulated FVPTC.[21]

CYSTIC PAPILLARY CARCINOMA

Approximately 15% of papillary carcinomas undergo cystic change[8] and at times the cystic change is marked enough to mimic a benign cystic lesion (Fig. 11.1). Because cystic

Table 11.2. Variants of PTC: Behavior compared to conventional PTC and diagnostic pitfalls

Subtype	Aggressiveness	Likely misdiagnosis
Microcarcinoma	Less	none
Encapsulated conventional	Less	none
Follicular variant, infiltrative	Similar	none
Follicular variant, encapsulated	Less	Follicular adenoma
Cystic	Similar	Benign cystic lesion
Tall cell	More	none
Columnar cell	More	Metastasis of G.I. or endometrial origin
Diffuse sclerosing	More	Chronic thyroiditis
Macrofollicular	Similar	Benign follicular lesion
Cribriform-morular	Similar	Poorly differentiated (insular) CA
Solid	Similar	Poorly differentiated (insular) CA
Oxyphil	Similar	Hurthle cell neoplasm
Multinodular follicular variant	More	Multinodular goiter
With fasciitis-like component	Similar	Primary mesenchymal neoplasm
Hobnail	More	Metastatic carcinoma

PTCs are commonly under-diagnosed on FNA, cystic thyroid nodules should be examined carefully on gross examination, even if the prior FNA was interpreted as benign. A cytoscrape preparation should be made of the residual solid component if it lacks the colloid-rich appearance of a benign adenomatous nodule, and a FS should be performed if the cytologic findings are equivocal.

OTHER VARIANTS OF PAPILLARY CARCINOMA

There are many variants of PTC[22–30] and most can be correctly recognized as PTC on FNA if a good sample is obtained. All of these variants are treated by total thyroidectomy. The extent of lymph node dissection, and whether or not perithyroid soft tissue is resected, are dictated by the stage of the disease and not the histologic sub-type. Mistaking one of these variants for some other type of thyroid malignancy has minor intraoperative consequences. Table 11.2 lists the variants of PTC, their behavior compared to conventional PTC and the diagnostic challenges they present intraoperatively. Some of these variants are illustrated in Fig. 11.8.

PAPILLARY LESIONS THAT MIMIC PAPILLARY CARCINOMA

It is well known that cytologic features are cardinal in the diagnosis of PTC and that papillary structures are not required for the diagnosis. Papillary structures are certainly helpful for the intraoperative recognition of PTC but it should be remembered that well-developed papillary structures are found in a minority of follicular adenomas and hyperplastic nodules (Fig. 11.9).

(a)

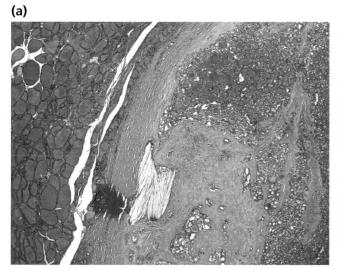

(b)

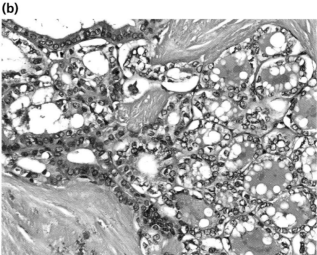

Fig. 11.7. Follicular variant of PTC (FVPTC). (a) The dense sclerosis is a clue to the diagnosis. (b) The cytologic features are those of conventional papillary carcinoma.

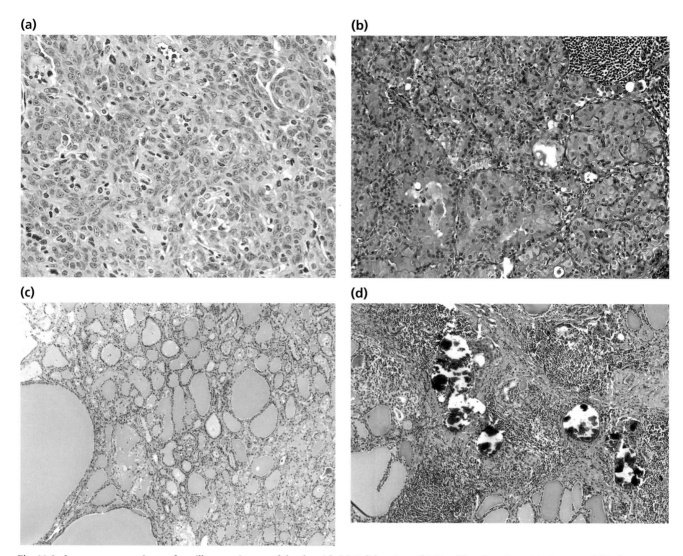

Fig. 11.8. Less common variants of papillary carcinoma of the thyroid: (a) Solid variant, (b) Hurthle cell variant, (c) the macrofollicular variant which may be very difficult to recognize intraoperatively, and (d) diffuse sclerosing variant.

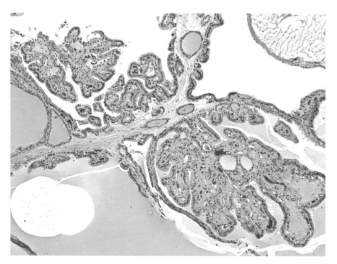

Fig. 11.9. Papillary structures in a benign adenomatous nodule. Clues to the correct diagnosis include: projection of the papillary structures into a cystic space, the lack of fibrous cores in the papillae and the presence of small, secondary follicles within the papillary structures.

Follicular neoplasms

Clinical issues

Follicular neoplasms are classified as follicular adenoma, minimally invasive follicular carcinoma, and widely invasive follicular carcinoma. Over 80% of follicular neoplasms are adenomas, and the majority of follicular carcinomas are minimally invasive. Widely invasive follicular carcinoma is rare in the United States but more common in iodine-deficient areas where it is frequently associated with MNG. Follicular adenoma (FA) and minimally invasive follicular carcinoma (miniFC) present as a solitary nodule; in contrast, widely invasive follicular carcinoma may present as an overt malignancy with local invasion and distant metastases, but may have a more subtle presentation.

Lobectomy or lobectomy/isthmusectomy is the appropriate surgical treatment for FA. Widely invasive follicular carcinoma is treated by total thyroidectomy. There is no consensus about the appropriate surgical treatment of miniFC; some surgeons feel that lobectomy is sufficient, whereas others prefer total thyroidectomy. This disagreement is partly due to varying thresholds for the diagnosis of miniFC, and the wide range in the reported incidence of local recurrences, metastases (5%–20%) and death from disease (0%–28% at 10 years, with capsular and vascular invasion, respectively).[31,32] If permanent sections reveal a miniFC with vascular invasion, it is very likely that a completion thyroidectomy will be performed. Completion thyroidectomy is not any more complicated than performing an initial total thyroidectomy, and there are no added risks above those associated with a second general anesthetic.

Pathologic findings

FNA cannot distinguish between FA, miniFC and widely invasive FC. Moreover, a significant percentage of lesions interpreted as "follicular neoplasm" on FNA are either hyperplastic (adenomatous) nodules with a microfollicular component or less commonly, the follicular variant of papillary carcinoma. The confident distinction between the different follicular neoplasms is based on architectural features and requires examination of a tissue specimen.

The diagnosis of grossly invasive FC may be evident or may be suspected on gross examination of the resected specimen, either because of an obvious infiltrative malignancy or because of a nodule with irregular margins (Fig. 11.10). The purpose of FS is to confirm that the lesion is a primary thyroid malignancy.

FA and miniFC present as an encapsulated nodule (Fig. 11.11). The capsule of miniFC is usually >1 mm in thickness,[33] a finding that is not specific but should alert the pathologist to the possibility of invasive carcinoma. The diagnosis of miniFC is made by identifying capsular and/or vascular invasion. This requires thorough examination of well fixed sections. Some pathologists attempt to make the distinction between FA and miniFC on FSs, but in our opinion, this should be deferred to permanent sections for the following reasons:

- At times, true capsular invasion is difficult to distinguish from an irregular interface of tumor with capsule, or secondary fibrosis due to degenerative changes. Furthermore, the interpretation of capsular invasion is confounded by lack of consensus on how to define capsular invasion. Some pathologists require penetration of the full thickness of the capsule, whereas others

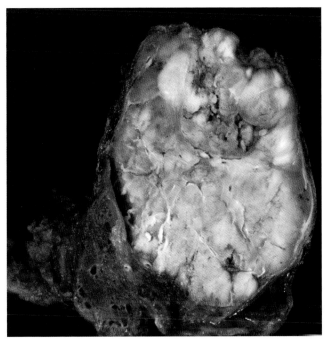

Fig. 11.10. Grossly invasive follicular carcinoma with an expansile growth pattern. Not all "grossly invasive" follicular carcinomas show widespread infiltration into the adjacent thyroid tissue. This thyroid mass has irregular margins, a clue to the diagnosis of invasive carcinoma. The patient presented with a bone metastasis, and the primary thyroid nodule was found only after the diagnosis of metastatic follicular carcinoma was made on biopsy of the bony lesion.

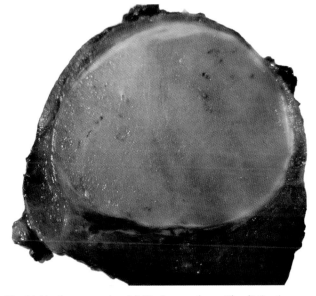

Fig. 11.11. An encapsulated follicular neoplasm. The distinction between follicular adenoma and follicular carcinoma cannot be made intraoperatively as this requires thorough examination of the capsule of the nodule. Some thyroid experts recommend gross examination only; an alternative approach is to render a preliminary diagnosis based on a cytoscrape preparation and a single FS.

(a) **(b)**

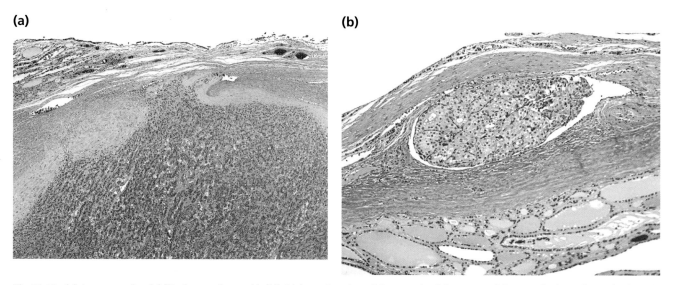

Fig. 11.12. (a) An encapsulated follicular neoplasm with full thickness invasion of the capsule. Other areas of the capsule showed vascular invasion, diagnostic of minimally invasive follicular carcinoma. (b) Another example of miniFC with vascular invasion.

will accept less than full thickness invasion of the capsule (Fig. 11.12). Occasionally, a miniFC penetrates the capsule, but evokes a new secondary capsule, making it difficult to decide if capsular invasion is really present. The situation is compounded by the fact that FNA can cause capsular disruption and mimic true capsular invasion.

- There is generally greater agreement about the criteria for vascular invasion but vascular invasion may be difficult to interpret on FSs. First, the affected vessels have to be in the capsule of the nodule or immediately outside the capsule – but not within the nodule. Second, the nidus of tumor cells that projects into the lumen of the vessel has to be covered by endothelium; third, if endothelial cells are lacking, the tumor cells have to be attached to the wall and there has to be an associated thrombus. One of the problems with evaluating vascular invasion is that clusters of follicular epithelial cells may abut onto the endothelium of vessels at the interface of tumor and capsule but this does not qualify as vascular invasion unless the neoplastic cells form a polypoid nodule that projects into the lumen of the vessel (Fig. 11.12). The degree of protrusion that qualifies as vascular invasion is subjective, and open to differences of opinion.
- In the series by Goldstein,[34] miniFC had an average of three foci of capsular invasion and 3 foci of vascular invasion. There is therefore, only a small chance of detecting convincing foci of invasion in a single

random section of the capsule. The opportunity of detecting capsular and vascular invasion intraoperatively will naturally increase with multiple FSs of the capsular area, but we do not support this approach because it is difficult to retain the integrity of the capsule and its relationship to the nodule when multiple sections are made into an unfixed encapsulated thyroid nodule. As a result, permanent sections may be difficult to interpret because of distortions of the capsule.

- There is high inter-observer variation in the interpretation of capsular and vascular invasion when well-fixed, paraffin-embedded sections are examined by thyroid experts, and it seems likely that this variance will be even greater on FS slides.

When all the above points are considered, it makes sense to take a minimalist approach to the intraoperative evaluation of an encapsulated thyroid nodule.[9] Our approach to this issue has been summarized above (p. 168).

If the permanent sections show a minimally invasive carcinoma, the diagnosis should be conveyed to the surgeon promptly because completion thyroidectomy is technically less challenging when performed within a few days of the first surgical procedure.

Hurthle cell neoplasms

The classification and intraoperative management of Hurthle cell neoplasms is the same as follicular neoplasms.

(a)

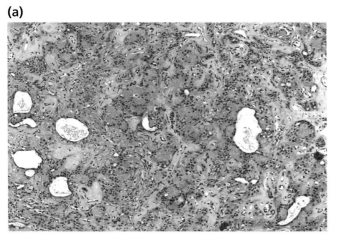

(b)

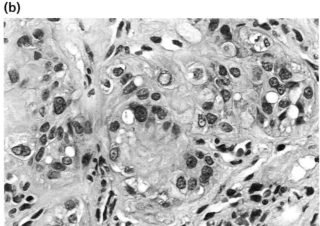

Fig. 11.13. (a) Hyalinizing trabecular adenoma, showing the characteristic trabecular pattern and diffuse sclerosis. (b) The nuclear features, including intranuclear inclusions, are similar to those of papillary carcinoma.

Hyalinizing trabecular neoplasms

Clinical issues

Hyalinizing trabecular neoplasms may be viewed as a variant of follicular neoplasms. Most are adenomas and should be treated by lobectomy. Rarely, a hyalinizing trabecular neoplasm has features of minimally invasive carcinoma[35] and should be treated in the same way as miniFC.

Pathologic issues

Hyalinizing trabecular adenoma may be misdiagnosed as papillary thyroid carcinoma because of the overlap in nuclear changes, including intranuclear inclusions (Fig. 11.13). However, if the diagnosis of hyalinizing trabecular adenoma is considered at the time of FNA, it can be confirmed by the identification of cytoplamic inclusion bodies and by the presence of membrane positivity for MIB-1 antigen.[36,37] This will allow the surgeon to approach the nodule as a probably benign neoplasm.

On gross examination, hyalinizing trabecular neoplasms are encapsulated. The intraoperative handling of the specimen is the same as outlined for follicular neoplasms above.

Poorly differentiated thyroid carcinoma

Clinical issues

Poorly differentiated thyroid carcinoma is an aggressive carcinoma of follicular origin that commonly produces regional lymph node and distant metastases.[38,39] Treatment consists of total thyroidectomy, and therapeutic regional lymph node dissection to remove all detectable disease.

Pathologic issues

If a specific diagnosis of poorly differentiated follicular carcinoma has been made on FNA, intraoperative diagnosis will be limited to evaluating regional lymph nodes for metastases. If a specific diagnosis has not been made pre-operatively, the following features should be sought to make the diagnosis: (i) an insular pattern of growth; (ii) the nuclei show more atypia than those of well-differentiated follicular carcinoma; (iii) mitoses are readily found; and (iv) necrosis is often present.

On FS, the neoplasm may be mistaken for the solid variant of PTC or one of the variants of medullary carcinoma, but the presence of microfollicles is a clue to the follicular nature of the neoplasm (Fig. 11.14). Fortunately, all the neoplasms that this carcinoma can be mistaken for are treated by total thyroidectomy. The specific diagnosis of poorly differentiated thyroid carcinoma will prompt the surgeon to be more aggressive about resecting cervical lymph nodes.

Anaplastic carcinoma

Anaplastic carcinoma usually presents as an obvious malignancy with rapid growth, invasion of soft tissues of the neck and metastases. The diagnosis is generally made by FNA. An incisional biopsy will be performed if the FNA is non-diagnostic and if the neoplasm is unresectable. In this situation, the surgeon will request a FS diagnosis to confirm adequacy of the biopsy. The majority of anaplastic carcinomas are unresectable, but resectable carcinomas are treated aggressively by total thyroidectomy and node dissection because complete resection offers the best chance of

(a)

(b)

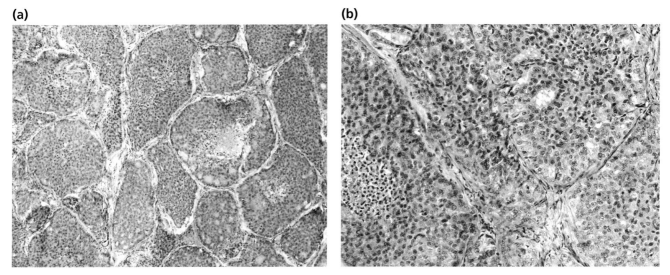

Fig. 11.14. Poorly differentiated thyroid carcinoma. (a) This particular neoplasm has an insular pattern. (b) The cytologic atypia, mitotic figures and necrosis distinguish this neoplasm from well differentiated follicular carcinoma. Microfollicles help to distinguish this neoplasm from medullary carcinoma.

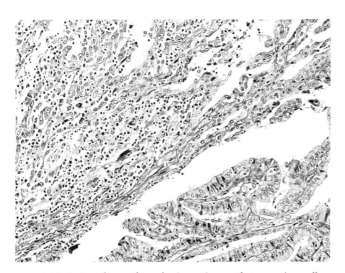

Fig. 11.15. A 1 cm focus of anaplastic carcinoma that arose in a tall cell variant of papillary carcinoma. The anaplastic component was overlooked and only identified on review of the thyroidectomy slides when the patient presented 2 months later with multiple liver metastases composed of anaplastic carcinoma. This illustration shows the transitional area of the neoplasm; the anaplastic carcinoma (upper left) was more pleomorphic elsewhere.

cure. Infrequently, a small focus of anaplastic carcinoma is found in association with a predominantly well-differentiated papillary or follicular carcinoma (Fig. 11.15). It is important to recognize the anaplastic component intraoperatively as this will prompt total thyroidectomy and an aggressive approach to neck dissection to remove all detectable disease.

Medullary carcinoma

Clinical issues

Eighty percent of medullary carcinomas of the thyroid (MCT) are sporadic and 20% are familial. Patients with familial disease either have familial MCT or one of the MEN 2 syndromes. Patients with a family history are usually fully evaluated by the time they come to surgery, and the appropriate surgical treatment is planned in advance. Total thyroidectomy is the appropriate surgical treatment for familial MCT because of the multifocal and bilateral nature of the carcinoma and its precursor lesion, C-cell hyperplasia. Family members who have the RET germline mutation responsible for MCT will undergo prophylactic total thyroidectomy for the same reasons.

Patients with sporadic MCT may or may not have a definitive diagnosis on prior FNA. Sporadic MCT is also treated by total thyroidectomy. The rationale for total thyroidectomy is that a minority of patients with sporadic disease have intrathyroid metastases to the opposite lobe, and total thyroidectomy is the best opportunity for cure. In addition, a seemingly "sporadic" case of MCT may turn out to be the index case for undiscovered familial MCT, and total thyroidectomy is the appropriate treatment. Prophylactic central neck dissection is performed if the primary tumor is greater than >1 cm because lymph node metastases are present in >60% of patients.

(a) **(b)**

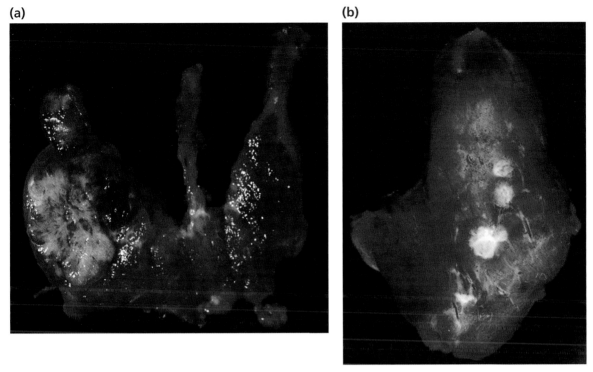

Fig. 11.16. (a) Medullary carcinoma of the thyroid (MCT) usually presents as a solid, pale mass with poorly defined margins. (b) Familial MCT is often multifocal, as in this case where the opposite lobe contained multiple smaller foci of MCT.

Pathologic issues

When there is a prior FNA diagnosis of MCT, intraoperative consultation will be requested on the thyroid gland if there is concern about the status of the surgical margins. Lymph nodes may also be submitted for FS to help plan the extent of lymph node dissection.

When there is no prior FNA diagnosis or chemical evidence of medullary carcinoma, the surgeon will submit a lobectomy specimen for IOD. The correct diagnosis can be made if the neoplasm has the characteristic gross and histologic features of medullary carcinoma. The prototypic MCT has a solid, pale appearance on gross examination, and microscopically, is characterized by solid growth of polygonal cells with granular cytoplasm (Figs. 11.16 and 11.17). Abundant stroma in the form of collagen, fibrovascular septa and amyloid are useful clues to the diagnosis. However, MCT may assume a wide range of microscopic patterns (Fig. 11.17), and when amyloid is absent in the FS, this neoplasm may be mistaken for some other type of thyroid carcinoma, especially in the sporadic setting where there are no clinical clues to the diagnosis. Table 11.3 lists the variants of MCT and the neoplasms with which they may be confused.[38,40] If the specific diagnosis of MCT is

not made intraoperatively, the pathologist should at least recognize the lesion as a carcinoma that requires total thyroidectomy and node dissection.

Metastatic neoplasms

A metastasis should be considered if a thyroid neoplasm has an unusual appearance, or if there are multiple colloid-poor tumor nodules in the gland. The first step is to review the clinical history with the surgeon. If the clinical history is not helpful and a firm diagnosis cannot be made, the pathologist should discuss the dilemma with the surgeon and leave the surgeon to decide whether a total thyroidectomy should be performed. If a lobectomy is performed and the neoplasm turns out to be an unusual primary malignancy that warrants total thyroidectomy, completion thyroidectomy can be performed at a later date. The most common malignancies to metastasize to the thyroid gland include lung carcinoma, melanoma and renal cell carcinoma (Fig. 11.18). Metastatic amelanotic melanoma may mimic medullary carcinoma, and metastatic renal cell carcinoma has to be distinguished from the clear cell variant of follicular carcinoma.

(a)

(b)

(c)

(d)

(e)

(f)

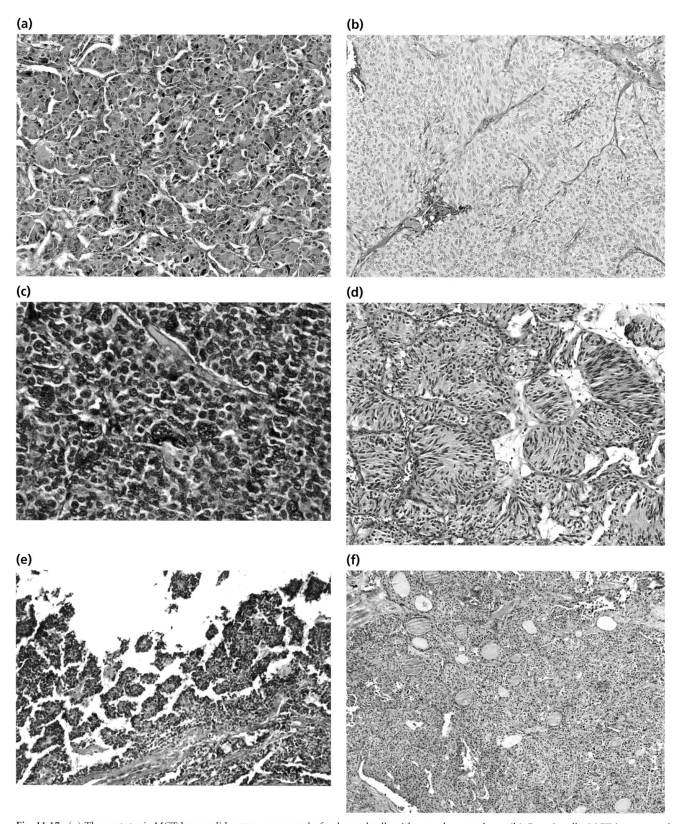

Fig. 11.17. (a) The prototypic MCT has a solid pattern composed of polygonal cells with granular cytoplasm. (b) Occasionally, MCT is composed predominantly of oval cells similar to the solid pattern of papillary carcinoma, or (c) small cells and giant cells that may be interpreted as anaplastic carcinoma (d). Infrequently, MCT may have a trabecular or (e) pseudopapillary pattern. (f) Entrapment of benign thyroid follicles at the periphery of the neoplasm may be mistaken for invasive follicular carcinoma.

Table 11.3. Variants of medullary carcinoma and lesions with which they may be confused

MCT Variant	Possible Misdiagnosis
Tubular/follicular	Follicular carcinoma
Papillary	Papillary carcinoma
Small cell	Lymphoma; poorly diff. carcinoma
Giant cell/pleomorphic	Anaplastic carcinoma
Clear cell	Clear cell follicular; metastasis
Oncocytic	Hurthle cell carcinoma
Squamous	Metastasis
Spindle cell	Mesenchymal neoplasm
Pigmented (melanocytic)	Metastatic melanoma
Carcinoid-like	Metastastic carcinoid tumor
Paraganglioma-like	Metastasis
Hyalinizing trabecular-like	Hyalinizing trabecular adenoma

Hashimoto's disease

Clinical issues

Surgery is seldom performed on uncomplicated Hashimoto's disease. However, surgical resection is performed for the following reasons. (a) The thyroid gland contains a nodule that is a FNA proven papillary carcinoma, warranting thyroidectomy. (b) A nodule is present and the FNA shows only chronic thyroiditis. A lobectomy will be performed to rule out a neoplasm. (c) A nodule is present and the FNA shows a follicular or Hurthle cell neoplasm. A lobectomy will be performed and the specimen will be sent for IOD. (d) A mass is present and the FNA shows a lymphoproliferative disorder. If a firm diagnosis cannot be made on FNA, an incisional biopsy or lobectomy will be performed, and the specimen will be sent for IOD, either for diagnosis or to determine specimen adequacy.

Pathologic issues

Nodules that occur in Hashimoto's disease are either nodular areas of Hashimoto's disease, hyperplastic Hurthle cell nodules (Fig. 11.19) or a thyroid malignancy of some kind. The approach towards a solitary follicular neoplasm, Hurthle cell neoplasm and PTC are the same as if they were unassociated with Hashimoto's disease. Malignant lymphomas that arise in Hashimoto's disease are discussed below. There is one cautionary note about evaluating nodules in Hashimoto's disease. Occasionally, the surgeon will encounter a nodule adjacent to the thyroid gland and submit this as lymph node when in fact it is tenuously pedunculated nodule of Hashimoto's

(a)

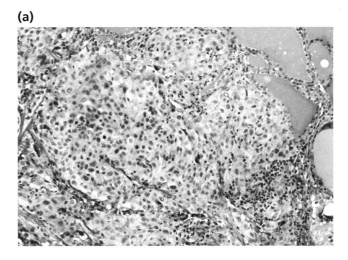

(b)

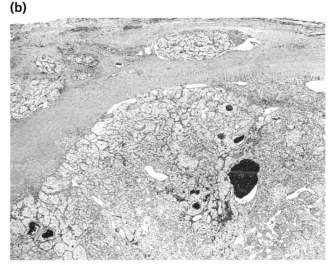

Fig. 11.18. Metastases to the thyroid gland may mimic primary carcinomas. (a) Metastatic melanoma can mimic medullary carcinoma when melanin pigment is absent in the FS slide. (b) Metastatic renal cell carcinoma may be mistaken for clear cell follicular carcinoma; in this example, there is a capsule with invasion of capsular vessels, further mimicking a clear cell follicular carcinoma. The presence of hemorrhage in glandular spaces is a clue to the diagnosis of metastatic renal cell carcinoma.

disease. If the pathologist is not aware that the patient has Hashimoto's disease, the nodule could be incorrectly interpreted as a lymph node containing metastatic thyroid carcinoma.

Lymphoma

Most lymphomas arise in association with Hashimoto's disease or chronic thyroiditis. Approximately 75% of primary thyroid lymphomas are diffuse large cell lymphoma, and a proportion of these have transformed from low grade extranodal marginal zone B-cell lymphoma of mucosa-associated lymphoid

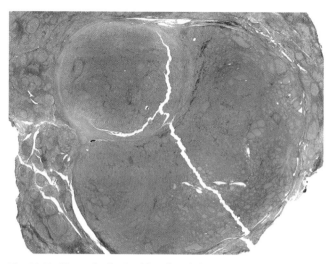

Fig. 11.19. Hyperplastic Hurthle cell nodule in Hashimoto's disease. Hyperplastic Hurthle cell nodules are usually multiple, lack a well formed capsule, and lack the prominent nucleoli of Hurthle cell carcinoma.

tissue type (MALTomas) (Fig. 11.20). MALTomas constitute most of the remaining lymphomas.

Large cell lymphoma can be suspected or recognized on touch or cytoscrape preparations, but the final diagnosis may have to be deferred to permanent sections. Care should be taken to distinguish lymphoma from other small cell malignancies such as small cell medullary carcinoma and poorly differentiated thyroid carcinoma to avoid unnecessary surgical treatment. Cytologic preparations should be made when lymphoma is suspected because the lymphoid nature of the neoplasm will be more evident, especially on Diff–Quik or Wright–Giemsa stained air-dried preparations.

Low grade lymphoma may be more difficult to diagnose with confidence because plasma cells and reactive lymphoid follicles may be present. The diagnosis should be deferred to permanent sections after sufficient material has been procured. Fresh tissue should be procured for flow cytometry analysis as this often helps in making a prompt diagnosis.

(a) **(b)**

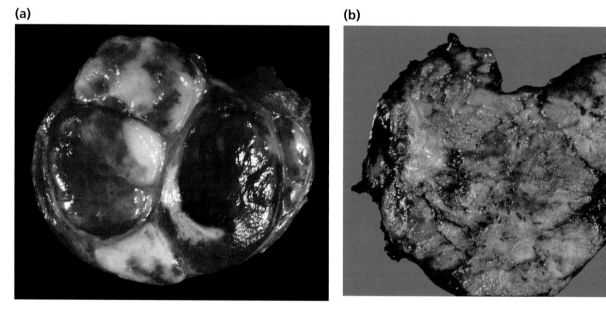

Fig. 11.20. (a) Large cell lymphoma of the thyroid gland forming a large fleshy mass, characteristic of lymphoma. (b) Small cell lymphoma of the thyroid gland producing diffuse infiltration of the gland, not dissimilar from Hashimoto's disease on gross examination.

REFERENCES

1. Stulak JM, Grant CS, Farley DR, *et al*. Value of preoperative ultrasonography in the surgical management of initial and reoperative papillary thyroid cancer. *Arch Surg* 2006; **141**: 489–494.

2. Kelly NP, Lim JC, DeJong S, Hermath C, Dudiak C, Wojcik EM. Specimen adequacy and diagnostic specificity of ultrasound-guided fine needle aspirations of nonpalpable thyroid nodules. *Diag Cytopathol* 2006; **34**: 188–190.

3. Barroeta JE, Wang H, Shiina N, Gupta PK, LiVolsi VA, Baloch ZW. Is fine-needle aspiration (FNA) of multiple thyroid nodules justified? *Endocr Pathol* 2006; **17**: 61–65.

4. Boostrom S, Richards ML. Total thyridectomy is the preferred treatment for patients with Graves' disease and a thyroid nodule. *Otolaryngol Head Neck Surg* 2007; **136**: 278–281.

5. Nguyen GK, Ginsberg J, Crockford PM, Villaneuva RR. Hashimoto's thyroiditis: cytodiagnostic accuracy and pitfalls. *Diagn Cytopathol* 1997; **16**: 531–536.

6. Baloch ZW, Tam D, Langer J, Mandel S, LiVolsi VA, Gupta PK. Ultrasound-guided fine-needle aspiration biopsy of the thyroid: role of on-site assessment and multiple cytologic preparations. *Diagn Cytopathol* 2000; **23**: 425–429.

7. Baloch ZW, Hendreen S, Gupta PK, *et al*. Interinstitutional review of thyroid fine-needle aspirations: impact on clinical management of thyroid nodules. *Diagn Cytopath* 2001; **27**: 231–234.

8. de los Santos ET, Keyhani-Rofagha S, Cunningham JJ, Mazzaferri EL. Cystic thyroid nodules. The dilemma of malignant lesions. *Arch Int Med* 1990; **150**: 1422–1427.

9. Udelsman R, Westra WH, Donovan PI, *et al*. Randomized prospective evaluation of frozen-section analysis for follicular neoplasms of the thyroid. *Ann Surg* 2001; **233**: 716–722.

10. Layfiedl LJ, Mohrmann RL, Kopald KH, *et al*. Use of aspiration cytology and frozen section examination for management of benign and malignant thyroid nodules. *Cancer* 1991; **68**: 130–134.

11. Ylagan LR, Farkas T, Dehner LP. Fine needle aspiration of the thyroid: a cytohistologic correlation and study of discrepant cases. *Thyroid* 2004; **14**: 35–41.

12. Tollin SR, Mery GM, Jelveh N, Fallon EF, Mikhail M, Blumenfeld W. The use of fine-needle aspiration biopsy under ultrasound guidance to assess the risk of malignancy in patients with multinodular goiter. *Thyroid* 2000; **10**: 235–241.

13. Nishida T, Nakao K, Hashimoto T. Local control in differentiated thyroid carcinoma with extrathyroidal invasion. *Am J Surg* 2000; **179**: 86–91.

14. McConahey WM, Hay ID, Woolner WB, van Heerden JA, Taylor WF. Papillary thyroid cancer treated at the Mayo Clinic, 1946 through 1970; initial manifestations, pathologic findings, therapy, and outcome. *Mayo Clinic Proc* 1986; **61**: 978–996.

15. Cooper DS, Doherty GM, Haugen B, *et al*. Management guidelines for patients with thyroid nodules and differentiated thyroid cancer. *Thyroid* 2006; **16**: 109–142.

16. Hay ID, Grant CS, van Heerden JA, Goellner JR, Ebersold JR, Bergstralh EJ. Papillary thyroid microcarcinoma: a study of 535 cases observed in a 50-year period. *Surgery* 1992; **112**: 1139–1146.

17. Chow SM, Law SC, Chan JK, Au SK, Yau S, Lau WH. Papillary microcarcinoma of the thyroid – Prognostic significance of lymph node metastasis and multifocality. *Cancer* 2003; **98**: 31–40.

18. Jain M, Khan A, Patwardhan N, Reale F, Safran M. Follicular variant of papillary carcinoma: a comparative study of histopathologic fatures and cytology results in 141 patients. *Endocr Prac* 2001; **7**: 79–84.

19. Hirokawa M, Carney JA, Goellner JR, *et al*. Obsever variation of encapsulated follicular lesions of the thyroid gland. *Am J Surg Pathol* 2002; **26**: 1508–1514.

20. Lloyd RV, Erickson LA, Casey MB, *et al*. Observer variation in the diagnosis of follicular variant of Papillary Thyroid Carcinoma. *Am J Surg Pathol* 2004; **28**: 1336–1340.

21. Chan JKC. Strict criteria should be applied in the diagnosis of encapsulated follicular variant of papillary thyrid carcinoma. *Am J Clin Pathol* 2002; **117**: 16–18.

22. Albores-Saavedra J, Gould E, Vardaman C, Vuitch F. The macrofollicular variant of papillary thyroid carcinoma: a study of 17 cases. *Hum Pathol* 1991; **22**: 1195–1205.

23. Beckner ME, Heffess CS, Oertel JE. Oxyphil papillary carcinoma. *Am J Clin Pathol* 1995; **103**: 280–287.

24. Berho M, Suster S. The oncocytic variant of papillary carcinoma of the thyroid: a clinicopathologic study of 15 cases. *Hum Pathol* 1997; **28**: 47–53.

25. Cameselle-Teijeiro J, Chan JKC. Cribriform-morular variant of papillary carcinoma: a distinctive variant representing the sporadic counterpart of familial adenomatous polyposis-associated thyroid carcinoma. *Mod Pathol* 1999; **13**: 363–365.

26. JKC Chan, Carcangiu ML, Rosai J. Papillary carcinoma of thyroid with exhuberant nodular fasciitis-like stroma. *Am J Clin Pathol* 1991; **95**: 309–314.

27. Ivanova R, Soares P, Castro P, Sobrinho-Simoes M. Diffuse (or multinodular) follicular variant of papillary thyroid carcinoma: a clinicopathologic and immunohistochemical analysis of ten cases of an aggressive form of differentiated thyroid carcinoma. *Virch Arch* 2001; **440**: 418–424.

28. Johnson TL, Lloyd RV, Thompson NW, Beierwaltes WH, Sisson JC. Prognostic implications of the tall cell variant of papillary carcinoma. *Am J Surg Pathol* 1988; **12**: 22–27.

29. Nikiforov YE, Erikson LA, Nikiforova MN, Caudill CM, Lloyd RV. Solid variant of papillary thyroid carcinoma: incidence, clinical-pathologic characteristics, molecular analysis, and biologic behavior. *Am J Surg Pathol* 2001; **25**: 1478–1484.

30. Wenig BM, Thompson LDR, Adair CF, Shmookler B, Heffess CS. Thyroid papillary carcinoma of columnar cell type. *Cancer* 1998; **82**: 740–753.

31. D'Avanzo A, Treseler P, Ituarte PHG, *et al*. Follicular thyroid carcinoma: histology and prognosis. *Cancer* 2004; **100**: 1123–1129.

32. Van Heerden JA, Hay AD, Goellner JR, *et al*. Follicular thyroid carcinoma with capsular invasion alone: a nonthreatening malignancy. *Surgery* 1992; **112**: 1130–1138.

33. Yamashina M. Follicular neoplasms of the thyroid. *Am J Surg Pathol* 1992; **16**: 392–400.

34. Goldstein NS, Czako P, Neill JS. Metastatic minimally invasive (encapsulated) follicular and Hurthle cell thyroid carcinoma: a study of 34 patients. *Mod Pathol* 2000; **13**: 123–130.

35. Molberg K, Albores-Saavedra J. Hyalinizing trabecular carcinoma of the thyroid gland. *Hum Pathol* 1994; **25**: 192–197.

36. Hirokawa M, Carney JA Cell membrane and cytoplasmic staining for MIB-1 in jyalinizing trabecular adenoma of the thyroid gland. *Am J Surg Pathol* 2000; **24**: 575–578.

37. Rothenberg HJ, Goellner JR, Carney JA. Hyalinizing trabecular adenoma of the thyroid gland: recognition and characterization of its cytoplasmic yellow body. *Am J Surg Pathol* 1999; **23**: 118–125.

38. Rosai J, Carcangiu ML, DeLellis RA. *Tumors of the Thyroid Gland Atlas of Tumor Pathology* Washington DC: Armed Forces Institute of Pathology, 1992.

39. Volante M, Collini P, Nikiforov YE, *et al.* Poorly differentiated thyroid carcinoma: the Turin proposal for the use of uniform diagnostic criteria and an algorithmic diagnostic approach. *Am J Surg Pathol* 2007; **31**: 1256–1264.

40. Chan JKC. Tumors of the thyroid and parathyroid glands. In *Diagnostic Histopathology of Tumors*, CDM Fletcher (ed) 3rd edn. Churchill Livingstone, 2007, pp. 1038–1046.

12 PARATHYROID GLAND

Mahendra Ranchod, John K.C. Chan, and Electron Kebebew

CHANGES IN THE MANAGEMENT OF PRIMARY HYPERPARATHYROIDISM

The pathologist's role in the management of primary hyperparathyroidism has changed significantly during the past few decades. These changes will be reviewed briefly because they illustrate the impact of technological advances as well as point to an embarrassing interlude in the management of this disease.

In the pre-1970s, a solitary adenoma was considered responsible for primary hyperparathyroidism in 80%–85% of cases, double adenomas in 2%–5%, carcinoma in 1%, and hyperplasia for the remaining 10%–12%. In the early 1970s, it was proposed that hyperplasia was under-recognized and responsible for >50% of cases of primary hyperparathyroidism, and as a result, many patients with a single enlarged gland were treated by subtotal parathyroidectomy. Furthermore, it was posited that hyperplasia frequently occurred in normal-sized glands and required histologic examination for its recognition. Thus, when a single enlarged gland was encountered, surgeons were encouraged to biopsy one or more normal-sized glands to determine if they were normal or hyperplastic. Frozen sections (FSs) on these biopsies were interpreted as normal or hyperplastic based on the cellularity of the parathyroid tissue. The distinction between normal and microscopic hyperplasia was often difficult and a variety of ancillary tests were developed, including density tests and rapid stains for intracellular fat.

This misguided era came to an end in the late 1970s when the concept of microscopic hyperplasia was challenged.[1–4] There were two reasons for the over-diagnosis of microscopic hyperplasia: (a) the proponents of microscopic hyperplasia had unwittingly included a disproportionate number of patients with familial hyperparathyroidism (and thus hyperplasia) in their studies, and (b) surgical pathologists who were persuaded by the concept of microscopic hyperplasia were not fully aware of the range of cellularity of normal parathyroid glands. Normal-sized glands with a high epithelial/fat ratio were interpreted as hyperplastic when in fact they were normal. This led to a return to the notion that an adenoma was responsible for most cases of primary hyperparathyroidism, and that the surgeon should determine if the patient has single or multiple gland disease based on the gross findings at surgery. Thus, if a single gland was enlarged, the patient had an adenoma and only the enlarged gland was excised; normal-sized glands were not subjected to biopsy. If the patient had multiple enlarged glands, the diagnosis was hyperplasia and an appropriate volume of parathyroid tissue was resected (usually 3–3½ glands). This approach required bilateral neck exploration and identification of all four parathyroid glands.

More recent advances in parathyroid surgery have been driven by the desire to limit surgical exploration to the abnormal gland/s. The technetium sestamibi scan (Fig. 12.1), with or without SPECT/CT, correctly identifies >90% of parathyroid adenomas, and allows the surgeon to initially perform a unilateral neck exploration. The enlarged gland is excised and the second gland on the ipsilateral side is examined with the naked eye to determine if the patient has single or multiple gland disease. The rapid intraoperative parathyroid hormone test has brought about an even more focused approach to parathyroidectomy because this biochemical test can determine the adequacy of surgical resection.

CURRENT SURGICAL APPROACH TO PRIMARY HYPERPARATHYROIDISM

The causes of primary hyperparathyroidism are listed in Table 12.1. The surgical management of primary hyperparathyroidism can be considered in three main categories: sporadic

Intraoperative Consultation in Surgical Pathology, ed. Mahendra Ranchod. Published by Cambridge University Press.

Table 12.1. Causes of primary hyperparathyroidism

Adenoma

Lipoadenoma (rare)

Sporadic hyperplasia

Familial hyperparathyroidism

    Isolated familial hyperparathyroidism

    MEN type 1

    MEN type 2a

    Hyperparathyroidism-jaw syndrome

Parathyroid carcinoma

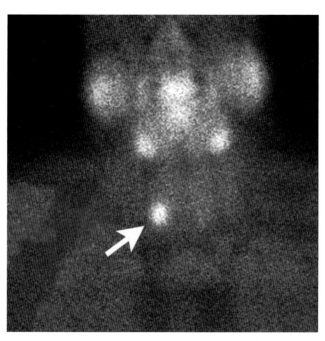

Fig. 12.1. Sestamibi scan showing persistent uptake on the right side of the neck, in keeping with a parathyroid adenoma (arrow). The paired structures in the upper neck are the submandibular salivary glands.

disease, familial disease, and persistent/recurrent hyperparathyroidism.

Sporadic primary hyperparathyroidism

A single adenoma is responsible for approximately 80% of cases of primary hyperparathyroidism. A sestamibi scan is performed routinely and this correctly predicts the location of an adenoma in >90% of cases.[5,6] When the sestamibi scan is negative, ultrasound examination is usually performed to localize an adenoma, and if a potential adenoma is identified, fine needle aspiration biopsy with evaluation of the aspirate for parathyroid hormone, will often confirm the parathyroid nature of the nodule. Some surgeons use radioguided surgery, with the aid of a parathyroid probe, to locate an adenoma.

If the rapid parathyroid hormone test is not available, the surgeon will explore the area of the positive sestamibi scan, remove the enlarged gland and identify the normal gland on the ipsilateral side. There is no reason to biopsy or remove the normal-sized gland. The disadvantage of this approach is that the contralateral side of the neck is not explored, and there is a small risk of missing a second adenoma or multiglandular disease. However, the risk of missing additional enlarged glands is reduced to <5% if pre-operative U/S examination confirms the location of the enlarged gland.

If the rapid parathyroid hormone test is available, the surgeon will focus on the enlarged gland and resect it. This procedure may be performed through a small, laterally placed incision, and can be done as an out-patient procedure under local anesthesia. Initially, no attempt is made to identify the other parathyroid glands. Instead, blood samples are drawn for rapid parathyroid hormone assay, and if the parathormone level drops by >50% of the baseline value 10 minutes after resection of the enlarged gland, it is assumed that the patient has a single adenoma. However, in about 20% of cases, the parathyroid hormone level fails to show the expected decrease after resection of an adenoma, in which case, the serum parathormone test is repeated 20 minutes after resection. If the serum parathormone remains elevated, both sides of the neck are explored for additional enlarged parathyroid glands. The use of intraoperative parathyroid assays thus allows a minimally invasive surgical approach to parathyroidectomy in approximately 80% of patients with an adenoma, and intraoperative pathologic confirmation is not required in this circumstance.

Familial and syndromic primary hyperparathyroidism

Seventy to eighty percent of patients who have familial or syndromic hyperparathyroidism have parathyroid gland hyperplasia. A sestamibi scan is performed even though it is recognized that this test is of limited value for detecting multiple enlarged glands. In the study by Perrier *et al.*, the sestamibi scan detected all the enlarged glands in only 25% of patients, and was potentially misleading by showing a single hot spot in 40% of patients.[6] Most patients with familial disease therefore require bilateral neck exploration.

Persistent or recurrent hyperparathyroidism

Persistent hyperparathyroidism is defined as an elevated serum calcium detected within 6 months of prior parathyroidectomy, and recurrent hyperparathyroidism refers to an elevation of serum calcium that first appears >6 months after the initial surgical procedure. The surgical treatment of persistent and recurrent hyperparathyroidism is generally more challenging because of altered tissue planes and scar tissue, and as a result, thorough pre-operative evaluation is necessary; this includes: whether the patient has sporadic or familial disease, the findings at the time of prior surgery, the extent of prior parathyroidectomy, the prior pathologic diagnosis, and the expertise of the surgeon who performed the prior procedure/s. Deciding whether to perform unilateral or bilateral neck exploration will depend on the specifics of the case. In the Mayo Clinic experience with re-exploration for persistent/recurrent disease, a single enlarged gland was removed in 87% of cases, and 76% of the adenomas were in a normal anatomic location. These adenomas were successfully managed by unilateral neck exploration.[7] This affirms that the challenge in parathyroid surgery is to *locate* the abnormal gland/s. In the current era, re-operation is best performed with the assistance of intraoperative parathormone assays. When multiple enlarged glands are resected and there is a risk of hypoparathyroidism, the surgeon may implant a portion of parathyroid tissue in the patient's forearm or submit part of the specimen for cryopreservation.

INFORMATION NEEDED BEFORE AND DURING IOC

Most parathyroid explorations are uncomplicated, yield a single adenoma, and can be handled without detailed clinical information. However, it is not always possible to anticipate the complexity of a case so it pays to be familiar with the clinical data in advance. The pathologist should obtain the following information: Is this the initial surgical procedure or re-exploration? Is there evidence of familial or syndromic disease? What are the results of imaging studies? Are there any unusual findings at the time of surgical exploration?

HANDING SPECIMENS INTRAOPERATIVELY

Accurate labeling of specimens

Although mundane, it is the pathologist's responsibility to make sure that the specimen is clearly labeled with regard to anatomic location. This becomes particularly important

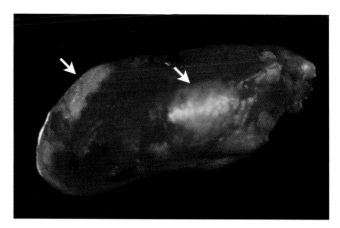

Fig. 12.2. Parathyroid adenoma with areas of visible fatty tissue on the surface (arrows). The fatty tissue represents residual normal parathyroid gland and should be included in the section taken for FS.

it the patient has to undergo re-exploration for persistent or recurrent hyperparathyroidism.

Gross examination

Every parathyroid gland received in the laboratory should be measured in three dimensions and weighed, and when appropriate, weighed to the closest milligram. A small amount of fatty tissue, representing residual normal parathyroid gland, may be visible on the surface of the gland (Fig. 12.2). This fatty area should be included in the sample taken for FS as it helps to recognize the specimen as parathyroid tissue if that becomes an issue. In most situations, the surgeon will submit the entire gland for IOD, but only part of a gland will be submitted if the specimen is used for auto-transplantation or sent for cryopreservation.

Inking the specimen

There is no reason to routinely ink an excised parathyroid gland, but the specimen should be inked if there is any suspicion of parathyroid carcinoma. Parathyroid carcinoma should be suspected if the gland was adherent to surrounding structures at the time of surgical excision, when the gland has a thick capsule, and when the specimen is an en bloc resection that includes other tissues such as soft tissue and thyroid gland.

Frozen section vs. cytologic preparations

Most enlarged parathyroid glands can be recognized on gross examination by their shape, consistency and color, and microscopic examination serves to confirm the gross impression of an enlarged parathyroid gland. The combination of FSs and cytologic preparations have the highest sensitivity and specificity for correctly identifying parathyroid tissue,[8] but as a single test, FSs are superior to cytologic preparations. Cytologic preparations tend to yield many bare nuclei that are non-diagnostic (Fig. 12.3) and they lack architectural features that are helpful in identifying parathyroid tissue in difficult situations.

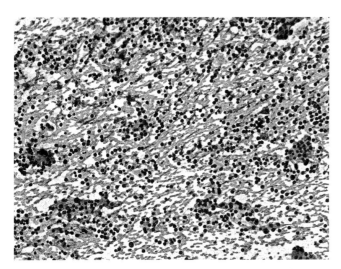

Fig. 12.3. Cytoscrape of a parathyroid adenoma. The smear shows mainly bare nuclei. Occasional small clusters are present and these reveal the delicate clear cytoplasm of the parathyroid chief cells.

CLINICOPATHOLOGIC ISSUES

The normal parathyroid gland

Each parathyroid gland weighs 30–50 mg, and a gland that weighs >60 mg should be considered abnormal. There is little reason to biopsy or remove a normal parathyroid gland in the current management of primary hyperparathyroidism. A normal parathyroid gland may be biopsied in only one circumstance: when the surgeon has difficulty finding an enlarged gland and can make a more directed search if a questionable structure is confirmed to be normal parathyroid gland; the search can then be directed elsewhere. If a biopsy of a normal gland is submitted for FS, the pathologist should ascertain the reason for the FS request. The only purpose of the FS is to confirm that the tissue is parathyroid tissue, and not to determine if the gland is normal or abnormal. Thirty to 50% of normal parathyroid glands have <10% stromal fat,[9,10] so cellularity of the biopsy cannot be used to distinguish normal from abnormal parathyroid gland (Fig. 12.4).

The chief cells of the normal parathyroid gland contain cytoplasmic lipid droplets that are visible on air-dried Romanowsky-stained smears as well as on FSs stained with oil red-O and Sudan IV stains. These lipid droplets decrease in size and quantity in most enlarged glands

(a)

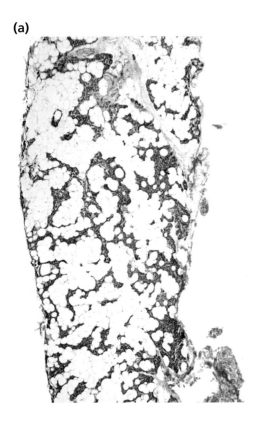

(b)

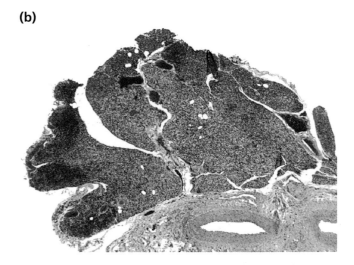

Fig. 12.4. Normal parathyroid glands showing variation in the amount of stromal fat. (a) Some glands have abundant stromal fat whereas others (b) have virtually no fat. Specimen (b) was removed inadvertently during thyroid lobectomy in a patient who was normocalcemic.

(adenoma and hyperplastic glands). Evaluating intracyto-plasmic lipid was in vogue during the era of "microscopic hyperplasia," but has no practical application in the current management of hyperparathyroidism. Small nodules composed of oncocytic cells may be present in the normal parathyroid gland of elderly patients; these are of no clinical significance and should not be over-interpreted as microadenomas.

Anatomic location of abnormal parathyroid glands

The task of finding abnormal parathyroid gland/s is facilitated by the availability of imaging techniques, but imaging is less reliable in patients with multiple enlarged glands. The surgeon has to be familiar with the usual and unusual locations of enlarged parathyroid glands. Approximately 85% of enlarged parathyroid glands are found in usual locations and 15% are in ectopic locations.[11] The upper parathyroid glands and the lateral lobes of the thyroid arise from the fourth branchial pouch, which explains why intra-thyroid adenomas are usually derived from one of the upper parathyroid glands. In contrast, the lower parathyroid glands are derived from the third branchial pouch and migrate with the thymus. During migration, the lower parathyroid glands dissociate themselves from this complex and remain in the neck, whereas the thymus gland continues its migration into the mediastinum. This association between the thymus and lower parathyroid glands explains why one or both of the lower parathyroid glands may be located within the thymus or elsewhere in the mediastinum. Furthermore, aberrations in the dissociation process during migration accounts for the occurrence of supernumerary glands and the occasional presence of small non-encapsulated foci of parathyroid tissue in the path of migration.

Parathyroid adenoma

Clinical issues

More than 90% of adenomas are single. The incidence of double adenomas is reported to be 2%–15%,[12–14] but it is probably <2% in non-tertiary medical centers. By convention, a patient with more than two enlarged parathyroid glands has hyperplasia. There is lack of a linear relationship between the level of serum parathormone and weight of an adenoma, but a significant elevation of parathormone is not likely to be explained by a minimally enlarged parathyroid gland.[15] The surgeon has to keep this in mind when searching for an elusive adenoma because a

minimally enlarged parathyroid gland is not likely to explain a marked elevation of serum parathyroid hormone. The surgeon may forgo intraoperative evaluation when a typical adenoma is excised and there is an appropriate decrease in the rapid serum parathormone level. The specimen may be submitted to the laboratory in formalin. The rapid parathyroid hormone assay has thus impacted the pathologist's role in the management of hyperparathyroidism, and this erosion will continue as the rapid parathormone test becomes more widely available.

Pathologic issues

A parathyroid adenoma is best defined by its weight. Most adenomas weigh 200 mg–1 g; less frequently, an adenoma will weigh 60–100 mg or >2 g. The appearance of most adenomas is characteristic enough to allow recognition by gross examination. The majority of adenomas are oval, but a minority are lobulated. The vast majority of adenomas have a thin capsule that is barely visible with the naked eye. A thick capsule should alert the pathologist to the possibility of carcinoma. Approximately 50% of adenomas contain residual normal parathyroid tissue, recognizable as a fatty area near the surface (so-called fatty hood or cap) (Fig. 12.2). It is worth looking for this fatty area and to include it in the sample taken for FS because the presence of normal parathyroid tissue helps to identify the specimen as parathyroid tissue. The cut surface is light tan (Fig. 12.5), a feature that distinguishes an adenoma from a thyroid nodule and lymph node.

A minor degree of cystic change is common in large adenomas; rarely, the cystic change is extensive, making it difficult to recognize the specimen as a parathyroid adenoma on gross examination (Fig. 12.6). Rarely, a parathyroid adenoma will undergo spontaneous infarction (Fig. 12.7).[16] Pain in the area of the affected gland, and a return of the serum calcium to normal or near normal are clues to the diagnosis. At surgery, the gland may be lightly adherent to the surrounding tissues because of a granulation tissue reaction to the infarction. Histologically, most of the adenoma may be infarcted, but a thin rim of residual non-infarcted parathyroid tissue is usually present at the periphery of the mass.

The vast majority of parathyroid adenomas are easily recognized on histologic examination. However, the following features may be challenging in the intraoperative setting:

▪ Parathyroid adenomas with a follicular pattern may be difficult to distinguish from thyroid nodules (Fig. 12.8).

This challenge is greatest when the parathyroid adenoma is located within the thyroid gland. The following features help to make the correct diagnosis: (a) the presence of normal fat-containing parathyroid tissue somewhere along the circumference of the nodule; (b) the presence of stromal fat cells in the adenoma itself; (c) well-circumscribed nests of oxyphil cells scattered between the dominant chief cells favor a parathyroid lesion because Hurthle cells in thyroid adenomas tend to blend with non-Hurthle follicular epithelial cells; (d) oxalate crystals in the follicles strongly favor thyroid tissue because oxalate crystals are only rarely found in parathyroid adenomas.

Fig. 12.5. Parathyroid adenoma with characteristic tan cut surface. The tan color distinguishes parathyroid adenomas from thyroid nodules and lymph nodes. Small foci of cystic change are present.

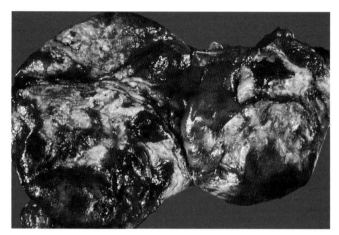

Fig. 12.6. Parathyroid adenoma with extensive cystic change. This is a view of the opened cyst. The lesion resembled a non-specific thin-walled benign cyst and was not recognizable as an abnormal parathyroid gland. However, parathyroid chief cells were present in the wall of the cyst. The patient was hypercalcemic and was rendered normocalcemic after excision of the lesion.

(a)

(b)

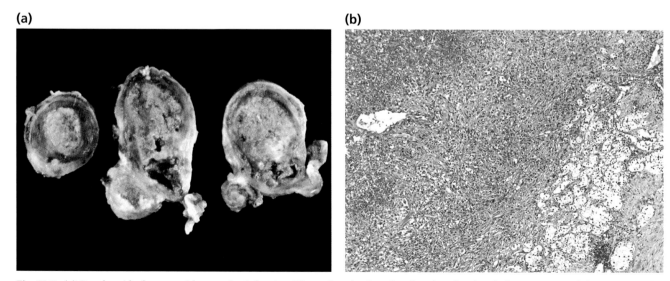

Fig. 12.7. (a) Parathyroid adenoma with extensive infarction. The patient developed neck pain a few days before surgery, and this was thought to be due to subacute thyroiditis. The patient's serum calcium was normal during routine testing the day prior to surgery but this finding was ignored. (b) A thin rim of residual, non-infarcted adenoma was present at the periphery of the excised gland (clear cells, lower right). The adenoma was adherent to the thyroid gland, requiring excision of part of the thyroid gland because of concern about malignancy.

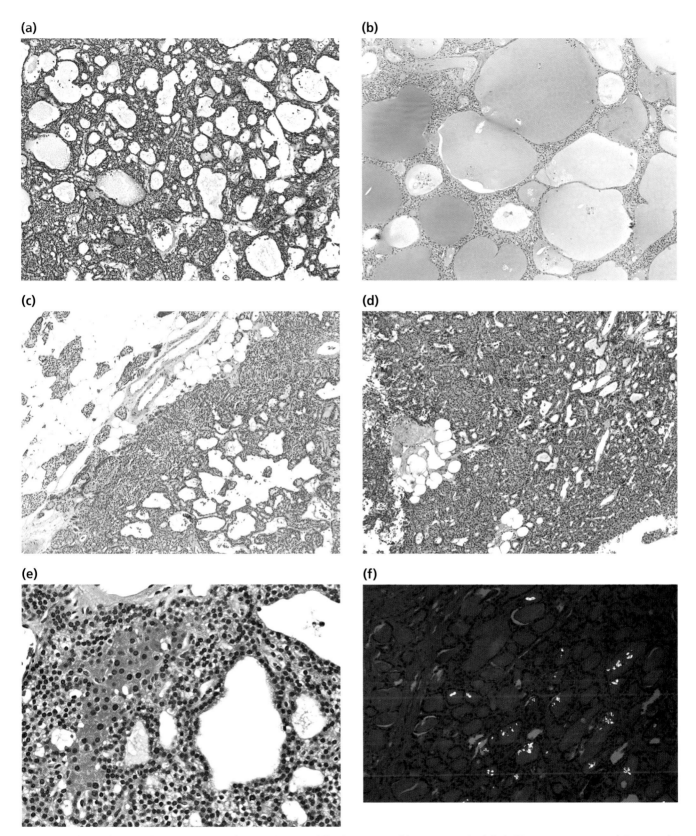

Fig. 12.8. (a) Parathyroid adenoma with a predominantly microfollicular pattern. (b) Sometimes the follicle-like structures are much larger and contain colloid-like material, strongly resembling thyroid tissue. (c) The presence of more typical solid areas elsewhere in the lesion, the presence of normal fat-containing parathyroid tissue adjacent to the adenoma, (d) fat cells within the adenoma, and (e) small islands of oxyphil cells permit the diagnosis of parathyroid adenoma. (f) Birefringent calcium oxalate crystals in the proteinaceous material strongly supports thyroid tissue as these rarely occur in parathyroid adenomas.

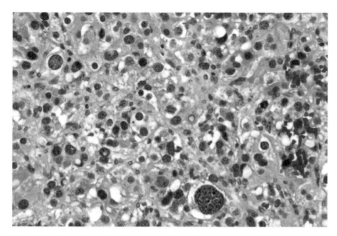

Fig. 12.9. Parathyroid adenoma with nuclear pleomorphism. In contrast to parathyroid carcinoma, the chief cells between the large cells do not show any atypia.

Table 12.2. Variants of parathyroid adenoma and differential diagnosis

Variant	Differential diagnosis
Microfollicular pattern	Follicular adenoma of thyroid
Oxyphil adenoma	Hurthle cell adenoma of thyroid
Lipoadenoma	Normal parathyroid gland (incisional biopsy)
Adenoma with pseudopapillary pattern	Papillary carcinoma of thyroid
Adenoma with chronic inflammation	Pedunculated nodule of Hashimoto's disease

- Occasional adenomas show marked nuclear pleomorphism (Fig. 12.9). This is of no clinical significance and should not be misconstrued as evidence of malignancy. The pleomorphism in adenomas is usually focal, in contrast to the diffuse, uniform atypia found in parathyroid carcinoma.

- Dense fibrous bands are present in a minority of adenomas and sometimes these are associated with hemosiderin, suggesting that the fibrous bands are ischemic in origin. Dense fibrous bands are more characteristic of carcinoma but they are of no significance when other features of carcinoma are lacking.

- Oxyphil adenomas account for 3% of functioning parathyroid adenomas.[17] Grossly, the lesion is characterized by a mahogany-brown cut surface, and microscopically, it is composed of uniform oxyphil cells (Fig. 12.10). When an oxyphil parathyroid adenoma is located within the thyroid gland, it can be difficult to distinguish from Hurthle cell adenoma of the thyroid gland. Clues to the diagnosis are similar to those listed for other intra-thyroid parathyroid adenomas with a follicular pattern (Table 12.2).

- Rarely, cystic change in an adenoma forms linear spaces imparting a pseudopapillary appearance to the lesion,[18,19] but this is unlikely to be mistaken for thyroid papillary carcinoma when the findings are taken in context.

- Rarely, parathyroid adenomas show chronic inflammation. The inflammation is usually focal and concentrated towards the periphery of the adenoma.[20] The inflammation is not dense enough to obscure the adenoma and should not present a challenge.

- Adenomas located in the thyroid gland may not be well encapsulated, and while the junction between adenoma

(a)

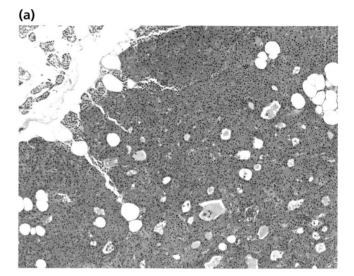

(b)

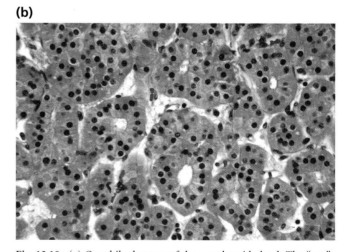

Fig. 12.10. (a) Oxyphil adenoma of the parathyroid gland. The "cap" of residual normal parathyroid gland and fat in the stroma of the adenoma readily distinguish an oxyphil parathyroid adenoma from a Hurthle cell adenoma of the thyroid gland. (b) Higher magnification of oxyphil cells.

(a) **(b)**

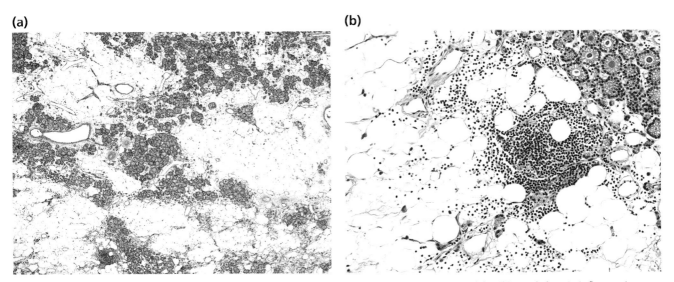

Fig. 12.11. (a) Lipoadenoma of the parathyroid gland showing an admixture of chief cells and stromal fat. (b) Focal chronic inflammation is often present. This neoplasm can be mistaken for normal parathyroid tissue if the surgeon submits an incisional biopsy, and if the pathologist is unaware of the surgical findings.

and thyroid tissue may be poorly defined, adenomas do not infiltrate the thyroid parenchyma; obvious infiltration of the thyroid parenchyma should suggest malignancy.

- FSs of lymph nodes with ice-crystal artifacts may be mistaken for parathyroid tissue, but the lymphoid nature of the specimen will be apparent if a cytologic preparation has been made.

Lipoadenoma of the parathyroid gland

Lipoadenoma of the parathyroid gland (parathyroid hamartoma) is a rare cause of hyperparathyroidism. It is characterized by a variable admixture of parathyroid chief cells and stromal fat;[21] stromal fat is the dominant component in large tumors (Fig. 12.11). Focal myxoid change and mild chronic inflammation may be present. Lipoadenomas may measure >10 cm in maximum dimension and weigh more than 5 g. Large, fat-rich lipoadenomas may cause consternation at the time of surgical exploration because they do not resemble the usual parathyroid adenoma; the surgeon may therefore, submit an incisional biopsy for diagnosis. If the pathologist is not aware of the size of the mass, the biopsy may be misinterpreted as normal parathyroid tissue because of the admixture of fat and parathyroid chief cells. This error can be easily averted by familiarity with the clinical and surgical findings.

Atypical adenoma

The term atypical parathyroid adenoma is applied to an enlarged parathyroid gland that has some but not all of

the features of parathyroid carcinoma (see Parathyroid carcinoma below). This term is useful because there are neoplasms that lack criteria for the diagnosis of carcinoma, but are sufficiently atypical to warrant close follow-up.[21]

Sporadic primary hyperplasia of the parathyroid glands

Clinical issues

Primary hyperplasia of the parathyroid glands is defined as enlargement of three or more parathyroid glands. By convention, synchronous enlargement of two glands is considered double adenomas. Occasionally, patients have metachronous enlargement of multiple parathyroid glands and in this situation, the diagnosis of hyperplasia can only made in retrospect. Sestamibi scans are not sensitive for detecting multiple enlarged glands, and as a result, the diagnosis of hyperplasia may be made for the first time during surgical exploration. Surgical explorations for known or suspected cases of hyperplasia are best performed with the help of rapid parathormone tests because some patients have more than four enlarged glands. In most patients however, the hyperparathyroidism is corrected after removal of three or three and a half glands.

Pathologic issues

The surgeon should determine if multiple parathyroid glands are enlarged based on naked eye examination of the glands. The pathologist can confirm this by weighing the specimens, but the diagnosis of hyperplasia should not be made by microscopic criteria alone; the gland should weigh >60 mg to qualify as abnormal, regardless of its cellularity. The pathologist cannot distinguish between an adenoma and a hyperplastic gland when a single enlarged parathyroid gland is examined out of context. Nodular versus diffuse pattern of growth, a rim of residual normal parathyroid tissue and cell types are all non-specific. The pathologist can confirm the diagnosis of hyperplasia only when three enlarged glands have been submitted, and when each gland weighs >60 mg. Microscopically, hyperplastic glands are usually composed entirely of chief cells. For reasons that are unclear, the entity of primary clear cell hyperplasia has virtually disappeared.

Familial primary hyperparathyroidism

Familial primary hyperparathyroidism consists of four main entities: Isolated Familial Hyperparathyroidism, MEN 1, MEN2a, and Hyperparathyroidism-jaw syndrome.

Isolated familial hyperparathyroidism (IFHP)

IFHP is rare. There is disagreement about its relationship to MEN1[22,23] and there is also disagreement about the frequency of hyperplasia in this disease; for example, Carneiro et al.[24] have reported that >90% of patients with IFHP have a single enlarged parathyroid gland. While the frequency of hyperplasia is unsettled, the surgical approach is clear. These patients should have a sestamibi scan to guide the initial neck exploration and the enlarged gland/glands should be removed with the help of intraoperative parathyroid hormone assays.

MEN type 1

Approximately 90% of patients with MEN1 have hyperparathyroidism and almost all have hyperplasia of the parathyroid glands. The mitogenic factors that drive parathyroid hyperplasia in MEN type1 cause hyperplasia of all the parathyroid tissue in the patient's neck, including supernumerary and ectopic glands. Furthermore, after subtotal parathyroidectomy, the residual parathyroid tissue may undergo hyperplasia and cause recurrent hyperparathyroidism years later. Since imaging studies are not helpful in detecting all the enlarged glands, the surgeon has to identify at least 4 parathyroid glands. The standard surgical treatment is subtotal parathyroidectomy (3½

gland resection), leaving the patient with approximately 50 mg of functional parathyroid tissue. Some surgeons routinely perform bilateral superior thymectomies as well.[25] When neck dissection is extensive and there is a risk of hypoparathyroidism (especially after re-exploration), the surgeon may transplant pieces of parathyroid tissue in the patient's forearm, or submit part of the specimen for cryopreservation, creating an option for delayed auto-transplantation.

The pathologist should weigh, measure and confirm that the excised tissue is parathyroid tissue. If part of the thymus gland is submitted, it should be sectioned at 3–4 mm intervals to ascertain if the specimen harbors an enlarged parathyroid gland. Intraoperative confirmation of the number and location of enlarged parathyroid glands may help to guide the surgeon's search for additional abnormal glands if the intraoperative serum parathormone levels remain elevated.

MEN 2a and 2b

About 30% of patients with MEN 2a develop hyperparathyroidism. These patients have hyperplasia but the disease is milder and more readily cured by surgical resection than MEN type 1. The enlarged glands are excised with the help of intraoperative parathormone levels. Patients with MEN 2b do not develop clinical hyperparathyroidism but the parathyroid glands fail to involute with age and remain cellular.[26] If a parathyroid gland is inadvertently removed during thyroidectomy for medullary carcinoma, its cellularity should not be misinterpreted as evidence of clinically significant hyperplasia.

Hyperparathyroidism-jaw tumor syndrome

In this rare syndrome, hyperparathyroidism is accompanied by benign fibro-osseous lesions of the jaw in about 30% of the cases.[27] These patients usually present with clinical evidence of hyperparathyroidism in adolescence and early adult life. Most patients have a parathyroid adenoma, but 10%–15% have parathyroid carcinoma. Treatment is based on the findings at surgery.

Carcinoma of the parathyroid gland

Clinical issues
The majority of parathyroid carcinomas are functional and cause hyperparathyroidism. The hyperparathyroidism

Table 12.3. Criteria for the diagnosis of parathyroid carcinoma

Primary features:
    Regional lymph node metastasis
    Invasion of soft tissue and thyroid gland
    Lymphatic/vascular invasion
    Perineural invasion
Secondary features:
    Solid, sheet-like growth pattern
    Diffuse nuclear atypia (nuclear enlargement and nucleoli)
    Mitotic count of >5/50HPF
    Necrosis
    Dense fibrous bands that traverse the neoplasm

is often profound, with marked hypercalcemia and hypophosphatemia.[25] These biochemical findings as well as a palpable mass and hoarseness, will alert the surgeon to the likelihood of parathyroid carcinoma. At the time of surgical exploration, parathyroid carcinoma is very likely if the enlarged gland is adherent to the surrounding tissues. Recognizing the possibility of parathyroid carcinoma at the outset is important because this should prompt en bloc resection of the mass with surrounding soft tissues and the ipsilateral lobe of the thyroid gland. Complete resection of parathyroid carcinoma with clear surgical margins offers the best chance of cure. Incisional biopsy is avoided because of the risk of implantation, and local recurrence.

Pathological issues

The specimen should be inked, and an attempt should be made to confirm the diagnosis of carcinoma intraoperatively. Approximately one-third of parathyroid carcinomas lack cytologic atypia and can be distinguished from adenoma only by an infiltrative pattern of growth. Table 12.3 lists the histologic criteria for the diagnosis of parathyroid carcinoma. Any single primary feature, regardless of cytologic atypia and mitotic activity, is sufficient to make the diagnosis of carcinoma (Fig. 12.12). If primary features are absent, at least three secondary features are required to make a firm diagnosis of carcinoma. The surgical margins should be evaluated as best as possible if the neoplasm is an obvious carcinoma with invasion of the surrounding soft tissue.

Sometimes, it is not possible to make a firm diagnosis of carcinoma intraoperatively; in this situation, it is appropriate to render a diagnosis of "atypical adenoma versus carcinoma" and to make sure that the surgical margins are clear.

Parathyromatosis

Clinical issues

Parathyromatosis refers to the rare situation when multiple small foci of hyperplastic parathyroid tissue are present in the neck and/or mediastinum, unrelated to the main parathyroid glands. Most patients present with recurrent hyperparathyroidism after previous parathyroid surgery, and the parathyromatosis is due to inadvertent implantation of parathyroid tissue during surgery. However, parathyromatosis may occur de novo, and in this situation, the hyperplastic parathyroid tissue is assumed to arise from nests of parathyroid cells deposited in the migratory pathway of the parathyroid glands.[28] Scstamibi scans and color Doppler sonography may help to locate these foci of parathyroid tissue. The diagnosis may be apparent to the surgeon when the nodules are grossly visible, but most surgeons will not have any experience with this entity and will very likely submit one or more of these nodules for FS evaluation.

Pathologic issues

Parathyromatosis consists of nodules of cellular benign parathyroid tissue in the soft tissue of the neck and/or mediastinum. The main distinction is from well differentiated parathyroid carcinoma that has invaded soft tissue. The following points help to make the diagnosis of parathyromatosis: awareness of this entity; the absence of a mass lesion with characteristic features of primary parathyroid carcinoma; the absence of cytologic atypia; the absence of lymphatic, vascular and perineural invasion; the absence of a fibrous reaction; and the distribution of the lesions.

Secondary and tertiary hyperparathyroidism

Secondary hyperparathyroidism occurs most often in patients with chronic renal failure. The need for surgical correction of secondary hyperparathyroidism has decreased with improved medical management of chronic renal failure. Occasionally, one of the glands in secondary hyperparathyroidism appears to function autonomously (tertiary hyperparathyroidism); surgical resection is undertaken if medical control fails.

(a)

(b)

(c)

(d)

(e)

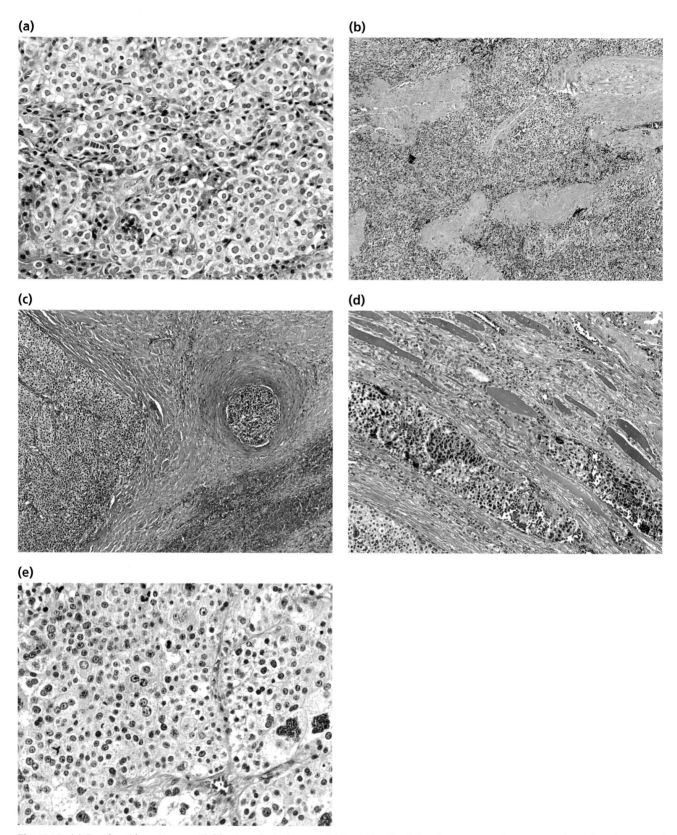

Fig. 12.12. (a) Parathyroid carcinoma with bland cytologic features. (b) Broad bands of fibrosis are present in many parathyroid carcinomas and are a clue to the diagnosis. (c) Invasion of soft tissue and venous invasion permit a confident diagnosis of carcinoma. (d) Another parathyroid carcinoma without significant cytologic atypia but the neoplasm invaded the throid gland. (e) The majority of parathyroid carcinomas show diffuse cytologic atypia.

REFERENCES

1. Attie JN, Wise L, Mir R, *et al.* The rationale against routine subtotal parathyroidectomy for primary hyperparathyroidism. *Am J Surg* 1978; **136**: 437–444.

2. Badder EM, Graham WP, Harrison TS. Functional insignificance of microscopic parathyroid hyperplasia. *Surg Gynecol Obstet* 1977; **145**: 863–868.

3. Edis AJ, Beahrs OH, van Heerden JA, *et al.* "Conservative" versus "liberal" approach to parathyroid neck exploration. *Surgery* 1977; **82**: 466–473.

4. Purnell DC, Scholz DA, Beahrs OH. Hyperparathyroidism due to single gland enlargement. *Arch Surg* 1977; **112**: 369–371.

5. Pellitteri PK. Directed parathyroid exploration: evolution and evaluation of this approach in a single-institution review of 346 patients. *Laryngoscope* 2003; **113**: 1857–1869.

6. Perrier ND, Ituarte PHG, Morita E, *et al.* Parathyroid surgery: separating promise from reality. *J Clin Endocrinol Metab* 2002; **87**: 1024–1029.

7. Thompson GB, Grant CS, Perrier ND, *et al.* Reoperative parathyroid surgery in the era of sestamibi scanning and intraoperative parathyroid hormone monitoring. *Arch Surg* 1999; **134**: 699–704.

8. Shidham VB, Asma Z, Rao RN, *et al.* Intraoperative cytology increases the diagnostic accuracy of frozen sections for the confirmation of various tissues in the parathyroid region. *Am J Clin Pathol* 2002; **118**: 895–902.

9. Dekker A, Dunsford HA, Geyer SJ. The normal parathyroid gland at autopsy: the significance of stromal fat in adult patients. *J Pathol* 1979; **128**: 127–133.

10. Dufour DR, Wilkerson SY. The normal parathyroid revisited. *Hum Pathol* 1982; **13**: 717–721.

11. Wang C-A. Parathyroid re-exploration. A clinical and pathological study of 112 cases. *Ann Surg* 1977; **186**: 140–145.

12. Bergson EJ, Heller KS. The clinical significance and anatomic distribution of parathyroid double adenomas. *J Am Coll Surg* 2004; **198**: 185–189.

13. Kebebew E. Hwang J, Reiff E, *et al.* Predictors of single-gland versus multigland parathyroid disease in primary hyperparathyroidism: a simple and accurate scoring model. *Arch Surg* 2006; **141**: 777–782.

14. Milas M, Wagner K, Easley MA, *et al.* Double adenomas revisited: nonuniform distribution favors enlarged superior parathyroids (fourth pouch disease). *Surgery* 2003; **134**: 995–1004.

15. Mozes G, Curlee KJ, Rowland CM, *et al.* The predictive value of laboratory findings in patients with primary hyperparathyroidism. *J Am Coll Surg* 2002; **194**: 126–130.

16. Kovacs KA, Gay JD. Remission of primary hyperparathyroidism due to spontaneous infarction of a parathyroid adenoma. Case report and review of the literature. *Medicine* 1998; **77**: 398–402.

17. Wolpert HR, Vickery AL, Wang C-A. Functioning oxyphil adenomas of the parathyroid gland. *Am J Surg Pathol* 1989; **13**: 500–504.

18. Ho K-J. Papillary parathyroid adenoma. *Arch Pathol Lab Med* 1996; **120**: 883–884.

19. Sahin A, Robinson RA. Papillae formation in parathyroid adenoma. *Arch Pathol Lab Med* 1988; **112**: 99–100.

20. Lawton TJ, Feldman M, LiVolsi V. Lymphocytic infiltrates in solitary parathyroid adenomas. *Int J Surg Pathol* 1998; **6**: 5–10.

21. Chan JKC. *The Parathyroid Gland in Diagnostic Histopathology of Tumors.* Fletcher CDM. (ed.), Churchill Livingston/Elsevier. 3rd edn. 2007.

22. Pannett AA, Kennedy AM, Turner JJ, *et al.* Multiple endocrine neoplasia type 1 (MEN 1) germline mutations in familial isolated primary hyperparathyroidism. *Clin Endocrinol* 2003; **58**: 639–646.

23. Simonds WF, Robbins CM, Agarwal SK, *et al.* Familial isolated hyperparathyroidism is rarely caused by germline mutation in HRPT2, the gene for the hyperparathyroidism-jaw tumor syndrome. *J Clin Endocrinol Metab* 2004; **89**: 96–102.

24. Carneiro DM, Irvin GL, Inabnet WB. Limited versus radical parathyroidectomy in familial isolated primary hyperparathyroidism. *Surgery* 2002; **132**: 1050–1054.

25. Fernandez-Ranvier GG, Khanafshar E, Jensen K, *et al.* Parathyroid carcinoma, atypical parathyroid adenoma, or parathyromatosis? *Cancer* 2007; **110**: 255–264.

26. Carney JA, Roth SI, Heath H, *et al.* The parathyroid glands in Multiple Endocrine Neoplasia Type 2b. *Am J Pathol* 1980; **99**: 387–398.

27. DeLellis RA, Lloyd RV, Heitz PU, Eng C. *World Health Organization Classification of Tumors, Pathology and Genetics: Tumours of Endocrine Organs.* Lyons: IARC Press, 2004.

28. Reddick RL, Costa JC, Marx SJ. Parathyroid hyperplasia and parathyromatosis. *Lancet* 1977; **1**(8010); 549.

13 BREAST

Mahendra Ranchod, Roderick R. Turner, and Carl A. Bertelsen

INTRODUCTION

The management of breast carcinoma has changed significantly during the past two decades and these changes have affected the pathologist's role in patient management. Open biopsy of a palpable mass for initial diagnosis, which was the standard approach in the past, is seldom employed today. Instead, fine needle aspiration (FNA) and needle core biopsies are used to make diagnoses on palpable lesions, and ultrasound guided and stereotactic needle core biopsies are performed to evaluate non-palpable, mammographically-detected lesions. Lumpectomy, followed by radiation to the breast, is now more common than total mastectomy for the local control of breast cancer, and sentinel lymph node biopsy is the procedure of choice for evaluating the status of axillary lymph nodes in patients with invasive mammary carcinoma as this spares the majority of patients from having axillary lymph node dissection.

INDICATIONS FOR INTRAOPERATIVE CONSULTATION (IOC)

1. Evaluation of surgical margins on lumpectomy specimens.
2. Occasionally, a suspicious area may be found outside of the planned lumpectomy field, and intraoperative diagnosis (IOD) may change surgical management. This may become less of an issue with more frequent use of MRI to detect subtle abnormalities away from the target lesion.
3. When breast carcinoma is treated with nipple-sparing mastectomy and immediate reconstruction, the surgeon may submit a subareolar shave biopsy for FS evaluation.

4. Evaluation of an excisional biopsy of a palpable or an ultrasound detected lesion for which there is no prior diagnosis.
5. Evaluation of a J-wire directed biopsy specimen to confirm that a small or subtle lesion detected by imaging (including MRI) is present in the specimen.

INFORMATION NEEDED BEFORE AND DURING IOC

Lumpectomy specimens

Before evaluating the margins on a lumpectomy specimen, it is helpful to know if the prior biopsy was a FNA, needle core biopsy or J-wire biopsy, even though this will become obvious after sectioning the specimen. A cavity will be present after a recent open biopsy, variable amounts of residual lesion will be present after needle core biopsy, and the entire lesion should be present following FNA.

It is helpful to know the histologic diagnosis rendered on the prior biopsy because this will help interpret the gross findings in a lumpectomy specimen. For example, if the prior biopsy showed an invasive lobular carcinoma, areas of induration close to the surgical margin should be viewed with suspicion, as lobular carcinomas are more likely to form poorly defined areas of induration instead of a discrete mass. Furthermore, if the prior diagnosis was duct carcinoma in situ (DCIS), the specimen is likely to lack a discrete lesion, and the evaluation of surgical margins is usually futile.

It is good practice to routinely examine the specimen radiographs and to read the radiologist's report on lumpectomy specimens as this will allow the pathologist to anticipate the gross findings in the specimen. In specimens

Intraoperative Consultation in Surgical Pathology, ed. Mahendra Ranchod. Published by Cambridge University Press.

with previous core biopsy, a metallic clip will mark the site of the prior biopsy. Occasionally, the metallic clip will migrate away from the biopsy site, a phenomenon that should be kept in mind if the target lesion is not found in the specimen.

Sometimes, the surgeon will deliver the specimen to the laboratory and help with orientation or point out an area of concern that may not be apparent by any other means, and at times, the surgeon will remove additional tissue from a margin of concern and help to orient its relationship to the main lumpectomy specimen. If there is any doubt about the orientation of a lumpectomy specimen, the surgeon should be asked to help with orientation before the specimen is inked and sectioned.

Excisional biopsy specimens

Excisional biopsy specimens are only occasionally submitted for initial IOD. The pathologist should be aware of the surgeon's operative plan, especially the consequences of rendering a diagnosis of malignancy.

SPECIFIC CLINICO-PATHOLOGIC ISSUES

Excisional biopsy specimens for initial diagnosis

Clinical issues
Excisional biopsy, once the most common technique for the initial evaluation of a palpable mass in the breast, has been supplanted by FNA and core biopsies. There are three situations however, when the surgeon may perform an open biopsy for a palpable lesion. (a) A lesion has the characteristic clinical features of fibroadenoma and the surgeon elects to excise the lesion without first performing a FNA or needle core biopsy. There is no reason for intraoperative diagnosis in this situation. (b) Occasionally, when a FNA diagnosis of "highly suspicious of carcinoma" has been rendered on a lesion that has clinical and mammographic features of carcinoma, the surgeon will proceed with definitive surgical treatment if the diagnosis of malignancy is confirmed intraoperatively. (c) The patient has a palpable lump and the surgeon chooses to perform an open biopsy either de novo or after a non-diagnostic FNA. The biopsy is usually for diagnostic purposes only, without immediate therapeutic consequences, and IOD is requested either to confirm that the lesion is present in the specimen or to appease patient anxiety.

Pathologic issues
When an excisional biopsy is submitted for IOD, it is important to know what is at stake. The stakes are high if the surgeon's intention is to perform immediate definitive surgery for carcinoma. Careful attention should be paid to the gross features of the specimen because discordance between gross and microscopic features should prompt re-evaluation of the diagnosis. A cytoscrape preparation should be made as this may be all that is necessary to make a definitive diagnosis but a FS should be performed if the prior FNA was indeterminate, or if there is any doubt about the diagnosis on the cytologic examination. There is one caveat to performing a FS: the target lesion has to be >1 cm in maximum dimension to ensure that sufficient lesional tissue is spared from the artifacts of freezing, a precaution that should be taken in the event that a firm diagnosis cannot be made intraoperatively.

If there is nothing at stake, the test that should be performed depends on the gross findings. Gross examination is all that is necessary if there is no discrete lesion; random FSs should not be performed. If there is a discrete lesion such as a fibroadenoma, gross examination alone or a cytoscrape preparation will suffice.

A phyllodes tumor may be encountered unexpectedly when a palpable mass is thought to be a fibroadenoma on clinical grounds. If the gross findings suggest a phyllodes tumor, a FS should be performed to confirm the diagnosis so that the surgeon may proceed with complete excision with adequate margins.

J-wire directed biopsy for initial diagnosis

Clinical issues
J wire-directed biopsy was once the standard way to make an initial diagnosis on non-palpable mammographic lesions, but it has been largely supplanted by ultrasound and vacuum-assisted stereotactic needle core biopsies. Needle core biopsies have the advantage of being less invasive and less expensive than J-wire biopsies, and they provide most of the information required to plan surgical management.

A wire-directed open biopsy is still the preferred technique for initial diagnosis in the following situations. (a) When a mammographically-abnormal lesion is close to the chest wall, it is best evaluated by J-wire biopsy instead of stereotactic needle core biopsy to avoid the risk of pneumothorax. (b) The design of the procedure table is such that it limits access to lesions close to the chest wall. (c) The target lesion is close to an implant and J-wire biopsy minimizes the chances of puncturing the implant. (d) When there is widespread calcification, J-wire provides a more reliable sample of the lesion. (e) J-wire is a better choice for patients who cannot lie in the prone position for the duration of a needle core biopsy procedure. (f) Some patients are anxious and prefer to have a general anesthetic or conscious sedation for the biopsy procedure, making J-wire biopsy the better option. (g) Some patients prefer to have the mammographically abnormal area excised because they are unwilling to deal with the uncertainties of sampling. (h) J-wire biopsy is performed when more complete evaluation is necessary for lesions such as ADH, LCIS, incompletely removed radial scars, and cellular intraductal papillary neoplasms diagnosed on a needle core biopsy.

Pathologic issues

It is highly unlikely that a surgeon will proceed with immediate definitive treatment following a diagnostic J-wire biopsy. Specimen mammography is used routinely to confirm that the target lesion is in the specimen, but the surgeon may request pathologic confirmation. The main medical reason for intraoperative evaluation is to confirm that the target lesion is present in the specimen. If there is a grossly visible lesion and the surgeon insists on a diagnosis, a cytoscrape preparation is sufficient for a preliminary diagnosis. If the target lesion is <1 cm, it should not be subjected to FS for fear of compromising the specimen. Random frozen sections should not be performed on J-wire biopsy specimens that lack a discrete lesion; it serves no purpose and may provide misleading information.

Evaluation of lumpectomy specimens for carcinoma

Clinical issues

Lumpectomy, followed by post-operative radiation therapy to the breast, is now the most common treatment for local control of in-situ and invasive carcinoma of the breast. Lumpectomy refers to complete excision of the index neoplasm with adequate margins of normal tissue. The term partial mastectomy is sometimes used interchangeably with a large lumpectomy, and quadrantectomy, which is more popular in Europe, refers to removal of an entire quadrant of the breast together with skin and deep fascia.

Lumpectomy is performed with or without the assistance of J-wires, depending on the ease of identifying the target area. The goal of lumpectomy is two-fold: to remove

the malignancy with adequate margins, and to do so with good cosmetic results. The extent of the lumpectomy depends on the size of the palpable or mammographic lesion, location of the lesion, size of the patient's breast, surgeon's experience, and size of the existing biopsy cavity – if the patient had a prior J-wire biopsy with positive or suboptimal margins.

There is a growing trend amongst breast surgeons to perform an adequate lumpectomy, and then remove additional marginal tissue from the lumpectomy cavity. The additional tissue may be removed only from areas of concern or they may be routine excisions from most of the cavity. There is data to suggest that this approach results in fewer positive margins and thus fewer second surgical procedures. The additional marginal tissue from the cavity is usually submitted in formalin for permanent sections,[1] but some surgeons request frozen sections on these specimens.[2]

Pathologic issues

WHEN DOES THE SURGEON REQUEST EVALUATION OF THE SURGICAL MARGINS?

Lumpectomy specimens are submitted in formalin when the surgeon is confident that the target lesion has been completely excised, or when the surgeon has maximized the amount of tissue that can be removed for a good cosmetic result. However, a lumpectomy is sent for IOD for the following reasons:

- When there is an area of concern at a margin in the lumpectomy specimen; for example, if a suspicious area is present at the anterior margin close to the skin, or the deep margin close to the chest wall, the specimen is sent for intraoperative evaluation because a positive margin would require removal of skin or part of the pectoralis muscle, respectively.
- When an abnormal area of breast tissue is palpated outside of the planned lumpectomy field, a biopsy of that area will be submitted for IOD because a diagnosis of carcinoma would alter the surgical approach. This experience should become less frequent with increasing use of MRI to evaluate the breast prior to tissue-conserving surgery.
- The surgeon may submit a lumpectomy specimen for evaluation of the surgical margins even when there is every reason to believe that the neoplasm has been adequately excised; this is done either to re-assure the surgeon or to appease an anxious patient.

ORIENTATION OF THE SPECIMEN

Most surgeons orient lumpectomy specimens with sutures. Two sutures are usually sufficient for orientation but more than two sutures may be used when orientation is complex. While orientation is important, retaining specimen orientation is not as precise as surgeons would like to believe. Gravity and specimen handling cause some flattening of the specimen so that the margins in the specimen may not perfectly match corresponding loci in the biopsy cavity. However, even if there is some distortion, orientation of the specimen is preferable to no orientation because a positive margin will still guide the surgeon to the appropriate area.

INKING THE SPECIMEN

We suggest using at least four colors of ink for specimens that have been oriented.[*] There are four challenges to inking:

- It is not possible to ink the margins accurately if a specimen is submitted in more than one piece. The surgeon should be asked to approximate the pieces of tissue – if possible – before inking the specimen, but if the pieces cannot be oriented, the pathologist should decide if one or more of the pieces should be inked.

- Inking has to be done with extra care when the specimen contains a biopsy cavity that is partially exposed on the surface of the specimen.

- Sometimes the surgeon may modify the plane of excision during lumpectomy and create a flap of tissue. The flap should be approximated to the main specimen, and the specimen should be inked with extra care to avoid inking a false margin.

- Some lumpectomy specimens are composed of friable fatty tissue, that when inked, allows ink to track into crevices between fatty lobules. This is an issue that the pathologist will have to wrestle with on permanent sections but it is mentioned here because inking often takes place in the FS suite. There are two clues to identifying the true margin: first, the ink is often bolder on the true margin than the false margin; and second, the outer contour of the tissue section represents the true margin, not the cleavage lines that extend from the

[*] Some pathologists prefer to use six different inks, but four colors are sufficient if the slices are kept in order and if all the sections are taken at right angles to the margins.

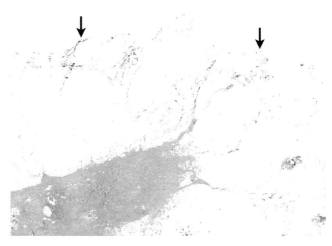

Fig. 13.1. Lumpectomy specimen showing ink that has tracked along clefts in the specimen. The true margin can be identified by following the outer contour of the section (arrows).

surface into the specimen (Fig. 13.1). Mordants such as Bouin's solution and white vinegar (acetic acid) increase the adhesion of ink to tissue, and should be used routinely on breast specimens. Use of a mordant also reduces the transfer of ink to the cut surfaces of the specimen during sectioning. The ink should of course, be thoroughly dried before the specimen is sprayed with a mordant solution.

SECTIONING THE SPECIMEN

The specimen should be cut only after the ink has dried completely. As stated above, a mordant will help to bind the ink to the surfaces of the specimen. It is much easier to cut parallel slices of tissue of even thickness with a long, straight-edged blade instead of a short, curved Bard–Parker blade, and ideally, the blade should be at least 2–3 times longer than the axis of the specimen (see Chapter 2, p. 15). When there is a distinct palpable mass, some pathologists prefer to make a single section through the equator of the lesion in an axis where the palpable mass is closest to the surgical margin (Fig. 13.2). This single section may be sufficient to evaluate the margin closest to the carcinoma, and because there is a single cut, little effort is required to retain orientation of the specimen. On the other hand, when a distinct mass is not palpable, the specimen should be cut at 3–5 mm intervals for proper evaluation. One way to keep the slices of tissue in order is to place them on white cards (Fig. 13.3). The protein in the tissue will cause the slices to adhere to the card, keeping the tissue flat during fixation and retaining the sequence of the tissue slices.

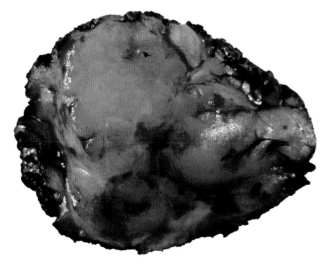

Fig. 13.2. Invasive ductal carcinoma in a lumpectomy specimen. Because the carcinoma was easily palpable, the pathologist made a single section into the specimen, perpendicular to the closest palpable margin. This single cut was good enough to evaluate the proximity of the carcinoma to the closest margin.

EVALUATION OF SURGICAL MARGINS

The issue of margin evaluation in breast specimens is not as simple as it appears at first glance,[3] and some of the problems are discussed below:

- There is no consensus on what constitutes an adequate margin. It is generally agreed that a wider margin is needed for DCIS because of "skip areas" that occur when preparing two dimensional tissue sections of a branching ductal system (Fig. 13.4), and as a result, 5 mm of normal tissue is considered the minimum margin for DCIS. Narrower margins are adequate for the majority of invasive carcinomas as most invasive carcinomas grow as an expansile mass; as shown in the study by Gage et al.,[4] invasive carcinomas with <1 mm margin had the same outcome as cases with a wider margin.

- It is difficult to compare data from different studies because there is no agreement on what constitutes a positive margin for invasive mammary carcinoma. Some pathologists require tumor to abut onto the inked margin,[4] whereas other groups consider the margin positive if the invasive carcinoma is within 2 mm of the inked margin.[5] We interpret a positive margin as carcinoma that extends to the inked surgical margin; an invasive carcinoma that approximates the surgical margin is reported as "close to the margin" and the distance of the carcinoma from the margin is

measured or estimated (e.g., "1.5 mm from the inked margin" or "within microns of the inked margin," etc.).

- The surgeon's ability to obtain adequate clear margins depends on the type of carcinoma. Invasive carcinomas with a minimal infiltrative pattern of growth are more easily excised with clear margins than carcinomas with highly infiltrating margins. A minority of carcinomas, especially invasive lobular carcinoma, grow in a skip fashion, with multiple small foci of carcinoma beyond the main neoplasm (Fig. 13.5). These foci, which presumably represent intramammary spread of carcinoma, are not palpable or visible on gross examination, and are only identified on microscopic examination. Clear margins may be difficult to achieve in this group of tumors.

- The important issue in the local control of breast carcinoma is what remains in the patient's breast *after* lumpectomy. In a minority of patients, small foci of undetected in-situ or invasive carcinoma remain in the breast after lumpectomy with clear margins, and these foci of carcinoma are expected to be ablated by postoperative radiation therapy.

- Invasive carcinomas accompanied by extensive intraductal carcinoma (EIC) are often more difficult to excise with clear margins,[6–9] even though EIC is not an independent prognostic factor for local recurrence if the DCIS is excised with adequate clear margins.[4] The issue of EIC is relevant to intraoperative consultation because the DCIS component is not visible on gross examination and this leads to a greater risk of rendering a false negative evaluation of the margins.*

- Most carcinomas occur as a single localized lesion but a minority are multiple** (Fig. 13.6). MRI, which

---

* There are two categories of EIC: a) extensive DCIS with multiple small foci of invasive carcinoma, including microcarcinomas; and b) the more common situation where an invasive carcinoma is accompanied by extensive DCIS (DCIS constituting >25% of the volume of the tumor), and where the DCIS is present in the breast tissue beyond the boundaries of the invasive carcinoma.
** The terms multifocal and multicentric are used to describe multiple foci of in situ and invasive carcinoma. Multifocal refers to multiple separate foci of carcinoma derived from a single clone; multifocal carcinomas are usually in the same region (quadrant) of the breast. Multicentric carcinomas are multiple independent in situ or invasive carcinomas; because they are derived from different clones of neoplastic cells, the lesions are often located in different quadrants of the breast and have varying histological appearances. However, the distinction between multifocal and multicentric is not always clear, either on scientific or clinical grounds. The situation is compounded by a lack of consistency in the use of these terms. In

(a) **(b)**

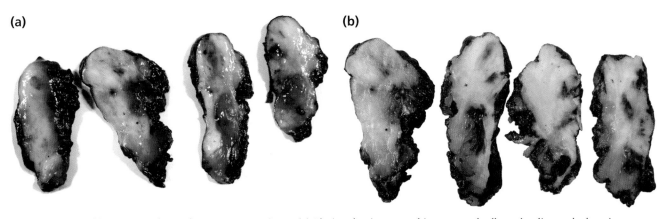

Fig. 13.3. Slices of breast tissue from a lumpectomy specimen. (a) Placing the tissue on white note cards allows the slices to be kept in sequence. (b) After overnight fixation, the slices of tissue are flat and easy to trim and sample for histologic examination.

(a) **(b)** **(c)**

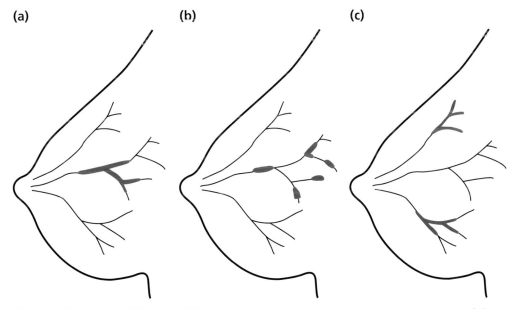

Fig. 13.4. (a) Unicentric DCIS: the DCIS is limited to a single ductal unit and grows in a continuous fashion. (b) Multifocal DCIS: DCIS limited to a single ductal unit of the breast but there are skip areas of growth within the duct, imparting the appearance of multiple separate foci. (c) Multicentric DCIS: Separate foci of DCIS arising in more than one ducal unit of the breast. It is difficult to distinguish between different segments of the breast in two dimensional histologic sections so distance between different foci of carcinoma (4–5 cm) is used as a surrogate marker of multicentricity.

is sometimes used to evaluate the breast prior to breast-conserving surgery, detects additional in situ and

the current management of breast carcinoma, what matters is the number of foci of carcinoma, their anatomic location, and whether they prohibit breast-sparing surgical treatment.

invasive carcinomas in approximately 20% of cases and these new findings change surgical management in approximately half of these patients.[10] Occasionally, an additional lesion is first encountered at the time of surgery, and this will be submitted for frozen section

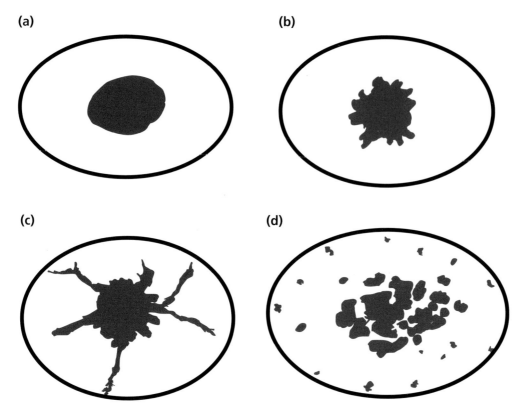

Fig. 13.5. Different growth patterns of invasive ductal carcinoma. (a), (b) The majority of carcinomas have a limited infiltrative pattern making it relatively easy to achieve clear margins of excision. (c) A proportion of invasive carcinomas have thin strands of neoplastic cells that extend well beyond the grossly visible neoplasm. (d) A subset of carcinomas form poorly defined areas of induration rather than a distinct mass. It is difficult to accurately evaluate the surgical margins intraoperatively in carcinomas with patterns (c) and (d).

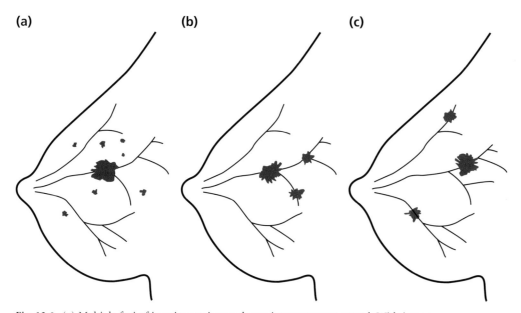

Fig. 13.6. (a) Multiple foci of invasive carcinoma due to intramammary spread. With intramammary spread, each of the foci should have the same histologic appearance. Multiple primary invasive carcinomas may be (b) multifocal or (c) multicentric, using the definitions of multifocal and multicentric as in Fig. 13.4. Features that favor separate primary invasive carcinomas over intramammary spread include one or more of the following: (i) a distance of at least 2 cm of benign breast tissue between the carcinomas; (ii) the carcinomas differ histologically and; (iii) the invasive carcinomas have a radial pattern of growth, show stromal elastosis and are accompanied by DCIS.

evaluation. The number and distribution of additional foci of carcinoma may cause the surgeon to modify the extent of surgical resection in order to obtain clear surgical margins.

IS GROSS EXAMINATION SUFFICIENTLY ACCURATE FOR EVALUATION OF SURGICAL MARGINS?

Gross examination of surgical margins is accurate enough in most cases of invasive carcinoma but has its limitations. Balch *et al.* reported false negative interpretation of margins in 25% of their cases, but it should be kept in mind that these authors interpreted margins as positive if the carcinoma was within 2 mm of the inked margin.[5] Fleming *et al.* correctly interpreted the margins in 97% of invasive carcinoma, but they required a minimum clear margin of 1 cm.[12] In our experience, gross examination is an imperfect but acceptable test. The intraoperative diagnosis should include a measure or estimate of the distance of the malignancy from the closest margin/s, giving the surgeon the opportunity to remove more marginal tissue if this is feasible. Because of the limitations of gross examination, the pathologist should be familiar with the clinical aspects of the case, as well as the findings in the original biopsy. For example, it is prudent to be circumspect about the margins in cases of invasive lobular carcinoma and invasive ductal carcinoma with EIC. Furthermore, gross examination is clearly unsuited for evaluating the margins in cases of DCIS. Experienced breast surgeons understand the limitations of intraoperative evaluation of surgical margins and will accept equivocation in certain situations.

WHEN SHOULD THE MARGINS BE EVALUATED BY FS AND CYTOLOGIC PREPARATIONS?

When the surgeon is concerned about an anatomically critical margin, the specimen will be submitted for IOD with a suture marking the area of concern. There are two ways to handle the specimen: In the first approach, a cytoscrape is made from the margin of concern before the specimen is inked and sectioned. If the cytoscrape is equivocal, the specimen is inked, and a single section is made perpendicular to the inked margin. We do not evaluate the margin with parallel sections as this is likely to give a false positive diagnosis in a proportion of cases.[13] In the second approach, the specimen is inked and sectioned serially in the conventional manner. Carefully directed cytoscrape preparations are made from suspicious areas close to the margins and a FS should be performed if

the cytology preparation is equivocal. We prefer this approach because the cytoscrape is made under direct visual guidance.

There are pathologists who routinely evaluate the entire surgical margin with touch preparations. We do not recommend this approach because it gives a false sense of security. Touch imprints cannot reliably distinguish between low grade DCIS and epitheliosis at the margins, and they cannot evaluate the closeness and volume of DCIS in relation to the margin. Valdes *et al.* report the use of touch preparations on all re-excised margins following positive or close margins in lumpectomy specimens, and their error rate of nearly 18%, both false positive and false negative, appears to be no better than gross examination.[14]

The FS evaluation of biopsies taken from the post-lumpectomy cavity is a challenge as the tissue is usually fatty. It is best to defer the examination of this tissue to permanent sections, but if the surgeon insists, a cytoscrape preparation can be prepared from the new marginal surface. If it becomes necessary to perform a FS on partially fatty tissue, the excess fat can be removed by firm compression or by gently scraping away the excess fat with a blade.

Newer techniques for evaluating completeness of excision

Gross examination of the surgical margins, supplemented with microscopic examination when necessary, has an accuracy rate of approximately 80%. This is not ideal but it is a limitation of intraoperative pathologic techniques that are currently available. As a result, non-morphologic techniques are being investigated, including PET-FDG scans and radiofrequency spectroscopy of the lumpectomy cavity using hand-held probes.[15]

Histological distinctions that matter in lumpectomy specimens

When there is an area of undue firmness at the surgical margin of a lumpectomy specimen, associated fibrocystic disease and reactive changes due to prior biopsy have to be distinguished from carcinoma. The following differential diagnoses can sometimes be challenging.

- The distinction of low grade carcinoma from benign lesions can be difficult when the tissue at the margin

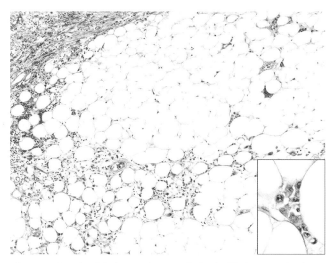

Fig. 13.7. Invasive lobular carcinoma admixed with fat necrosis close to a surgical margin. The invasive carcinoma (upper right) is masked by reactive changes but the cytologic features are evident on higher magnification (inset).

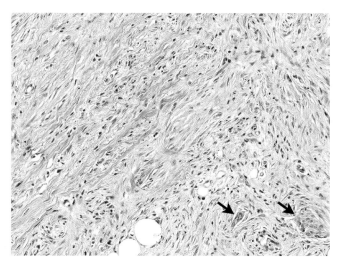

Fig. 13.8. Invasive ductal carcinoma with a fibromatosis-like spindle cell component. The spindle cells may be mistaken for reactive fibroblasts, especially if the lesion is encountered in an area of prior biopsy. In this case, the diagnosis could be made on H&E stained sections because conventional invasive ductal carcinoma was present focally (arrows), and because the spindle cell proliferation was away from the prior biopsy site.

shows thermal artifactual changes. A diagnosis of DCIS should not be made in areas of thermal artifact unless the evidence is compelling.

- Invasive carcinoma is usually readily distinguished from cellular areas of granulation tissue and fat necrosis but invasive lobular carcinoma may be subtle when it has a skip pattern of growth and is admixed with granulation tissue and fat necrosis (Fig. 13.7). Careful attention should be paid to cords or groups of cells with scanty cytoplasm. The histiocytoid variant of invasive lobular carcinoma is particularly difficult to identify in areas of granulation tissue and fat necrosis because the neoplastic cells have abundant vacuolated cytoplasm.

- Metaplastic carcinoma with a fibromatosis-like spindle cell component can be difficult to distinguish from post-biopsy fibrosis (Fig. 13.8), and the diagnosis may have to be deferred to permanent sections and cytokeratin immunohistochemical stains if the lesion is encountered at a critical surgical margin.

- The distinction of low grade DCIS from ADH and epitheliosis can be challenging on FS. However, familiarity with the previous biopsy findings may be helpful. The absence of DCIS in the previous biopsy would make the diagnosis of DCIS at the margins less likely. If the previous biopsy information is not available, an extensive intraductal lesion is more likely to be DCIS because ADH is usually limited in extent; however, there are exceptions, and the

surgeon should be encouraged to remove additional tissue if the diagnosis is in doubt.

Phyllodes tumors

Clinical issues

Phyllodes tumor almost always presents as a palpable mass, with an average size of 4–5 cm in diameter, although the neoplasm may be 10 or > cm in size. The diagnosis may be suspected in larger tumors but small lesions are not clinically distinguishable from fibroadenomas. The treatment of phyllodes tumors is complete surgical excision with a margin of normal tissue around the neoplasm.[16] The choice between lumpectomy and total mastectomy depends on the size of the neoplasm, histologic grade, location within the breast, patient's preference, and size of the patient's breast; small neoplasms are adequately treated with lumpectomy, whereas large neoplasms may require total mastectomy to accomplish complete excision.

All categories of phyllodes tumors are at risk for local recurrence after lumpectomy, and margin status is the single most important factor that determines local recurrence. The local recurrence rate is approximately 15% for "benign" phyllodes tumors, and 25%–30% for borderline and malignant phyllodes tumors. Lymph nodes are only

Table 13.1 Criteria for the diagnosis of phyllodes tumors

Benign phyllodes tumor (15% recurrence rate; 0 risk of metastasis)

    Circumscribed margins (mainly)

    Cellular stroma without significant atypia

    < 2 mitoses/10HPF

Borderline phyllodes tumor (25%–30% local recurrence rate; no metastases)

    Moderate stromal cellularity and atypia but not frankly sarcomatous

    Infiltrative margins

    2–5 mitoses/10HPF

    No stromal overgrowth or necrosis

Malignant phyllodes tumor (25%–30% local recurrence; 20%–30% metastatic rate)

    Stroma has features of frank sarcoma with:

      Infiltrative margins

      Usually >10 mitoses/10HPF

      Moderate to marked atypia

      Stromal overgrowth (>1 x40 field without epithelium)

      Metaplastic features (e.g., cartilaginous)

      Necrosis

rarely involved by phyllodes tumors so there is no reason to perform a sentinel lymph node biopsy.

Pathologic issues

Phyllodes tumors are divided into 3 categories: benign with a potential for local recurrence, borderline and malignant. There is a great deal of variance in the criteria used for classifying phyllodes tumors, and as a result, there is a wide range in the reported rates of local recurrence and metastasis. Table 13.1 summarizes our classification of phyllodes tumors based on the studies published by Moffat *et al.* and Putti *et al.*[17,18]

The diagnosis of phyllodes tumor may be suspected on FNA, but core biopsy is better suited to making a firm or provisional diagnosis (see below). There is a risk of underestimating the malignant potential of phyllodes tumors in needle core biopsies because of histologic heterogeneity within the neoplasm and the inability to confidently evaluate stromal overgrowth in thin cores. Consequently, tumors diagnosed as borderline may be upgraded to frankly malignant on subsequent excision.

When a lumpectomy specimen is submitted with a definite or provisional diagnosis of phyllodes tumor, the specimen should be inked and then sectioned serially

for gross evaluation of the lesion and evaluation of the margins (Fig. 13.9). One or two FSs should be taken from areas where the neoplasm is close to the margin, but comprehensive evaluation should be deferred to permanent sections. Benign phyllodes are usually circumscribed but the stromal cells of borderline and malignant tumors often extend beyond the grossly visible lesion making it difficult to confidently evaluate surgical margins with limited sampling.

Evaluation of mastectomy specimens

Conventional total mastectomy specimens do not require intraoperative evaluation except in the rare situation when the surgeon is concerned about the deep margin and may excise a portion of the pectoralis muscle if the margin is interpreted as positive. The area of concern should be inked and the section should be taken perpendicular to the inked margin.

Nipple-sparing mastectomies and skin-sparing mastectomies are beginning to come into vogue. The surgeon may submit a shave biopsy for FS from the subareolar area in a nipple sparing-mastectomy, and from the anterior surface overlying the carcinoma in a skin-sparing mastectomy.[19]

Evaluation of reduction mammoplasties

Some surgeons submit reduction mammoplasty specimens to the laboratory for the specimen to be weighed in the fresh state. These patients would have had prior negative mammograms so there is usually no reason for routine intraoperative evaluation. Occasionally, the surgeon may encounter a nodular area and submit a biopsy for FS to confirm that it is benign. Microscopic malignancies, especially lobular carcinoma in situ, are found infrequently on permanent sections but this has no bearing on intraoperative evaluation.

SENTINEL LYMPH NODE BIOPSY

Clinical issues

When mammary carcinoma metastasizes to axillary lymph nodes, the sentinel lymph node is the first to be involved in almost all cases.[20,21] Examination of the sentinel node is therefore, a reliable way to evaluate the status of the axillary lymph nodes.[22–24] One major advantage of sentinel

(a) **(b)**

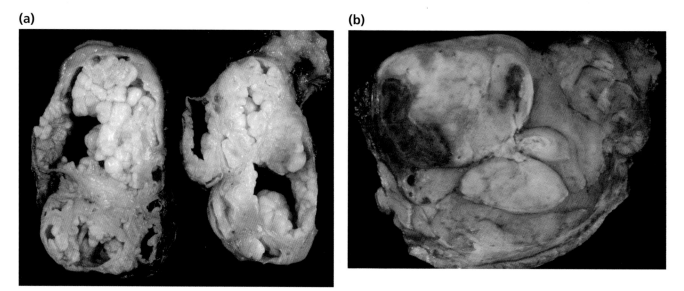

Fig. 13.9. (a) Benign phyllodes tumor with well formed clefts and (b) malignant phyllodes tumor showing a large fleshy neoplasm. The malignant phyllodes tumor in (b) appears circumscribed but the lesion extended beyond the grossly visible lesion.

lymph node biopsy (SLNB) is that 70%–75% of patients have negative sentinel lymph nodes and they are spared the potential morbidity of axillary lymph node dissection. When a macrometastasis (>2 mm) is present, axillary lymph node dissection is justified because the non-sentinel nodes will show metastatic carcinoma in 40%–63% of cases.[25–27] Thirty-three to sixty percent of sentinel node metastases are macrometastases,[26–28] and the large majority (81%–98%) will be successfully detected at the time of intraoperative examination, either by FS or cytologic examination.[28–33] It is no surprise that only 21%–28% of micrometastases (0.2–2 mm) are detected intraoperatively.

The sentinel node is identified either with isosulphan blue, labeled technetium (^{99m}Tc-labeled sulfur colloid), or both. One to three sentinel nodes are usually identified but there may be more. The sentinel node may not be successfully identified in up to 5% of cases, and this may be due to surgical technique or changes in lymphatic drainage caused by previous breast surgery, such as reduction mammoplasty, mastopexy and transaxillary breast augmentation.[23] In addition, a sentinel lymph node may not take up dye or technetium if it is completely replaced by metastatic carcinoma, but the surgeon will very likely recognize the lymph node as abnormal and remove it for IOD.

There is on-going controversy about the role of SLNB for duct carcinoma in situ (DCIS). DCIS should not produce nodal metastases but sentinel node metastases are reported in 1.8%–13% of cases,[34–37] suggesting that an invasive carcinoma has been overlooked in the breast specimen. There are three possible reasons for failing to identify invasive carcinoma in the breast specimen: (a) it may be difficult to recognize small foci of invasive carcinoma in cases of high grade DCIS that show extensive periductal fibrosis, duct distortion and cancerization of lobules; (b) some types of invasive carcinoma (e.g., cribriform and solid patterns) mimic in situ carcinoma on H&E stained sections because they grow as small circumscribed nests with "pushing" margins; and (c) breast tissue that shows widespread DCIS may not be sampled thoroughly enough to exclude small foci of invasion.

Many surgeons feel that sentinel node biopsy should not be performed in all cases of DCIS, but the surgeon's dilemma is to determine which patients to select for sentinel node biopsy, thus avoiding a second surgical procedure if invasive carcinoma is found in the excised specimen. This is relevant because DCIS in needle core biopsy is upstaged to invasive carcinoma on subsequent excision in 8%–38% of cases.[*,34,38–40] The surgeon will naturally take clinical and mammographic data into account to reach a decision; the presence of a palpable

---

* There is a wide range in the reported percentage of cases upstaged from DCIS to invasive carcinoma. This is at least partly related to the amount of lesional tissue removed at the time of core biopsy (number of cores, gauge of needle etc.).

or mammographic mass lesion and widespread mammographic abnormalities will prompt SLNB because of the increased risk of an invasive carcinoma. Patients with DCIS who are treated with total mastectomy are also likely to undergo SLNB because total mastectomy precludes SLNB at a later date.

Pathologic issues

SHOULD THE SENTINEL LYMPH NODE BE SENT FOR INTRAOPERATIVE EVALUATION?

There is currently no consensus on how to handle sentinel lymph nodes. Practices have changed in the last few years, with a shift towards performing IOD selectively. Current practices include the following:

- The surgeon sends the sentinel lymph node for IOD in selected cases, only if they are suspected of harboring metastatic carcinoma. As a result, the majority of sentinel nodes are submitted to the laboratory in formalin.
- The sentinel nodes are sent to the laboratory in the fresh state routinely and the pathologist is left to decide on the intraoperative tests that will be performed. IOD is limited to gross examination if the node is small and unremarkable, and by FS or cytologic examination if the node is abnormal by gross examination.
- The surgeon requests microscopic evaluation on all sentinel lymph nodes, and the pathologist decides on whether to examine the node by FS or cytologic examination.

Because there is no consensus, the pathologist and surgeon should agree on how sentinel lymph node biopsies will be handled intraoperatively.[22] There should be agreement on which test/tests will be performed, and there should be a clear understanding of the limitations of intraoperative diagnosis.

If the sentinel node is subjected to microscopic examination intraoperatively, the pathologist should be familiar with the findings in the prior breast biopsy to help interpret subtle changes in the sentinel node. When the case is approached with an informed mind, histiocyte-like cells in the sinuses are less likely to be of concern if the primary carcinoma is high grade, but these same cells warrant scrutiny if the patient has invasive lobular carcinoma.

RADIATION EXPOSURE FROM HANDLING SENTINEL NODES

The exposure dose to the gamma rays of labeled technetium is so low that there is no need for special handling of the specimen.[41,42]

GROSS EXAMINATION OF SENTINEL NODES

The lymph node/s should be dissected away from the surrounding fat. If FSs are performed, excess fat in the hilar area of the node can be removed but this should be done with care to avoid removing nodal parenchyma. The number of nodes and their sizes should be recorded. Each lymph node should be cut at 2–3 mm intervals. Pathologists differ in their preference for cutting the node along its short axis or long axis. Sectioning the lymph node along its long axis makes it easier to make cytologic preparations as there are fewer pieces of tissue to sample. Longitudinal sections also reflect the maximum dimension of metastases more accurately.

FROZEN SECTIONS ON SENTINEL LYMPH NODES

The advantage of FSs is that nodal architecture is retained and the pathologist can pay extra attention to the subcapsular sinus for subtle nodal metastases because this is where metastases first make their appearance. However, FSs have their disadvantages: it is difficult to obtain high quality FSs on lymph nodes with fatty infiltration, and tissue is lost during trimming of the FS block. This tissue loss would seem be an issue if a search is made later for micrometastases and isolated tumor cells with the aid of immunohistochemical stains.[43]

CYTOLOGIC PREPARATIONS ON SENTINEL NODES

Cytologic preparations have the following advantages over FSs: (a) they allow sampling of the specimen without significant loss of tissue; (b) they are free from the technical challenges of preparing FSs on fatty lymph nodes and; c) the tissue is spared from the artifacts of freezing. Touch preparations and cytoscrape preparations work equally well and they are similar in sensitivity and specificity to FSs,[31,44,45] but touch preparations are obviously easier to prepare on small lymph nodes. About two-thirds of metastases are macrometastases (>2 mm) and the large majority of these will be detected by cytologic techniques. Most micrometastases (<2 mm) will not be detected by intraoperative evaluation but this does not invalidate the use of cytologic preparations.

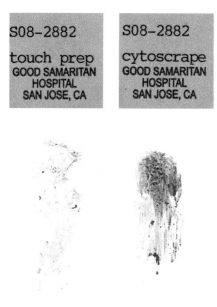

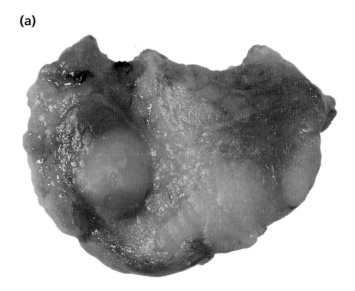

(a)

Fig. 13.10. Touch preparation (left) and cytoscrape preparation (right) of the same sentinel lymph node. The cytoscrape preparation is more cellular and produces a concentrated sample.

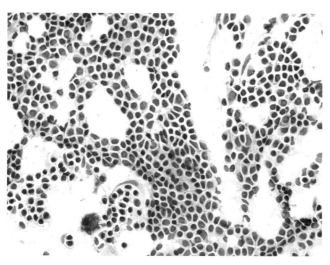

Fig. 13.11. Touch preparation of a benign sentinel lymph node with air drying artifact. Enlargement and angulation of lymphocytes may cause concern about metastatic lobular carcinoma but the peripheral distribution of these changes is a clue to air-drying artifact.

(b)

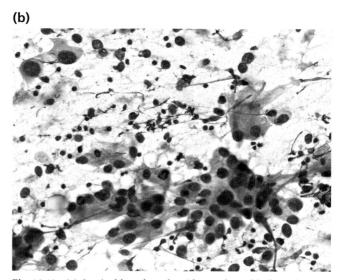

Fig. 13.12. (a) Sentinel lymph node with grossly visible foci of metastatic carcinoma. The diagnosis can be readily made with any type of cytologic preparation. (b) In this case, a cytoscrape was made and it showed metastatic carcinoma.

Cytoscrape smears provide more concentrated cellular samples whereas touch imprints produce more uniform monolayer preparations (Fig. 13.10). When a sentinel node shows extensive adipose infiltration, cytoscrape preparations yield more lymphoid tissue because the scraping can be directed to the residual rim of lymphoid tissue. Some degree of air-drying is usually present at the periphery of touch imprints, causing enlargement and angulation of lymphocytes, a finding that may be a source of consternation

(Fig. 13.11). Touch imprints and cytoscrape preparations are both fine; the choice depends on the pathologist's preference as well as the size and gross appearance of the lymph node.

OUR RECOMMENDATION FOR EVALUATING SENTINEL LYMPH NODES

If the surgeon requests IOD, we recommend making touch and/or cytoscrape preparations. We see no reason to perform frozen sections – unless there is a disparity between the gross and cytologic findings (negative cytology and a grossly suspicious lymph node). Our rationale for this approach is that the goal of IOD, using conventional light microscopic techniques, is to detect the majority of macrometastases (Fig. 13.12), and by serendipity, a small proportion

(a)

(b)

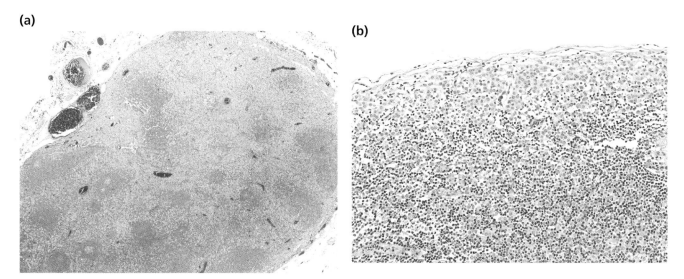

Fig. 13.13. (a) Invasive lobular carcinoma infiltrating the sinuses of a sentinel lymph node. The expanded sinuses warrant close attention when the primary carcinoma is invasive lobular carcinoma. (b) Higher magnification shows the epithelial nature of the cells in the peripheral sinus.

of micrometastases. The goal of IOD is not to detect minute metastases because that demands more than the test can deliver. It seems inappropriate to routinely embed all the nodal tissue for FS, and to cut multiple levels, searching for minute metastases.

HISTOLOGIC AND CYTOLOGIC DISTINCTIONS THAT MATTER

The cells of conventional lobular carcinoma are bland and may be confined to the sinuses of the node, mimicking reactive sinus histiocytosis (Fig. 13.13). The cells in expanded sinuses should be scrutinized for cohesiveness, intracytoplasmic lumina and minor degrees of nuclear atypia. Metastatic lobular carcinoma also has a tendency to produce diffuse infiltrates in the lymph node parenchyma instead of a distinct nodule. While the cytologic changes may be subtle, the pallor of the nodal parenchyma on low magnification is a clue to the diagnosis.

Nevus cells occur in axillary lymph nodes in <0.5% of patients with breast carcinoma, and they should not pose a problem when they are located within the capsule or fibrous trabeculae of a lymph node (Fig. 13.14).[46] Rarely, however, nevus cells occur in the parenchyma of the lymph node and they may then be mistaken for metastatic lobular carcinoma.[47] Errors can be avoided by considering nevus cells in the differential diagnosis, and by comparing these cells to the patient's primary carcinoma. The presence of intranuclear inclusions and the occasional presence of melanin pigment are additional clues to the correct

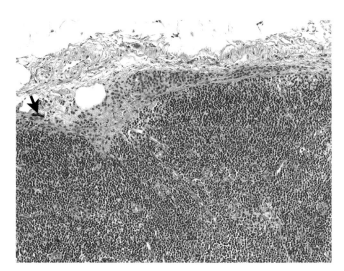

Fig. 13.14. Nevus cells in the capsule of an axillary sentinel lymph node in a patient with breast carcinoma. The capsular location, and scanty melanin pigment (arrow) are clues to the diagnosis.

diagnosis. Nevus cells are not identified in cytologic preparations because of the small size of the cellular groups and the fact that they are not readily dislodged from their capsular location.

Benign mammary epithelial cells are only rarely present in axillary lymph nodes.[48,49] They occur in capsular and subcapsular locations and may be mistaken for micrometastases (Fig. 13.15). Distinct gland formation, bland cytology and discordance with the histologic appearance of the primary carcinoma (e.g., the primary carcinoma is high grade and non-gland forming) should prompt consideration of this diagnosis. The presence of myoepithelial cells on subsequent

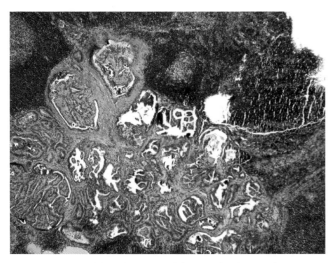

Fig. 13.15. Sentinel lymph node with benign glandular inclusions in a patient with carcinoma of the breast. This image is from case 1 of the series reported by Peng et al.[49] The authors are grateful to Dr. Yan Peng, Department of Pathology, University of Texas Southwestern Medical Center, Dallas, Texas, for providing this image.

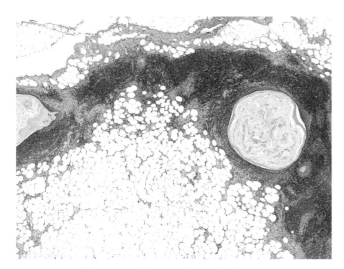

Fig. 13.16. Axillary sentinel lymph node with a benign squamous inclusion.

immunohistochemical examination will confirm the diagnosis. Rarely, squamous epithelial inclusion cysts occur in sentinel nodes,[49] but these do not offer any challenge (Fig. 13.16).

REFERENCES

1. Cao D, Lin C, Woo S-H et al. Separate cavity margin sampling at the time of initial breast lumpectomy significantly reduces the need for re-excisions. Am J Surg Pathol 2005; 29: 1625–1632.
2. Olson TP, Harter J, Munoz A et al. Frozen section analysis for intraoperative margin assessment during breast-conserving surgery results in low rates of re-excision and local recurrence. Ann Surg Oncol 2007; 14: 2953–2960.
3. Schnitt SJ. Evaluation of microscopic margins in patients with invasive breast cancer: technical and interpretive considerations. Breast J 1998; 4: 204–208.
4. Gage I, Schnitt SJ, Nixon AJ et al. Pathologic margin involvement and the risk of recurrence in patients treated with breast-conserving therapy. Cancer 1996; 78: 1921–1928.
5. Balch GC, Mithani SK, Simpson J et al. Accuracy of Intraoperative gross examination of surgical margins in women undergoing partial mastectomy for breast malignancy. Am Surgeon 2005; 71: 22–28.
6. Holland R, Connolly J, Gelman R et al. The presence of an extensive intraductal component (EIC) following a limited excision correlates with prominent residual disease in the remainder of the breast. J Clin Oncol 1990; 8:113–118.
7. Goldstein NS, Kestin L, Vicini F. Factors associated with ipsilateral breast failure and distant metastases in patients with invasive breast carcinoma treated with breast-conserving therapy. Am J Clin Pathol 2003; 120: 500–527.
8. Osteen RT, Connolly JL, Recht A et al. Identification of patients at high risk for local recurrence after conservative surgery and radiation therapy for stage I and stage II breast cancer. Arch Surg 1987; 122: 1248–1252.
9. Schnitt SJ, Connolly JL, Khettry U et al. Pathologic findings on re-excision of the primary site in breast cancer patients considered for treatment by primary radiation therapy. Cancer 1987; 59: 675–681.
10. Bilimoria KY, Cambic A, Hansen NM, et al. Evaluating the impact of preoperative breast magnetic resonance imaging on the surgical management of newly diagnosed breast cancers. Arch Surg 2007; 142: 441–445.
11. Faverly DRG, Burgers L, Bult P, et al. Three dimensional imaging of mammary ductal carcinoma in situ: clinical implications. Sem Diagn Pathol 1994; 11: 193–198.
12. Fleming FJ, Hill ADK, McDermott EW et al. Intraoperative margin assessment and re-excision rate in breast conserving surgery. Eur J Surg Oncol 2004; 30: 233–237.
13. Guidi AJ, Connolly JL, Harris JR et al. The relationship between shaved margin and inked margin status in breast excision specimens. Cancer 1997; 79: 1568–1573.
14. Valdes EK, Boolbol SK, Cohen J-M et al. Intra-operative touch preparation cytology: does it have a role in re-excision lumpectomy? Ann Surg Oncol 2007; 14: 1045–1050.
15. Karni T, Pappo I, Sandbank J et al. A device for real-time, intraoperative margin assessment in breast-conservation surgery. Am J Surg 2007; 194: 467–473.
16. Reinfuss M, Mitus J, Duda K, Stelmach A, Rys J, Smolak K. The Treatment and prognosis of patients with Phyllodes Tumor of the Breast. Cancer 1996; 77: 910–916.
17. Moffat CJC, Pinder SE, Dixon AR et al. Phyllodes tumors of the breast: a clinicopathologic review of thirty-two cases. Histopathology 1995; 27: 205–218.
18. Putti TC, Pinder SE, Elston WW et al. Breast pathology practice: most common problems in a consultation service. Histopathology 2005; 47: 445–457.
19. Cao D, Tsangaris TN, Kouprina N et al. The superficial margin of the skin-sparing mastectomy for breast carcinoma: factors predicting involvement and efficacy of additional margin sampling. Ann Surg Oncol. 2008; 15: 1330–1340.
20. Giuliano AE, Dale PS, Turner RR et al. Improved axillary staging of breast cancer with sentinel lymphadenectomy. Ann Surg 1995; 222: 394–401.

21. Turner RR, Ollila DW, Krasne DL *et al*. Histopathologic validation of the sentinel lymph node hypothesis for breast carcinoma. *Ann Surg* 1997; **226**: 271–278.

22. Lyman GH, Giuliano AF, Somerfield MR *et al*. The American Society of Clinical Oncology guideline recommendations for sentinel lymph node biopsy in early-stage breast cancer. *J Clin Oncol* 2006; **24**: 210–211.

23. Schwartz GF, Giuliano, Veronesi U. Proceedings of the consensus conference on the role of sentinel lymph node biopsy in carcinoma of the breast April 19 to 22, 2001 Philadelphia, *Pennsylvania Human Pathol* 2002; **33**: 579–588.

24. Weaver DL. Sentinel lymph nodes and breast carcinoma. *Am J Surg Pathol* 2003; **27**: 842–845.

25. Fan YG, Tan YY, Wu CT *et al*. The effect of sentinel node tumor burden on non-sentinel node status and recurrence rates in breast cancer. *Ann Surg Oncol* 2005; **12**: 705–711.

26. Rutledge H, Davis J, Chiu R *et al*. Sentinel node micrometastasis in breast carcinoma may not be an indication for complete axillary dissection. *Mod Pathol* 2005; **18**: 762–768.

27. Viale G, Maiorano E, Pruneri G *et al*. Predicting the risk for additional axillary metastases in patients with breast carcinoma and positive sentinel lymph node biopsy. *Ann Surg* 2005; **241**: 319–325.

28. Dabbs DJ, Fung M, Johnson R. Intraoperative cytologic examination of breast sentinel lymph nodes: test utility and patient impact. *The Breast J* 2004; **10**: 190–194.

29. Cao Y, Rajan PB. Sentinel node status and tumor characteristics: a study of 234 invasive breast carcinomas. *Arch Path Lab Med* 2005; **129**: 82–84.

30. Creager AJ, Geisinger KR, Shiver SA *et al*. Intraoperative evaluation of sentinel lymph nodes for metastatic breast carcinoma by imprint cytology. *Mod Pathol* 2002; **15**: 1140–1147.

31. Henry-Tillman RS, Korourian S, Rubio IT *et al*. Intraoperative touch preparation for sentinel lymph node biopsy: a 4-year experience. *Ann Surg Oncol* 2002; **9**: 333–339.

32. Turner RR, Hansen NM, Stern SL *et al*. Intraoperative examination of the sentinel lymph node for breast carcinoma staging. *Am J Clin Pathol* 1999; **112**: 627–634.

33. Weiser MR, Montgomery LL, Susnik B *et al*. Is routine intraoperative frozen-section examination of sentinel lymph nodes in breast cancer worthwhile? *Ann Surg Oncol* 2000; **7**: 651–655.

34. Cox CE, Nguyen K, Gray RJ *et al*. Importance of lymphatic mapping in ductal carcinoma in situ (DCIS): Why map DCIS? *Am Surgeon* 2001; **67**: 513–519.

35. Klauber-DeMore N, Tan LK, Liberman L *et al*. Sentinel node biopsy: Is it indicated in patients with high-risk ductal carcinoma-in-situ and ductal carcinoma-in-situ with microinvasion? *Ann Surg Oncol* 2000; **7**: 636–642.

36. Pendas S, Dauway E, Giuliano R *et al*. Sentinel node biopsy in ductal carcinoma in situ patients. *Ann Surg Oncol* 2000; **7**: 15–20.

37. Veronesi P, Intra M, Vento AR *et al*. Sentinel lymph node biopsy for localized ductal carcinoma in situ. *The Breast* 2005; **14**: 520–522.

38. Goyal A, Douglas-Jones A, Monypenny I *et al*. Is there a role of sentinel lymph node biopsy in ductal carcinoma in situ? Analysis of 587 cases. *Breast Cancer Res Treat* 2006; **98**: 311–314.

39. Huo L, Sneige N, Hunt KK *et al*. Predictors of invasion in patients with core-needle biopsy-diagnosed ductal carcinoma in situ and recommendations for the selective approach to sentinel lymph node biopsy in ductal carcinoma in situ. *Cancer* 2006; **107**: 1760–1768.

40. Rutstein LA, Johnson RR, Poller WR *et al*. Predictors of residual invasive disease after core needle biopsy diagnosis of ductal carcinoma in situ. *Breast J* 2007; **13**: 251–257.

41. Fitzgibbons P, LiVolsi VA. Recommendations for handling radioactive specimens obtained by sentinel lymphadectomy. *Am J Surg Pathol* 2000; **24**: 1549–1551.

42. Stratmann SL, McCarty TM, Kuhn JA. Radiation safety with breast sentinel node biopsy. *Am J Surg* 1999; **178**: 454–457.

43. Arora N, Martins D, Huston TL *et al*. Sentinel node positivity rates with and without frozen section for breast cancer. *Ann Surg Oncol* 2008; **15**: 256–261.

44. Motomura K, Inaji H, Komoike Y *et al*. Intraoperative sentinel lymph node examination by imprint cytology and frozen sectioning during breast surgery. *Brit J Surg* 2000; **87**: 597–601.

45. Teal CB, Tabbara S, Kelly TA. Evaluation of intraoperative scrape cytology for sentinel lymph node biopsy in patients with breast cancer. *Breast J* 2007; **13**: 155–157.

46. Bautista NC, Cohen S, Anders KH. Benign melanocytic cells in axillary lymph nodes. A prospective incidence and immunohistochemical study with literature review. *Am J Clin Pathol* 1994; **102**: 102–108.

47. Biddle DA, Evans HL, Kemp BL *et al*. Intraparencymal nevus cell aggregates in lymph nodes: possible diagnostic pitfall with malignant melanoma and carcinoma. *Am J Surg Pathol* 2003; **27**: 673–681.

48. Fisher CJ, Hill S, Millis RR. Benign lymph node inclusions mimicking metastatic carcinoma. *J Clin Pathol* 1994; **47**: 245–247.

49. Peng Y, Ashfaq R, Ewing G *et al*. False-positive sentinel lymph nodes in breast cancer patients caused by benign glandular inclusions. *Am J Clin Pathol* 2008; **130**: 21–27.

14   THE FEMALE GENITAL TRACT

Teri A. Longacre, Jonathan S. Berek, and Michael R. Hendrickson

The pathologist's role in the intraoperative management of female genital tumors in the United States has changed considerably in the last decade. While ovarian masses continue to be the leading indication for frozen section in gynecological surgery, intraoperative evaluation of the uterus, cervix, vulva, and lymph nodes now plays a smaller role. New high resolution imaging techniques, the widespread use of fine needle aspiration (FNA), and sophisticated methods for direct examination of the cervix and uterine cavity have redesigned the landscape of intraoperative consultation. In some instances, the implementation of new standardized treatment regimens has resulted in a change of emphasis of the consultation; for example, the recommendation for placement of an intraperitoneal catheter to administer chemotherapy for ovarian cancer has changed the stakes of the "ovarian cancer" diagnosis: exclusion of metastasis, correct assignment of primary site within the mullerian tract (i.e., uterus versus non-uterus) and appropriate deferral to permanent sections have become more pivotal to the management of the gynecologic cancer patient, since ports are placed depending on the pathologist's intraoperative diagnosis (IOD).

To optimize patient care, the pathologist should have a thorough understanding of the surgeon's management plan. The probability of a successful intraoperative consultation is maximized when the pathologist has a good grasp of the rationale and indications for major surgical procedures and an understanding of those pathologic findings that should (or could) activate or abort extensive surgical procedures. Although regional variations exist, in most cases, these critical decision points reflect standard practices across the country, and these are addressed in this chapter.

OVARY

General clinical issues

The majority of ovarian masses are benign, and the majority of benign ovarian masses are cystic. The diagnosis of a malignancy of the ovary is certain when an ovarian mass is accompanied by malignant ascites, but in most cases the suspicion of malignancy is indirect, based on clinical, imaging (U/S and CT scan) and serologic findings (elevated CA-125, etc.). Fine needle aspiration of the ovary is contraindicated because of the risk of spillage of neoplastic cells into the peritoneal cavity, and as a result, open laparotomy is performed when a malignancy is suspected.

When a diagnosis of primary ovarian malignancy is confirmed, the surgeon will remove all grossly visible tumor if feasible – because debulking improves the response to post-operative chemotherapy.

Indications for intraoperative consultation

The main indications for intraoperative evaluation for a suspected ovarian malignancy are to:

1. Render an initial diagnosis on an ovarian mass.
2. Evaluate extraovarian disease to determine if an ovarian malignancy is primary or metastatic.
3. Procure tissue for ancillary studies.

General pathologic issues

When an ovarian mass is submitted for IOD, it is important to initially think in broad diagnostic categories: functional, inflammatory, vascular, neoplastic, metaplastic

Intraoperative Consultation in Surgical Pathology, ed. Mahendra Ranchod. Published by Cambridge University Press.
© Cambridge University Press 2010.

Table 14.1. Serum markers in evaluation of the ovarian mass

Serum marker	Tumor
CA-125	Gynecologic cancer, but elevations seen in variety of benign processes, including endometriosis; mucinous and clear cell ovarian tumors often have minimally elevated CA-125; colorectal carcinoma may also have elevated CA-125, but CEA is usually comparatively more elevated
CEA	Colorectal cancer, other GI cancer (modest elevations may be seen in gynecologic cancer, but CA-125 is usually comparatively more elevated)
AFP	Yolk sac tumor
hCG	Choriocarcinoma, other gestational trophoblastic diseases, dysgerminoma (mild elevation)
LDH	Dysgerminoma, lymphoma
Inhibin	Sex cord-stromal tumors

(e.g., endometriosis, endosalpingiosis), etc. Many errors in frozen section (FS) diagnosis occur because the initial differential diagnostic set is too narrow (e.g., primary ovarian neoplasms only). In addition, clinical correlation is essential. The minimum data required for evaluation of an ovarian mass are: age, clinical history, whether the neoplasm is unilateral or bilateral, and whether there is disease outside the ovary. For obvious reasons, the nature of an ovarian neoplasm is highly dependent on patient age, e.g., germ cell tumors are more likely to occur in children and young adults, whereas high-grade surface epithelial carcinoma is exceedingly rare in the pediatric patient. Inflammatory processes are often associated with fever, leukocytosis, and tenderness. Adnexal torsion presents with acute abdomen, and in adult patients, is often due to a benign neoplasm (50%), a non-neoplastic cystic process such as paraovarian cyst, corpus luteum, or endometrioma (30%), normal ovary (20%), and only rarely a carcinoma (1%–2%). Serum markers may suggest a diagnosis of germ cell malignancy, sex cord-stromal tumor, or a primary mullerian surface epithelial neoplasm (Table 14.1). Laterality provides useful information since many primary tumors are unilateral, whereas metastases are more often bilateral. Similarly, the presence of extra-ovarian tumor is useful in distinguishing between primary and metastatic malignancy. Each of these data should be considered because they supplement pathologic examination. Careful gross examination and intelligent sectioning are required preconditions for accurate FS diagnosis. The external surface of an ovarian mass should always be examined for the presence of

surface excrescences, rupture, and/or adhesions, and possible sites of surface involvement should be inked to ensure correct interpretation on subsequent microscopic examination. The ovarian mass should be serially sectioned and areas of necrosis and hemorrhage should be noted, since these findings usually indicate a malignancy. If an ovarian mass is predominantly cystic, attention should be focused on the solid or papillary components. The fallopian tube, including the fimbriae should also be carefully examined, particularly if the patient is a known BRCA1/2 mutation carrier or if there is a prior history of breast cancer.

Cytoscrape preparations should be used liberally to complement FS. They provide greater cellular detail and are free of the artifacts of freezing; however, cytoscrapes are not as reliable as FS when the diagnosis depends on architectural features, as in the distinction between primary and metastatic carcinoma.

Normal structures and non-neoplastic processes in the ovary may sometimes be mistaken for malignancy (Table 14.2), usually during FS evaluation of the adnexa in a patient with uterine carcinoma; they are usually correctly interpreted on permanent sections but pose challenges when they are scrutinized on FS in the setting of a known malignancy.

Once non-neoplastic disorders have been excluded, neoplasms of the ovary should be considered in two broad groups: tumors seemingly confined to a single anatomic site versus tumors involving more than one anatomic site (e.g. an ovarian mass in association with either uterine carcinoma or disseminated peritoneal disease) (Table 14.3). In addressing the extensive list of possible differential diagnoses for these two broad groups of tumors, the pathologist should consider patient age, laterality (Table 14.4) and direction of differentiation: is it epithelial, gonadal stromal, germ cell, or metastatic? If metastatic, both gynecologic and non-gynecologic sites have to be considered.

If the patient is of reproductive age or younger, consideration is given to reproductive conservation if the clinical situation warrants conservation, an issue that the pathologist should recognize as a high stake situation when rendering a diagnosis. All surface epithelial neoplasms that are diagnosed as low malignant potential (borderline) or carcinoma require staging. The extent of staging will depend on (a) the pathologic diagnosis and (b) whether the patient is a candidate for reproductive conservation (Table 14.5). The diagnosis of serous tumor of low malignant potential in a patient who is a candidate for reproductive conservation will generally result in cystectomy

Table 14.2. Ovarian findings that mimic malignancy

Non-neoplastic process	Process most commonly mimicked	Diagnostic clue(s)
Hilus cells around ovarian hilar nerves	Metastatic germ cell neoplasm	Hilar location, no LVSI
Rete ovarii	Metastatic adenocarcinoma	Located in the hilum of the ovary, no atypia, absence of mitotic figures, no LVSI
Surface inclusion cysts	Metastatic adenocarcinoma	Cortical location. Bland tubal-type epithelium.
Stromal hyperplasia – stromal hyperthecosis	Sex cord-stromal tumor (steroid cell tumor, luteinized thecoma), endometrioid stromal sarcoma	Bilateral involvement (may be asymmetric). Struma hyperplasia: diffuse or nodular, scant cytoplasm, may have Leydig cell hyperplasia; Struma hyperthecosis: large rounded cells with eosinophilic or vacuolated cytoplasm, may have Leydig cell hyperplasia
Corpus luteum with degenerative change	Steroid cell tumor	Small size, reproductive age
Nests of stromal lutein cells	May appear epithelial and mimic metastatic carcinoma.	Postmenopausal ovaries
Tangentially cut follicular structures	Undifferentiated carcinoma (mitotically active)	Call-Exner bodies, bilaminar architecture, deeper level sections
Decidual reaction	Large cell non-keratinizing carcinoma	Surface of ovary, large cells with large nuclei. Gestational setting.
Endometriosis with cytological atypia	Adenocarcinoma (primary or metastatic)	Endometriosis elsewhere, reproductive age

LVSI = lymphovascular space involvement.

Table 14.3. Ovarian masses presenting in association with disease elsewhere

Extraovarian site(s)	Comment
Uterus	Concurrent uterine tumor may be a separate primary or the ovarian tumor may be a metastasis from endometrium or rarely, cervix
Omentum	Usually ovarian primary, but consider stomach, pancreas, biliary tract, colon, and appendix if histology not classic for mullerian serous differentiation
Colonic	Mucosal involvement favors colon primary; serosal-based disease favors metastasis to colon
Appendix	Pseudomyxoma peritonei or mucinosis peritonei (abundant intraperitoneal mucin, appendiceal low-grade mucinous neoplasm), goblet cell carcinoid

diagnosis; this may lead to a second operative procedure, either for complete staging and/or for placement of an intraperitoneal catheter if a diagnosis of carcinoma is made on permanent sections.

Specific clinico-pathological issues

Serous tumors
Clinical issues
Serous tumors of low malignant potential are managed differently than serous carcinomas, particularly in reproductive aged patients. If there is any doubt about whether the tumor is a carcinoma, the diagnosis should be deferred to permanent sections.

When the primary site is uncertain (i.e., ovary vs. fallopian tube vs. surface peritoneum), the diagnosis of "pelvic serous carcinoma" is sufficient. This diagnosis provides the surgeon with the necessary information for further surgical staging without committing to a definite site of origin. If there is concern that the tumor may be arising in the uterus, this should be stated.

Pathologic issues
Serous carcinoma is the most common histologic subtype of ovarian carcinoma. Grossly, they are solid or solid and cystic with foci of necrosis (Fig. 14.1). Although serous carcinoma is distinguished by destructive stromal invasion, the intraoperative diagnosis is usually based on the presence of slit-like spaces, complex papillae, and marked cytologic atypia (Fig. 14.2); psammoma bodies are often present. Serous tumors of low malignant potential (LMP)

with preservation of ovarian tissue whenever possible. In contrast, a diagnosis of serous carcinoma or clear cell carcinoma will usually lead to a full staging procedure without reproductive conservation, regardless of the patient's age.

The surgeon will often insert an intraperitoneal port for adjuvant chemotherapy when a diagnosis of carcinoma is rendered.[1] When a diagnosis of carcinoma cannot be made with confidence, it is best to err on the side of under-

Table 14.4. Ovarian tumors: unilateral versus bilateral involvement

Tumor	Age, years (range)	Comment
Unilateral		
Epithelial		
Clear cell – carcinoma, esp. low stage (benign and low malignant potential very rare)	Mean = 57 (35–80)	Pelvic and/or ovarian endometriosis (50–60%); Involvement of contralateral ovary, when present, typically small and in context of high stage disease. Exclude yolk sac tumor in young women.
Mucinous, intestinal type -benign, low malignant potential and carcinoma	Mean = 45 (14–84)	Often quite large (>15 cm), multicystic. Benign mucinous tumors may be bilateral (10–15%).
Transitional – benign and low malignant potential	Mean = 55 (26–79)	Solid, microcysts, calcifications.
Sex cord-stromal		
Adult granulosa cell tumor	Mean = 52 (15–80)	Estrogenic manifestations. Steroid content may impart yellow appearance, solid or solid and cystic or rarely, purely cystic hemorrhagic mass. If numerous mitotic figures, consider undifferentiated carcinoma. Potential to recur, esp. high stage.
Juvenile granulosa cell tumor	Mean = 13 (0.5–67) 95% less than 30	Isosexual pseudoprecocity. Steroid content may impart yellow appearance, solid or solid and cystic or rarely, purely cystic mass. May have nuclear atypia and high mitotic index. Most benign (90%).
Sclerosing stromal tumor	Mean = 28 (10–51) 80% less than 30	Solid, hypercellular and hypocellular pseudolobulated areas. Benign.
Steroid cell tumor	Mean = 43 (2.5–80) 75% greater than 30	Androgenic manifestations.
Sertoli–Leydig cell tumor	Mean = 25 (2–75) 90% less than 50	Androgenic manifestations. Solid, yellow. May have heterologous elements: mucinous, carcinoid, cartilage, embryonic skeletal muscle.
Fibroma–Thecoma Group	Mean = 46 (17–90)	May have estrogenic manifestations. Luteinized thecoma may be androgenic. Solid, firm or lobulated. May be assoc with Meig's syndrome (ascites and pleural effusion). Most are benign.
Germ cell		
Dysgerminoma (10% grossly bilateral)	Mean = 21 (8–41) 80% less than 30	Solid, fleshy mass. Two-thirds FIGO stage I. Bilateral tumors often assoc with gonadoblastoma.
Yolk sac tumor (most)	Mean = 18 (5–45) 95% less than 30	Exclude clear cell carcinoma in young women.
Immature teratoma	Mean = 19 (1–40) 95% less than 30	Solid and cystic, necrosis, hemorrhage
Other		
Small cell carcinoma, hypercalcemic type	Mean = 24 (<1–46)	Extraovarian involvement (50%). Two-thirds have hypercalcemia.
Female adnexal tumor of wolffian origin	Mean = 50 (15–83)	Broad ligament, rarely ovarian.
Bilateral (%)		
Epithelial		
Serous low malignant potential (40–60%)	Mean = 45 (12–90)	Extraovarian involvement (40–60%)
Serous carcinoma (40–60%)	Mean = 55 (15–95)	Low-grade serous carcinoma may occur at younger age
Endometrioid – low malignant potential and carcinoma (30–40%)	Mean = 52 (25–85)	Simultaneous tumors in uterus, fallopian tube (20%); Pelvic and/or ovarian endometriosis (40%)
Mucinous, endocervical-like – low malignant potential (30%–40%)	Mean = 39 (21–79)	Pelvic and/or ovarian endometriosis (50%); Extraovarian implants (20%)
Transitional cell carcinoma (40%)	Mean = 56 (33–94)	Often mixed with serous carcinoma.

continued on next page

Table 14.4. *(continued)*

Tumor	Age, years (range)	Comment
Germ cell		
Gonadoblastoma (mixed germ cell-stromal) (30%)	Children and young adults	Calcification common (40%). Dysgerminoma assoc. with Y chromosome and maldeveloped gonads (50%). Requires complete removal of all gonadal tissue.
Mature teratoma (15%–20%)	Any age, but most common in reproductive years	Exclude somatic tumor arising in teratoma (mucinous tumors, carcinoid, struma). Squamous carcinoma most common somatic malignancy, but wide variety), typically in post-menopausal women.
Other		
Metastases (40%–60%)	Mean = 50 (20–90)	Colon, breast, stomach, appendix, pancreatobiliary, most common – but *anything* can metastasize to the ovary. Metastatic gastric signet ring may occur at younger age range.

Table 14.5. Current recommended surgical treatment for common ovarian neoplasms

Neoplasm	Cystectomy/ oophorectomy/ adnexectomy	Cystectomy/oophorectomy/ adnexectomy + staging	TAH-BSO + Staging
Epithelial			
Benign	X		
Low malignant potential		X (Pediatric & Reproductive)	X (Post-menopausal)
Carcinoma*			X
Germ cell			
Mature teratoma	X		
Malignant germ cell tumor: Yolk sac, Dysgerminoma, Embryonal, Immature teratoma		X	
Sex cord-stromal			
Adult granulosa cell tumor		X	X (Post-menopausal)
Juvenile granulosa cell tumor	X		
Sclerosing stromal tumor	X		
Fibroma/thecoma	X		
Sertoli–Leydig cell tumor		X	
Steroid cell tumor			X

* A conservative approach is frequently used for reproductive age women with well differentiated carcinomas, since many of these tumors present as stage IA tumors and have a very favorable prognosis.

are predominantly cystic with papillary excrescences which may be present inside the cyst lining or covering the surface of the ovary (Fig. 14.3). The papillary excrescences should be sampled for IOD; these show branching papillae, lined by columnar epithelium with minimal to moderate cytologic atypia; mitotic figures are sparse (Fig. 14.4). Micropapillary architecture may be present (Fig. 14.5). Serous cystadenomas are generally smaller and composed of simple cysts.

The pathologist should try to distinguish high-grade serous carcinoma from low-grade (grade 1) serous carcinoma since the extent of staging may differ in a reproductive aged patient with apparent low stage disease. Low-grade serous carcinoma is uncommon and in most cases, cannot be reliably diagnosed in the intraoperative setting due to morphologic overlap with serous tumors of LMP. The distinction between serous tumor of LMP and serous cystadenoma with focal proliferation may be difficult in the intraoperative setting, since it is based on a single sampling and an estimate percent volume of epithelial proliferation; when in doubt, the surgeon should be notified that the tumor may be of LMP and the diagnosis should be deferred

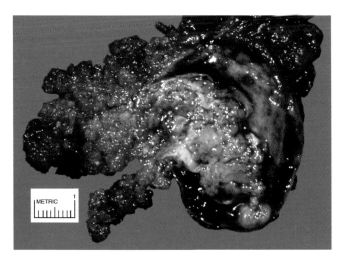

Fig. 14.1. Ovarian serous carcinoma is solid or solid and cystic with necrosis. Most high grade serous carcinomas are high stage at presentation.

(a)

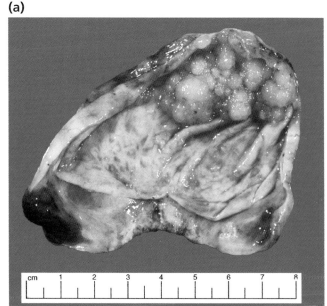

(b)

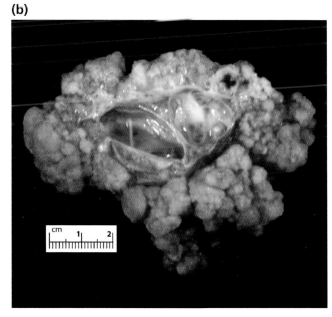

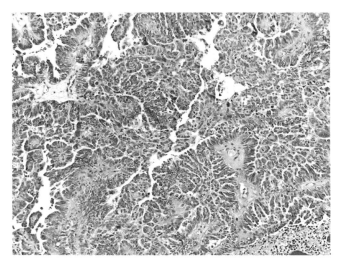

Fig. 14.2. Serous carcinoma is recognized by complex papillary structures, glands with slit-like spaces and marked cytologic atypia. Psamomma bodies are often present, but are not specific.

Fig. 14.3. Ovarian serous tumors of low malignant potential are typically cystic, but can exhibit a range of architectural complexity. (a) Simple cyst lined by small papillary excrescences. If the papillary excrescences make up 10% or less of the cyst volume, the tumor is a serous cystadenoma with focal proliferation. (b) Coalescent papillary structures stud the surface of the ovary, simulating a malignant neoplasm.

to permanent sections; this allows the surgeon to consider a limited staging procedure, if clinically indicated.

Mucinous tumors, intestinal type
Clinical issues

Primary mucinous tumors of the ovary present diagnostic challenges for the gynecologic oncologist and pathologist.[2,3] Mucinous tumors of low malignant potential (LMP) comprise approximately 15% of all ovarian mucinous neoplasms and can be subdivided into intestinal and endocervical-like types, with the intestinal type comprising about 85%–95%. Intestinal mucinous tumors of LMP usually present as a large (>10 to 15 cm), smooth-surfaced, unilateral, multiloculated cystic adnexal mass (Fig. 14.6). Bilaterality, which occurs in less than 10% of cases, is sufficiently uncommon that it should prompt consideration of a metastasis. Necrosis is unusual, and this too, should suggest a metastasis. Unlike serous LMP, almost all are stage 1.

(a)

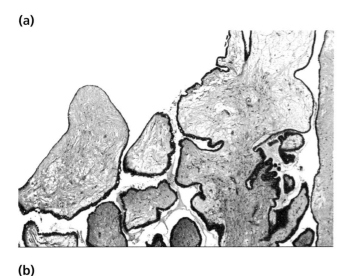

(b)

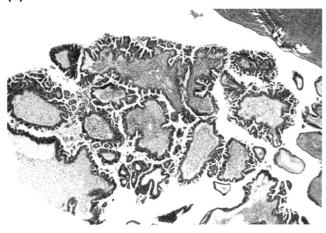

Fig. 14.4. (a) Papillary excrescences in serous tumors may be composed of coarse papillae with simple serous epithelium (serous cystadenofibroma). (b) Papillae with more complex branching and epithelial tufting warrant diagnosis of at least serous tumor of low malignant potential (borderline tumor).

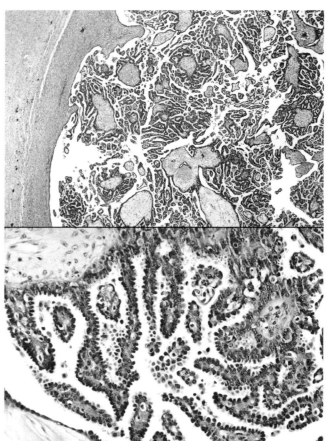

Fig. 14.5. Serous tumor of low malignant potential (borderline tumor) with micropapillary features. The papillae are elongated, at least x5 in length as in width. In absence of stromal invasion, these tumors are managed the same as the usual type of serous tumor of low malignant potential.

Mucinous carcinoma, which accounts for less than 15% of all primary ovarian mucinous neoplasms, usually presents as a large, complex, solid, and cystic mass. Approximately 80% are unilateral. Necrosis and solid mural nodules are characteristic. Surface ovarian involvement is not present in most cases, although larger tumors may exhibit areas of rupture and/or adhesions. Ascites may be present, even though the tumor is confined to the ovary at presentation.

Pathologic issues

Most mucinous cystadenomas are readily diagnosed on the basis of simple cystic architecture and a single, uniform layer of cytologically bland epithelium. However, mucinous tumors with proliferative changes, stratification and gland complexity pose significant problems. Because of intraoperative sampling limitations, it is difficult, and sometimes impossible, to make the distinction between mucinous LMP, mucinous carcinoma and sometimes even a benign mucinous tumor. Mucinous carcinomas are often heterogeneous on microscopic examination, showing the full range from benign to LMP to frank carcinoma within the same neoplasm (Figs. 14.7 and 14.8). Careful gross examination is essential; this includes thorough sectioning and a search for solid areas. Solid areas should be sampled for FS, and this is one situation where multiple FS blocks may have to be prepared to identify the highest grade neoplasm. FS examination can be supplemented with cytoscrape preparations because the latter allows examination of a larger surface area of the neoplasm. Solid areas may show: (a) conventional mucinous carcinoma; (b) anaplastic carcinoma arising in an otherwise typical LMP or mucinous carcinoma; (c) pseudosarcomatous mural nodule; and/or (d) stromal mucin and mucin granulomas due to

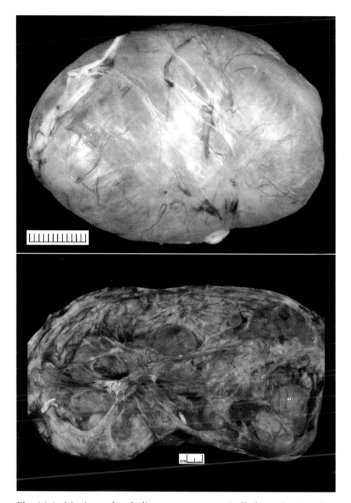

Fig. 14.6. Mucinous borderline tumors are typically large (>15 cm), unilateral, and multicystic. These tumors must be extensively sampled (at least 1 section per cm) in order to exclude carcinoma. If suspicious areas (i.e., severe cytological atypia or possible stromal invasion) are present on initial sectioning, additional sections should be submitted. Since the diagnosis of primary mucinous carcinoma requires thorough sampling, most complex mucinous neoplasms are diagnosed as "mucinous tumor, at least borderline, cannot exclude carcinoma" in the intraoperative setting.

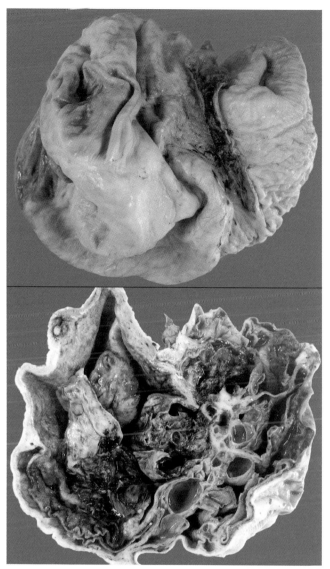

Fig. 14.7. External and cut surface of a mucinous carcinoma arising in the ovary. The macroscopic appearance may be indistinguishable from mucinous borderline tumor, but the presence of more complex cysts with or without solid nodules should prompt extensive sampling.

ruptured benign mucinous glands (Fig. 14.9). The diagnosis should be deferred to permanent sections if a firm decision cannot be made.

Metastatic mucinous carcinoma should be considered whenever both ovaries are involved, when there is grossly visible necrosis, and when there is accompanying extra-ovarian tumor because most bona fide primary mucinous carcinomas are limited to the ovary or show minimal pelvic involvement at the time of diagnosis. In addition, the presence of pseudomyxoma peritonei (mucinosis peritonei) is almost certainly evidence of an extra-ovarian primary. When any of these conditions are present, the surgeon should be asked to search for an extra-ovarian primary, with particular focus on the appendix, pancreas, and colon. When the biological nature of a mucinous neoplasm is in doubt in a patient who wishes to retain her reproductive capacity, unilateral adnexectomy with conservation of the contralateral adnexa and uterus is appropriate.

Clear cell carcinoma
Clinical issues
Clear cell carcinoma (CCC) is a high-grade carcinoma that occurs more frequently in younger women compared to other high-grade carcinomas of the ovary, shows a greater

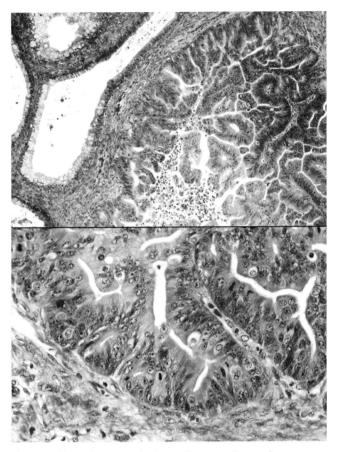

Fig. 14.8. Tumor heterogeneity in mucinous ovarian carcinoma. Benign cystadenoma and mucinous adenocarcinoma in the same field. The mucinous carcinoma shows an expansile growth pattern interpreted as stromal invasion.

propensity for nodal metastases, and responds poorly to standard platinum-based chemotherapy. CCC is treated by aggressive surgical resection and debulking of all grossly visible disease. Association with ovarian or pelvic endometriosis is not uncommon.

Pathologic issues

CCC is the most commonly misdiagnosed ovarian carcinoma on FS.[4,5] The distinction from other primary ovarian carcinomas is not important intraoperatively, but care should be taken to avoid misinterpreting CCC as a mucinous or serous tumor of low malignant potential. CCC may be solid, or solid and cystic with fleshy papillary excrescences, and may arise in association with an endometriotic cyst (Fig. 14.10).

CCC exhibits three main architectural patterns: dilated glands lined by hobnail cells, papillae, and solid sheets of cells (Fig. 14.11), and most tumors show mixture of all three patterns. Diagnostic errors occur because the sample

selected for FS may not show features that are pathognomonic of CCC. The main pitfalls are as follows.

(a) Clear cells may be absent, and instead, the neoplasm may be composed of non-descript cells with granular cytoplasm. Formalin fixation of the FS slide may enhance the detection of clear cytoplasm and papillary architecture.[6]

(b) Cytologic atypia, one of the hallmarks of CCC, may be subdued in the area sampled; and

(c) Mitotic figures may not be prominent.

Unlike serous tumors, CCC is often unilateral; bilateral disease occurs in high stage disease, with the contralateral ovary containing small surface or cortical tumor deposits that are usually detected only on microscopic examination. The papillary pattern of CCC is different from serous carcinoma in that the branching of the papillae is non-hierarchical (Fig. 14.11). The presence of associated pelvic and/or ovarian endometriosis should also prompt consideration of CCC.[7] Clear cell carcinoma differs from mucinous tumors by having a more prominent adenofibromatous stroma (Fig. 14.11).

A variety of other primary ovarian tumors may also exhibit clear cytoplasm, usually due to glycogen or lipid accumulation (Table 14.6). On very rare occasions, renal cell carcinoma may present as a metastasis to the ovary, and when this diagnosis is considered, it is simple enough to ask the surgeon to palpate the kidneys or check if the patient has had a prior nephrectomy.

Endometrioid carcinoma
Clinical issues

Benign and LMP endometrioid tumors are uncommon, and almost all are adenofibromas. They typically occur in perimenopausal and postmenopausal patients and present as a unilateral ovarian mass.

Endometrioid carcinomas occur most commonly in the fifth to seventh decade, and many patients have associated pelvic endometriosis and/or endometriosis involving the ovary. Low-grade endometrioid carcinomas are often associated with synchronous low-grade endometrioid carcinoma of the endometrium, and in this setting, the ovarian tumors may be bilateral. Various molecular approaches have been used to determine whether these concurrent tumors are independent primary tumors or metastases from one organ to the other, with conflicting results. However, if these tumors are low-grade and limited

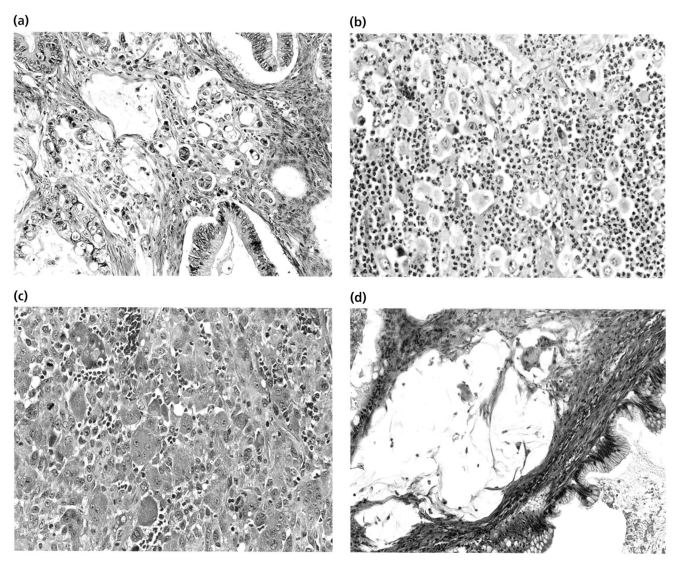

Fig. 14.9. Solid areas in primary ovarian mucinous cystic tumors may show (a) conventional invasive mucinous carcinoma; (b) anaplastic carcinoma arising in an otherwise typical LMP or mucinous carcinoma; (c) pseudosarcomatous mural nodule; or (d) stromal mucin and mucin granulomas due to ruptured benign mucinous glands.

to the ovary and uterus, the prognosis is similar to that of low-grade carcinoma limited to one or the other organ, and is driven by the depth of myometrial invasion.

Pathologic issues

Squamous metaplasia is very common in endometrioid carcinomas, as are other metaplastic changes (secretory, ciliated cell, oxyphilic); a minor component of mucinous differentiation may be present, similar to that seen in the homologous carcinoma arising in the endometrium. Endometrioid carcinomas exhibit a wide range of patterns, including spindled, tubular, insular, trabecular, microglandular, adenoid basal, and adenoid cystic (Fig. 14.12). When these patterns are prominent, they may mimic a sex

cord-stromal tumor, carcinoid tumor, or Brenner tumor. A diagnosis of sex cord-stromal tumor or endometrioid carcinoma will usually motivate surgical staging, whereas a diagnosis of carcinoid tumor may or may not initiate staging. Benign Brenner tumors are not staged. Careful gross examination will often assist in the latter differential diagnosis (Fig. 14.13). When the spindle cell component is prominent, endometrioid carcinoma may be mistaken for a carcinosarcoma,[8] a problem that is heightened when the carcinoma also shows stromal hyalinization, osteoid-like collagen, or frankly chondroid or osteoid elements (Fig. 14.14). Clues to the correct diagnosis include: (a) the endometrioid component is no more than grade 2; (b) the spindle cell component is not markedly atypical;

poorly differentiated (or undifferentiated) surface epithelial carcinoma, metastatic carcinoma, primitive germ cell neoplasms, granulosa cell tumor (adult or juvenile), undifferentiated gonadal stromal neoplasm, mesenchymal neoplasms (primary or metastatic), and hematolymphoid malignancies (Fig. 14.16). Less commonly encountered primary ovarian neoplasms include small cell carcinoma, hypercalcemic type, small cell carcinoma, pulmonary type, and non-small cell neuroendocrine carcinoma.

Patient age, anatomic distribution of disease, including laterality (unilateral versus bilateral ovarian involvement), and clinical history may provide important clues to the diagnosis (e.g., prior history of lymphoma).

Pathologic issues
Cytologic preparations should be examined because they may offer useful clues.

The characteristic nuclear features of adult granulosa cell tumor (nuclear grooves, open chromatin, small nucleoli), carcinoid tumor, and lymphoma are often more easily recognized on cytoscrape preparations, and goblet cells may be more apparent on cytologic preparation than in the frozen tissue section, permitting distinction between endometrioid carcinoma and metastatic colorectal carcinoma.

If a firm diagnosis cannot be made, the diagnosis should be deferred to permanent sections, and tissue should be procured for appropriate ancillary studies. The surgeon should be given license to perform surgical staging if high-grade carcinoma and malignant germ cell tumor are in the differential diagnosis, and an enlarged lymph node should be sampled if lymphoma is likely. The surgeon should be reminded to obtain a blood sample intraoperatively for serum markers (e.g., hCG and alpha-fetoprotein) if a germ cell malignancy is possible; this will not only aid in diagnosis but will be helpful in following the response to treatment.

Metastases to the ovary
Clinical issues
The distinction between primary ovarian carcinoma and metastases to the ovary is not always clear pre-operatively, so the surgeon relies on the pathologist to discriminate between these two, a distinction that is important because of differences in surgical management. Approximately 5%–10% of ovarian masses that present as primary ovarian neoplasms are eventually interpreted as metastases. Common primary sites include colorectum, breast, stomach, appendix, pancreas, and biliary tract.

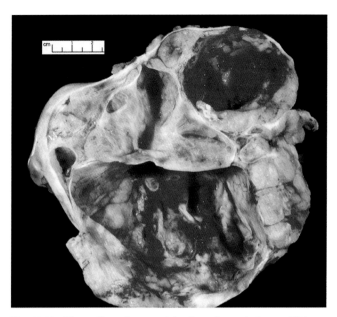

Fig. 14.10. Clear cell carcinoma arising in endometriotic cyst. This tumor has a cystic appearance with papillary excrescences, simulating a serous tumor. However, clear cell carcinoma is typically unilateral and more frequently associated with endometriosis.

(c) squamous metaplasia with keratin formation is frequently present, and this blends imperceptibly with the spindle cell component. In contrast, carcinosarcoma should contain high-grade epithelial and mesenchymal elements.

Endometrioid differentiation is recognized by rounded gland contours, cribriform or villoglandular structures and squamous or morular metaplasia. When present, an adenofibromatous component and better differentiated foci resembling endometrioid LMP are additional supporting features. Poorly differentiated carcinomas that lack squamous or mucinous differentiation are more likely to be high-grade serous carcinomas.

Metastatic colon cancer should always be considered because it closely resembles endometrioid carcinoma (Fig. 14.15). Extensive "dirty cell" necrosis with abundant karyorrhectic debris, a garland-like glandular pattern and an absence of squamous differentiation are clues to the diagnosis (see discussion of metastases below). The colon carcinoma may be antecedent or concurrent, and if there is no prior history, the surgeon should be asked to palpate the entire colon, and examine the small intestine if the colon does not harbor a mass.

Undifferentiated malignant neoplasms
Clinical issues
Undifferentiated malignant neoplasms of the ovary are relatively uncommon. The differential diagnosis includes

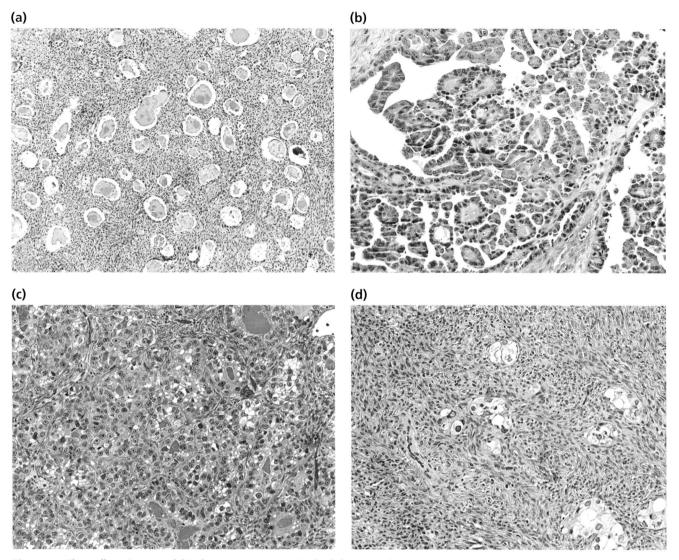

Fig. 14.11. Clear cell carcinomas exhibit three main patterns: (a) glandular or tubulocystic; (b) papillary; and (c) solid. Most tumors show a mixture of patterns. (d) An ovarian tumor with prominent adenofibromatous stroma should prompt consideration for clear cell carcinoma.

Table 14.6. Clear cell change in ovarian tumors

Primary ovarian neoplasms

    Clear cell carcinoma

    Endometrioid carcinoma

    Mucinous carcinoma

    Steroid cell tumors

    Sertoli–Leydig cell tumor

    Yolk sac tumor

Metastases

    Renal cell carcinoma

Since most metastatic mucin-producing adenocarcinomas originate in the gastrointestinal tract, a disproportionate elevation of CEA especially when combined with a normal or near-normal CA-125, should suggest a gastrointestinal primary.

Pathologic issues

The following gross and histologic features should raise the possibility of metastatic carcinoma.

- A metastasis should be considered whenever a mucinous neoplasm is encountered, no matter how bland the histologic findings. Metastatic mucinous carcinomas often show a range of differentiation, with some areas mimicking a benign mucinous cystadenoma. The ovarian mass should be subjected to careful gross examination, seeking solid areas and grossly visible necrosis as these areas are likely to harbor the frankly malignant component of the neoplasm. Both FS and cytoscrape preparations should be made as they are complementary. The pathologist should know if the ovarian mass is unilateral or bilateral, and if there is

(a)

(b)

(c)

(d)

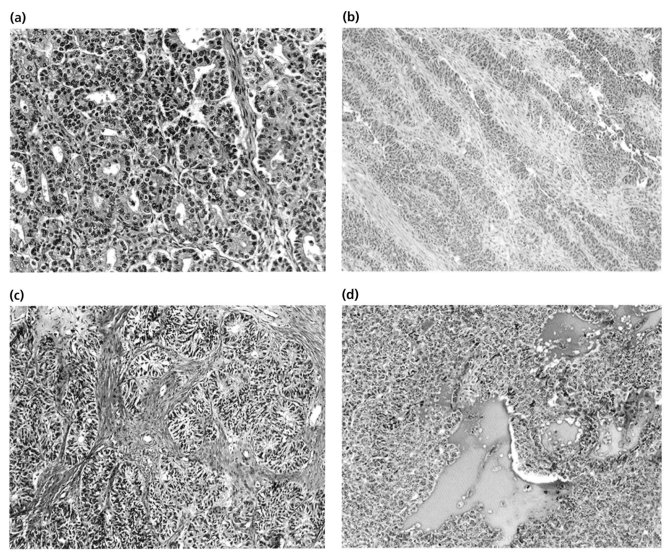

Fig. 14.12. Well-differentiated endometrioid carcinoma may exhibit (a) tubular, (b) trabecular, or (c) insular growth pattern. (d) In addition, cystic follicle-like spaces may simulate adult granulosa cell tumor. The presence of squamous elements helps in establishing the diagnosis, but this may be sparse or absent. If the diagnosis is uncertain in a patient of reproductive age, deferral to permanent sections is appropriate.

accompanying extra-ovarian disease, such as peritoneal metastases, because bilaterality and peritoneal disease favor an extra-ovarian primary.

- When handling an apparent endometrioid carcinoma of the ovary, one of the first steps is to exclude a colonic metastasis. Clues to a colorectal metastasis include the following: (a) bilaterality; (b) absence of squamous or morular differentiation; (c) a cribriform pattern; (d) glandular structures with a garland pattern; (e) incomplete glands due to necrosis; and (f) "dirty necrosis" (Fig. 14.15).

- Metastatic carcinoma of mammary origin usually produces bilateral metastases. Unlike other metastases that form nodular masses in the ovary, breast carcinoma often produces uniform enlargement with a smooth external surface. Metastatic breast carcinoma may be ductal (predominantly gland-forming) or lobular. When gland-forming, the pattern of gland formation, although usually dissimilar to mullerian carcinoma, may be difficult to distinguish from a primary ovarian serous carcinoma on FS. The pattern of spread, i.e., bilateral ovarian involvement without omental involvement, should be a red flag, since most high-grade serous carcinomas are high stage at presentation. Metastatic lobular carcinoma raises a different problem: ovarian involvement may be subtle since

(a)

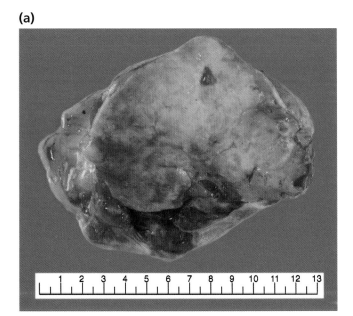

(b)

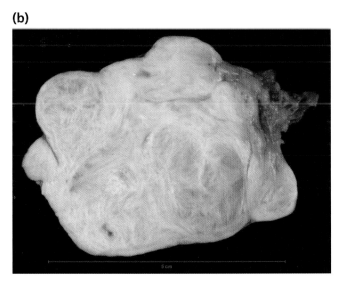

Fig. 14.13. (a) Benign Brenner tumor is recognized on gross examination by the presence of small cysts (due to the presence of mucinous epithelium) set in a solid, dense fibromatous stroma. Calcification is often present and will impart a gritty sensation on cutting the specimen. (b) Ovarian fibroma is also solid, but typically has no cysts.

(a)

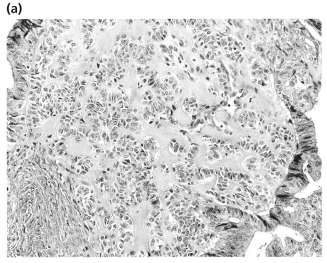

(b)

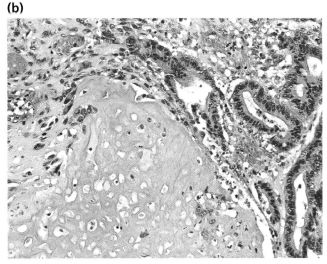

Fig. 14.14. (a) The presence of spindled cell elements or (b) osteoid-like or chondroid-like matrix in low grade endometrioid tumors may be mistaken for carcinosarcoma, but the glandular and spindle cell elements in endometrioid carcinoma are low grade, while in carcinosarcoma both glandular and stromal components are high grade.

the neoplasm stimulates proliferation of ovarian stroma, and cursory examination may lead to misdiagnoses such as fibroma and fibrothecoma (Krukenberg tumor).[9]

▪ An adenocarcinoma with a signet ring cell pattern should be interpreted as a metastasis because this pattern is rarely seen in primary ovarian carcinomas. Likely sites include stomach, appendix (goblet cell carcinoid), and breast (mucinous lobular carcinoma). If a history of prior malignancy was not forthcoming pre-operatively, this should be re-visited intraoperatively, and the surgeon should be asked to explore the abdomen for an alternative primary site. In a small proportion of cases, an extraovarian primary may not be found at the time of surgery, and these patients require additional imaging studies after surgery, to completely exclude a primary tumor of sites such as pancreas and/or biliary tract. Metastatic signet ring cancer may elicit pronounced ovarian stromal hyperplasia, simulating a stromal tumor (Fig. 14.17).

▪ Patients who have a mucinous ovarian tumor and intraperitoneal mucin (pseudomyxoma peritonei or

(a)

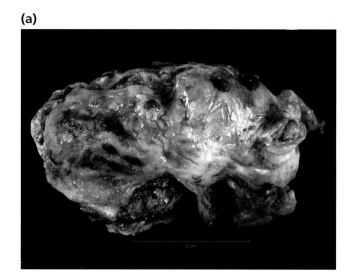

(b)

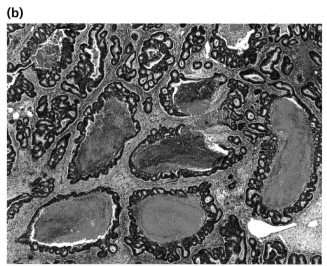

Fig. 14.15. (a) Metastatic colorectal carcinoma may simulate primary ovarian cancer. The capsule is predominantly smooth, but surface nodules are present in this example. (b) Metastatic colorectal carcinoma can be recognized on frozen section (FS) by the presence of large, dilated cribriform glands forming a garland pattern with central "dirty" necrosis. "Dirty" necrosis consists of necrotic tumor cells, fibrin, and inflammatory cells and may be seen in other tumors.

mucinosis peritonei) should be considered to have a primary appendiceal neoplasm with ovarian metastases (Fig. 14.18). These patients require appendectomy, regardless of the appearance of the appendix (see chapter on GI tract, p. 114). Rarely, the appendix is normal, and some of these patients have a mucinous ovarian tumor arising in association with an ovarian mature teratoma[10,11] or a mucinous neoplasm arising in the urachus or other site, each of which may give rise to pseudomyxoma peritonei (more appropriately named mucinosis peritonei) (Table 14.7).

(a)

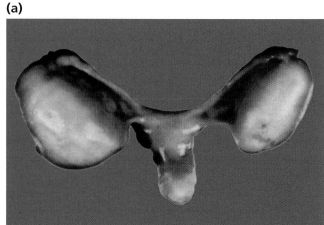

(b)

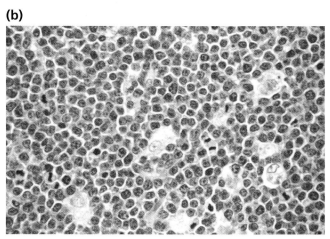

Fig. 14.16. (a) Bilateral ovarian involvement is not unusual in Burkitt's lymphoma. (b) Starry sky appearance of Burkitt's lymphoma in the ovary. (Courtesy of Dr. Ronald Dorfman).

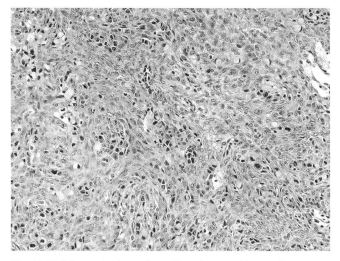

Fig. 14.17. Metastatic signet ring cell carcinoma with prominent stromal hyperplasia. When diffuse, this lesion may mimic a fibroma or fibrothecoma. Bilateral fibroma-like ovarian tumors should suggest the possibility of metastasis and prompt careful search for small gland-like structures or signet ring cells.

(a)

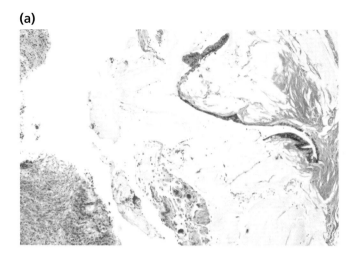

(b)

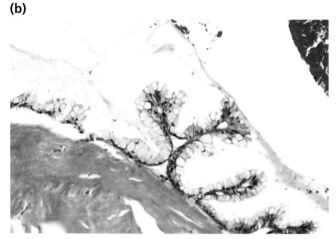

Fig. 14.18. (a) Ovarian mass due to low grade mucinous tumor of appendiceal origin. The characteristic features are pools of mucin in the stroma in which there are cytologically bland strips or fragments of columnar mucinous epithelium. (b) The mucinous epithelium often exhibits an undulating appearance. In the absence of an appendiceal tumor, the ovary should be extensively sampled to exclude a mucinous neoplasm arising in an ovarian teratoma.

A variety of clinical and pathologic strategies have been proposed to be of value in differentiating primary from metastatic carcinoma in the ovary (Table 14.8).[12,13] Many of these strategies increase the probability of a primary versus a metastasis, but they do not provide certainty and in many instances their relative importance has been over-emphasized. For example, while the presence of bilateral disease may help differentiate a primary neoplasm from a metastasis in some scenarios, a consideration of prior probability indicates that unilaterality only slightly favors a primary tumor (1:2.5). In the problematic case, the diagnosis often rests on a constellation of clinical, histologic, and management decisions. When the pathologist is faced with an unusual appearing neoplasm, it is important to remember that practically any tumor can metastasize to the ovary

Table 14.7. Pseudomyxoma peritonei (mucinosis peritonei) syndrome

Anatomic Site of Involvement	Pathologic Features
Peritoneum	Mucinous ascites associated with fibrosis; may be localized, although this does not fall under the umbrella of classic pseudomyxoma peritonei (mucinosis peritonei)
Appendix	May not be clinically obvious. Cytologically bland mucinous epithelium with simple or villous, undulating architecture. Goblet cells and distended mucin-filled columnar cells. Mucinous dissection through wall of appendix often present. If no such lesion present on microscopic examination, consider other sites: urachus, primary ovarian mucinous tumor arising in association with teratoma, etc.
Ovary	Cytologically bland mucinous epithelium with simple or villous, undulating architecture. Goblet cells and distended mucin-filled columnar cells. May be no more atypical than mucinous adenoma. Pools of stromal mucin (pseudomyxoma ovarii or mucinosis ovarii). May have appearance of mucinous borderline tumor, intestinal type (usually focal)

(Fig. 14.19). Clinical history of a prior malignancy, however remote, should always be taken under consideration.

Lesions of the ovary and peritoneum in pregnancy

There are several pregnancy related changes that occur in the ovaries and peritoneum and these can be divided into two main groups: (a) lesions that are unique to pregnancy, and (b) secondary, hormone-related changes that occur in pre-existing neoplasms. Lesions that are unique to pregnancy, and the neoplasms they may be mistaken for, are listed in Table 14.9.

Luteinization in granulosa cell tumors may produce histologic changes that are confusing (Fig. 14.20), but the neoplasm is still likely to be recognized as a sex cord-stromal tumor, and not confused for a malignancy.

Pregnancy-induced changes in serous borderline tumors can be confusing. Peritoneal implants that accompany an ovarian serous LMP may induce a florid mesothelial proliferation as well as a stromal decidual change, simulating invasive implants or invasive carcinoma.

Because pregnancy-induced changes can be confusing, a diagnosis of an ovarian or peritoneal malignancy should

Table 14.8. Evaluation of ovarian mucinous cystic neoplasms: features that distinguish primary from metastasis

Feature	Primary	Metastatic
Macroscopic		
Surface implants	−/+	++++
Surface mucin	−/+	++
Bilaterality	+	+++
Extraovarian spread	−/+	+++
Multinodular growth pattern	−/+	++
Smooth external surface	+/−	−/+
Large size (> 10 cm)*	++	+
Microscopic		
'Dirty' necrosis	+	+++
Colloid pattern	−/+	+++
Heterogeneous nodular stromal invasion	−/+	+++
Infiltrative stromal invasion	−/+	++
Hilar involvement	+	++
Lymphovascular involvement	+	++
Expansile invasion	+++	+
Mullerian histology	+++	+
Mural nodule	++++	−
Associated primary tumor (e.g., teratoma, Sertoli–Leydig cell tumor, Brenner tumor)	++++	−/+

* The likelihood that a unilateral mucinous ovarian tumor is primary increases with increasing size (i.e., a tumor that is >15 cm is more likely to be primary than one that is only 10 cm in size).

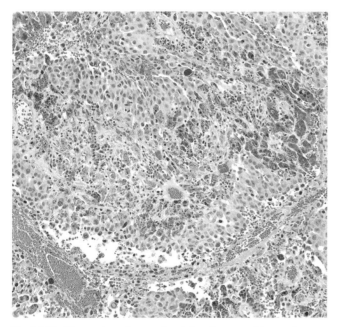

Fig. 14.19. Metastatic melanoma involving the ovary. Metastasis should always be considered when any ovarian tumor has an unusual appearance. In this example, the presence of melanin pigment strongly favors melanoma.

Table 14.9. Gynecologic processes typically encountered during pregnancy

Process	Process most commonly mimicked	Diagnostic clue(s)
Pregnancy luteoma	Steroid cell tumor Metastatic melanoma	Well-demarcated nodule (s) in cortex of ovary. Central degenerative changes. Mitotic figures may be present.
Hyperreactio luteinalis – ovarian hyperstimulation syndrome	Granulosa cell tumor	Multiple thin-walled cysts, often bilateral. History of molar pregnancy, ovulation induction.
Solitary luteinized cyst of pregnancy and peurperium	Unilocular granulosa cell tumor	Luteinized cells in wall of cyst often atypical with degenerative features. Absence of follicle formation.
Clear cell hyperplasia of fallopian tube epithelium	Clear cell carcinoma	Mitotically inactive Bland cytology. May occur in tubal ectopic gestation
Decidual change	Peritoneal carcinomatosis Squamous cell carcinoma	History of pregnancy. Bland cytology.
Arias-Stella reaction	Clear cell carcinoma	Smudged chromatin
Granulosa cell proliferations of pregnancy	Granulosa cell tumor. Sertoli cell tumor	Small size. Multiple foci. Association with atretic follicles.
Disseminated peritoneal leiomyomatosis	Peritoneal carcinomatosis	Circumscribed, small nodules distributed over surface of peritoneum. Bland smooth muscle – may have foci of endometriosis, decidual change.

be made with great caution, because it is more likely that the lesion is a pseudomalignancy rather than a true malignancy.

Ovarian lesions in the pediatric and post-pubertal patient
Clinical issues
Ovarian tumors are uncommon in pediatric and post-pubertal patients. At least one-third of all ovarian masses occurring in this age group are non-neoplastic or functional (usually follicular) cysts. Approximately 60% of

(a)

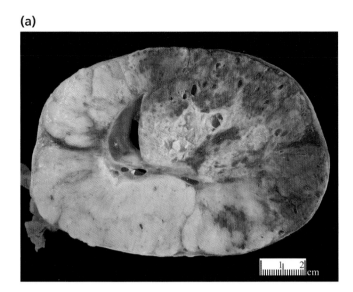

(b)

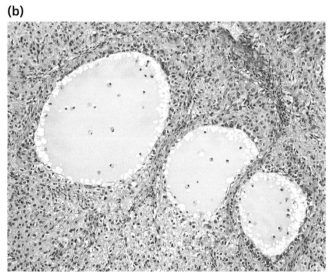

Fig. 14.20. (a) Juvenile granulosa cell tumor with prominent luteinization. Sex cord-stromal tumors often exhibit yellow coloration because of stromal luteinization. (b) Luteinization may mask the characteristic features of granulosa cell tumors.

neoplasms are germ cell tumors, followed by surface epithelial and sex cord-stromal tumors. Most germ cell tumors are benign. The most common malignant germ cell tumors, in order of frequency are: dysgerminoma, immature teratoma, and yolk sac tumor. Surface epithelial tumors tend to exhibit serous or mucinous histology and are often benign; serous carcinomas are almost always low grade, whereas mucinous carcinomas tend to behave in an aggressive fashion.

Adnexal torsion presents a unique management issue in the pediatric and adolescent patient. Most cases of torsion occur in association with a normal ovary, follicular cysts, or a benign neoplasm, and <1% are associated with a

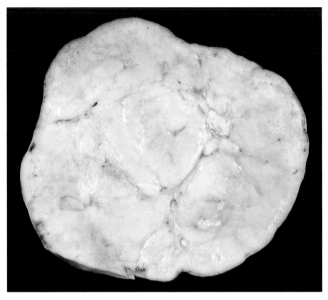

Fig. 14.21. Dysgerminoma. Solid, pale tan to yellow homogeneous appearance is characteristic of dysgerminoma, but lymphoma may have a similar appearance. Scrape preparations are useful in distinguishing lymphoma from dysgerminoma.

malignant neoplasm, usually a germ cell tumor. Both adnexae undergo torsion in up to 15% of cases. When torsion affects a benign appearing ovary, there is a premium on preserving ovarian tissue; after detorsion, oophoropexy will very likely be performed on the affected ovary as well as on the contralateral normal ovary, and a biopsy will be submitted for FS evaluation if there is any suspicion of an underlying malignant neoplasm.

The surgical treatment of malignant neoplasms depends on the stage of the disease. Patients with non-hematolymphoid tumors are treated in the same way as adult patients, and patients with hematolymphoid neoplasms usually have a diagnostic oophorectomy, and if the nature of the neoplasm is recognized intraoperatively, no further surgery is performed.

Pathologic issues
The correct diagnosis can be made by gross examination in the majority of benign functional cysts and mature cystic teratomas, and FS is usually not necessary. Frozen section and a cytoscrape preparation should be made of all solid or solid/cystic neoplasms. Dysgerminoma (Fig. 14.21) and lymphoma share many gross and microscopic features, and cytologic preparations, especially air dried smears, are useful for recognizing lymphoma. When lymphoma is suspected, a sample should be selected for flow cytometry.

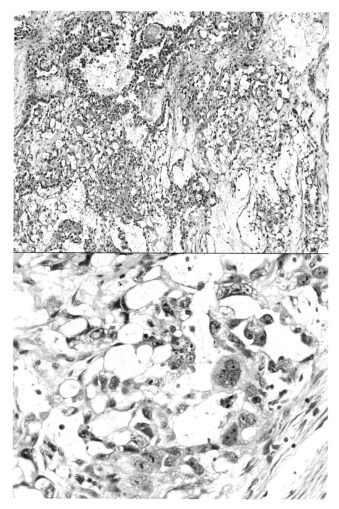

Fig. 14.22. Typical yolk sac tumor with a reticular or microcystic pattern. The neoplastic cells often have enlarged, moderately pleomorphic, hyperchromatic nuclei that contain one or more distinct nucleoli.

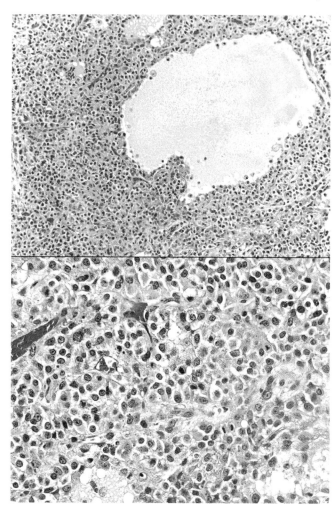

Fig. 14.23. Juvenile granulosa cell tumor has large, irregular follicular structures set in a solid cellular background. The cells are generally more hyperchromatic and mitotically active than those in adult granulosa cell tumor.

Distinguishing juvenile granulosa cell tumor from yolk sac tumor may pose difficulties because they occur in the same age group, are usually unilateral, and both have a solid or solid/ cystic gross appearance with foci of necrosis and hemorrhage. The presence of a reticular or microcystic pattern on FS favors yolk sac tumor (Fig. 14.22), while large, irregular follicular structures set in a solid cellular background favors a juvenile granulosa cell tumor (Fig. 14.23).

The hemorrhagic ovarian cyst

The differential diagnosis of a hemorrhagic ovarian cyst includes endometriosis, hemorrhagic functional cyst, and rarely, *unilocular* granulosa cell tumor (Fig. 14.24). Clear cell carcinoma often arises within the wall of an endometriotic cyst (Fig. 14.10). Other neoplasms commonly associated with endometriotic cysts include low-grade endometrioid neoplasms and endocervical-like mucinous tumors (often bilateral), but any tumor may co-exist with endometriosis.

Most endometriotic cysts are unilateral with a relatively smooth interior wall, although adherent blood may be present (Fig. 14.25). Any excrescences or mural nodules should be viewed with suspicion and sampled for FS evaluation. Occasionally, endometriosis may form larger, more complex cysts with polypoid masses, which may be difficult to distinguish from adenosarcoma with limited sampling. When in doubt, the diagnosis should be deferred, and the surgeon should be encouraged to remove any other areas of bulky endometriosis in order to make a full evaluation.

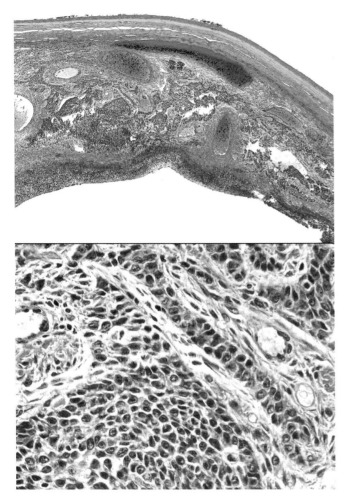

Fig. 14.24. Unilocular adult granulosa cell tumor may mimic an endometriotic or functional follicular cyst on gross examination. However, the large size and presence of a more pronounced granulosa cell proliferation in the cyst wall should suggest the diagnosis.

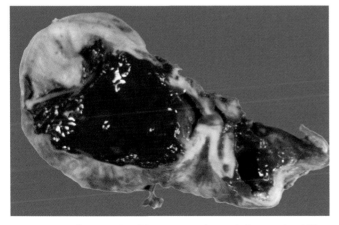

Fig. 14.25. Endometriosis of the ovary. Endometriotic cysts should be carefully examined to exclude occult clear cell carcinoma. Papillary excrescences or other solid areas should be submitted for frozen section.

UTERUS

Indications for intraoperative diagnosis

1. To evaluate the uterus for grade, depth of myometrial invasion, and cervical stromal involvement in patients with biopsy documented endometrial carcinoma.
2. To evaluate whether carcinoma is present, and whether it is myoinvasive, in a patient with a prior biopsy diagnosis of atypical complex hyperplasia.
3. To evaluate an unusual intrauterine mass (uncommon);
4. To evaluate endometrial curettings for chorionic villi.
5. To evaluate endometrial curettings in patients who have massive hemorrhage.

Specific clinico-pathological issues

The hysterectomy specimen in patients with endometrial carcinoma
Clinical issues

The current management of endometrial carcinoma depends heavily on surgicopathologic staging, and the pathologist may play a key role in this process, depending on the institution and the individual surgeon's threshold for performing a full staging procedure. In some centers, all patients with a pre-operative diagnosis of endometrial carcinoma are treated by a full staging procedure and the pathologist plays no role in intraoperative management. In other centers, full staging is performed only when one of the following features is present: (a) high-grade carcinoma; (b) high risk special variant carcinoma (e.g., serous or clear cell histology); (c) obvious adnexal involvement by carcinoma; (d) grossly suspicious pelvic or para-aortic nodes; and (e) cervical stromal involvement. When these features are absent or equivocal, intra-operative consultation is indicated, since up to 25% of clinical stage I carcinomas are upstaged after complete staging. To help the surgeon decide on the need for surgical staging, the pathologist is expected to evaluate the following.

- Whether or not there is myoinvasion, and if myoinvasion is present, the depth of invasion. The depth of myometrial invasion that will prompt full staging varies depending on the grade, the presence of lymphovascular space involvement and the presence or absence of lower uterine segment involvement.

- Whether or not there is evidence of involvement of the cervix. Gross examination is adequate in the vast majority of cases.
- The extent of endometrial surface involvement by carcinoma by gross examination (i.e., > 4 cm).

Pathologic issues
Evaluation of the uterus and cervix

The uterus should be opened along its lateral margins, and if the uterus is distorted, a probe can be used to sound the uterus to guide the blade of the scissors. The endometrial surface is then examined and a grossly visible carcinoma > 4 cm in surface dimension – even without myometrial invasion- warrants staging since tumors of this size are associated with a poorer prognosis. Transverse cuts should then be made from fundus to cervix to look for gross evidence of myometrial invasion. If myometrial invasion is visible on gross examination, a sample should be taken for FS to document the area of deepest invasion; if gross invasion is absent, a sample of the uterine wall should be sampled for FS where the myometrium is different in appearance because some carcinomas invade the myometrium as small nests, without forming a visible mass (Fig. 14.26).[14] The evaluation of myometrial invasion may pose the following challenges:

- It is sometimes difficult to distinguish an irregular endometrial/myometrial junction from superficial myoinvasion, but this is usually of little clinical consequence.
- Involvement of adenomyosis by non-invasive carcinoma may be difficult to distinguish from invasive carcinoma; this is often clinically significant because it may involve the deep myometrium. Irregular glands with a granulation tissue host response should be required before making a firm diagnosis of myoinvasion, but the absence of a host reaction does not exclude myometrial invasion. If the issue cannot be resolved on FS, a search should be made for lymphovascular invasion, as the latter will usually trigger lymph node sampling. Caution should be exercised when evaluating lymphovascular invasion in laparoscopic-assisted hysterectomy specimens since the intracavitary balloon may cause artefactual displacement of neoplastic tissue into uterine vessels; the presence of extensive vascular involvement in uteri that contain minimally invasive, low-grade adenocarcinoma is a clue to correct interpretation.

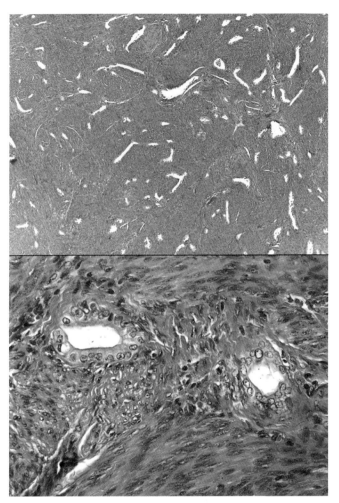

Fig. 14.26. Low grade endometrial carcinoma with extensive, diffuse myometrial invasion. This pattern of invasion may not form a visible mass on gross examination and may be overlooked on initial examination. With this pattern of invasion, the cervix should be carefully examined to exclude cervical stromal invasion.

- When evaluating the cornual portion of the uterus, direct extension of non-invasive carcinoma into the intramural portion of the fallopian tube should not be misconstrued as myoinvasive carcinoma. This error can be avoided by knowing where the FS sample was taken from, a non-trivial issue when microscopic evaluation is done by a pathologist who has not examined the gross specimen.

A thorough examination of the lower uterine segment and the cervix is also required (Fig. 14.27). The cervix should be serially sectioned along the longitudinal plane to the level of the peritoneal reflection, even if it is grossly normal in order to exclude the presence of an endometrial cancer that is burrowing into the underlying cervical stroma; this provides a more accurate assessment of extension into the

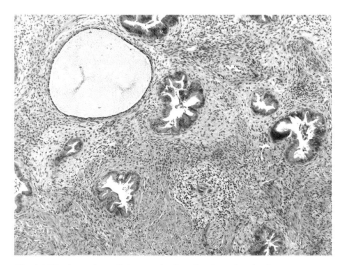

Fig. 14.27. A section of the cervix showing invasion by low grade endometrial carcinoma. Cervical stromal invasion is best recognized on frozen section by a stromal response around the infiltrating glands.

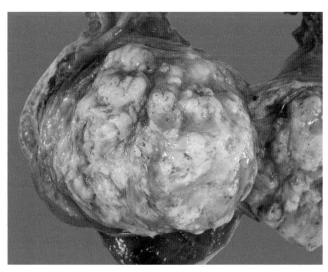

Fig. 14.28. Uterine leiomyoma with degenerative changes. Because of the variety of degenerative appearances that can be seen in benign uterine smooth muscle tumors, caution should be exercised in the intraoperative evaluation of these neoplasms. Only tumors with severe cytologic atypia, tumor cell necrosis, and increased mitotic index should be diagnosed as sarcoma on frozen section.

cervical tissue than examination of the unsectioned cervix and keeps the specimen relatively intact. If grossly uninvolved, FS is not indicated.

Evaluation of the adnexa

Gross involvement of the ovary and/or fallopian tube by neoplasm is usually due to a simultaneous primary adnexal neoplasm in the setting of low-grade (Grade I or II) non-myoinvasive endometrial carcinoma. In contrast, adnexal involvement by uterine papillary serous carcinoma may be extensive even in the absence of gross abnormalities within the uterus. In most situations, gross examination of bivalved ovaries (two sections can be made if the ovaries are enlarged) is sufficient to exclude the presence of neoplasm. If there is uncertainty about involvement of the ovaries, a FS can be performed, although in most instances, a FS diagnosis of metastatic endometrial carcinoma will not significantly alter patient management because these patients have other identifiable risk factors that warrant a staging procedure. When evaluating the adnexa, it is important to keep in mind that there are a variety of normal and benign lesions that may be mistaken for carcinoma (Table 14.2).

The unusual uterine mass

A request may be made for intraoperative evaluation of an unusual uterine mass encountered during myomectomy or when an unexpected or unusual mass is encountered during hysterectomy.

Myomectomy

Most patients who undergo myomectomy are infertile, premenopausal women interested in retaining their uterus, and a diagnosis of malignancy should be made with great caution if the surgeon is likely to proceed with hysterectomy. We sound this cautionary note because of the many diagnostic pitfalls in distinguishing unusual leiomyomas from leiomyosarcoma.

Most uterine masses that strike the surgeon or pathologist as grossly unusual (Fig. 14.28) are clinically benign smooth muscle tumors exhibiting one or more patterns of degeneration. Some of these patients may have been treated with hormonal preparations, and the presence of an increased mitotic index (i.e., mitotic figures per ten high power fields) and necrosis have been attributed to these agents. Moreover, many cytologic changes that would warrant a diagnosis of malignancy in other organ systems do not correlate with clinically malignant behavior in uterine smooth muscle neoplasms. Accordingly, unless the smooth muscle tumor is blatantly malignant histologically – extensive tumor cell necrosis, diffuse severe atypia, frequent and abnormal mitotic figures – the diagnosis should be deferred for permanent sections. It is quite rare to make a diagnosis of leiomyosarcoma on a myomectomy specimen – one more reason to exercise great caution in making the diagnosis of sarcoma in this clinical setting.

HYSTERECTOMY

The surgeon will usually submit the hysterectomy specimen for IOD when the mass is unusually large and has grown rapidly. In most cases, a rapidly growing mass is a conventional leiomyoma. The mass should be serially sectioned and carefully examined for infiltrative margins or intravascular extension. When examining the mass, it is important to remember that uterine smooth muscle tumors can exhibit epithelioid, highly cellular, or myxoid features, which may mimic an epithelial, stromal, or sarcomatous process (Fig. 14.29). The differential diagnosis of a myometrial mass with poorly defined margins includes adenomyosis, adenomatoid tumor, stromal sarcoma, leiomyosarcoma, and diffuse leiomyomatosis. Intravascular tumor growth may be due to a high-grade sarcoma, low-grade stromal sarcoma and intravenous leiomyomatosis. Intravascular growth may be simulated by a variety of processes, e.g., retraction of otherwise typical leiomyomas from the surrounding myometrium, leiomyomas with perinodular myxoid degeneration, and extension of adenomyosis into vascular channels (Fig. 14.30). When the diagnosis cannot be made on FS, the surgeon should be informed that there are atypical features that have to be resolved on permanent sections, and that a hysterectomy is all that should be performed.

In some instances, the distinction between a stromal and smooth muscle tumor may be difficult; since criteria for malignancy differ for these two mesenchymal processes, the diagnosis should be deferred to permanent section in these instances. However, whenever stromal sarcoma or intravenous leiomyomatosis is a serious possibility, the surgeon should be urged to assess the patient for extrauterine disease. Occasionally the surgeon will report that the "myoma won't shell out" in the expected way. This finding is almost diagnostic of localized adenomyosis and the diagnosis is obvious on frozen section. Rarely, adenomatoid tumors may present in this fashion (Fig. 14.31).

Evaluation for possible intrauterine pregnancy
Clinical issues
The management of patients with suspected ectopic pregnancy has undergone significant change in the last two decades. Ultrasound examination has proved to be highly reliable in the diagnosis of ectopic pregnancy, and in conjunction with serial hCG determinations (which now has a rapid turn-around-time), has become the diagnostic method of choice in most large centers.

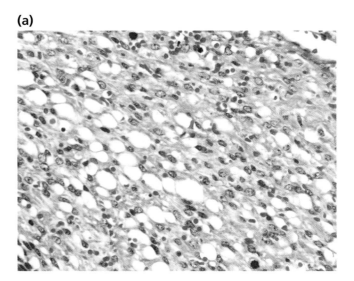
(a)

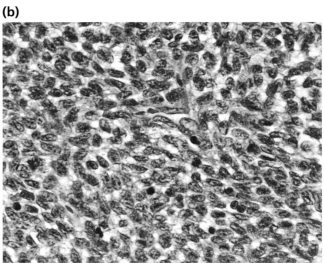
(b)

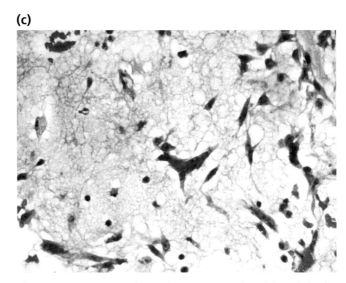
(c)

Fig. 14.29. Uterine smooth muscle tumors may show (a) epithelioid, (b) cellular, and (c) myxoid changes. In most instances, confirmation that the mass is a mesenchymal neoplasm is sufficient in the intraoperative setting.

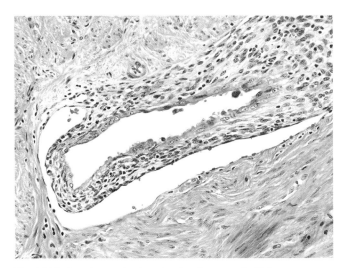

Fig. 14.30. Pseudovascular invasion in adenomyosis. This finding should be interpreted with caution in the absence of a mass lesion.

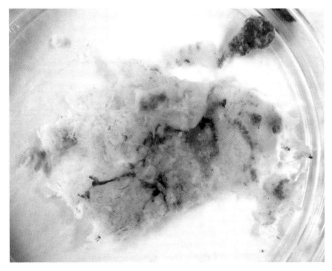

Fig. 14.32. Saline float test for chorionic villi. The villous tissue will float to the surface, forming sea anemone-like structures.

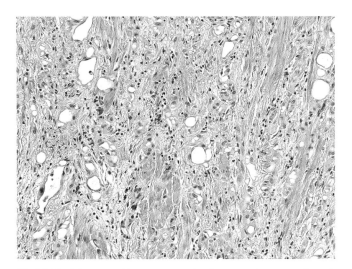

Fig. 14.31. Adenomatoid tumors may simulate a uterine mesenchymal process. The lesions feature distinctive thin, cellular bridges that help in establishing the diagnosis.

Removal of the ectopic pregnancy may not even occur, as methotrexate is adequate therapy in early tubal gestations. However, frozen sections of uterine curettings are still performed in centers with less expertise in ultrasonography, whenever ultrasonography is not immediately available, or when the diagnosis remains in doubt. If the FS is negative for an intrauterine pregnancy, the surgeon will need to decide whether to perform laparoscopic visualization of the fallopian tubes, followed by salpingostomy or salpingectomy if a tubal ectopic is identified.

Pathologic issues

There is a significant false-negative rate with FS analysis of endometrial curettings for products of conception when only occasional villi are present.[15,16] When the specimen is scanty and can be embedded in one block, the entire specimen should be submitted for FS evaluation, and more than one level should be examined if the initial FS slide is negative. The hemorrhagic areas of the FS slides should be examined carefully, because necrotic villi ("ghost villi") tend to be embedded in blood clot.

If the specimen is abundant and bloody, the saline float test should first be performed because villous tissue will stand out against the bloody background and these pieces can be selected for FS (Fig. 14.32). The saline float test should be performed under sterile conditions if the clinician requests chromosome analysis. The float test will be negative if chorionic villi are very scanty, and the pathologist should then use her judgment about the number of FS blocks to prepare.

Massive uterine hemorrhage
Clinical issues

Rarely, women require an emergency curettage for massive uterine bleeding that requires immediate diagnosis and prompt treatment. In most instances, the treating clinician has a general idea of etiology and needs confirmation: Is this a gestational event gone awry? Is this a malignant process, requiring immediate surgical and/or radiation therapy? In most cases, a temporizing approach with a preliminary FS diagnosis (or differential diagnosis) will suffice to direct immediate patient management, until the patient is stabilized and permanent sections can be evaluated.

Pathologic issues

A specific diagnosis should be made whenever possible but some distinctions are difficult to make on FS, requiring deferral to permanent sections. Fortunately, the stakes are low because definitive surgery can usually be delayed until permanent sections are examined. Frozen section should not be expected to distinguish well differentiated endometrial carcinoma from complex hyperplasia and atypical polypoid adenomyoma; similarly, distinguishing disintegrating benign endometrium from a neoplastic glandular or endometrial stromal neoplasm may sometimes be difficult. In most cases however, a specific diagnosis can be made, including intra-uterine pregnancy, high-grade carcinoma, carcinosarcoma, or sarcoma. If a diagnosis of adenocarcinoma is made, the surgeon should be prompted to perform differential curettage if the origin of the carcinoma is obscure.

CERVIX

Clinical issues

There is lack of uniformity in the way surgeons approach cervical carcinoma. In many institutions, initial examination under anesthesia is performed to determine the presence or absence of paracervical or parametrial disease. If no abnormality is detected, the abdomen is explored for gross parametrial disease or grossly positive para-aortic lymph nodes. The presence of either, confirmed by FS, is sufficient reason for stopping the planned hysterectomy. Since the presence of multiple or bilateral pelvic lymph node metastases is also an indication for stopping, FS may be requested on suspicious pelvic lymph nodes. If the pelvic lymph nodes are grossly normal, most surgeons will perform a complete lymphadenectomy but not request intraoperative evaluation. At other centers, routine lymphadenectomy is performed and all the lymph nodes are submitted for intraoperative evaluation; if any positive nodes are found, the hysterectomy is not performed. Still other centers will proceed with radical hysterectomy regardless of the lymph node status and treat with post-operative radiation if lymph nodes are positive.

Although radical abdominal hysterectomy with pelvic lymphadenectomy forms the mainstay of treatment for early-stage cervical carcinoma, fertility preserving radical trachelectomy with pelvic lymphadenectomy is an option

for women with early-stage disease.[17–20] This procedure is gaining in popularity and appears to be an acceptable and safe alternative to the standard radical hysterectomy for some patients. The general eligibility criteria for radical vaginal trachelectomy include: women less than 40 years of age who have a strong desire to preserve fertility, no clinical evidence of impaired fertility, FIGO stages IA–IB1* (tumors <2 cm are eligible for vaginal trachelectomy, whereas tumors between 2 cm and 4 cm are treated by abdominal trachelectomy), no involvement of the upper endocervical canal, and negative regional lymph nodes. Women with a history of prior large cervical conization or repeated conization, abnormal anatomy, and in some instances, tumor size greater than 2 cm may benefit more from radical abdominal trachelectomy. Both procedures aim at resecting the cervix, upper 1–2 cm of the vagina, and parametrium. A critical component of these procedures involves FS evaluation of the superior (endo-cervical/lower uterine segment) margin, which should include measuring the distance of the carcinoma from this margin. The pathologist should ink the parametrial soft tissue one color and the proximal margin a separate color. The proximal 1 cm of the specimen should then be removed from the main trachelectomy specimen, sectioned serially at 3 mm to 5 mm intervals in the longitudinal axis, and submitted for FS. Ideally, the carcinoma should be at least 5 mm from the inked margin. Since this is often a labor intensive procedure, the surgeon should inform the pathologist at least a day in advance to allow adequate staffing of the FS suite. The interpretation of the FS is usually non-problematic for squamous cell carcinoma, but more challenging for cervical adenocarcinoma, when endometrial tissue from the lower uterine segment may be mistaken for cervical adenocarcinoma by the inexperienced pathologist. For this reason, it is essential for the pathologist to be familiar with the case history prior to performing the intraoperative consultation, and to examine prior pathologic material if the slides are available. A patient with negative margins on a pre-trachelectomy cone biopsy is unlikely to have positive margins in the trachelectomy specimen. Radical trachelectomy should be discouraged for adenoma malignum, since distinguishing adenoma malignum from benign endocevical glands may be next to impossible.

---

* Stage 1A: Invasive cervical carcinoma limited to the cervix, measuring <5 mm in thickness and <7 mm in maximum surface dimension. Stage 1B1: Invasive cervical carcinoma limited to the cervix, measuring <4 cm in any dimension.

Table 14.10. Uterine findings that mimic malignancy

Non-neoplastic process	Process most commonly mimicked	Diagnostic clue(s)
Adenomyosis	Invasive adenocarcinoma	Endometrial stroma and glands confined to irregular junction or dispersed in rounded contours with associated uterine smooth muscle hypertrophy (as opposed to irregular, haphazard infiltration by malignant glands).
Gland-poor adenomyosis	(Low-grade) endometrial stromal sarcoma	Stroma may appear atrophic. Often only focal finding. Concentric uterine smooth muscle hypertrophy.
Stromal-poor adenomyosis	Invasive adenocarcinoma	Noncomplex glands with rounded contours. Concentric uterine smooth muscle hypertrophy.
Adenomatoid tumors	Metastatic adenocarcinoma	Subserosal location. Bland cytologic features.
Decidual reaction	Large cell non-keratinizing carcinoma	Gestational setting.
Endometriosis (serosa)	Metastatic adenocarcinoma	Endometrial stroma & hemosiderin deposition. May have atypical, smudged chromatin with degenerative changes.
Benign intravascular menstrual or nonmenstrual tissue	Lymphovascular involvement by adenocarcinoma or stromal sarcoma	Absence of carcinoma or mass lesion elsewhere.

There are limited indications for performing FS on a cervical biopsy for initial diagnosis. When a patient has a clinically obvious cervical carcinoma, the surgeon may wish to proceed with radical hysterectomy at the same sitting when it has not been possible to make the diagnosis as an office procedure, or when a diagnosis of invasive carcinoma has been made at another institution but the slides are not available for review. Frozen sections on grossly invasive cervical carcinoma are usually easy to interpret.

We think it is unwise to perform FS on cone biopsies, and we feel that FS should not be used to distinguish between microinvasive and grossly invasive carcinoma. It is far better to make these assessments on cone biopsies that are processed routinely.

Pathologic issues

The most common mimics of cervical carcinoma are: decidual stromal reaction (cervical squamous carcinoma) and endometriosis, endocervical glandular hyperplasia, tuboendometrioid metaplasia, Arias–Stella reaction, and lower uterine segment on deep cones (cervical adenocarcinoma). Attention to clinical setting and uterine location will prevent most misdiagnoses.

FALLOPIAN TUBE

There are very few management-related indications for FS evaluation of the fallopian tube. A fallopian tube harboring a primary carcinoma may be submitted for IOD; usually peritoneal metastases are present and identification of the primary site helps to confirm a primary gynecological malignancy. There is no reason for intraoperative examination of the fallopian tubes in high risk patients (such as germline BRCA1/2 mutations) who have risk-reducing TAHBSO – unless one of the fallopian tubes is grossly abnormal and found to contain carcinoma. Intraoperative confirmation of the diagnosis of carcinoma will almost certainly prompt surgical staging.

On occasion, a tubo-ovarian abscess with an atypical presentation may be submitted for frozen section to exclude a malignancy. Suspected tubal pregnancies are only rarely submitted for intraoperative evaluation, and only if the surgeon is uncertain that the fallopian is the site of implantation.

LYMPH NODES

The indications for intraoperative evaluation of lymph nodes in gynecologic surgery have changed substantially in the past decade. PET scan has replaced the need for intraoperative evaluation of most lymph node dissections in cervical cancer in many centers, and although lymphatic mapping with sentinel lymph node biopsy has been evaluated in gynecological surgery, intraoperative evaluation of sentinel lymph nodes is not standard practice. The current, most common indications are: (a) sentinel node evaluation (controversial), and (b) evaluation of a

Table 14.11. Lymph node findings that mimic malignancy

Non-neoplastic process	Process most commonly mimicked	Diagnostic clue(s)
Decidual reaction	Metastatic large cell non-keratinizing carcinoma	Subcapsular sinuses and cortex but deeper lymph node involvement can also occur. Foci of endometriosis or endosalpingiosis elsewhere in the lymph nodes.
Endosalpingiosis	Metastatic adenocarcinoma or involvement by serous borderline tumor, esp. if psammoma bodies and fibrous reaction present	Capsular, subcapsular or interfollicular location within the cortex, but extension into the deep portions of the node may occur. Smooth outer contour but may feature simple intraluminal papillary configurations. Mix of ciliated, secretory, and intermediate cuboidal or columnar cells. Small nucleoli may be present.
Endometriosis with or without cytological atypia	Metastatic adenocarcinoma, esp. if endometrioid, mucinous epithelium of müllerian type (endocervical), or metaplastic squamous epithelium	Subcapsular location, absence of a desmoplastic stromal response, absence of cytologic atypia. Endometriosis elsewhere. Reproductive age.
Extramedullary hematopoiesis	Undifferentiated carcinoma, lymphoma, melanoma	History of myeloproliferative disorder or a myelodysplastic syndrome. Megakaryocytes.
Lymphangioleiomyomatosis (LAM)	Benign metastasizing leiomyoma, metastatic low-grade endometrial stromal sarcoma	Reproductive years. Presence of diffuse cystic pulmonary disease. Prominent involvement of lymph vascular channels.

suspicious lymph node to determine possible recurrent or metastatic disease in selected clinical settings, and at some centers, initial evaluation of pelvic nodes in cervical cancer.

When the outcome of nodal status affects the extent of surgical resection, there is no reason to intentionally spare tissue for permanent sections; the goal of intra-operative evaluation is to make the correct diagnosis when it matters most. If the lymph node is grossly abnormal, a cytoscrape preparation may be all that is needed, but in normal sized nodes we prepare five to six levels routinely.

A variety of processes may mimic carcinoma during intraoperative evaluation of lymph nodes (Fig. 14.33); these are listed in Table 14.11.

VULVA

There are few indications for intraoperative evaluation of the vulva. In the past, FS was often performed to evaluate margins of excision for Paget's disease because of the difficulty of determining the extent of the disease on clinical examination. However, FS evaluation of margins has fallen out of favor because of tumor multifocality and the early success with non-surgical forms of treatment. The examination of surgical margins during a skinning vulvectomy procedure for multifocal vulvar intraepithelial

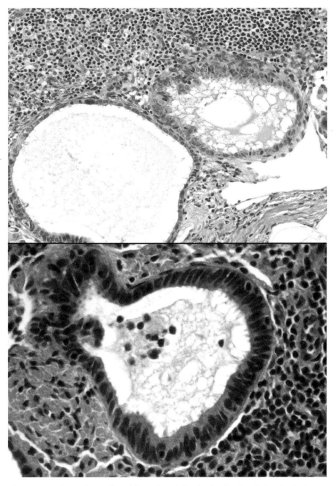

Fig. 14.33. Lymph node with endosalpingiosis. Endosalpingiosis is recognized by simple gland architecture, absence of cytologic atypia, infrequent mitotic figures, and (3) ciliated cells.

neoplasia is also not indicated, since margin status does not appear to be predictive of risk for recurrence.

Current indications for FS on vulvar lesions include: (a) margin status for local excision of basal cell carcinoma or squamous cell carcinoma, particularly if the lesion extends close to midline structures such as urethra, anal mucosa or vagina; and (b) margin status of excisions of mesenchymal neoplasms when the neoplasm is close to bone or a vital structure.

The extent of surgery for vulvar squamous cell carcinoma is determined by the following factors: (a) size and location of the neoplasm; (b) depth of invasion; and to a lesser extent, (c) pattern of invasion; (d) lymphovascular space invasion; (e) clinical status of the groin nodes; (f) condition of the vulvar skin away from the carcinoma; (g) the presence of dysplasia elsewhere on the vulva; and (h) the presence of comorbidities. For clinical stage 1 carcinomas >1 mm in thickness, a margin of at least 2 cm is desirable.

Wide local excision is considered to be adequate surgical treatment for microinvasive squamous cell carcinoma,* provided that the surrounding skin is normal. If the surrounding skin is dysplastic, the microinvasive carcinoma is excised and the associated dysplastic skin is either treated by laser vaporization or wider excision with evaluation of margins. Malignant neoplasms that cross the midline obviously require radical surgery.

When margins are evaluated on excision specimens, sections should be taken perpendicular to the margin, so as to evaluate the distance of neoplasm from the margin.

VAGINA

There are limited indications for evaluation of vaginal lesions. Biopsies may be submitted for evaluation of margins during surgical procedures for primary cervical or vulvar squamous cell carcinoma. On occasion, an incisional biopsy is submitted to determine specimen adequacy for diagnosis, either for a suspected primary vaginal malignancy (e.g., embryonal rhabdomyosarcoma

---

* Vulvar squamous carcinomas measuring up to 2.0 cm in diameter with 1 mm or less stromal invasion (measured from the epithelial-stromal junction of the closest adjacent dermal papilla to the deepest point of invasion) and no evidence of lymphovascular space invasion are labeled microinvasive vulvar carcinoma at Stanford University Hospital and Clinics; these neoplasms are associated with a very low incidence (≤1%) of nodal metastases.

or yolk sac tumor in the pediatric patient), or suspected metastatic or recurrent cervical, endometrial or ovarian malignancies involving the vagina. In these situations, the purpose of the test is to ensure that sufficient diagnostic tissue is present for routine and ancillary tests. Whenever possible, tissue should be procured for cytogenetic studies in the pediatric-malignancies.

PERITONEUM

Indications for intraoperative diagnosis

The indications for IOD are to:

1. Establish the diagnosis of suspected metastatic ovarian/fallopian tube carcinoma.
2. Exclude metastasis from a non-gynecological primary tumor.
3. Exclude metastasis from another gynecological site, such as uterine corpus or cervix.
4. Establish the diagnosis of a primary peritoneal process.
5. Establish a diagnosis when the intraoperative findings are inconclusive and/or unexpected.

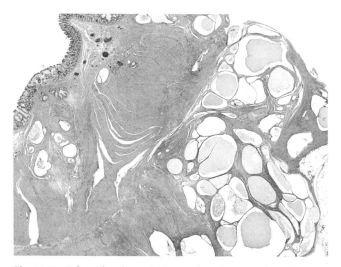

Fig. 14.34. Polypoid endometriosis may form large, cystic and polypoid masses in the bowel wall. The glands have bland cytologic features, are surrounded by endometrial-type stroma, and they are uniformly distributed within the mass. In the presence of glandular atypia or stromal predominance, the possibility of carcinoma, adenosarcoma, or stromal sarcoma should be considered. If there is doubt about the diagnosis, the surgeon should remove all grossly visible mass lesions and the diagnosis should be deferred to permanent sections to avoid an unwarranted staging procedure.

Table 14.12. Peritoneal findings that mimic Mullerian malignancy

Non-neoplastic process	Process most commonly mimicked	Diagnostic clue(s)
Endometriosis	Metastatic adenocarcinoma	Periglandular endometrial stroma. Endometriosis elsewhere. May have grey-white plaques, adhesions or polypoid masses simulating a malignant neoplasm. Pseudoxanthomatous endometriosis may have zones of central necrosis surrounded by histiocytes. Hyperplastic, metaplastic or atrophic changes may be present.
Endosalpingiosis	Metastatic adenocarcinoma Serous borderline tumor	Ciliated cells, "peg" cells and secretory type cells. Psammoma bodies.
Endocervicosis	Metastatic adenocarcinoma	Located in posterior uterine serosa and cul-de-sac peritoneum. Bland epithelium.
Mesonephric remnants	Metastatic adenocarcinoma	Vicinity of fallopian tube. Cuff of smooth muscle. Bland epithelium.
Decidual reaction	Metastatic squamous carcinoma.	Typically a microscopic finding, visible grey-white masses, plaques or polyps over the peritoneal surfaces may be present, simulating carcinoma. Associated with pregnancy, persistent corpus luteum or exogenous progestin.
Histiocytic and foreign body reactions, – e.g., keratin granulomas	Undifferentiated carcinoma Metastatic carcinoma (if mitotically active)	Keratinous material in association with ruptured mature cystic teratoma or endometrial proliferations with prominent squamous metaplasia. Reaction to endometriosis.
Mesothelial hyperplasia	Metastatic adenocarcinoma Serous borderline tumor	Predominantly uniform cuboidal cells, superficial, non-invasive peritoneal involvement, psammoma bodies may be present.
Well-differentiated papillary mesothelioma	Metastatic adenocarcinoma Serous borderline tumor Serous carcinoma	Uniform cuboidal cells, non-hierarchical branching papillae, psammoma bodies may be present.
Gliomatosis	Disseminated carcinoma Metastatic immature teratoma	Associated ovarian teratoma – often with immature elements. However, when the peritoneal implants are mature, this does not adversely affect prognosis.
Melanosis	Melanoma	Associated mature cystic teratoma. No cytologic atypia.
Splenosis	Lymphoma or leukemia, esp. if associated with extramedullary hematopoiesis	History of prior trauma.
Squamous metaplasia	Large cell non-keratinizing carcinoma	Typically focal, incidental finding. Minimal or no cytologic atypia.
Disseminated peritoneal leiomyomatosis	Carcinomatosis Metastatic leiomyosarcoma	Circumscribed, small nodules distributed over surface of peritoneum. Bland smooth muscle – may have foci of endometriosis, decidual change.

General pathologic issues

- Endometriosis sometimes has an unusual presentation, forming one or more polypoid, mass-forming lesions involving the peritoneum, bladder serosa, bowel wall as well as ovary (Fig. 14.34). There are two possible challenges with these lesions: First, foci of atypia may be present and these are at risk of being misinterpreted as carcinoma, leading to an unwarranted staging procedure. Second, mullerian malignancies arise from these endometriotic lesions and may be missed with limited sampling (Table 14.12);

careful gross examination will help to sample the correct area.

- On occasion, smooth muscle neoplasms present as adnexal, retroperitoneal, or intraperitoneal masses. When encountered in extrauterine sites, the differential diagnosis includes the extrauterine component of intravenous leiomyomatosis, lymphangioleiomyomatosis, and a primary pelvic or retroperitoneal smooth muscle neoplasm (Table 14.13). Retroperitoneal smooth muscle neoplasms require special attention because the histological criteria of malignancy are

Table 14.13. Differential diagnosis of smooth muscle proliferations in the female genital tract

	DPL	BML	IVL	LAM	LMS
Age (years)	Reproductive (mean, 31)	Late reproductive (mean, 45)	Peri-menopausal (mean, 47)	Reproductive (mean, 35)	Peri-menopausal (mean, 50)
Clinical features	Pregnancy, steroid hormone exposure	Prior benign uterine smooth muscle tumor	Uterine leiomyoma with intravascular protrusion	Tuberous sclerosis complex may be present	Uterine or retroperitoneal leiomyosarcoma
Site	Throughout abdomen, subperitoneum	Uterus, lung, lymph nodes, abdomen	Uterus, pelvic veins, inferior vena cava, right heart	Lymphatic channels, lung, lymph nodes of mediastinum, pelvis, retroperitoneum	Pelvis or retroperitoneum
Size	Usually <2 cm, but larger tumors have been reported	Variable, but often >2 cm	Worm-like venous intrusions vary, but may be quite large	Usually <2 cm, but larger lesions have been reported	May be large
Behavior	Usually regress	Recurrence and metastases with prolonged course	Intravenous extension	Slowly progressive pulmonary dysfunction	Recurrences & metastases common with rapid course
Mitotic index	Low	Low	Low	Low	May be high (<10/10 hpf)
Cellular atypia	Absent	Absent or minimal	Absent – similar to smooth muscle tumors of uterus	Spindle and epithelioid (clear) cells	Usually severe
Necrosis	Absent	Absent	Absent	Absent	Present

DPL, disseminated peritoneal leiomyomatosis; BML, benign metastasizing leiomyoma; IVL, intravenous leiomyomatosis; LAM, lymphangioleiomyomatosis; LMS, leiomyosarcoma.

different, as even bland neoplasms may behave aggressively. It is our practice to defer the diagnosis in these cases and ensure that the surgeon clearly determines the anatomic origin of the neoplasm.

- Disseminated peritoneal leiomyomatosis, leiomyosarcoma, and benign metastasizing leiomyoma should be distinguished because of differences in management.

  Metastatic leiomyosarcoma is characterized by large, fleshy necrotic tumor masses with significant cytologic atypia and mitotic activity (Fig. 14.35) and is treated by surgical debulking.

  Disseminated peritoneal leiomyomatosis is usually not treated by debulking because these lesions often regress without treatment. However, the surgeon should be encouraged to remove all nodules larger than 2 cm to exclude metastatic leiomyosarcoma (Table 14.13).

  Benign metastazing leiomyoma is treated by debulking because these lesions do not regress.

- Some peritoneal lesions, while associated with tumor elsewhere in the gynecological tract, do not have

any impact on the overall prognosis of the primary tumor. For example, the presence of multiple nodules of mature glial tissue (gliomatosis peritonei) is not associated with any adverse outcome beyond that of the primary ovarian teratoma (Fig. 14.36). Similarly, the presence of keratin granulomas secondary to retrograde extrusion of keratin from an endometrial carcinoma with prominent squamous differentiation does not upstage the patient in absence of malignant cells (Fig. 14.37). However, all such nodules should be carefully examined on permanent sections to exclude a more ominous finding.

- Primary peritoneal mesothelioma is uncommon, but should be considered whenever a papillary tumor predominantly involves the surfaces of the peritoneum and ovaries. Well-differentiated papillary mesotheliomas are composed of papillary structures that are generally less complex than serous tumors (Fig. 14.38), and the neoplasm is composed of a uniform, non-stratified population of cuboidal cells. As with serous tumors, psammoma bodies may be present.

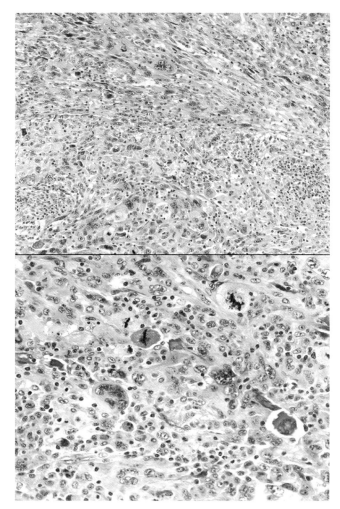

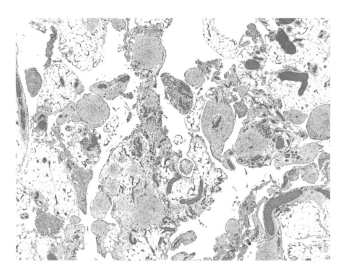

Fig. 14.35. Typical uterine leiomyosarcoma with marked cellularity, severe cytological atypia, and numerous mitotic figures. Tumor cell necrosis is also often present.

Fig. 14.36. Gliomatosis peritonei consists of multiple nodules of mature glial tissue involving the peritoneum. This lesion is found in association with mature and immature teratomas, and may be mistaken by the surgeon for peritoneal carcinomatosis; It does not adversely affect prognosis even when associated with grade 2 ovarian immature teratomas.

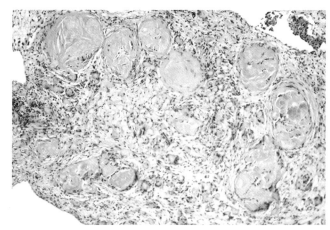

Fig. 14.37. Keratin granuloma of the peritoneum are secondary to extruded keratin from uterine endometrial carcinoma. This finding does not upstage the tumor if neoplastic epithelial cells are absent.

(a)

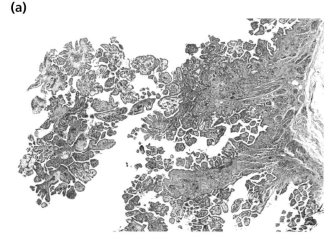

(b)

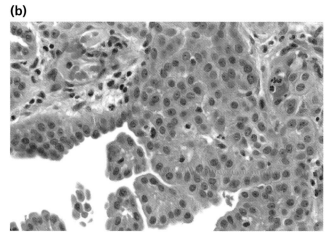

Fig. 14.38. Well-differentiated mesothelioma. (a) The papillary architecture and psammoma bodies mimic mullerian serous differentiation. (b) The neoplastic cells are uniform, cuboidal in shape, and non-stratified.

REFERENCES

1. Armstrong DK, Bundy B, Wenzel L, *et al.* Intraperitoneal cisplatin and paclitaxel in ovarian cancer. *N Engl J Med* 2006; **354**: 34–43.

2. Brun JL, Cortez A, Rouzier R, *et al.* Factors influencing the use and accuracy of frozen section diagnosis of epithelial ovarian tumors. *Am J Obstet Gynecol* 2008; **199**: 244 e241–247.

3. Ilvan S, Ramazanoglu R, Ulker Akyildiz E, Calay Z, Bese T, Oruc N. The accuracy of frozen section (intraoperative consultation) in the diagnosis of ovarian masses. *Gynecol Oncol* 2005; **97**: 395–399.

4. Stewart CJ, Brennan BA, Hammond IG, Leung YC, McCartney AJ, Ruba S. Intraoperative assessment of clear cell carcinoma of the ovary. *Int J Gynecol Pathol* 2008; **27**: 475–482.

5. Longacre TA, Teng NN, Hendrickson MR. The female genital tract. *Pathology (Phila)* 1996; **3**: 427–492.

6. Patel K, Schreiber Z, Kane PB, *et al.* Intraoperative frozen section fixation with formalin improves diagnostic accuracy of tumors with clear cells, papillary architecture, or micropapillary type of invasion. *Mod Pathol* 2008; **21**: 368A.

7. Sangoi AR, Soslow RA, Teng NN, Longacre TA. Ovarian clear cell carcinoma with papillary features: a potential mimic of serous tumor of low malignant potential. *Am J Surg Pathol* 2008; **32**: 269–274.

8. Tornos C, Silva EG, Ordonez NG, Gershenson DM, Young RH, Scully RE. Endometrioid carcinoma of the ovary with a prominent spindle-cell component, a source of diagnostic confusion. A report of 14 cases. *Am J Surg Pathol* 1995; **19**: 1343–1353.

9. Kiyokawa T, Young RH, Scully RE. Krukenberg tumors of the ovary: a clinicopathologic analysis of 120 cases with emphasis on their variable pathologic manifestations. *Am J Surg Pathol* 2006; **30**: 277–299.

10. McKenney JK, Soslow RA, Longacre TA. Ovarian mature teratomas with mucinous epithelial neoplasms: morphologic heterogeneity and association with pseudomyxoma peritonei. *Am J Surg Pathol* 2008; **32**: 645–655.

11. Vang R, Gown AM, Zhao C, Barry TS, Isacson C, Richardson MS, Ronnett BM. Ovarian mucinous tumors associated with mature cystic teratomas: morphologic and immunohistochemical analysis identifies a subset of potential teratomatous origin that shares features of lower gastrointestinal tract mucinous tumors more commonly encountered as secondary tumors in the ovary. *Am J Surg Pathol* 2007; **31**: 854–869.

12. Yemelyanova AV, Vang R, Judson K, Wu LS, Ronnett BM. Distinction of primary and metastatic mucinous tumors involving the ovary: analysis of size and laterality data by primary site with reevaluation of an algorithm for tumor classification. *Am J Surg Pathol* 2008; **32**: 128–138.

13. Young RH, Scully RE. Metastatic tumors in the ovary: a problem-oriented approach and review of the recent literature. *Semin Diagn Pathol* 1991; **8**: 250–276.

14. Longacre TA, Hendrickson MR. Diffusely infiltrative endometrial adenocarcinoma: an adenoma malignum pattern of myoinvasion. *Am J Surg Pathol* 1999; **23**: 69–78.

15. Al-Ramahi M, Nimri C, Bata M, Saleh S. The value of frozen section Pipelle endometrial biopsy as an outpatient procedure in the diagnosis of ectopic pregnancy. *J Obstet Gynaecol* 2006; **26**: 63–65.

16. Heller DS, Hessami S, Cracchiolo B, Skurnick JH. Reliability of frozen section of uterine curettings in evaluation of possible ectopic pregnancy. *J Am Assoc Gynecol Laparosc* 2000; **7**: 519–522.

17. Einstein MH, Park KJ, Sonoda Y, *et al.* Radical vaginal versus abdominal trachelectomy for stage IB1 cervical cancer: a comparison of surgical and pathologic outcomes. *Gynecol Oncol* 2009; **112**: 73–77.

18. Ismiil N, Ghorab Z, Covens A, *et al.* Intraoperative margin assessment of the radical trachelectomy specimen. *Gynecol Oncol* 2009; **113**: 42–46.

19. Olawaiye A, Del Carmen M, Tambouret R, Goodman A, Fuller A, Duska LR. Abdominal radical trachelectomy: success and pitfalls in a general gynecologic oncology practice. *Gynecol Oncol* 2009; **112**: 506–510.

20. Rob L, Charvat M, Robova H, *et al.* Less radical fertility-sparing surgery than radical trachelectomy in early cervical cancer. *Int J Gynecol Cancer* 2007; **17**: 304–310.

21. Hendrickson MR, Longacre TA. Problems in uterine corpus pathology: In *Gynecologic Cancer: Controversies in Management*, Gershenson DM, Gore M, McGuire WP, Thomas G, and Quinn MA, eds. Elsevier, Philadelphia, PA, 2004.

22. Longacre TA, Atkins KA, Kempson RL, Hendrickson MR. The uterine corpus. Evaluation of endometrial and myometrial specimens. In *Sternberg's Diagnostic Surgical Pathology*, Mills SE, ed, 5th edn, New York, NY: Lippincott Williams and Wilkins, 2009.

15 URINARY TRACT AND MALE GENITAL SYSTEM

Steven S. Shen, Luan D. Truong, Seth P. Lerner, and Jae Y. Ro

URINARY BLADDER, URETER, AND URETHRA

Introduction

Urothelial carcinoma (transitional cell carcinoma) constitutes >90% of bladder carcinomas in the United States. Squamous cell carcinoma, adenocarcinoma, and neuroendocrine carcinomas are much less common but similar principles of management apply to these neoplasms. The diagnosis of bladder carcinoma is usually suspected when patients have hematuria, sometimes combined with other urinary symptoms such as dysuria and urgency, but the diagnosis is only made after cystoscopic examination and transurethral resection (TUR) of the lesion. Almost all neoplastic lesions of the bladder are resected or biopsied before intravesical therapy or definitive surgery, but intraoperative diagnosis (IOD) remains important in selected situations.[1-3] The issues in IOD are mirrored by changes in the management of urinary tract neoplasia, but there are also differences in practice between institutions and between urologists.

Information needed before and during intraoperative consultation

The pathologist should be familiar with the clinical history, the imaging findings when necessary, the prior biopsy findings, history of prior treatment, and the surgeon's operative plan. The following examples will illustrate the value of clinicopathologic correlation.

- Familiarity with the clinical aspects of the case and prior biopsy findings may help to anticipate the chances of finding invasive carcinoma or carcinoma in-situ (CIS) at the surgical margins, e.g., imaging data may suggest a neoplasm in one of the ureters, or there may be extensive biopsy-proven CIS.

- Familiarity with the prior transurethral resection (TUR) findings may help to interpret unusual findings in a biopsy of an extravesical nodule; for example, a spindle cell lesion will not be dismissed as reactive fibroblastic tissue if the patient is known to have a sarcomatoid urothelial carcinoma.

- It is important to know the surgeon's operative plan especially if the frozen section (FS) diagnosis has high stakes, e.g., if a nodal or visceral metastasis will cause the surgeon to abandon radical cystectomy.

Indications for intraoperative diagnosis

1. Evaluation of surgical margins including ureteral, urethral, and soft tissue margins during radical cystectomy.
2. Evaluation of surgical margins in partial cystectomy specimens.
3. Occasionally, to make an initial diagnosis on a transurethral biopsy or resection of a bladder lesion.
4. Evaluation of incidentally found extravesical nodules during cystectomy.
5. Evaluation of pelvic lymph nodes for metastatic carcinoma.

Specific clinico-pathologic issues

Evaluation of the surgical margins during radical cystectomy or cystoprostatectomy
Clinical issues

Cystectomy, combined with pelvic lymph node dissection, is the standard treatment for muscle invasive bladder

Intraoperative Consultation in Surgical Pathology, ed. Mahendra Ranchod. Published by Cambridge University Press.
© Cambridge University Press 2010.

carcinoma, high grade non-muscle invasive urothelial carcinomas that are resistant to conventional intravesical therapy, tumors with adverse prognostic features such as extensive lymphovascular invasion, and aggressive histologic variants of urothelial carcinoma such as micropapillary urothelial carcinoma. Intraoperative evaluation of ureteral, urethral, and perivesical soft tissue margins during radical cystectomy or cystoprostatectomy are important because negative margins decrease the risk of tumor recurrence and may influence decision-making regarding choice of urinary diversion.[4–6] The incidence of high-grade dysplasia/ carcinoma in situ of the ureteral margins ranges from 4.8% to 9%,[5–7] whereas the apical urethral margin is rarely positive.[8] As a result, the distal ureteral margins are routinely submitted for FS, and the urethral margin much less frequently. However, a FS diagnosis of the urethral margin may be requested if biopsies of the prostatic urethra were not performed prior to cystectomy. If there are changes of concern in the perivesical soft tissue, a biopsy will be submitted for FS evaluation as this may influence whether cystectomy is undertaken.

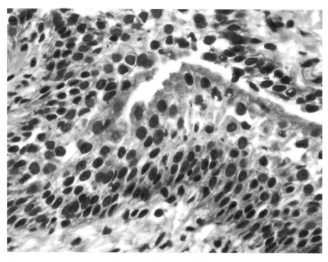

Fig. 15.1. Reactive atypia of urothelium. This frozen section was prepared from the proximal ureteral margin in a patient undergoing radical cystectomy. There is preservation of cellular polarity and surface umbrella cells; the cells have slightly enlarged nuclei, open chromatin, and small nucleoli.

Pathologic issues
Evaluation of the ureteral margin

When a short segment (<0.5 cm) of ureter is submitted, the entire specimen should be embedded for FS evaluation, taking care to embed the tissue on end. For longer segments of ureter, the true margin is usually designated by the surgeon with a suture or with ink, and this end should be amputated from the specimen and embedded for FS.

The changes at the surgical margin should be reported as (a) non-dysplastic (normal or reactive), (b) atypia not further classified, and (c) high grade dysplasia/carcinoma in situ or invasive carcinoma. Reactive atypia is relatively common in patients with bladder cancer and is often associated with inflammation, edema or fibrosis of the lamina propria (Fig. 15.1). The diagnosis of low grade dysplasia should be avoided because of poor reproducibility and the uncertainty about how this lesion should be treated. The diagnosis of high grade dysplasia/CIS is based on both architectural and cytologic features (Fig. 15.2), but full thickness atypia is not required to make the diagnosis; partial involvement or pagetoid spread is sufficient for the diagnosis of CIS (Fig. 15.3). Dilatation of the ureter, vascular proliferation and chronic inflammation of the subepithelial connective tissue are often present, accompanied by complete or partial sloughing of neoplastic urothelial cells (Fig. 15.4); when this is encountered, deeper levels should be prepared as these

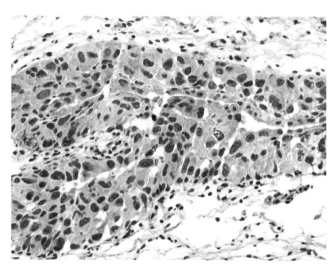

Fig. 15.2. Frozen section showing urothelial carcinoma in-situ in a ureteral margin. The urothelium shows disordered cellular polarity, nuclear pleomorphism, hyperchromasia and mitoses. Nuclear enlargement is best appreciated by comparing the atypical cells with residual normal basal urothelial cells.

may show diagnostic changes. The differential diagnosis for high grade dysplasia/CIS includes reactive atypia and atypia induced by prior chemotherapy.

Evaluation of the urethral margin

Because of retraction of the urethral mucosa, multiple levels may be necessary to identify the mucosa. Pagetoid spread with a few high grade malignant cells is sufficient for the diagnosis of urothelial carcinoma in-situ (Fig. 15.5). The urethral mucosa is often denuded because

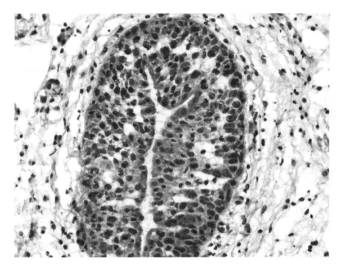

Fig. 15.3. Carcinoma in situ of the ureter with partial involvement of the urothelium. Some of the cells show enlarged, irregular nuclei, increased N/C ratio, hyperchromasia, apoptosis and mitoses. The umbrella cell layer is still maintained.

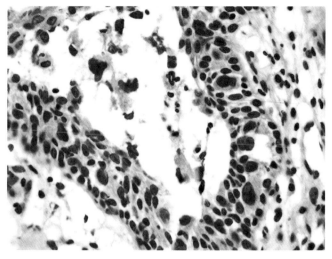

Fig. 15.5. Urethra with pagetoid spread of urothelial carcinoma in situ. Single large atypical cells are scattered between normal urothelial cells.

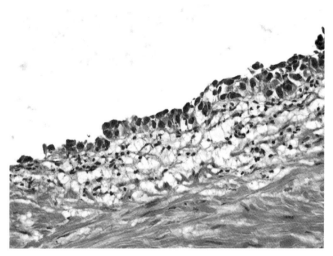

Fig. 15.4. Clinging urothelial carcinoma in situ at the surgical margin of the ureter. The urothelium is largely denuded but the residual cells have enlarged, hyperchromatic nuclei.

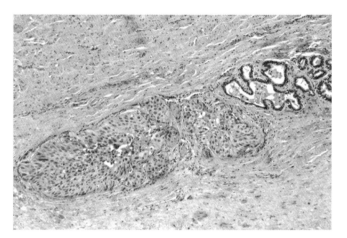

Fig. 15.6. Peri-urethral gland with focal involvement by urothelial dysplasia in a radical cystectomy specimen removed for invasive urothelial carcinoma. Most of the surface urethral epithelium was denuded but the peri-urethral glands were preserved and showed dysplasia.

of intravesical therapy or intubation, so special attention should be paid to the periurethral glands or ducts as these may harbor diagnostic changes (Fig. 15.6).

Perivesical soft tissue margins

A biopsy of perivesical fat may be submitted for FS evaluation to determine if there is invasion of the extravesical soft tissue. Fat necrosis and associated fibrosis is not uncommonly seen in the perivesical soft tissue and is usually not difficult to distinguish from carcinoma. Reactive endothelial cells can sometimes be problematic, especially when they are altered by cautery (Fig. 15.7)

Evaluation of the surgical margins during partial cystectomy
Clinical issues

Partial cystectomy is reserved for localized malignancies, including localized urothelial carcinoma, carcinoma arising in a bladder diverticulum and urachal adenocarcinoma.[9]

Pathologic issues

The diagnosis would have been established on prior biopsy, so the purpose of IOD is to evaluate the surgical margins. This is one situation where it is helpful to examine the specimen with the surgeon, both for orientation and to ascertain which margins are of concern to the surgeon.

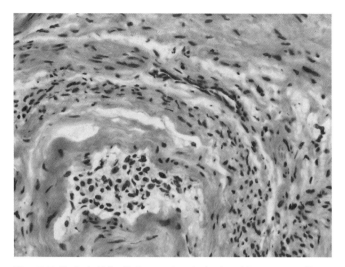

Fig. 15.7. Endothelial cells in a peri-vesical vein with cautery artifact simulating urothelial carcinoma.

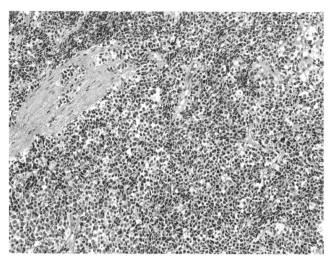

Fig. 15.8. High-grade endocrine cell carcinoma of the bladder. This neoplasm had an unusual cystoscopic appearance, prompting the urologist to submit a biopsy for FS. A diagnosis of high grade urothelial carcinoma was made on FS; although this diagnosis was incorrect, the error was of no consequence for immediate intraoperative management. This image is from the subsequent transurethral resection which showed invasion of the muscularis propria.

The margins should be inked with different colors, and whether they are evaluated with sections taken parallel or perpendicular to the margins will depend on the gross findings. If a visible lesion is present within 5 mm of the margin, we recommend taking multiple serial sections perpendicular to that margin; on the other hand, if the grossly visible carcinoma is >5 mm from the margin, sections may be taken parallel to that margin (en face). Before taking sections parallel to the margin, the tissue layers should be lined up so that all layers are represented in the FS block.

It is much easier to interpret the FS findings when the pathologist is familiar with the histologic characteristics of the malignancy. For example, mucin pools at the surgical margin in a patient with mucinous carcinoma would be interpreted as carcinoma even if epithelial cells are absent, and a spindle cell process would be viewed with suspicion in a patient who has a biopsy diagnosis of spindle cell carcinoma.

Serosal nodules of the bladder and extravesical lesions
Clinical issues
During radical cystectomy, the surgeon may encounter nodules, areas of thickening, or areas of discoloration on the peritoneal surface of the bladder or in the perivesical fat, usually prompting a request for FS diagnosis. The diagnosis may not alter the surgical procedure if it is in close proximity to the bladder, but extensive extravesical spread of invasive carcinoma may cause the surgeon to abandon radical cystectomy.

Pathologic issues
The most commonly encountered lesions include mesothelial hyperplasia, fibrous nodules, chronic inflammation, calcification, endometriosis, endocervicosis, endosalpingiosis, and rarely metastatic carcinoma of non-vesical origin.

Initial diagnosis of bladder lesions
Clinical issues
Rarely, FS diagnosis will be requested on a bladder lesion that has an unusual appearance on cystoscopic examination, or when attempts at prior biopsy have been unsuccessful. The surgeon's goal is to confirm that the specimen contains diagnostic tissue, and when appropriate, to ensure that muscularis propria is present in the specimen for purposes of staging.

Pathologic issues
If the first specimen is a small biopsy, the entire specimen should be embedded for FS; if the specimen is a TUR specimen and contains multiple pieces of tissue, the firmer areas should be selected as they are more likely to contain muscularis propria. A specific diagnosis should be made when possible, but a "good enough" diagnosis such as "high grade carcinoma with invasion of muscularis" is sufficient for immediate management (Fig. 15.8). Under no circumstances should definitive radical surgery be performed on the basis of a FS diagnosis;

malignant neoplasms such as lymphoma and metastasis, neoplasms that do not warrant radical surgery, should be excluded, and this is best done on permanent sections with ancillary tests.

Evaluation of the pelvic lymph nodes during cystectomy

Clinical issues

Pelvic lymph node dissection is performed routinely during radical cystectomy because removal of these nodes provides prognostic information and also appears to offer therapeutic benefits. Furthermore, there are data to suggest that patients who have an extended lymphadenectomy have a better outcome than patients who have a more limited lymph node dissection. Some urologists will there-fore, perform an extended pelvic lymph node dissection routinely and submit the specimens in formalin for evalu-ation on permanent sections, whereas other urologists will perform a limited dissection, request intraoperative evalu-ation of the specimen, and extend the node dissection if the lymph nodes contain metastases.

Pathologic issues

The pathologist should know what is at stake when asked to examine pelvic lymph nodes in a patient with bladder carcin-oma. If the extent of lymph node dissection will be influenced by IOD, then every effort should be made to determine if there are nodal metastases. If one or more of the lymph nodes are grossly abnormal, a cytoscrape preparation should be made, and this is all that is necessary if the node shows metastatic carcinoma. If, however, the cytologic preparations are negative, the lymph nodes should be embedded in their entirety for FS evaluation, and multiple levels should be prepared in an attempt to identify metastases. Metastatic urothelial carcinoma is usually easy to identify on cytologic preparations or FS, but the changes may be more difficult to interpret in patients who have received neoadjuvant therapy, and when the neoplastic cells are scanty (Fig. 15.9).

KIDNEY

General clinical issues

The diagnosis of a space-occupying lesion in the kidney is usually indirect, based on clinical and imaging data. The majority of solitary solid lesions of the kidney in adults are renal cell carcinomas (RCCs), and the diagnosis can

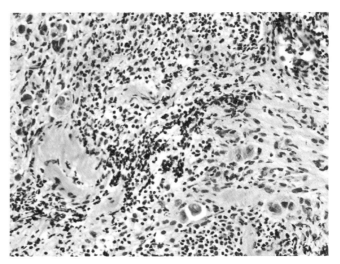

Fig. 15.9. Lymph node with metastatic high grade urothelial carcinoma. The carcinoma was present mainly as single cells, and can be overlooked, especially in a poorly prepared FS.

usually be made with confidence based on clinical and imaging characteristics.[10] The vast majority of cystic lesions are benign, although secondary changes such as hemorrhage, fibrosis or calcifications may make it difficult to distinguish a benign cyst with secondary changes from an extensively cystic renal cell carcinoma. Most urothelial carcinomas of the kidney are recognized pre-operatively, but infrequently, a high-grade urothelial carcinoma may form a large mass, mimicking RCC. Similarly, clinical and imaging data provide important clues to the diagnosis of less common lesions such as angiomyolipoma and xanthogranulomatous pyelo-nephritis. In most instances therefore, a urologist will plan definitive treatment of a renal mass without a pre-operative biopsy because the clinical and imaging information provide a near-specific diagnosis, and the mass has to be removed because of the high risk of malignancy; furthermore, when the diagnosis is unclear, fine needle aspiration and needle core biopsy are usually not performed because they may not provide a definitive diagnosis. In most situations there-fore, the pathologic diagnosis is made after the definitive surgical procedure has been performed. However, there are situations when the pathologist's help is needed to decide on the correct surgical procedure.

Indications for intraoperative diagnosis

The most common indications for IOD are as follows.

1. To evaluate an incisional biopsy of a renal mass when the FS diagnosis may influence whether the surgeon

performs a radical nephrectomy or a partial nephrectomy.

2. To evaluate the margins on a partial nephrectomy specimen.

3. To distinguish between RCC and urothelial carcinoma when this distinction cannot be made pre-operatively.

4. To evaluate an excisional biopsy on a patient who has multiple renal masses, unilateral or bilateral, because the FS diagnosis may influence immediate surgical management.

5. To offer a preliminary diagnosis on a radical nephrectomy specimen, either to satisfy the surgeon's curiosity or to appease the patient or patient's family.

Specific clinico-pathologic issues

Evaluation of radical nephrectomy specimens
Clinical issues

Most RCCs are treated by radical nephrectomy. Large neoplasms are sometimes pre-treated with renal artery embolization in an attempt to reduce the vascularity of the tumor and to reduce blood loss during surgery, a procedure that usually results in extensive infarct type necrosis of the neoplasm. In patients for whom radical nephrectomy carries high risks, the carcinoma can be successfully ablated by cryosurgery or radiofrequency treatment, delivered either by the laparoscopic or percutaneous route. A needle core biopsy of the mass is usually performed prior to

ablation to document the nature of the neoplasm, but there is no reason for IOD.

Oncocytomas behave in a benign fashion, and a minority are recognized pre-operatively by the characteristic central scar; unfortunately, a central scar is neither frequent nor specific. In contrast, the majority of angiomyolipomas are recognized pre-operatively because the fatty component can be recognized on CT scan.

Pathologic issues

Since radical nephrectomy is the definitive surgical treatment for RCC and its mimics, there are no immediate management issues at stake. If the surgeon requests an IOD, gross examination is all that is necessary. If the gross findings are equivocal (e.g., cystic RCC versus cystic mixed stromal and epithelial tumor versus complex benign cyst with secondary hemorrhage and fibrosis), it is best to defer the diagnosis to permanent sections instead of performing multiple FSs to make a diagnosis because it may be difficult to make these distinctions with limited sampling (Fig. 15.10). Similarly, oncocytomas are characterized by circumscription, a mahogany brown cut surface, absence of necrosis and sometimes a focal area of scarring (Fig. 15.11), but the diagnosis of oncocytoma should be provisional, with an understanding that the final diagnosis will be made on permanent sections.

There are two situations when FS on a radical nephrectomy can be justified. First, when the clinical and imaging

(a) 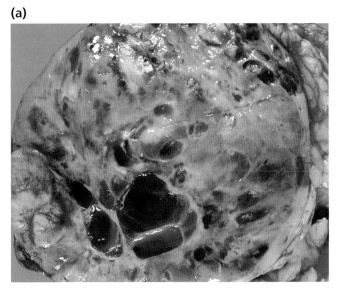 **(b)**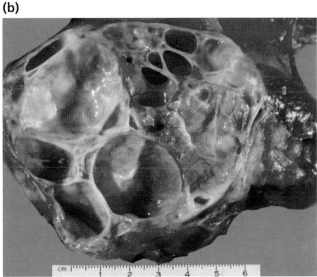

Fig. 15.10. (a) Cystic renal cell carcinoma. Renal cell carcinomas that undergo extensive cystic change may be difficult to distinguish from other cystic lesions of the kidney such as (b) the cystic mixed epithelial stromal tumor of the kidney.

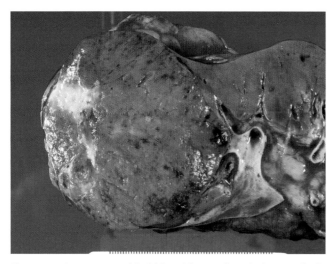

Fig. 15.11. Oncocytoma of the kidney. The neoplasm is circumscribed, has a characteristic brown cut surface, and shows a focal scar; the latter is a characteristic but infrequent finding.

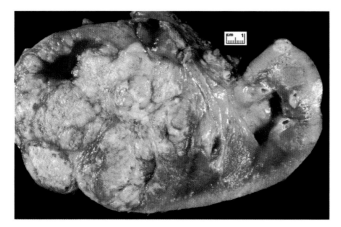

Fig. 15.12. High grade renal cell carcinoma with sarcomatoid change. Clinical and imaging studies could not confidently discriminate between high grade RCC and high grade urothelial carcinoma. The urologist requested a FS to distinguish between these two neoplasms. This distinction is relevant since the urologist will resect the entire ipsilateral ureter and a cuff of bladder tissue if a FS diagnosis of urothelial carcinoma is rendered. Sections from the periphery of the mass as well as the pelvis of the kidney are often helpful for identifying high grade urothelial carcinoma.

studies do not allow clear discrimination between RCC and urothelial carcinoma (Fig. 15.12); it is important to make this distinction because the surgeon will perform a nephroureterectomy if a diagnosis of urothelial carcinoma is rendered. Second, some surgeons will perform an extended lymph node dissection if the RCC is high grade or if there are other poor prognostic features – even though there is still uncertainty about the value of extended lymphadenectomy. If a FS is requested to grade the carcinoma, the surgeon should be informed that there is a risk of under-grading because of tumor heterogeneity.

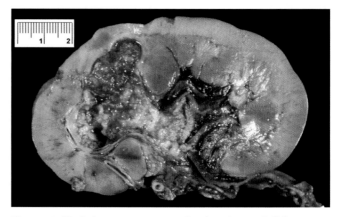

Fig. 15.13. Typical gross appearance of an invasive urothelial carcinoma involving the calyces and pelvis of the kidney. There is no reason for a FS diagnosis when the gross appearance is characteristic of urothelial carcinoma.

Evaluation of nephrectomy specimens with urothelial carcinoma
Clinical issues

The diagnosis of urothelial carcinoma of the kidney is made on the basis of clinical, imaging and sometimes cytologic data. When the diagnosis is conclusive, the surgeon will perform a nephroureterectomy, with complete removal of the ureter as well as a cuff of bladder, thus eliminating any potential foci of neoplasia on the ipsilateral side. There are situations when the diagnosis is not clear; for example, a urothelial carcinoma that involves the medulla of the kidney may be difficult to distinguish from variants of RCC that affect the medulla, such as collecting duct carcinoma. In this situation, the surgeon may choose to perform ureteropyeloscopy or proceed with a nephrectomy and have the pathologist examine the specimen intraoperatively to make this distinction, a distinction that is important because a diagnosis of urothelial carcinoma will lead to nephroureterectomy.

Pathologic issues

The nephroureterectomy specimen consists of kidney, perirenal adipose tissue, Gerota's fascia, the entire ureter, and a cuff of bladder wall. The kidney should be bivalved through the pyelocalyceal system with the help of a probe. If the gross features are characteristic of urothelial carcinoma, there is no reason to perform confirmatory FSs of the neoplasm (Fig. 15.13). If, on the other hand, the nature of the neoplasm is not clear on gross examination, sections should be taken from the periphery of the mass as well as calyceal tissue that shows mucosal abnormalities because the latter areas are the most likely to show recognizable urothelial carcinoma if the main mass is a poorly differentiated carcinoma.[11]

The ureter and bladder cuff of a nephroureterectomy specimen should also be examined, and if there is a lesion of concern at or close to the distal margin, the distal margin should be evaluated by FS.

Frozen section to evaluate a cystic renal mass
Clinical issues
Up to 15% of renal tumors are predominantly cystic. Cystic change is easily recognized on imaging and is graded using the Bosniak classification.[12,13] Treatment will vary, depending on the favored radiologic diagnosis, and when parenchymal sparing is important, the surgeon may request a FS diagnosis to guide the extent of resection.

Pathologic issues
The specimen submitted for FS is usually a wedge biopsy of the cyst wall. The entire specimen should be embedded for FS. The differential diagnosis includes a simple cyst with superimposed hemorrhage or infection, cystic nephroma, RCC with marked cystic change, and mixed stromal and epithelial tumor. The distinction between these entities may be difficult at the time of IOD and may have to be deferred to permanent sections.

Partial nephrectomy specimens
Clinical issues
Partial nephrectomy has become a more frequent procedure for treating renal mass lesions because of the increased detection of small, asymptomatic lesions during imaging for other reasons, as well as to preserve long-term renal function.[14] Patients who are candidates for this procedure include: (a) patients with a solitary kidney; (b) patients with bilateral renal carcinomas; (c) patients who have a genetic predisposition to multiple synchronous or metachronous tumors as in von Hippel–Lindau disease, tuberous sclerosis, hereditary papillary renal carcinoma syndrome and Birt–Hogg–Dube syndrome; and (d) patients with benign renal tumors such as angiomyolipoma, cystic nephroma and mixed epithelial and stromal tumor of the kidney that are amenable to partial nephrectomy. Two types of specimens are submitted for FS evaluation:

- An incisional biopsy of the lesion will be submitted for diagnosis if the decision about partial nephrectomy versus radical nephrectomy depends on the pathologic diagnosis (i.e., partial nephrectomy for a benign neoplasm, and radical nephrectomy for carcinoma). In this situation, the entire biopsy should be embedded for FS, and multiple levels should be prepared if the diagnosis is in doubt.

- A partial nephrectomy is considered the definitive treatment regardless of the diagnosis, and the specimen is submitted for evaluation of the surgical margins. A 1 cm margin of normal tissue is optimal for RCC but narrower margins do not appear to affect outcome – provided that the margins are clear of malignancy. Benign neoplasms can be excised with very narrow margins.

Pathologic issues
The surgical margin should be inked; sampling of the surgical margin will depend on the distance of the neoplasm from the margin, and the specimen should be sectioned perpendicular to the surgical margin to determine the relationship of the tumor to the margin (Fig. 15.14). When the tumor is >1 cm from the margin, a section should be taken parallel to the surgical margin from an area closest to the neoplasm. If the neoplasm is <1 cm from the margin, we recommend taking one or more sections perpendicular to the inked margin, recognizing that carcinomas may show microscopic extension beyond the grossly visible lesion; sections taken perpendicular to the margin will also allow the pathologist to measure and report the distance of the carcinoma from the margin.

The following pitfalls may be encountered when evaluating margins on a partial nephrectomy specimen:

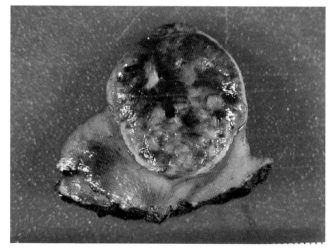

Fig. 15.14. Partial nephrectomy specimen containing a well circumscribed renal cell carcinoma, clear cell type. The carcinoma is well away from the inked surgical margin; at most, a section should be taken parallel to the surgical margin and submitted for FS.

(a)

(b)

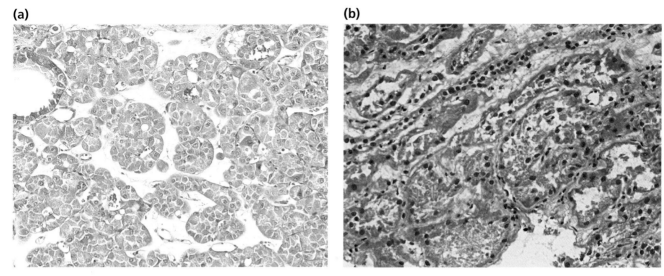

Fig. 15.15. (a) Oncocytoma of the kidney. Although tubules occur in oncocytomas, a nested pattern and edematous stroma should be sought as these features are characteristic of oncocytomas. (b) Frozen section of non-neoplastic proximal renal tubules adjacent to an oncocytoma. Cytologic features cannot be relied upon to make the distinction between oncocytoma and non-neoplastic proximal renal tubules. However, the parallel arrangement of tubular structures is a clue to non-neoplastic renal tubules; normal or hyalinized glomeruli between the tubules will clinch the diagnosis. In a partial nephrectomy specimen, the distinction of oncocytoma from non-neoplastic proximal renal tubules becomes an issue mainly when the pathologist examining the FS is unaware of the gross findings; since oncocytomas are well circumscribed, examination of the gross specimen will readily resolve any problems with interpretation of the FS.

- Normal proximal renal tubules are difficult to distinguish from the tubular growth pattern in oncocytoma (Fig. 15.15), a problem that is more likely to occur when the FS is examined by a pathologist who is unfamiliar with the gross aspects of the specimen. Since oncocytomas are well circumscribed, a correlation of the gross and microscopic findings should resolve this problem in most cases (Figs. 15.11 and 15.15).
- Compressed, atrophic renal tubules at the periphery of a RCC may be distorted and show reactive nuclear atypia, changes that may suggest the possibility of low grade RCC at the surgical margin; the presence of glomeruli provides evidence for the non-neoplastic nature of these changes.

PROSTATE

The widespread use of screening and early detection with serum prostatic specific antigen (PSA) has led to a marked increase in the diagnosis of carcinomas confined to the prostate gland. Organ-confined prostatic carcinoma is treated mainly by external radiation therapy, brachytherapy or radical prostatectomy, and the latter may be by conventional open surgery or by robotic-assisted laparoscopic surgery. The long-term outcome for these treatment modalities is comparable, and the choice of treatment is based on a variety of clinical and pathologic factors, as well as patient preference. Patients who are offered radical prostatectomy are carefully selected to minimize the chances of finding extra-prostatic disease, and most of these patients will have nerve-sparing surgery, either unilateral or bilateral, to minimize the chances of post-operative impotence.

When a radical prostatectomy is performed, the anatomical planes of dissection are predictable, and when these are altered, the surgeon will suspect extra-prostatic extension of carcinoma. The apical margin is the most challenging for the urologist for two reasons: (a) there is no clear tissue plane that defines the apex, and in fact, benign prostatic tissue is often admixed with skeletal muscle; and (b) the apical area is anatomically compact so good surgical technique is needed to remove all the prostatic tissue, yet preserve sphincteric function and continence.

Indications for intraoperative diagnosis

The two most common indications for FS are:

(i) evaluation of a surgical margin during radical prostatectomy.
(ii) evaluation of pelvic lymph nodes for metastatic carcinoma.

Evaluation of surgical margins in prostate carcinoma

Clinical issues

The goal of radical prostatectomy is to remove the entire prostate gland and remove the carcinoma with clear surgical margins. With the use of various nomograms, patients who undergo radical prostatectomy are expected to have organ-limited disease, without any extra-prostatic extension, and as a result, the majority of prostatectomies are performed without recourse to evaluating surgical margins. When performing the resection, the known extent and distribution of the carcinoma – based on the results of prior biopsies- will guide the surgeon's dissection of the apical area, and determine whether the nerves can be spared on one or both sides. If there is any doubt about these areas, biopsies will be performed during the resection for FS evaluation.

Pathologic issues

With the current approach to surgery, almost all specimens that are submitted for FS diagnosis consist of small biopsies; it is rare for the urologist to ask the pathologist to sample margins from the resected prostate gland. The three most common sites that are biopsied, and the reasons for these biopsies, are as follows:

- A biopsy is submitted from the apex to determine if there is carcinoma in the specimen. The entire specimen should be embedded for FS, recognizing that the specimen cannot be oriented, and that carcinoma anywhere in the specimen should be considered a positive margin. If carcinoma is present, the urologist will attempt to remove additional apical tissue. One of the pitfalls in diagnosis of biopsies from the apex is that benign prostatic glands are intimately associated with skeletal muscle fibers in this location, and the mere presence of glands "infiltrating" skeletal muscle should not be taken to mean carcinoma (Fig. 15.16).
- A biopsy is submitted from the bladder neck to make sure that this area is clear of carcinoma. The specimen is usually much larger than biopsies from other locations, often in excess of 1cm, and should be sectioned if necessary, and submitted in toto for FS. These biopsies are usually easy to interpret and consist of smooth muscle only or of smooth muscle and benign prostatic glands.
- When a nerve-sparing procedure is planned, the urologist may submit a biopsy from one of the lateral areas

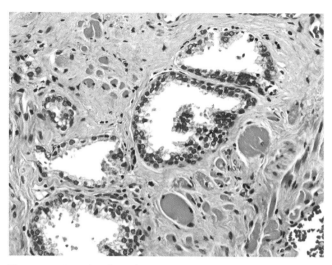

Fig. 15.16. A section from the apex of a radical prostatectomy specimen showing the intimate relationship of benign prostatic glands with skeletal muscle. The apex of normal prostate glands may show an admixture of glands with skeletal muscle; the FS diagnosis of carcinoma at the apical margin should be made with caution, and requires the presence of architectural and cytologic features of carcinoma.

of the prostate gland – in the area of the neurovascular bundle – to ascertain if carcinoma is present. The presence of carcinoma in the biopsy will result in abandonment of a nerve-sparing resection on that side. The biopsy is usually small and should be embedded in its entirety for FS. Multiple levels should be prepared routinely because cautery artifact may complicate interpretation. One pitfall is to mistakenly interpret clusters of ganglion cells and nerves as adenocarcinoma with perineural invasion, an error that may occur because ganglion cells and some prostatic adenocarcinomas have prominent nucleoli.

Evaluation of pelvic lymph nodes during radical prostatectomy

Clinical issues

Nodal metastases are a sign of disseminated carcinoma, and radical prostatectomy is not performed when there is obvious nodal disease. However, lymph node dissection helps with staging the carcinoma, and it is potentially therapeutic in patients who are found to have subclinical nodal disease. In recent years, there has been a significant decrease in the rate of nodal metastases because of stricter criteria in selecting patients for radical prostatectomy. A number of nomograms based on serum PSA, Gleason score and clinical tumor stage have been developed to predict the risk of lymph node metastasis;[15] patients at low risk for nodal metastases may not be subjected to node dissection, or if they have node dissection, the lymph nodes may not be submitted for intraoperative evaluation.[16] At some institutions, radical prostatectomy is offered to patients who are at higher risk for nodal metastasis (high PSA, Gleason score 7 or higher, or abnormal digital rectal examination); these patients will have node dissection, and the lymph nodes will very likely be submitted for FS evaluation because a diagnosis of nodal metastasis may cause the surgeon to abandon radical prostatectomy.[17]

Pathologic issues

The choice of FS versus gross examination of lymph nodes will depend on the surgeon's operative plan, an issue that is readily settled by discussion between the urologist and pathologist. The lymph nodes should be thoroughly examined if a diagnosis of metastatic carcinoma will cause the surgeon to abandon radical prostatectomy. In this situation, all the lymph nodes should be identified, and if they are enlarged, they should be serially sectioned at 3–4 mm intervals. All the lymph nodes should be submitted for FS evaluation; some pathologists also make cytologic preparations, either touch imprints or cytoscrape smears, before embedding the nodes for FS.

Metastatic carcinoma is usually easy to recognize on FS, but minute foci of carcinoma may be overlooked. False-positive diagnoses are rare, but an extensive infiltrate of foamy histiocytes, as in patients who have had a hip joint replacement, may be mistaken for metastatic foamy cell carcinoma (Fig. 15.17).[18]

TESTIS

More than 90% of testicular mass lesions are malignant germ cell tumors. When the tumor is limited to the testis, the diagnosis is made by physical examination, scrotal ultrasound, and serum markers such as lactate dehydrogenase (LDH), α-fetoprotein (AFP) and human chorionic gonadotropin (hCG). The diagnosis is less certain when the serum markers are negative (which occurs in 40% of patients), but if the physical examination and imaging findings are compelling, even these patients will undergo radical orchiectomy. In the majority of situations therefore, the definitive surgical procedure is performed without a pre-operative cytologic or tissue diagnosis; it is not appropriate to perform fine needle aspiration and needle core

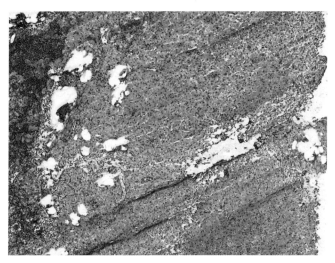

Fig. 15.17. Lymph node with sheets of histiocytes simulating metastatic high grade foamy cell carcinoma. The histiocytic infiltrate in this case was attributable to this patient's prior hip joint arthroplasty.

biopsies of the testis because of the risk of implanting malignant cells in the scrotum.

If there is a request for IOD, gross examination is all that is necessary, as there are no immediate management issues at stake (Fig. 15.18). There is no reason to perform a FS on the proximal margin of the spermatic cord because metastases to the cord are so rare in current day practice. There are three exceptions to one-step radical orchiectomy:

- Infrequently, when an adenomatoid tumor of the testis is suspected – small size, immediate subcapsular location, long history, slow growth and negative serum markers – the surgeon may externalize the testis as for a conventional radical orchiectomy, perform an incisional biopsy for FS interpretation, and limit the surgical procedure to complete but limited excision if the diagnosis of adenomatoid tumor (benign mesothelioma) is confirmed.

- Occasionally, the clinical and imaging features will suggest a neoplasm with a more benign natural history such as Leydig cell tumor, Sertoli cell tumor, epidermoid cyst or teratoma in a child. The urologist may attempt a partial orchiectomy, especially if the patient has a single testis. The partial orchiectomy specimen will be submitted for diagnosis and evaluation of the surgical margins.

- It is rare for urologists to consider partial orchiectomy in malignant germ cell tumors because of the lack of circumscription, potential multifocality, and frequent occurrence of intratubular germ cell tumor distant

(a) 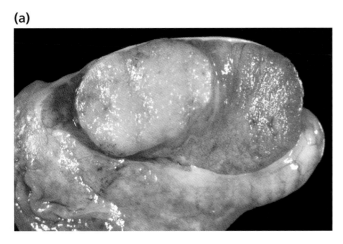 **(b)**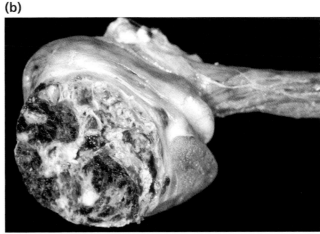

Fig. 15.18. (a) Radical orchiectomy specimen showing the characteristic gross appearance of a seminoma, with its solid tan cut surface. (b) In contrast, non-seminomatous malignant germ cell tumors tend to have a more heterogeneous appearance. Gross examination is sufficient to confirm the presence of a germ cell neoplasm in radical orchiectomy specimens; the definitive surgical procedure has been performed so there is no need to perform a FS.

from the main neoplasm. However, partial orchiectomy will be considered if the patient has a single testis, the lesion is small and the patient insists on preserving testicular tissue. The specimen will be submitted for IOD, with a request for diagnosis and evaluation of surgical margins.

Retroperitoneal lymph node dissection in patients with testicular neoplasms
Clinical issues
Retroperitoneal lymph node dissection for non-seminomatous testicular cancer may be performed for accurate staging and for therapeutic purposes in low volume disease, or for salvage after chemotherapy. In selected cases of metastatic seminoma, residual masses may be resected after radiation treatment. Because retroperitoneal nodal spread of germ cell tumors generally proceeds in an orderly anatomic fashion, FS may be requested to guide the extent of node dissection.

Pathologic issues
If multiple nodes are submitted, the largest or most abnormal lymph node should be submitted for FS evaluation. The type of germ cell should be reported if this is clear, but the type of neoplasm will not influence the extent of nodal dissection. In patients who have salvage surgery after chemotherapy, FS of the retroperitoneal mass may show only necrotic or fibrotic tissue, findings that should be

reported to the urologist with the caveat that foci of viable neoplasm may be found on permanent sections.

PENIS

Squamous cell carcinoma (SCC) is by far the most common malignancy of the penis. Partial or total penectomy is the usual treatment for invasive SCC of the penis, with the goal of adequate resection with a negative surgical margin. Tumor location, tumor size, tumor subtype, histologic grade and depth of invasion determine the extent of resection of the primary carcinoma as well as the need for nodal dissection. The histologic diagnosis of SCC is almost always made on a routinely processed incisional biopsy.[19,20] The most common indications for IOD are to:

(i) evaluate the surgical margins on partial or total penectomy specimen.
(ii) evaluate regional lymph nodes for metastatic SCC.

Evaluation of surgical margins in penectomy specimens
Clinical issues
Partial or total penectomy is the first line of treatment for invasive SCC of the penis. The goal is to achieve complete excision with adequate clear margins, usually defined as a margin of 1.5 to 2.5 cm of normal tissue. Most SCCs are located in the glans, prepuce, or coronal sulcus, and

adequate excision can be achieved with either partial or total penectomy, depending on the size of the lesion. It is easier to obtain adequate clear margins for carcinomas that grow in an expansile fashion, such as verrucous carcinoma or papillary squamous cell carcinoma, but more of a challenge with carcinomas that are highly infiltrative, or when the invasive carcinoma is associated with extensive carcinoma in situ (CIS).

Pathologic issues

The pathologist should be aware of the clinical aspects of the case and the prior biopsy findings, particularly the grade of the carcinoma, whether it is highly infiltrative, and if there is associated CIS.

The proximal margin of the specimen should be inked, and transverse sections should be made into the proximal part of the specimen to determine the distance of the carcinoma from the proximal margin by gross examination. If the carcinoma is distant from the margin by gross examination, a single circumferential section should be taken from the proximal margin and embedded for FS. On the other hand, if the carcinoma has an infiltrative pattern of growth and is within <1 cm of the margin, we recommend making serial longitudinal sections of the proximal 2 cm of the specimen and embedding the entire proximal margin for FS evaluation. With highly infiltrative carcinomas, the corpora should be scrutinized for vascular invasion as this can sometimes be subtle.

Occasionally, if the initial biopsy was superficial, the surgeon may request intraoperative FS evaluation of the carcinoma for grade and depth of invasion to help decide on the need for lymph node dissection. In this situation, sections should be made into the neoplasm, and using gross examination as a guide, more than one section might be taken from an area likely to provide the necessary information. In this situation, the pathologist should be aware of the less common patterns of invasive squamous cell carcinoma as the histologic features may be puzzling; these include verrucous, warty, papillary, pseudohyperplastic, and pseudoglandular variants of squamous carcinoma.

Evaluation of lymph nodes during penectomy

Clinical issues

Patients with clinical evidence of metastatic carcinoma in inguinal lymph nodes are treated with bilateral inguinal lymphadenectomy, but the best approach to clinically negative lymph nodes is still unresolved. Approximately 20% of patients with clinically negative lymph nodes have metastases.[21] but lymphadenectomy is done selectively because of the morbidity of inguinal node dissection. Lymph node dissection is not performed for low stage (T1[*]), low grade SCC, but is usually performed for T2[**] or poorly differentiated SCC.[22] Sentinel lymph node biopsy has been used successfully as a means of triaging patients for inguinal lymph node dissection, using a combination of dye and technetium, and this may become the standard of care in institutions where this technology is available.

Pathologic issues
Non-sentinel lymph nodes

Frozen section evaluation is only necessary if a positive lymph node will lead the surgeon to proceed with more extensive lymph node dissection. If the lymph node is grossly abnormal, cytological preparations should be made, and if these are negative, the lymph node should be submitted entirely for FS evaluation.

Sentinel lymph node biopsy

A standard protocol for examining inguinal sentinel lymph nodes for patients with penile carcinoma has not been established, but we section the lymph node into thin slices, make touch and cytoscrape preparations, and if these are negative, we embed the entire lymph node for FS. Intraoperative evaluation of a sentinel node is valid only if the surgeon will proceed with lymph node dissection if metastatic carcinoma is reported.

REFERENCES

1. Oneson RH, Minke JA, Silverberg SG. Intraoperative pathologic consultation. An audit of 1,000 recent consecutive cases. *Am J Surg Pathol* 1989; **13**: 237–243.
2. Whitehair JG, Griffey SM, Olander HJ, Vasseur PB, Naydan D. The accuracy of intraoperative diagnoses based on examination of frozen sections. A prospective comparison with paraffin-embedded sections. *Vet Surg* 1993; **22**: 255–259.
3. Gephardt GN, Zarbo R J. Interinstitutional comparison of frozen section consultations. A college of American Pathologists Q-Probes study of 90,538 cases in 461 institutions. *Arch Pathol Lab Med* 1996; **120**: 804–809.
4. Schoenberg MP, Walsh PC, Breazeale DR, Marshall FF, Mostwin JL, Brendler CB. Local recurrence and survival following nerve sparing radical cystoprostatectomy for bladder cancer: 10-year followup. *J Urol* 1996; **155**: 490–494.

[*] T1 = invasion of lamina propria.
[**] T2 = invasion of corpus cavernosum or corpus spongiosum.

5. Schumacher MC, Scholz M, Weise ES, Fleischmann A, Thalmann GN, Studer UE. Is there an indication for frozen section examination of the ureteral margins during cystectomy for transitional cell carcinoma of the bladder? *J Urol* 2006; **176**: 2409–2413; discussion 13.

6. Raj GV, Tal R, Vickers A, *et al.* Significance of intraoperative ureteral evaluation at radical cystectomy for urothelial cancer. *Cancer* 2006; **107**: 2167–2172.

7. Silver DA, Stroumbakis N, Russo P, Fair WR, Herr HW. Ureteral carcinoma in situ at radical cystectomy: does the margin matter? *J Urol* 1997; **158**(3 Pt 1): 768–771.

8. Stein JP, Clark P, Miranda G, Cai J, Groshen S, Skinner DG. Urethral tumor recurrence following cystectomy and urinary diversion: clinical and pathological characteristics in 768 male patients. *J Urol* 2005; **173**(4): 1163–168.

9. Ashley RA, Inman BA, Sebo TJ, *et al.* Urachal carcinoma: clinicopathologic features and long-term outcomes of an aggressive malignancy. *Cancer* 2006; **107**(4): 712–720.

10. Krishnan B, Lechago J, Ayala G, Truong L. Intraoperative consultation for renal lesions. Implications and diagnostic pitfalls in 324 cases. *Am J Clin Pathol* 2003; **120**(4): 528–535.

11. Perez-Montiel D, Wakely PE, Hes O, Michal M, Suster S. Highgrade urothelial carcinoma of the renal pelvis: clinicopathologic study of 108 cases with emphasis on unusual morphologic variants. *Mod Pathol* 2006; **19**(4): 494–503

12. Miller MA, Brown J J. Renal cysts and cystic neoplasms. *Magn Reson Imaging Clin N Am* 1997; **5**(1): 49–66.

13. Todd TD, Dhurandhar B, Mody D, Ramzy I, Truong LD. Fineneedle aspiration of cystic lesions of the kidney. Morphologic spectrum and diagnostic problems in 41 cases. *Am J Clin Pathol* 1999; **111**(3): 317–328.

14. Uzzo RG, Novick A C. Nephron sparing surgery for renal tumors: indications, techniques and outcomes. *J Urol* 2001; **166**(1): 6–18.

15. Partin AW, Kattan MW, Subong EN, *et al.* Combination of prostate-specific antigen, clinical stage, and Gleason score to predict pathological stage of localized prostate cancer. A multi-institutional update. *J Am Med Assoc* 1997; **277**(18): 1445–1451.

16. Kakehi Y, Kamoto T, Okuno H, Terai A, Terachi T, Ogawa O. Per-operative frozen section examination of pelvic nodes is unnecessary for the majority of clinically localized prostate cancers in the prostate-specific antigen era. *Int J Urol* 2000; **7**(8): 281–286.

17. Beissner RS, Stricker JB, Speights VO, Coffield KS, Spiekerman AM, Riggs M. Frozen section diagnosis of metastatic prostate adenocarcinoma in pelvic lymphadenectomy compared with nomogram prediction of metastasis. *Urology* 2002; **59**(5): 721–725.

18. Schned AR, Gormley E A. Florid xanthomatous pelvic lymph node reaction to metastatic prostatic adenocarcinoma. A sequela of preoperative androgen deprivation therapy. *Arch Pathol Lab Med* 1996; **120**(1): 96–100.

19. Hoffman MA, Renshaw AA, Loughlin KR. Squamous cell carcinoma of the penis and microscopic pathologic margins: how much margin is needed for local cure? *Cancer* 1999; **85**(7): 1565–1568.

20. Zhu Y, Ye DW, Chen ZW, Zhang SL, Qin X J. Frozen section-guided wide local excision in the treatment of penoscrotal extramammary Paget's disease. *BJU International* 2007; **100**(6): 1282–1287.

21. Abi-Aad AS, deKernion J B. Controversies in ilioinguinal lymphadenectomy for cancer of the penis. *Urol Clin of N Am* 1992; **19**(2): 319–324.

22. Ornellas AA, Seixas AL, de Moraes J R. Analyses of 200 lymphadenectomies in patients with penile carcinoma. *J Urol* 1991; **46**(2): 330–332.

16 LYMPH NODES, SPLEEN, AND EXTRANODAL LYMPHOMAS

Patrick A. Treseler and Mahendra Ranchod

INTRODUCTION

Pathologists are frequently called upon to provide intraoperative assistance in surgical procedures involving lymphoid tissues such as lymph nodes, spleen and extranodal lymphomas, either to procure fresh tissue for ancillary studies or to provide an intraoperative diagnosis (IOD) that may guide the course of the operation. As with all intraoperative consultations, clear communication between surgeon and pathologist is essential for a successful outcome.

LYMPH NODES

Clinical issues

The clinical approach to lymphadenopathy depends on a variety of factors such as patient age, duration of symptoms, rapidity of growth, number and location of nodes, lymph node mobility, pain and tenderness, systemic symptoms, various laboratory abnormalities, and a history of prior malignancy. Enlarged lymph nodes are more often reactive than neoplastic, and inflammatory lymphadenopathy is often treated empirically with antibiotics. However, a biopsy will be performed when the adenopathy persists, or if the clinical findings are worrisome for malignancy. Clinical and imaging studies can narrow the differential diagnosis but a biopsy is required to make a specific diagnosis in most situations. Four main procedures are used to obtain pathologic samples and the choice of procedure depends on the clinical situation.

Fine needle aspiration

Fine needle aspiration biopsy (FNA) has the advantage of being minimally invasive, and when combined with imaging studies such as ultrasound and CT scans, can be used to sample nodes in relatively inaccessible sites such as the retroperitoneum, and thus avoid a major surgical procedure. The adequacy of the specimen can be assessed with rapid stains, allowing the procedure to be repeated until an adequate sample is obtained. Some institutions use FNA as a screening tool,[1,2] but FNA can often yield a definitive diagnosis of malignant lymphoma when cytologic examination is supplemented with immunophenotyping by flow cytometry.[1,3] However, false-negative results occur, either because the node is partially involved (e.g., early involvement by Hodgkin's lymphoma)[4] or the lymphoma is cytologically bland and lacks a distinctive immunophenotypic profile (e.g., many peripheral T-cell lymphomas).[5] In addition, FNA samples cannot assess nodal architecture, an important feature in the diagnosis and classification of malignant lymphomas. FNA of lymph nodes is only rarely performed in the intraoperative setting.

Needle core biopsy

Needle core biopsy is particularly useful for evaluating deep-seated lymph nodes in the abdomen or retroperitoneum, because like FNA, it spares the patient an open surgical procedure. As with FNA, needle core biopsies only sample a portion of the node, and a negative result does not entirely exclude malignancy. Core biopsies are superior to FNA samples because they provide sufficient tissue for immunohistochemical stains, and often provide information about the architecture of the lesion. Needle core biopsies are occasionally submitted for IOD.

Incisional biopsy

An incisional biopsy is usually performed on large nodes that are difficult to excise safely because they are matted together or intimately associated with important structures

Intraoperative Consultation in Surgical Pathology, ed. Mahendra Ranchod. Published by Cambridge University Press.
© Cambridge University Press 2010.

such as large blood vessels and nerves. Incisional biopsies generally provide excellent specimens, but they too have the limitation of partial sampling.

Excisional biopsy

An excisional biopsy is performed when an intact lymph node is easy to remove in its entirety. This is the best of all lymph node biopsies because it permits the entire node to be examined histologically, and provides the best assessment of lymph node architecture.

Proper handling of lymph node specimens

Lymph nodes are more sensitive than most tissues to cautery, crush artifact, drying, and poor fixation, conditions that can adversely affect the ability to render a definitive diagnosis. Lymph nodes should therefore, be handled with care, beginning in the operating room. The following precautions should be taken.

- The surgeon should avoid unnecessary crush and cautery when removing the specimen, a problem that is encountered most often with incisional biopsies.
- Air drying should be avoided by placing small specimens on a telfa pad immersed in a small volume of saline, particularly when there is likely to be a delay in specimen delivery to the laboratory. Small biopsies should not be placed on dry gauze because the specimen will adhere to the gauze, desiccate, and be difficult to remove without crushing or tearing the tissue.
- When lymphoma is suspected, the specimen should be sent the laboratory promptly in the fresh state to ensure optimal fixation, as well as allow procurement of tissue for various ancillary studies (see below).
- Enlarged lymph nodes should be sectioned into thin (2–3 mm) slices with a sharp blade, and this should be done under sterile conditions if tissue has to be submitted for microbiologic culture (see below). Tissue selected for routine histologic examination should be fixed promptly.

Intraoperative diagnostic techniques

Gross examination

The lymph node should first be examined by gross examination, and large nodes should be sectioned at 2–3 mm intervals to detect focal lesions. Foci of necrosis may be due to necrotizing granulomas, coagulative tumor

necrosis or lymph node infarction,[6,7] and discrete white nodules may be due to metastases. Many lymphomas have a pale, "fish flesh" appearance, but this is not always present. Some lymphomas, including mediastinal and retroperitoneal lymphomas, and nodular sclerosing Hodgkin's lymphoma, may have extensive fibrosis, and in an incisional biopsy, it may not be obvious that the specimen is derived from a lymph node. Adipose infiltration, a common finding in axillary lymph nodes, is seen most often in sentinel node biopsies for breast carcinoma, but it may also cause adenopathy, prompting lymph node biopsy (Fig. 16.1).

Cytologic examination

Incisional and excisional biopsies should first be examined with a cytologic technique and not by frozen section (FS). There are four reasons for this approach:

- Cytologic preparations are adequate for triaging purposes (Fig. 16.2).
- Cytologic preparations are superior to FSs for cytologic detail (Fig. 16.3).
- There is no loss of tissue or freeze-thaw artifact, changes that are inevitable with preparing FSs.[8]
- They avoid contamination of the FS work area, and exposure of laboratory personnel to an infectious agent if the lesion proves to be infectious disease such as tuberculosis (Fig. 16.4).

The cytologic techniques that are employed should be customized to the specific situation. Touch preparations (touch imprints) work well for small specimens that are too small to scrape, and they are also more likely to yield monolayer cellular preparations. When the specimen is large enough, however, cytoscrape preparations should also be performed because of the higher yield of cellular material. Squash preparations are best for suspected lymphomas of the CNS approached by stereotactic biopsy.

Frozen section examination

When cytologic preparations are non-contributory for whatever reason, or when IOD will influence immediate surgical management, we recommend that one (or more) FSs be prepared to maximize the opportunity of making the correct diagnosis. The main benefit of FS is that it provides architectural information that is lacking in cytologic preparations.

(a)

(b)

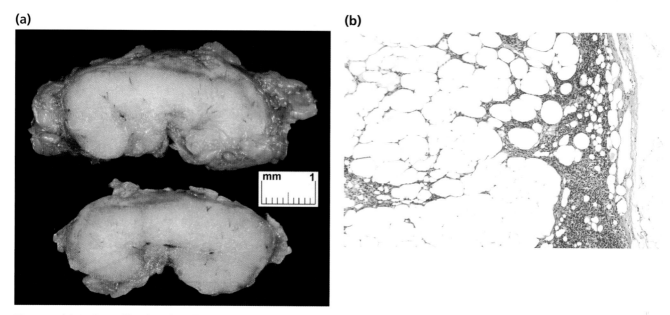

Fig. 16.1. (a) Benign axillary lymph node with adipose infiltration. The lymph node was enlarged and presented as a palpable mass. A narrow rim of residual lymphoid tissue is present at the periphery of the node. (b) Histologically, the adipose tissue extended into the cortex of the lymph node.

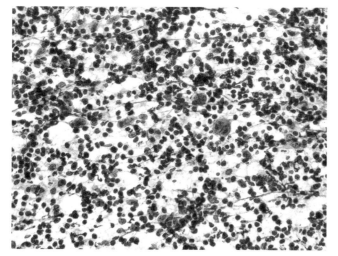

Fig. 16.2. Cytoscrape of an enlarged cervical lymph node. The background of small lymphocytes with scattered atypical large cells are highly suggestive of Hodgkin's lymphoma. These findings are sufficient for purposes of triaging the specimen; a FS is not necessary.

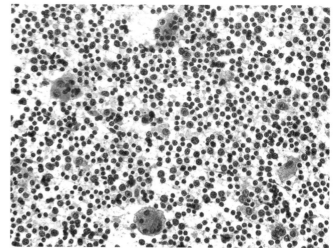

Fig. 16.3. Cytoscrape preparation showing one of the features of Rosai-Dorfman disease. The diagnosis of "benign lymph node" is a perfectly adequate intraoperative diagnosis, but this slide illustrates the ease with which emperipolesis can be seen in cytologic preparations.

Sampling of lymph nodes for ancillary studies

A wide variety of ancillary studies can be employed to aid the pathologic interpretation of lymphoproliferative lesions. Many such studies, including immunohistochemistry and fluorescence in situ hybridization (FISH), can be performed on formalin-fixed, paraffin-embedded tissue, and do not require special handling. Other studies require either living tissue or fresh frozen tissue, and these specimens need special attention.

Immunophenotyping by flow cytometry

When lymphoma is suspected, fresh tissue should be sent for immunophenotyping by flow cytometry if the specimen is large enough to yield enough tissue. While immunohistochemical staining on formalin-fixed, paraffin-embedded tissue is adequate for the diagnosis of many lymphomas, immunohistochemistry cannot detect certain immunophenotypic features such as the monoclonal expression of surface immunoglobulin, a characteristic that

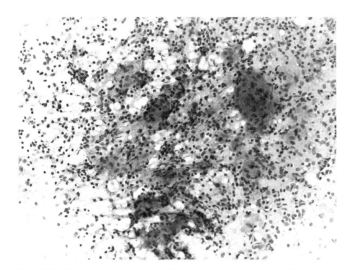

Fig. 16.4. Cytoscrape of a cervical lymph node showing the histiocytes and a multinucleate giant cell characteristic of granulomatous inflammation. Necrosis was also present, in keeping with an infection. Cytologic preparations are suited to screening lymph nodes for potential communicable infections.

can be detected by flow cytometry and which may be crucial to the diagnosis.[3,9–12]

B-cell and T-cell gene rearrangement studies

If a lymph node is of adequate size, and malignant lymphoma is in the differential diagnosis, a portion of the fresh specimen should be snap frozen and set aside for B-cell or T-cell gene rearrangement studies, because these tests can be extremely helpful in confirming the presence of a clonal – and probably malignant- lymphoid cell population.[13] Gene rearrangement studies can be performed on formalin-fixed paraffin-embedded tissue using polymerase chain reaction (PCR), but these PCR-based techniques employ consensus primers which are capable of detecting some, but not all, B-cell and T-cell gene rearrangements, resulting in a false negative rate of 10%–30%.[13] Thus, when the morphologic and immunophenotypic features are equivocal, a negative PCR-based study should be followed by more sensitive clonality studies using the Southern blot technique on fresh frozen tissue.

Cytogenetic studies

Fresh tissue may be sent for cytogenetic analysis as several non-Hodgkin's lymphomas have characteristic translocations or other cytogenetic abnormalities, such as the t(8;14) of Burkitt's lymphoma or the t(2;5) of anaplastic large cell lymphoma, information that can be helpful in establishing a diagnosis in cases with equivocal features.[14,15] However, the need for cytogenetic karyotyping has been greatly reduced with the advent of commercially available FISH testing on paraffin-embedded tissue.

Microbiologic cultures

When the differential diagnosis includes an infection, fresh tissue should be sent for appropriate microbiologic cultures. It is best if these samples are collected in the operating room to ensure that they are collected under sterile conditions, but this is an issue that should be decided in advance of surgery – another reason for close communication with the surgeon.

Information needed before and during intraoperative diagnosis

Clear communication between surgeon and pathologist is essential when a lymph node biopsy is submitted for IOD, because proper handling of the specimen depends on the clinical issues at stake. A few examples will illustrate this point.

- There is no need for IOD when the surgeon has completely removed the only enlarged lymph node in a patient with unexplained lymphadenopathy, and if the course of the operation will not be altered by IOD. Cytologic examination should be performed to triage tissue for ancillary studies, and this will also yield sufficient information to appease the surgeon who insists on a provisional diagnosis. There is no reason to perform a FS because any additional information that is forthcoming serves no immediate purpose, utilizes additional resources, and consumes tissue.
- When a patient with suspected lymphoma has multiple enlarged lymph nodes or matted nodes, the surgeon is likely to excise the most accessible, superficially-located lymph node because of the risks associated with excising a deep lymph node wrapped around major vessels and nerves. Often, the superficial lymph nodes will show only reactive changes, with malignant lymphoma lurking in the larger, more deeply seated lymph nodes (Fig. 16.5).[16] Familiarity with the clinical findings will allow the pathologist to recognize a sampling problem and encourage the surgeon to perform a biopsy of a deeper lymph node.
- Mediastinal and retroperitoneal lymphomas often show extensive fibrosis, sometimes obscuring the neoplastic cells. Examination of the biopsy in isolation may lead to the incorrect diagnosis of a benign inflammatory or fibrotic process, but the clinical and imaging findings should prompt the pathologist to request additional tissue, until such time that the biopsy findings account for the mass.

(a)

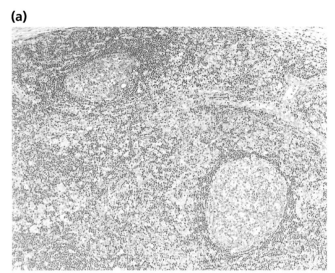

(b)

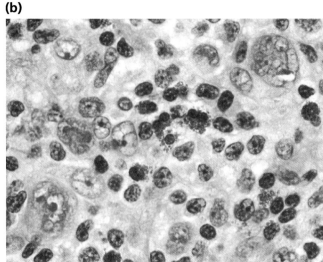

Fig. 16.5. (a) In this patient with classical Hodgkin's lymphoma, initial excision of a small superficial cervical lymph node showed only reactive hyperplasia. (b) Because this did not explain the patient's enlarged matted lymph nodes, biopsy of a deeper lymph node was performed and this showed Hodgkin's lymphoma.

- When a patient with known chronic lymphocytic leukemia/small lymphocytic lymphoma (CLL/SLL) undergoes lymph node biopsy for suspected Richter's transformation, the pathologist should know the reason for the surgical procedure. An IOD of "atypical lymphoid infiltrate, suspicious for lymphoma," which would suffice in other situations, will be inadequate in this situation because the purpose of the biopsy is to document transformation to a large cell lymphoma. If the biopsy shows only small cell lymphoma, the surgeon is likely to perform additional biopsies.

- In the case of a young patient with a mediastinal mass and worsening superior vena cava syndrome, where lymphoblastic lymphoma is suspected, every effort should be made to confirm the diagnosis of lymphoblastic lymphoma as this will allow the clinicians to proceed with immediate post-operative radiation and chemotherapy. Air dried cytologic preparations are likely to provide the best material for diagnosis, with the neoplastic cells showing their characteristic nuclear and cytoplasmic features (Fig. 16.6). This is one more situation where the surgeon will expect the pathologist to offer a specific or near-specific diagnosis, instead of a non-commital diagnosis of "probable lymphoma, final diagnosis pending immunophenotyping studies."

- Lymph node biopsies performed for suspected metastatic carcinoma are sent for IOD in two main situations, and it is important to know which applies.

  - In the first situation, the IOD will have no influence on immediate surgical management, and is performed to satisfy the surgeon's curiosity, assuage patient anxiety, or expedite referral to a radiation therapist or oncologist. If tissue conservation is an issue, we recommend performing cytologic examinations only, and not subject the tissue to FS.[8]

  - In the second situation, IOD will have a profound influence on immediate surgical management, and a diagnosis of carcinoma will either invoke the "stopping rule," causing the surgeon to abandon a planned major resection (e.g., a Whipple's resection for pancreatic carcinoma), or invoke the "go ahead rule," giving the surgeon license to extend the surgical resection (e.g., cervical lymph node dissection in a patient with salivary gland carcinoma). In these high-stake situations, the entire lymph node should be embedded for FS, and multiple levels should be prepared, without attempting to save tissue for permanent sections. There is no reason to submit tissue for ancillary studies, such as flow cytometry, unless the cytologic and histologic features are those of an unsuspected lymphoma.

The special case of sentinel lymph node biopsy

The purpose of IOD on sentinel lymph node biopsies is to identify those patients who have a metastasis, allowing the surgeon to proceed with completion lymphadenectomy during the same operation; conversely, patients who have a negative sentinel node are spared from having unnecessary surgery. Sentinel lymph node biopsy has become standard

(a)   **(b)**

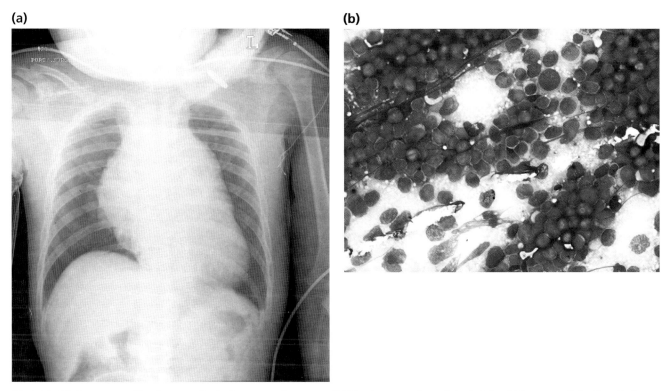

Fig. 16.6. (a) A teenager with a large mediastinal mass on chest x-ray. (b) Touch preparations of the incisional biopsy revealed cells with fine blastic chromatin and scanty cytoplasm, characteristic of lymphoblastic lymphoma. (Images courtesy of Dr. Megan Dishop, Children's Hospital, Aurora, Colorado).

of care for staging patients with breast carcinoma and melanoma, and its use is under investigation for other malignancies as well. However, the best way to handle sentinel nodes is still a work in progress.[17]

There is general agreement that grossly suspicious sentinel nodes should be examined intraoperatively, by cytologic touch or scrape preparations initially, and by FS if necessary. There is little agreement however, on how sentinel nodes should be examined if they appear to be normal on gross examination. An argument can be made that the surgeon should simply submit grossly normal sentinel nodes in formalin, because of the high false negative rates that occur with intraoperative evaluation.[8,17–20] An alternative approach, which we support, is to section the lymph node at 2–3 mm intervals, and make cytologic preparations from one or both surfaces of each slice. This should detect most metastases >2–3 mm, yet preserve nearly all of the nodal tissue for permanent sections.[17] The surgeon should understand that this approach will not detect tiny metastases, including metastases that are evident only with immunohistochemical stains. We do not see the point in routinely subjecting grossly normal sentinel nodes to FS evaluation with multiple step sections

because even this approach has a relatively low yield for detecting micrometastases.[17] The brouhaha about the intraoperative evaluation of sentinel nodes dissipates if we accept the limitations of current intraoperative techniques; the goal is to detect larger metastases, not minute lesions. While it is inconvenient and costly to have the patient return for a second surgical procedure after the detection of a metastasis on permanent sections, the health and well-being of the patient is not adversely affected by a delay in completion lymphadenectomy. (See Chapter 13, p. 201 for additional discussion of sentinel lymph node biopsy.)

Indications for intraoperative diagnosis

1. To determine the likely cause of an enlarged lymph node, so that tissue may be triaged for appropriate ancillary tests, such as microbiologic culture, flow cytometry, gene rearrangement studies, and cytogenetics.
2. To determine the adequacy of an incisional biopsy specimen performed for unexplained lymphadenopathy ("rule out lymphoma").

(a)   **(b)**

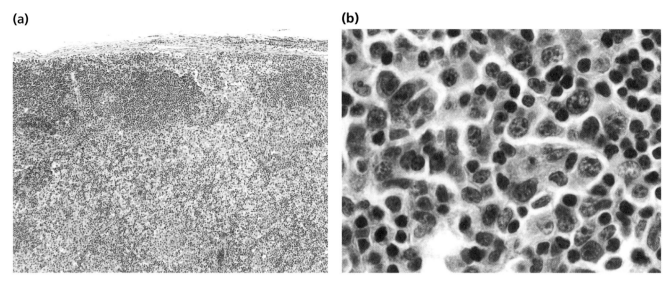

Fig. 16.7. (a) A lymph node showing a reactive immunoblastic proliferation. (b) Clusters of large lymphoid cells may be mistaken for a diffuse large cell lymphoma.

3. To stage a patient with a known or suspected carcinoma to determine if the primary tumor should be resected (e.g., Whipple's resection for pancreatic carcinoma).

4. To stage a patient with a known carcinoma to determine if a node dissection should be performed (e.g., cervical lymph node dissection in a patient with salivary gland carcinoma).

5. To render a preliminary diagnosis that will influence immediate post-operative management, e.g., a young patient with a mediastinal mass and severe superior vena cava syndrome presumed to be due to lymphoblastic lymphoma.

Reporting the results of intraoperative diagnosis

We referred to two situations earlier in this chapter where an attempt should be made to classify the lymphoma at the time of IOD, but it is prudent to be cautious about rendering a specific diagnosis in most other situations. We suggest offering a provisional diagnosis, tailoring the specific language to the clinical situation, and deferring the specific diagnosis to permanent sections and ancillary studies. A few examples will illustrate the reason for this position:

- A lymph node that shows apparent architectural effacement and many large lymphoid cells may well be a large cell lymphoma, but a similar appearance can occur in cases of reactive immunoblastic hyperplasia,

infectious mononucleosis being the best known example. (Fig. 16.7).[21]

- A lesion that appears to be a large cell lymphoma on intraoperative evaluation may later prove to be some other large cell malignancy, such as histiocytic sarcoma or metastatic melanoma, after appropriate immunohistochemical stains are performed.[22]

- A lymph node that appears to be composed almost entirely of small mature lymphocytes may be a small cell lymphoma, but could also be a quiescent lymph node that simply lacks significant reactive hyperplasia (Fig. 16.8).[23] Immunophenotyping on permanent sections may be necessary to make the distinction.

- A lymph node may show only follicular hyperplasia in one section and overt lymphoma in other areas.[24,25] Thus, a benign appearance on a single FS or a single cytologic sample does not completely exclude lymphoma.

- Some lymphomas, such as classical Hodgkin's lymphoma, can have a subtle interfollicular pattern in a lymph node dominated by reactive hyperplasia, and the lymphoma may only become apparent when permanent sections and special stains are examined.[23]

Thus, when a lymph node is excised for possible lymphoma, a specific diagnosis should not be offered unless the evidence is overwhelming; instead terms such as the following may be used: "atypical large cell proliferation, suspicious for large cell lymphoma" or "monotonous small

(a)　　　　　　　　　　　　　　　　　　**(b)**

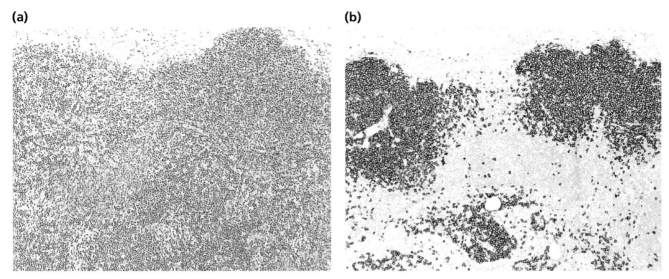

Fig. 16.8. (a) This quiescent lymph node is composed of a monotonous population of mature small lymphocytes that may suggest a small cell lymphoma on routine H&E-stained sections. (b) These lymph nodes are usually small, the clue to a benign diagnosis. Immunohistochemical stains on permanent sections show the normal pattern of CD20 positive B-cells restricted to primary follicles, while the interfollicular lymphocytes were CD3 positive T-cells (not shown).

lymphoid population, cannot exclude small cell lympho-proliferative disorder." Such "good enough" diagnoses will appease the surgeon, yet indicate that the final diagnosis has to await permanent sections and appropriate ancillary studies.

SPLEEN

General clinical issues

Most splenectomy specimens are not sent for intraoperative diagnosis. The majority of splenectomies are performed for post-traumatic bleeding or immune thrombocytopenic purpura (ITP), and these specimens are not usually submitted for IOD. Metastatic malignancies are uncommon, and usually occur in the setting of widespread metastases. Although a number of lymphomas and other lymphoproliferative disorders can involve the spleen and present with splenomegaly, only splenic B-cell marginal zone lymphoma and hepatosplenic T-cell lymphoma can be considered true primary splenic lymphomas.[26]

Splenic B-cell marginal zone lymphoma is not uncommon. It resembles other marginal zone lymphomas morphologically, immunophenotypically, and in terms of its indolent clinical course. Hepatosplenic T-cell lymphoma is rare and clinically aggressive; peripheral lymphocytosis and bone marrow involvement provide important clues to the diagnosis. Splenectomy is performed when there is a need to debulk

the disease, provide symptomatic relief, or provide tissue to confirm the clinical diagnosis.

Specimen handling and intraoperative diagnosis

When a lymphoproliferative disorder is suspected, the spleen should be submitted to the pathologist in the fresh state to allow procurement of tissue for ancillary studies such as flow cytometry, gene rearrangement studies, and cytogenetics. Air-dried cytologic preparations should be made for later examination. The spleen should be cut into thin slices to optimize fixation, and it is helpful to place a few thinly sectioned pieces of tissue in a separate container of formalin, or other appropriate fixative, to ensure optimal fixation.

If the surgeon requests an IOD, it is helpful to know the reason for the request. In the case of a lymphoproliferative lesion, it is unlikely that the diagnosis will affect immediate surgical management, and for this reason, making a cytologic preparation should be sufficient to confirm the diagnosis of a lymphoproliferative disease. There should be no reason to perform a FS, but since tissue is plentiful, the pathologist should perform a FS if the gross findings are unusual, and if there is a chance that the neoplasm is non-lymphoid and will influence immediate management.

Both splenic marginal zone lymphoma and hepatosplenic T-cell lymphoma are composed of monotonous

(a)

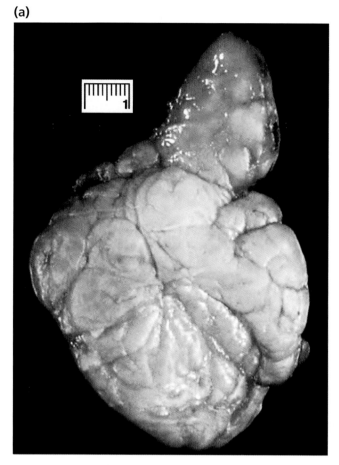

(b)

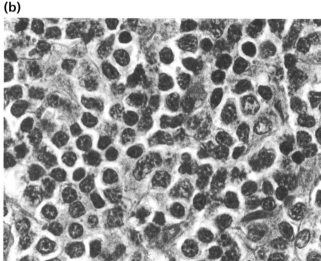

Fig. 16.9. Marginal cell lymphoma of the thyroid gland. (a) A thyroid lobectomy was performed for a dominant mass in a patient with Hashimoto's disease. (b) In MALT lymphomas, touch preparations and frozen sections show a monotonous population of mature small lymphocytes. (Images courtesy of Dr Raja Seethala, University of Pittsburgh School of Medicine).

populations of small to intermediate lymphoid cells, but ancillary studies are essential to confirm the diagnosis in most cases.

EXTRANODAL LYMPHOMA

General clinical issues

Approximately one-third of non-Hodgkin's lymphomas present in sites other than lymph node, spleen or bone marrow.[27] Extranodal B-cell marginal zone lymphoma, plasmablastic lymphoma, primary effusion lymphoma, intravascular large B-cell lymphoma, nasal-type extranodal NK/T-cell lymphoma, enteropathy-associated T-cell lymphoma, and a variety of cutaneous lymphomas occur almost exclusively in extranodal sites at least initially, and in addition, an extranodal presentation is not uncommon for a variety of other lymphomas, including Burkitt's lymphoma, diffuse large B-cell lymphoma, and mantle cell lymphoma.[28,29] Given the variety of histologic types

and the wide range of clinical presentations, the diagnosis of extranodal lymphoma can be challenging.

Extranodal B-cell marginal zone lymphoma (MALT lymphoma) is the most common form of extranodal lymphoma. It is composed mainly of mature small lymphocytes, and often occurs in association with dense chronic inflammation, either due to chronic infection or an autoimmune disorder, making it difficult to distinguish the lymphoma from the underlying chronic inflammation.[28] MALT lymphomas most often involve the stomach, but can arise in many other body sites, including salivary glands, ocular adnexa, skin, intestine, and thyroid gland (Fig. 16.9).[28]

Specimen handling and intraoperative diagnosis

Many extranodal lymphomas are initially diagnosed on small outpatient biopsies (e.g., gastric MALT lymphoma), or are resected but not sent for IOD because lymphoma was not suspected clinically (e.g., MALT lymphoma of the thyroid gland in a patient with Hashimoto's thyroiditis). Ideally, all biopsies that are large enough should be submitted fresh so that appropriate ancillary studies can be performed, as with lymph node biopsies. Extranodal lymphomas are sent for IOD for three main reasons:

- When a provisional diagnosis of a lymphoproliferative lesion is made on FNA, and a subsequent excision is performed to provide tissue for definitive diagnosis (e.g., a salivary gland or thyroid lobe).

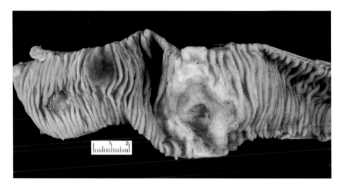

Fig. 16.10. Primary large cell lymphoma of the small intestine in a patient who presented with intestinal obstruction. Cytoscrape and frozen sections were performed, permitting a provisional diagnosis of large cell lymphoma.

- When the lymphoma presents as a mass in an anatomic site that is not usually sampled by FNA or incisional biopsy, and when IOD could affect immediate surgical management, as in lymphoma of the ovary.
- When there is an acute event, such as uncontrolled gastric bleeding, intestinal obstruction or perforation of the gastrointestinal tract that requires prompt surgical intervention, and a suspicious mass is found as the source of the problem (Fig. 16.10).

If IOD will not influence immediate surgical management (e.g., the perforated segment of small bowel has been resected), it is sufficient to determine that the lesion is a lymphoproliferative disorder by cytologic examination and FS, and not make a more specific diagnosis. Tissue should be sampled for appropriate ancillary studies, such as flow cytometry and gene rearrangement studies.

In some situations, it is important to distinguish between lymphoma and other malignancies because of differences in immediate surgical management. As an example, lymphoma of the ovary should be distinguished from primary small cell carcinoma of the ovary as this will allow the gynecologic oncologist to forgo standard staging for ovarian carcinoma, saving the patient from having unnecessary surgery (Fig. 16.11).

(a)

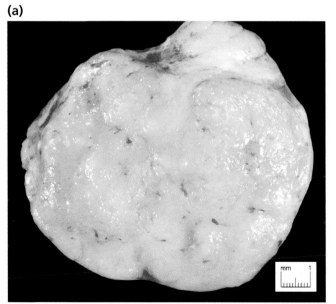

(b)

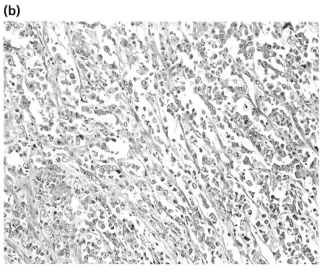

Fig. 16.11. Primary large cell lymphoma of the ovary in a patient who underwent laparotomy with a provisional clinical diagnosis of ovarian carcinoma. (a) The ovarian mass was solid and measured 9 cm in maximum dimension. (b) In lymphoma of the ovary, the neoplastic lymphocytes sometimes infiltrate between stromal cells, raising the possibility of a non-lymphoid malignancy.

There is reason to be cautious about rendering a firm diagnosis of lymphoma when there are no surgical issues at stake. Dense infiltrates of small lymphocytes may be benign or malignant, and even collections of large cells may prove to be benign or of non-lymphoid origin.

ACKNOWLEDGMENT

The authors thank Dr. Carl A. Bertelsen, Department of Surgery, Good Samaritan Hospital, San Jose, CA for reading this chapter.

REFERENCES

1. Dunphy CH, Ramos R. Combining fine-needle aspiration and flow cytometric immunophenotyping in evaluation of nodal and extranodal sites for possible lymphoma: a retrospective review. *Diagn Cytopathol* 1997; **16**: 200–206.
2. Wolf JS, Jr., Cher M, Dall'era M, *et al*. The use and accuracy of cross-sectional imaging and fine needle aspiration cytology for detection of pelvic lymph node metastases before radical prostatectomy. *J Urol* 1995; **153**: 993–999.
3. Swart GJ, Wright C, Brundyn K, *et al*. Fine needle aspiration biopsy and flow cytometry in the diagnosis of lymphoma. *Transfus Apher Sci* 2007; **37**: 71–79.
4. Doggett RS, Colby TV, Dorfman RF. Interfollicular Hodgkin's disease. *Am J Surg Pathol* 1983; **7**: 145–149.
5. Cotta CV, Hsi ED. Pathobiology of mature T-cell lymphomas. *Clin Lymphoma Myeloma* 2008; **8** Suppl 5: S168–S179.
6. Cleary KR, Osborne BM, Butler JJ. Lymph node infarction foreshadowing malignant lymphoma. *Am J Surg Pathol* 1982; **6**: 435–442.
7. Maurer R, Schmid U, Davies JD, *et al*. Lymph-node infarction and malignant lymphoma: a multicentre survey of European, English and American cases. *Histopathology* 1986; **10**: 571–588.
8. Van Diest PJ, Torrenga H, Borgstein PJ, *et al*. Reliability of intraoperative frozen section and imprint cytological investigation of sentinel lymph nodes in breast cancer. *Histopathology* 1999; **35**: 14–18.
9. Kaleem Z. Flow cytometric analysis of lymphomas: current status and usefulness. *Arch Pathol Lab Med* 2006; **130**: 1850–1858.
10. Stetler-Stevenson M. Flow cytometry in lymphoma diagnosis and prognosis: useful? *Best Pract Res Clin Haematol* 2003; **16**: 583–597.
11. Sheikholeslami MR, Jilani I, Albitar M. The use of the antibodies in the diagnosis of leukemia and lymphoma by flow cytometry. *Methods Mol Biol*. 2007; **378**: 53–63.
12. Demurtas A, Accinelli G, Pacchioni D, *et al*. Utility of flow cytometry immunophenotyping in fine-needle aspirate cytologic diagnosis of non-Hodgkin lymphoma: a series of 252 cases and review of the literature. *Appl Immunohistochem Mol Morphol* 2009.
13. Arber DA. Molecular diagnostic approach to non-Hodgkin's lymphoma. *J Mol Diagn* 2000; **2**: 178–190.
14. Campbell LJ. Cytogenetics of lymphomas. *Pathology* 2005; **37**: 493–507.
15. Hartmann EM, Ott G, Rosenwald A. Molecular biology and genetics of lymphomas. *Hematol Oncol Clin North Am* 2008; **22**: 807–823, vii.
16. Butler JJ. Non-neoplastic lesions of lymph nodes of man to be differentiated from lymphomas. *Natl Cancer Inst Monogr* 1969; **32**: 233–255.
17. Treseler P. Pathologic examination of the sentinel lymph node: what is the best method? *Breast J* 2006; **12**: S143–S151.
18. Veronesi U, Paganelli G, Galimberti V, *et al*. Sentinel-node biopsy to avoid axillary dissection in breast cancer with clinically negative lymph-nodes [see comments]. *Lancet* 1997; **349**: 1864–1867.
19. Turner RR, Hansen NM, Stern SL, *et al*. Intraoperative examination of the sentinel lymph node for breast carcinoma staging [see comments]. *Am J Clin Pathol* 1999; **112**: 627–634.
20. Ku NN. Pathologic examination of sentinel lymph nodes in breast cancer. *Surg Oncol Clin N Am* 1999; **8**: 469–479.
21. Ramsay AD. Reactive lymph nodes in pediatric practice. *Am J Clin Pathol*. 2004; **122** Suppl: S87–97.
22. Ioachim HL, Ratech H. *Ioachim's Lymph Node Pathology*. Philadelphia: Lippincott Williams & Wilkins, 2002.
23. Schwartz MR, Ramzy I. Lymph nodes. *Clinical Cytopathology and Aspiration Biopsy*. San Francisco: McGraw-Hill Professional, 2000, pp. 409–440.
24. Hansmann ML, Fellbaum C, Hui PK, *et al*. Progressive transformation of germinal centers with and without association to Hodgkin's disease. *Am J Clin Pathol* 1990; **93**: 219–226.
25. Hicks J, Flaitz C. Progressive transformation of germinal centers: review of histopathologic and clinical features. *Int J Pediatr Otorhinolaryngol* 2002; **65**: 195–202.
26. Isaacson PG. Primary splenic lymphoma. *Cancer Surv* 1997; **30**: 193–212.
27. Zucca E. Extranodal lymphoma: a reappraisal. *Ann Oncol* 2008; **19** Suppl 4: iv77–80.
28. Ferry JA. Extranodal lymphoma. *Arch Pathol Lab Med* 2008; **132**: 565–578.
29. Skoog L, Tani E. Extranodal lymphomas. *Monogr Clin Cytol* 2009; **18**: 60–63.

17   CENTRAL NERVOUS SYSTEM

Fausto J. Rodriguez, Bernd W. Scheithauer, and John L. Atkinson

INTRODUCTION

Intraoperative consultations for lesions of the central nervous system (CNS) are often daunting to general surgical pathologists since most lesions are unique to the CNS, and differ markedly from those occurring in other body sites. In addition, optimal performance depends heavily upon incorporating information from multiple sources, including clinical data, previous pathologic material, prior treatment, radiographic findings, and the anatomic compartment (s) involved. Thus, we emphasize the importance of open communication between pathologist and neurosurgeon, and argue that the pathologist who fails to correlate pathologic data with clinical and imaging data cannot function reliably as a consultant.

The frozen section (FS) technique has proven its usefulness for providing accurate intraoperative diagnoses, but in the CNS artifacts created by freezing tissue may produce changes that compromise pathologic interpretation, and it is for this reason that we strongly advocate the liberal use of cytologic preparations. The information obtained by cytologic techniques is as accurate, and usually more accurate, than FS, and moreover, spares the bulk of the specimen from the artifacts of freezing.

As discussed in the introductory chapter of this book, the surgical pathologist who evaluates CNS specimens should keep in mind the difference between managerial and scientific diagnoses, and recognize that what the neurosurgeon needs is information that will guide immediate surgical management. Fine points in nomenclature and grading can be deferred to permanent sections, with or without the aid of ancillary tests and/or expert consultation.

A broad spectrum of neoplasms, tumor-like lesions and medical diseases affect the CNS, and it is not possible to discuss every entity that may present for intraoperative evaluation. This chapter focuses on the management of common lesions of the CNS that general surgical pathologists are likely to encounter in their practices.

GENERAL CLINICAL ISSUES

Major advances in diagnostic imaging and surgical techniques have dramatically changed the approach to diagnosis and treatment of tumors of the CNS. The aggressiveness of surgical management is guided by the differential diagnosis, patient age, functional eloquence of the target site, and the patient's pre-operative status. Pre-operative imaging techniques may help to identify white matter tracks[1] as well as predict the risk of recurrence for low grade tumors.[2] A variety of operative techniques are now available, including outpatient biopsy,[3] awake craniotomy,[4] intraoperative motor mapping,[5] fluorescence guided tumor resection,[6] image guided stereotactic surgery, and intraoperative MRI,[7,8] contributing to more precise tissue sampling, and maximizing surgical resection, while considerably diminishing patient morbidity and mortality. More refined post-operative adjuvant therapies[9,10] have further added to optimism in the management of gliomas.

It is good practice for general surgical pathologists to review the imaging studies on all CNS neoplasms pre-operatively, and to discuss complex cases with the surgeon in an attempt to understand the surgeon's intraoperative needs and to be familiar with the surgeon's operative plan. Unlike tumors in other anatomic sites, the evaluation of surgical margins is generally not an issue in tumors of the CNS, as resection is guided by imaging characteristics, intraoperative evaluation of functional activity, and visual/tactile information obtained during the course of the

Intraoperative Consultation in Surgical Pathology, ed. Mahendra Ranchod. Published by Cambridge University Press.
© Cambridge University Press 2010.

surgery. The critical issue during surgery is to make the appropriate managerial diagnosis because this will determine the course of further surgical management.

The following surgical procedures are relevant to intraoperative diagnosis:

Stereotactic biopsy

The purpose of stereotactic biopsy is to obtain diagnostic tissue. The procedure, which is performed under imaging guidance, is undertaken when surgical resection is inappropriate or not feasible. The surgeon's goal is to obtain a representative sample of the target lesion with the minimum number of biopsies, thus avoiding intracranial bleeding that some lesions are susceptible to. The surgeon will therefore submit the first set of core biopsies for intraoperative evaluation, because the presence of lesional tissue will allow the surgeon to terminate the surgical procedure.

Subtotal resection

Subtotal resection is undertaken when resection is limited by critical structures in close proximity to the lesion, such as blood vessels, cranial nerves and eloquent brain tissue that cannot be sacrificed. Various pre-operative and intraoperative techniques are used to achieve maximal resection with minimal patient deficit in low-grade tumors; high grade tumors are debulked to diminish the mass effect of the tumor as well as improve the response to adjuvant therapy. Tissue will be sent for IOD to confirm the surgeon's pre-operative diagnosis, and in general this does not change the surgeon's operative plan – unless the pathologist's diagnosis is completely different from the surgeon's pre-operative working diagnosis, such as a fungal infection when a high-grade malignancy was expected.

Complete surgical resection

Complete surgical resection is performed for resectable extra-parenchymal neoplasms such as meningiomas and schwannomas, as well as for relatively benign, circumscribed gliomas, such as pilocytic astrocytoma, ganglioglioma and xanthoastrocytoma when they are located in non-eloquent areas of the brain. As stated earlier, tissue is not submitted for evaluation of margins; instead, imaging data and the findings at the time of surgery are used to judge the completeness of resection. The surgeons'

intraoperative assessment of complete "image resection," is confirmed by post-operative MRI, which serves as a baseline for future management.[11]

INDICATIONS FOR INTRAOPERATIVE DIAGNOSIS

1. In the case of stereotactic biopsies, intraoperative diagnosis is performed to ensure that lesional tissue has been obtained, and that the pathologic changes are representative of the imaging abnormalities, e.g., appropriate grade in a diffuse glioma.
2. To confirm the provisional clinical diagnosis when the surgeon's plan is to completely excise a radiographically circumscribed mass, e.g. meningioma, schwannoma, and ependymoma.
3. To confirm the provisional clinical diagnosis when debulking is planned, e.g., metastatic carcinoma and glioblastoma.
4. To facilitate immediate post-operative treatment when an infectious process is suspected, e.g., abscess.
5. To confirm that diagnostic tissue has been obtained when stereotactic or open biopsy are performed for a medical disease, e.g., demyelinating disease.
6. To procure tissue for ancillary studies such as culture and molecular tests.

INFORMATION REQUIRED BEFORE AND DURING INTRAOPERATIVE CONSULTATION

Clinical and imaging information are extremely important in evaluating most lesions of the CNS, and we would like to stress that it is inappropriate to render an intraoperative diagnosis without this information.[12] Table 17.1 summarizes how clinical information can narrow the differential diagnosis, and Table 17.2 underscores how the anatomic compartment in the CNS can limit the differential diagnosis, and sometimes allow an almost specific diagnosis.[13] A pathologist who turns a blind eye to these very helpful sources of information is more likely to make errors.

In addition to location, imaging characteristics can provide clues to the diagnosis. For example, a mass lesion with edema and peripheral enhancement is characteristic of a malignant glioma and not a low grade glioma, and

Table 17.1. Key clinical questions in the evaluation of surgical specimens

Feature	Question	Example
Age and gender	Pediatric patient?	Pilocytic astrocytomas, PXA, gangliogliomas, and medulloblastomas favor pediatric patients
	Female sex?	Spinal meningioma
Associated symptoms	History of chronic seizures?	DNET, ganglioglioma, angiocentric glioma
Past medical history	Immunosuppression?	Post-transplant lymphoproliferative disorder, toxoplasmosis, PML
Family/genetic history	Family or past medical history of NF1?	Predominantly pilocytic astrocytomas in CNS
Time course	Slowly evolving lesion with recent accelerated growth?	Progression from low- to high-grade infiltrative glioma
Anatomic location	Dural based lesion?	Dural based lesions are predominantly meningioma subtypes of varying grade.
	Intracortical lesion?	DNET
	Intraventricular lesion?	Ependymal tumors
Imaging features	Calcified lesion?	Oligodendroglioma, craniopharyngioma
	Well circumscribed process?	Less likely diffusely infiltrating astrocytoma
	Cyst with mural nodule?	Pilocytic astrocytoma, PXA, ganglioglioma, hemangioblastoma
Intraoperative appearance	Purulent? necrotic?	Abscess, glioblastoma, metastasis
Previous pathology	Primary resection or irradiation?	Changes due to prior surgery or radiation
Pre-operative treatment	Corticosteroids administered?	Lymphoma cells may completely disappear after a course of steroids or mimic demyelinating disease.

PXA = pleomorphic xanthoastrocytoma; DNET = Dysembryoplastic neuroepithelial tumor.; PML = progressive multifocal leukoencephalopathy; NF1 = neurofibromatosis type 1; CNS = central nervous system.

Table 17.2. Differential diagnosis of CNS tumors by anatomic location

Location	Specific entities
Cerebral cortex (superficial)	DNET, angiocentric glioma, oligodendroglioma
Intraventricular	
Lateral ventricles	Choroid plexus tumors, ependymoma, subependymoma
Third ventricle	Choroid glioma, ependymoma, papillary craniopharyngioma
Fourth ventricle	Ependymoma, subependymoma, choroid plexus tumors
Foramen of Monro	Colloid cyst, SEGA, central neurocytoma
Periventricular	Demyelination, lymphoma
Corpus callosum	Diffusely infiltrating glioma, lymphoma, demyelinating disease
Cerebellopontine angle	Schwannoma, meningioma, pilocytic astrocytoma (exophytic), epidermoid cyst, choroid plexus tumors, ATRT
Brain stem	Diffusely infiltrating astrocytoma, pilocytic astrocytoma (exophytic)
Pineal region	Pineal parenchymal tumors, germ cell tumors, papillary tumor of the pineal region
Spinal cord	
Intramedullary	Ependymoma, pilocytic and diffuse astrocytomas, hemangioblastoma
Extramedullary/nerve root involvement	Meningioma, schwannoma, paraganglioma, melanocytoma
Sellar/suprasellar region	Pituitary adenoma, germ cell tumors, craniopharyngioma, pilocytic astrocytoma, pituicytoma, granular cell tumor, spindle cell oncocytoma, metastases
Dura	Meningioma, mesenchymal tumors e.g., hemangiopericytoma, solitary fibrous tumor, etc.; marginal zone lymphoma, inflammatory pseudotumor

DNET = Dysembryoplastic neuroepithelial tumor.; SEGA = subependymal giant cell astrocytoma; ATRT = atypical teratoid-rhabdoid tumor.

HANDLING SPECIMENS

Gross examination

Gross examination plays a limited role in the evaluation of CNS lesions. In resections, a firm consistency is a clue to meningioma, schwannoma, a mesenchymal neoplasm or to a fibrous component in a glial neoplasm. Necrosis is a clue to malignancy, and a hemorrhagic appearance may suggest a vascular neoplasm or a neoplasm with prominent vascularity. The main issue with gross examination is that it guides sampling of the specimen, both for IOD and for ancillary tests.

additional tissue should be requested if the biopsy shows only a low grade neoplasm. Similarly, a cystic lesion with a mural nodule brings up a limited differential diagnosis, and evaluating a glial neoplasm without this information may lead to the incorrect diagnosis.

It is always helpful to know the surgeon's operative plan, and to know what is at stake. This information can be obtained quite easily by discussing the case with the surgeon.

Frozen sections

As a rule we do not perform FSs on stereotactic biopsies because of freezing artifacts that are present even after routine paraffin processing. We strongly recommend using cytological preparations, and in our department, this is the first step in the evaluation of all needle biopsies.

Frozen sections do, however, play a role in the evaluation of solid extra-axial lesions, such as meningiomas, schwannomas, and mesenchymal tumors because these specimens tend to produce poor quality cytologic preparations, they are better at withstanding the artifacts of freezing, and they are generally of sufficient volume to ensure that the bulk of the specimen is spared from freezing.[14]

One additional precautionary note about FSs on brain tissue: ice crystals formed in the tissue may mimic microcysts, a finding that may be mistaken for one of the characteristic features of pilocytic astrocytoma and oligodendroglioma (Fig. 17.1).

Cytologic preparations

Cytologic preparations are superior to FSs because the tissue is free of freezing artifact, and they provide a level

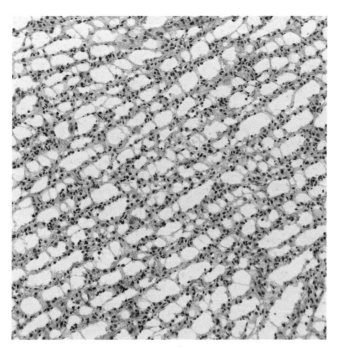

Fig. 17.1. Ice crystal artifact in a FS of an infiltrating astrocytoma. The spaces formed by ice crystals may be mistaken for microcysts, and cause the pathologist to consider pilocytic astrocytoma and oligodendroglioma, two neoplasms that frequently have microcysts.

of detail that cannot be achieved with FSs. Glial fibrils, Rosenthal fibers, granular bodies, ganglion cells, and cytologic atypia are all readily seen in glial neoplasms, and the cytologic features of metastatic carcinoma, metastatic melanoma, germ cell neoplasms, and lymphomas can be readily distinguished from malignant gliomas (Table 17.3; Fig. 17.2). In young patients with lesions in the pituitary area, cytologic preparations are ideal for recognizing lesions such as Langerhans cell histiocytosis and germinoma.

In a study of 5000 stereotactic biopsies, Tilgner et al. reported 90% correlation of intraoperative cytologic diagnoses with final histologic diagnoses,[15] and similar results have been reported by others.[16,17] Cytologic preparations do, however, have limitations: cellularity of glial neoplasms is more difficult to evaluate, architectural features are not as well seen as in FSs, mitoses are more difficult to find, some neoplasms such as some meningioma and schwannomas do not yield good monolayer preparations, and as with cytologic preparations from other anatomic sites, poorly prepared smears are difficult to interpret.

Of the three methods for making cytologic preparations, squash and smear preparations are by far the most favored in neuropathology because touch imprints tend to be paucicellular, and stereotactic biopsies are not suited to making scrape preparations. The way that the tissue sample smears often provides clues to the diagnosis (Table 17.4).

For stereotactic needle biopsies, we take a 1 mm piece from each end of the core, place them adjacent to one another on a glass slide, firmly squash both pieces of tissue simultaneously with a second slide, and then gently smear the material in the conventional way. Both slides are immediately placed in 95% alcohol and stained with H&E or hematoxylin and phloxine. In our practice we prefer phloxine because it highlights glial processes and provides better nuclear–cytoplasmic contrast.

Additional points about specimen handling

The pathologist who renders an IOD should triage the specimen for appropriate ancillary tests and make sure that these specimens are handled correctly. This includes collecting: (a) uncontaminated tissue for bacterial, fungal and viral cultures when infection is a consideration; (b) fresh tissue for flow cytometry when lymphoma and leukemia are considered; (c) fresh tissue for DNA/RNA studies, and to snap freeze the specimen to the appropriate temperature

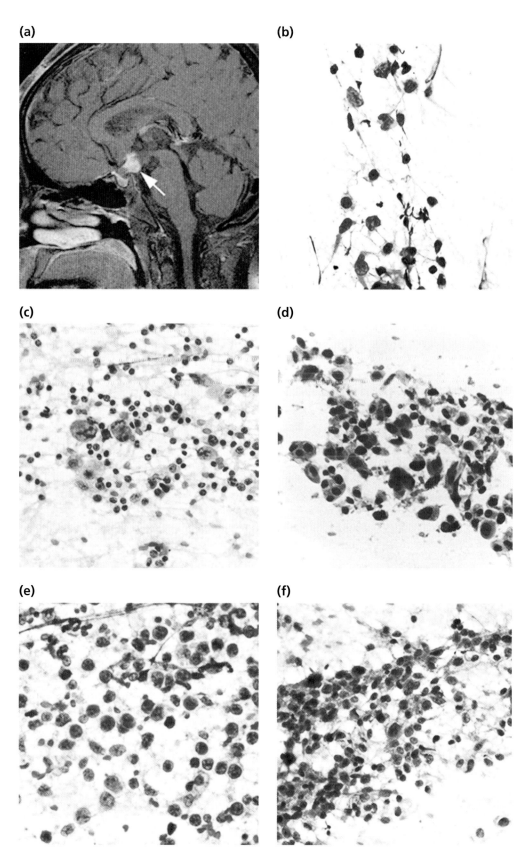

Fig. 17.2. Cytologic smear preparations. (a) Contrast enhancing lesion in the neurohypophysis in a child. (b) The cytology preparation of this lesion shows histiocytes with nuclear folds, characteristic of Langerhans cells. (c) Cytologic smears are also useful in the evaluation of germinomas, (d) metastatic carcinoma, (e) large B-cell lymphoma, and (f) melanoma. Note that pigment is frequently absent in metastatic melanoma to the CNS, but large epithelioid cells with atypical nuclei and a single macronucleolus are characteristic.

for future use; (d) placing tissue in a carrier medium for cytogenetics; (e) placing 1mm fragments of fresh tissue in gluteraldehyde for electron microscopy; (f) ordering immunohistochemical stains and unstained sections in advance to expedite the diagnosis.

Table 17.3. Useful cytologic clues in smears of CNS lesions

Microscopic feature	Differential diagnosis
EGB	Ganglioglioma, pilocytic astrocytoma, PXA, (coarse and fine EGBs)
Rosenthal fibers	Pilocytic astrocytoma, piloid gliosis
Macrophages	Demyelinating disease, infarct, treated lymphoma
Rhabdoid cells	ATRT, rhabdoid meningioma, rarely high-grade astrocytoma
Small cells (high nuclear/cytoplasmic ratio, scant processes)	Small cell astrocytoma, central PNET, Ewing sarcoma/PNET, medulloblastoma
Tight cell clusters	Metastatic carcinoma, meningioma
Ghost cells	Craniopharyngioma
Papillae	Choroid plexus tumor, ependymoma, metastatic carcinoma
Pigment	Melanin (melanoma, melanocytoma), lipofuscin (schwannoma, ependymoma)

PXA = plemorphic xanthoastrocytoma; EGB = eosinophilic granular bodies; ATRT = atypical teratoid-rhabdoid tumor; PNET = primitive neuroectodermal tumor.

SPECIFIC CLINICO-PATHOLOGIC ISSUES

Distinguishing normal from abnormal tissue

Because the architecture and cellular components of the CNS vary so much from site to site, the normal histology for the biopsy site should always be considered before concluding that the tissue is abnormal (Fig. 17.3). The following points should be kept in mind:

- There are differences in cell density between gray and white matter, with oligodendrocytes imparting a more cellular appearance to white matter; this feature is even

Table 17.4. Tissue consistency during smear preparations

Property	Tumor entities
Do not smear well	Schwannomas, desmoplastic or mesenchymal tumors, some meningiomas (fibrous variant), hemangioblastoma, normal pituitary
Smears well, but with slight effort	Most gliomas, pituitary adenoma, some meningiomas (meningothelial variant), craniopharyngiomas, choroid plexus tumors, some metastases
Smears smoothly	Normal brain, medulloblastoma, ATRT, lymphoma, abscess content, demyelinating diseases, melanoma

ATRT = atypical teratoid-rhabdoid tumor.

(a)   **(b)**

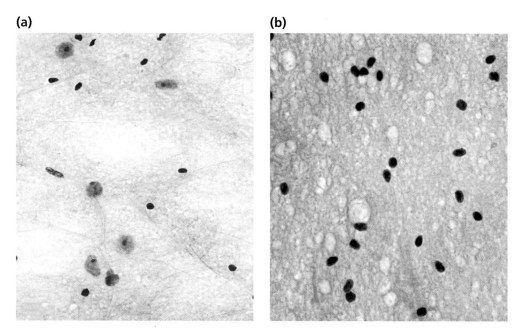

Fig. 17.3. Cytologic smears of normal CNS tissue. (a) Stripped neurons in smears of the cortex may be misinterpreted as neoplastic cells because of the large nucleus and prominent nucleolus. (b) Oligodendrocytes are more plentiful in white matter and should not be mistaken for neoplastic cells.

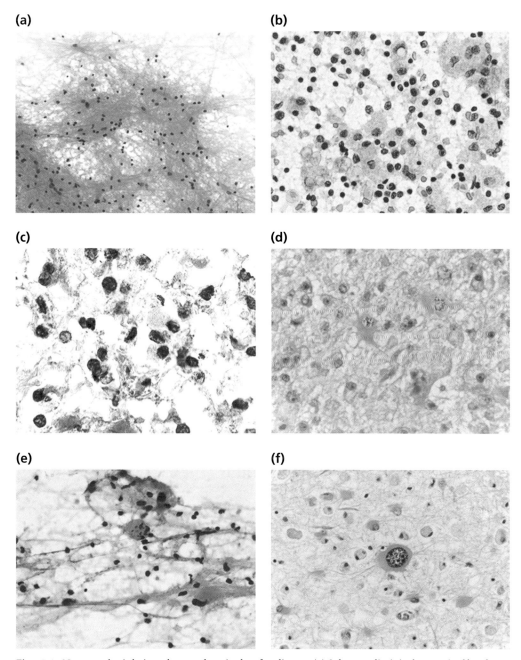

Fig. 17.4. Non-neoplastic lesions that may be mistaken for gliomas. (a) Subacute gliosis is characterized by plump astrocytes with numerous fine radiating processes, and with even spacing between cells. (b) Macrophages are readily seen in smear preparations and should suggest a non-neoplastic process. (c) In active demyelination, macrophages and reactive astrocytes may appear atypical in FSs and be mistaken for neoplastic cells. (d) Granular mitoses and (e) Creutzfeldt cells are frequently found in reactive conditions, particularly in demyelination. (f) Enlarged bizarre astrocytes, accompanied by macrophages, are typical of progressive multifocal encephalopathy.

more pronounced in patients with chronic seizures because of oligodendroglial hyperplasia.

- Normal cells may cause concern when they are altered by artifact. As an example, when neurons are stripped of their cytoplasm in cytologic preparations, their large bare nuclei with prominent nucleoli may be alarming when viewed out of context.

The highly cellular granular layer of the cerebellum may be misinterpreted as a small cell malignancy, such as medulloblastoma or lymphoma, if the pathologist does not pay attention to the biopsy site. However, when the anatomic site is taken into account, it will become abundantly clear that the tissue is normal because of the uniform distribution of the small cells, their round nuclei – each with a small centrally located nucleolus – and the presence of Purkinje cells.

Reactive conditions: gliosis and macrophage-rich lesions

Clinical issues

Most reactive and inflammatory conditions have characteristic clinical and radiographic findings, and are not confused for neoplasms. However, the clinical and imaging findings are atypical in a minority of cases; for example, active demyelination may cause mass effect with ring enhancement (i.e., "tumefactive multiple sclerosis") and mimic a neoplasm. Stereotactic biopsy is performed to make this distinction.

Pathologic issues

Reactive lesions can be challenging because they may resemble glial neoplasms; in addition, if the lesion is recognized as reactive intraoperatively, the pathologist has to decide if the biopsy is representative of the lesion, or if it is from reactive tissue adjacent to a neoplasm. This explains why clinico-pathologic correlation is so important, and why additional biopsies should be requested if there is any doubt about the adequacy of the specimen. Reactive/inflammatory processes have diverse appearances, mimicking different types of neoplasms. A few of the main patterns are discussed below (Fig. 17.4).

Subacute gliosis is a non-specific reaction to a variety of CNS injuries, but also occurs as a secondary reaction to primary neoplasms and at the periphery of metastatic neoplasms. Key features that distinguish subacute gliosis from low grade infiltrating astrocytomas include the even spacing of astrocytes, an increase in the size of astrocytes but not their number, finely radiating pericellular processes, lack of mitotic activity, and absence of significant nuclear atypia on frozen sections and cytologic preparations. In contrast, the presence of cell clustering, cytologic atypia, microcysts, calcifications and mitoses favor a glioma.

Piloid gliosis is a chronic reaction to long-standing non-neoplastic processes such as spinal cord syrinx and slow growing tumors such as craniopharyngioma and hemangioblastoma. The lesion is characterized by gliosis with an accumulation of Rosenthal fibers, so the main distinction is from pilocytic astrocytoma. Piloid gliosis lacks microcysts and cytologic atypia, but clinical and radiologic data are critical to making the correct diagnosis.

Macrophage-rich lesions. Macrophages in a cytologic smear should prompt consideration of a non-neoplastic condition. Macrophages are more easily identified in cytologic smears than on FS, underscoring the importance of making cytologic preparations routinely. *Creutzfeldt cells* and *granular mitoses*, although not limited to reactive lesions, are especially common in active demyelination, and their presence should suggest some type of demyelinating process. Progressive multifocal leukoencephalopathy, a distinct, macrophage-rich demyelinating disorder caused by the JC virus, occurs in immunosuppressed patients and results in enlarged, often bizarre-appearing astrocytes that mimic a glial neoplasm. The presence of macrophages, and viral inclusions in oligodendrocytes, are clues to the diagnosis.

Infarcts are encountered in stereotactic biopsies only when the imaging findings are atypical, and a neoplasm cannot be excluded on clinical grounds. Early infarcts may show endothelial hyperplasia, which could be mistaken for vascular proliferation associated with gliomas. However, red hypoxic neurons and/or neutrophils are usually present, and are useful clues to the diagnosis. Older infarcts will have gliosis and aggregates of macrophages. Again, the presence of macrophages is strongly suggestive of a non-neoplastic process.

The heterogeneity of gliomas in stereotactic needle biopsies

Clinical issues

Diffusely infiltrating gliomas comprise the majority of primary brain tumors. All are considered malignant, ranging from low to high grade (WHO grade II–IV), with glioblastoma multiforme, the most frequent neoplasm in this group, representing the highest grade. Most glioblastomas occur in older patients who present with a short clinical history and without a histologically identifiable low grade precursor ("*de novo* glioblastoma"). A minority of glioblastomas are secondary and occur after transformation of lower grade (grade II–III) infiltrating astrocytomas. Oligodendrogliomas are either low grade (WHO grade II) or anaplastic (WHO grade III); in addition, mixed gliomas with oligodendroglial and astrocytic morphology (oligoastrocytomas) are often encountered and are graded in the same way as oligodendrogliomas.

Given the heterogeneity of glial neoplasms, the surgeon's goal is to biopsy the imaging abnormality that represents the highest grade region within the neoplasm, as this will determine post-operative treatment as well as reflect the patient's prognosis. Imaging studies are relied

(a)

(b)

(c)

(d)

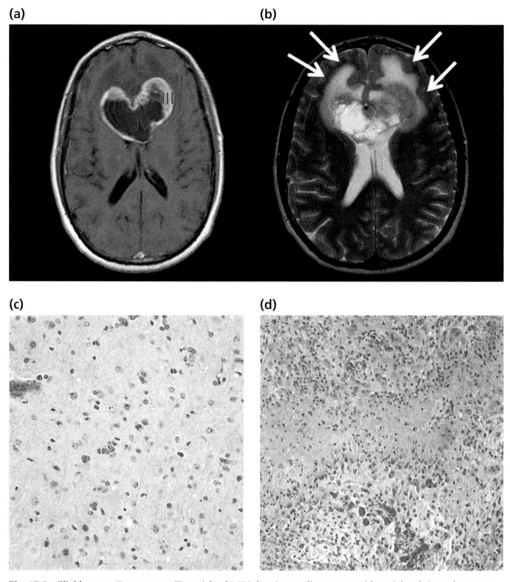

Fig. 17.5. Glioblastoma. Post-contrast T1-weighted MRI showing a solitary mass, with peripheral ring enhancement, extending across the corpus callosum. (a) Stereotactic biopsies may show grades II, III or IV glioma depending on the area sampled. (b) The T2 weighted MRI demonstrates increased signal beyond the limit of enhancement noted in (a); this is due to a mixture of peritumoral edema and infiltrating tumor of varying cellularity (arrows). (c) Biopsy samples from the periphery of a glioblastoma may lack mitotic activity, necrosis and endothelial proliferation, look deceptively bland, and be mistaken for a grade II astrocytoma if interpreted out of context. (d) Other areas of the same tumor show diagnostic features of glioblastoma, including pseudopallisading and necrosis.

upon to guide the biopsy site and are an integral part of planning stereotactic biopsy (Fig. 17.5).

Pathologic issues
While imaging studies are helpful in guiding the precise site of stereotactic biopsy, the surgeon depends on the pathologist to confirm that the highest grade component of the neoplasm has been sampled. The pathologist can offer this service only if she is familiar with the clinical and imaging aspects of the case, and is familiar with the surgeon's goals.

When there is discordance between the imaging and the pathologic findings in the initial stereotactic biopsy, the pathologist should report this discrepancy to the surgeon and make a request for additional biopsies.

Issues regarding high-grade neoplasms in adults

Clinical issues
The most frequently encountered high-grade tumors in the CNS are glioblastoma, metastases, and lymphoma. It is

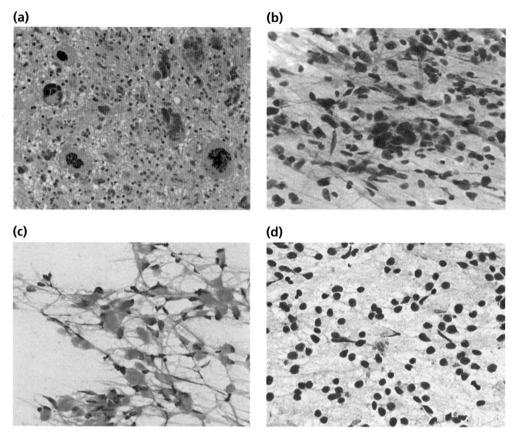

Fig. 17.6. Glioblastoma, showing the wide range of cell types that may appear in pure form or in combination: (a) giant cell, (b) fibrillary, (c) gemistocytic, and (d) small cell patterns.

important to distinguish lymphoma from other malignancies because it is treated with irradiation and/or chemotherapy, and debulking is contraindicated. High grade gliomas may be resected aggressively, especially in young patients, and when the neoplasm is located in accessible, non- eloquent locations such as the frontal lobe. The role of aggressive surgical resection of metastases has shifted as radiosurgery has gained favor as a way to treat these lesions.

Pathologic issues
If the specimen is a stereotactic biopsy, the purpose of IOD is to confirm that adequate diagnostic tissue is present in the specimen; precise classification of the malignancy is of secondary importance. On the other hand, if the surgeon does an open procedure and is planning a subtotal resection, then distinguishing lymphoma from other high grade malignancies is the main goal of IOD. The presence of glial processes facilitates the identification of glioblastoma in smears, although glioblastomas demonstrate remarkable histologic variation, including the presence of fibrillary, gemistocytic, small

and giant cells (Fig. 17.6). Even a partly neuronal immunophenotype or malignant mesenchymal components ("gliosarcoma") may be seen. These cell and tissue variations are generally not of prognostic importance but the pathologist should be familiar with these variants to avoid misdiagnosis. The cytologic and histologic features of lymphoma and metastases are discussed below under specific sections.

Oligodendrogliomas

Oligodendrogliomas are a subset of diffusely infiltrating gliomas that have a better prognosis than their astrocytic counterparts and therefore are important to recognize.

Most arise superficially, involve the cerebral cortex and are composed of round cells with delicate chromatin, small nucleoli, a small skirt of cytoplasm and scanty cytoplasmic processes (Fig. 17.7). Perinuclear halos, an artifact of fixation, are either absent or inconspicuous in cytologic preparations as well as on FSs. Anaplastic oligodendrogliomas (WHO grade III) are more cellular, demonstrate brisk mitotic activity and endothelial hypertrophy, and

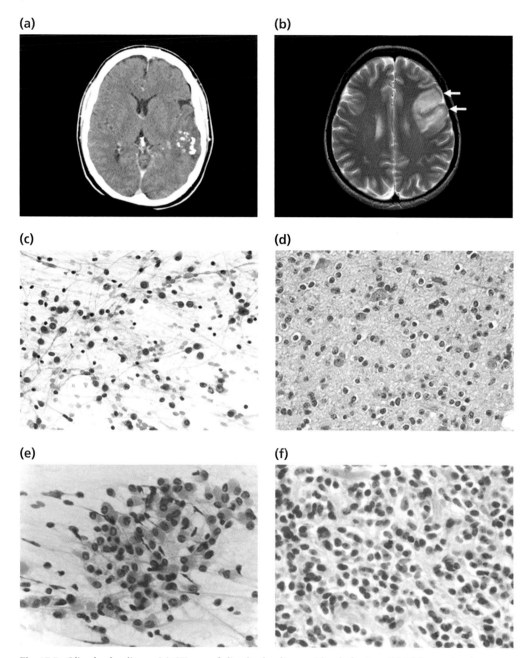

Fig. 17.7. Oligodendroglioma. (a) CT scan of oligodendroglioma with calcification. (b) MRI scan that shows two common features of oligodendrogliomas : superficial location and cortical thickening (arrows). (c) In cytologic smears, the cells have round nuclei, fine nuclear chromatin, and small nucleoli, with scanty cytoplasm and cell processes. (d) Perineuronal satellitosis is a hallmark of oligodendroglioma. (e) Minigemistocytes, which are common in oligodendroglioma, may be confusing because the dense cytoplasm and eccentrically placed nuclei may bring other neoplasms to mind, but they have the characteristic nuclear features of oligodendroglioma. (f) Endothelial hypertrophy and brisk mitotic activity are features of anaplastic oligodendroglioma.

are generally more cellular than their low-grade (grade II) counterparts. At times, it is difficult to distinguish oligodendroglioma from astrocytoma, and this is particularly difficult on FSs because freezing masks the usual morphologic hallmarks of oligodendroglioma, including nuclear roundness, delicate chromasia, and perinuclear halos (Fig. 17.8). The intraoperative distinction, however, is not

crucial as the surgical approach to oligodrendroglioma is the same as for infiltrating astrocyoma of similar grade.

The distinction from astrocytoma is more important on permanent sections because of the favorable prognosis attributed to co-deletion of chromosome arms 1p and 19q,[20] a test that can be performed by FISH on routinely processed, paraffin embedded sections.

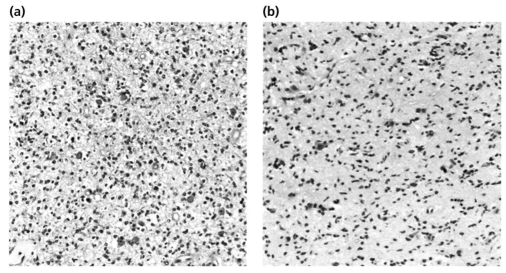

Fig. 17.8. Frozen section artifact in oligodendroglioma. (a) Non-frozen material shows the classical cytologic features of a grade II oligodendroglioma in particular round nuclei and perinuclear halos. (b) Same case after being frozen: the freezing process obscures the cytological features of oligodendroglioma by producing nuclear distortion and hyperchromasia, features that mimic an astrocytic neoplasm.

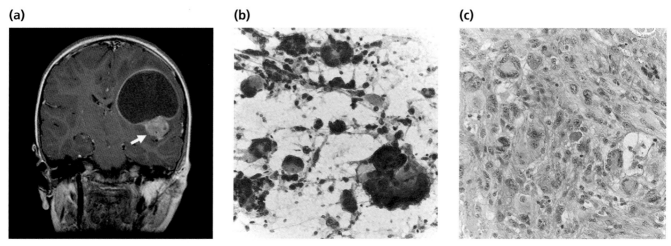

Fig. 17.9. Pleomorphic xanthoastrocytoma (PXA). (a) A cyst with enhancing mural nodule (arrow) is characteristic of tumors with a favorable prognosis, such as PXA. (b) The smear cytology preparation shows marked pleomorphism, mimicking a high grade glioma but (c) granular bodies, xanthic cells and paucity of mitoses are clues to the correct diagnosis.

Circumscribed gliomas and glioneuronal tumors

Clinical issues

There is a group of glial and glioneuronal neoplasms that are circumscribed, have very low likelihood of aggressive behavior or progression to anaplastic glioma, and are generally amenable to cure by surgical resection. This category includes *pilocytic astrocytoma, pleomorphic xanthoastrocytoma* and *ganglioglioma*. All show a predilection for children and young adults, and on imaging, show circumscription, contrast enhancement, and in many instances, are cystic with a mural nodule (Fig. 17.9).

Pathologic issues

Pilocytic astrocytoma (WHO grade I) occurs at any level of the neuraxis, but shows a predilection for the cerebellum, optic nerve/chiasm, and hypothalamic region. It occurs with increased frequency in neurofibromatosis type 1. Histologic hallmarks include compact bipolar cells with brightly eosinophilic processes and Rosenthal fibers (Fig. 17.10). Loose-textured areas with microcysts and eosinophilic granular bodies are found in the second main pattern. The two patterns are often seen in combination.

Pilomyxoid astrocytoma, a recently described variant of pilocytic astrocytoma, shows a predilection for the

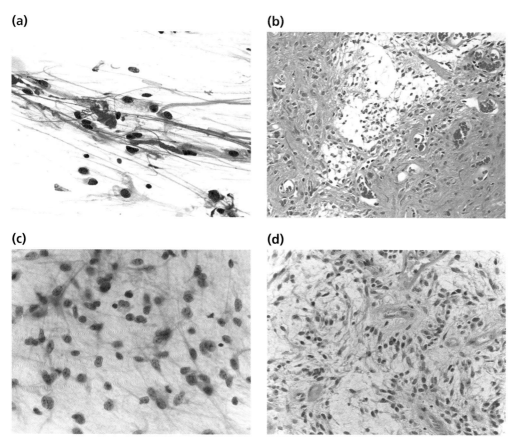

Fig. 17.10. Pilocytic astrocytoma. (a) Smear preparation showing pilocytic cells and Rosenthal fibers. (b) Histologically, a biphasic pattern is characteristic, with alternating compact and loose areas with microcysts. (c) Pilomyxoid astrocytoma demonstrates similar cytologic features, featuring bipolar cells with elongated processes, but lacks Rosenthal fibers and granular bodies. (d) Histologically, pilomyxoid astrocytoma has a monophasic architecture, with conspicuous perivascular pseudorosettes.

hypothalamic region of young children and behaves more aggressively than conventional pilocytic tumors.[22] The current WHO classification assigns it grade II status. The lesion is characterized by monomorphic, elongated cells, often disposed in perivascular arrays; Rosenthal fibers and granular bodies are absent (Fig. 17.10). A firm distinction from ordinary pilocytic astrocytoma is not possible intraoperatively, but can be suspected when accompanied by a "drop metastasis."

Ganglioglioma is a low grade tumor that shows a predilection for the temporal lobe and is typically associated with chronic seizures. It is a biphasic tumor, with a bland glial component admixed with dysmorphic ganglion cells. Eosinophilic granular bodies and Rosenthal fibers are often conspicuous (Fig. 17.11). This neoplasm has to be distinguished from astrocytoma with entrapped neurons, a distinction that is made by finding clusters of dysmorphic ganglion cells (including binucleated forms) and intracytoplasmic filamentous whorls.

Pleomorphic xanthoastrocytoma is a pleomorphic astrocytoma that may be mistaken for a high-grade malignant glioma because of marked cellular pleomorphism (Fig. 17.9). This neoplasm is distinguished from high grade astrocytoma by the presence of eosinophilic granular bodies, combined with the lack of necrosis, endothelial cell proliferation and significant mitotic activity. The clinical history and imaging findings are very important. Relatively young age, superficial location, and a cyst with a mural nodule, strongly support this diagnosis, no matter how much pleomorphism is present. When the imaging findings are characteristic, the surgeon will approach the lesion by open craniotomy, with the intent of achieving complete resection. Distinguishing this neoplasm from high grade astrocytoma is important.

Recurrent gliomas and treatment effect

Clinical issues

High grade gliomas (WHO grade III and IV) are usually treated by radiation therapy with or without adjuvant chemotherapy. Radiation necrosis, which has a latency period

(a)

(b)

(c)

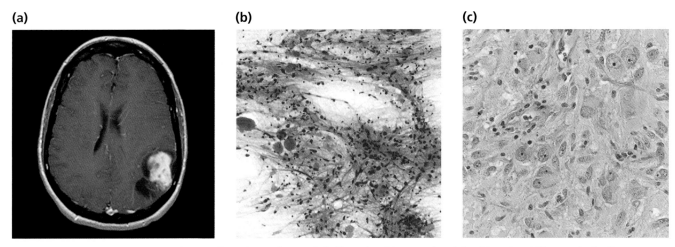

Fig. 17.11. (a) Ganglioglioma is another neoplasm that is characteristically cystic with a mural nodule. (b) Eosinophilic granular bodies are more conspicuous in ganglioglioma than in other tumors in the differential diagnosis tumors, a feature that is readily identified in smears. (c) Clusters of dysmorphic cells, binucleate cells and eosinophilic granular bodies are typical of this neoplasm.

of 6 months to 2 years, may result in a mass, as well as produce symptoms, and it then becomes necessary to distinguish radiation necrosis from recurrent tumor.[23] PET scans aid in the distinction by demonstrating far higher metabolic activity in tumors, but is not always definitive, and biopsy is often required. Radiation necrosis may be encountered in stereotactic biopsy or specimens obtained by open craniotomy. A variable degree of residual tumor is nearly always present – the greater the extent, the less favorable the prognosis.

Pathologic issues
A distinction has to be made between (a) radiation change in non-neoplastic tissue, (b) radiation-altered neoplasm, and (c) recurrent, actively growing glioma, distinctions that may be difficult to make intraoperatively, and sometimes require deferral to permanent sections. When the specimen is a stereotactic needle biopsy, the purpose of IOD is to determine if the sample is adequate. The following points require attention intraoperatively.

- Radiation necrosis has to be distinguished from the necrosis of glioblastoma. Unlike the sharply defined, abrupt areas of necrosis with palisading that is typical of glioblastoma, radiation necrosis is geographic and affects parenchyma as well as blood vessels, sometimes with recognizable fibrin impregnation or fibro-obliterative changes in blood vessels. If the initial core biopsy is composed predominantly of necrotic tissue, the surgeon should be asked to obtain additional biopsies.

- It may not be possible to make the distinction between quiescent, radiation-treated neoplastic tissue and actively proliferating, recurrent glioma

intraoperatively because the differences are subtle. The cells in quiescent glioma tend to have more cytoplasm, lack mitotic activity, and on permanent sections, show a low proliferation index as evaluated with MIB-1 staining. When the changes suggest quiescent glioma, the pathologist should consult with the surgeon to determine if the biopsies are representative of the imaging abnormality or if additional biopsies should be obtained.

- Radiation-induced reactive astrocytes have enlarged nuclei and abundant cytoplasm, and while atypical, they can be distinguished from neoplastic, proliferative glial cells (Fig. 17.12)

- The pathologist is expected to document tumor progression in a treated glioma, a task that may have to be deferred to permanent sections. The necrosis of radiation therapy should not be used to upgrade a glioma; conversely, necrosis with pseudopalisading is evidence of high grade glioma and not radionecrosis.

Meningiomas

Clinical issues
Meningiomas represent 25%–30% of intracranial neoplasms. Most affect middle-aged and elderly patients and show a female predominance, especially in the spinal dura. Meningiomas have very characteristic imaging findings (Fig. 17.13), and as a rule of thumb, a solitary mass lesion attached to the dura is a meningioma until proven otherwise. Additional imaging features include homogeneous, low T2 signal on MRI, and marked homogeneous

(a) (b)

(c) (d)

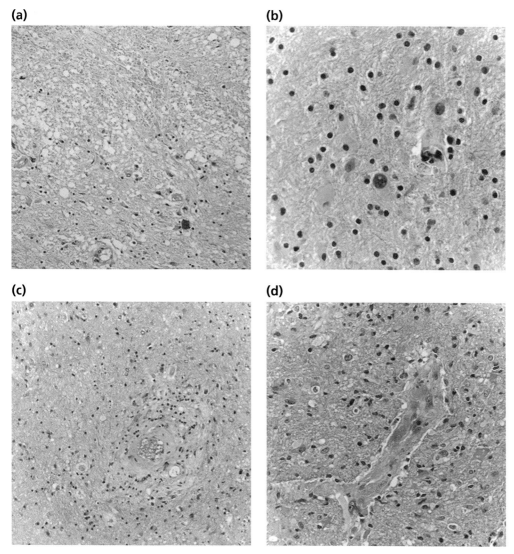

Fig. 17.12. Radiation changes in a high grade glioma. The changes include (a) radiation necrosis and (b) quiescent glioma, characterized by cytomegaly and nucleomegaly. Vascular changes include (c) vascular hyalinization and (d) prominent endothelial cells.

enhancement. The surgical approach to meningioma is open craniotomy with complete removal, including involved dura, when feasible. The surgical treatment of atypical meningioma is not any different, but this is a moot point because the diagnosis of atypical meningioma is done more reliably on permanent sections.

Pathologic issues

The vast majority of meningiomas have a characteristic solid, whorled appearance, composed of spindle or oval cells with frequent intranuclear inclusions (Fig. 17.13). Unless overtly anaplastic, meningiomas may be difficult to grade on the basis of FS since mitoses, the most important parameter, may be difficult to identify. The assessment of atypia or anaplasia, therefore is best made on permanent sections.

Brain invasion is a significant prognostic factor in otherwise low-grade meningiomas. In general, there is poor correlation between the surgeon's impression of brain invasion and its histologic demonstration; the evaluation of brain invasion is best done on permanent sections by sampling the tumor/brain interface. The presence of brain invasion alone qualifies for the diagnosis of grade II or "atypical meningioma."

While conventional meningioma is easily recognized, less common variants may cause considerable diagnostic difficulty, and the best way to make the correct diagnosis is to be familiar with these variants. Chordoid meningioma may be mistaken for chordoma; *clear cell, microcystic,* and *angiomatous* meningiomas may be interpreted as metastatic renal cell carcinoma, *secretory* and *papillary*

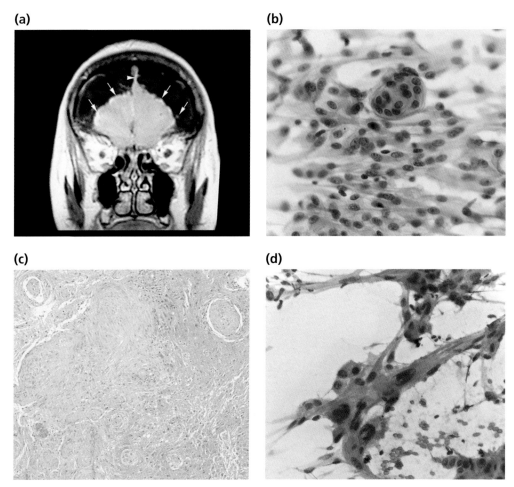

Fig. 17.13. (a) Large bifrontal meningioma (arrows) with typical broad enhancing dural tail on the falx, a highly characteristic finding (arrowhead) (b) Cytologic preparations often show the typical architectural features of meningioma, including whorls, but smears are not useful for grading. (c) Brain invasion may be identified on FS and is of prognostic significance. (d) Nuclear pleomorphism by itself does not affect the prognosis of meningiomas.

meningioma mimic metastatic adenocarcinoma, *fibrous* meningiomas resemble solitary fibrous tumor, and *lymphoplasmacytic* meningioma may be misdiagnosed as a lymphoproliferative process. Familiarity with the clinical and imaging findings will help to correctly interpret uncommon variants of meningioma because a solitary dura-based mass is highly likely to be a meningioma. In contrast, metastases to the dura are usually multiple and occur in patients who have a known malignancy

Primary versus metastatic neoplasm

Clinical issues

Metastatic tumors that involve the parenchyma of the CNS are primarily metastases from lung, breast, and kidney, or melanomas. Choriocarcinoma is rare, but is highly neurotropic. Brain metastases usually occur in patients with a known primary but occasionally, the primary is occult, or the history is overlooked, as with a cutaneous melanoma removed in the distant past. The diagnosis of metastatic neoplasm is readily made when there is a supportive clinical history, and when there are multiple lesions with disproportionate edema (Fig. 17.14). Clinical uncertainty occurs when the patient has a solitary lesion, and imaging characteristics do not allow discrimination between a metastasis and a high grade primary malignancy. In this situation, the diagnosis could be made either by stereotactic biopsy or open resection – depending on the clinical and imaging findings.

Pathologic issues

The diagnosis of metastasis is easily made when the neoplasm shows distinct non-glial differentiation such as gland formation, squamous differentiation and melanin pigment

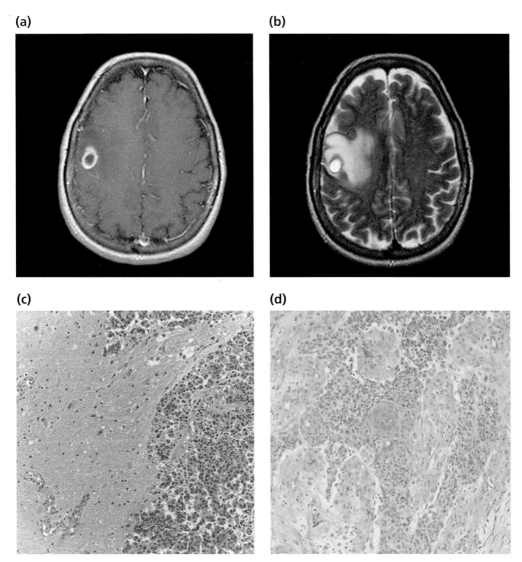

Fig. 17.14. Metastatic carcinomas frequently exhibit (a) ring enhancement and (b) massive edema, disproportionate to the size of the lesion. (c) A sharp interface with brain parenchyma is characteristic. Metastatic carcinoma has to be distinguished from (d) epithelioid glioblastoma.

production. Glioblastoma may be difficult to distinguish from metastatic carcinoma in some instances, especially the adenoid variant in which tumor cells appear small and cohesive, epithelioid, or even show true epithelial differentiation (Fig. 17.14). The presence of convincing, single tumor cell invasion of the parenchyma away from the main lesion is a useful clue to the diagnosis of glioblastoma (Fig. 17.5).

Metastatic renal cell carcinoma can be a problem because it often presents with a clinically occult primary tumor. When metastatic clear cell renal carcinoma occurs in the posterior fossa, it may be difficult to distinguish from hemangioblastoma, as both neoplasms are vascular and contain cytoplasmic lipid. The precise diagnosis

may have to be deferred to permanent sections; fortunately, both neoplasms are treated by complete resection.

Lymphoproliferative lesions

Clinical issues

The vast majority of primary lymphomas of the CNS are diffuse large B-cell lymphomas. They are usually multifocal and often periventricular in location. Ring enhancement, a reflection of necrosis, is typical of primary CNS lymphomas occurring in patients who are immunocompromised. Key imaging features include hyperdensity on CT scans, and homogeneous enhancement after contrast administration.

(a)

(b)

(c)

(d)

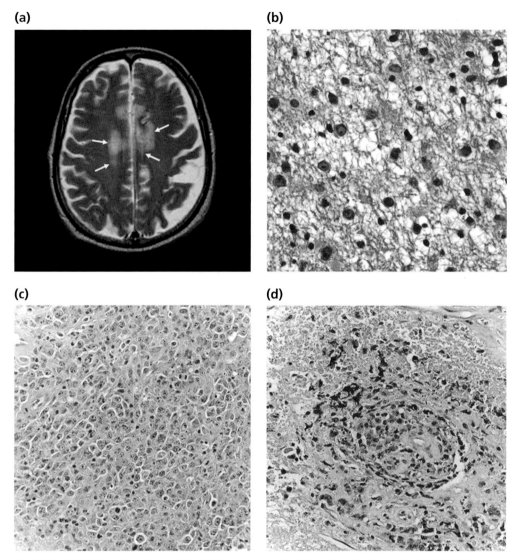

Fig. 17.15. (a) Primary lymphoma of the CNS usually involves the periventricular region of the brain. (b) Occasionally, lymphoma cells infiltrate the adjacent brain as isolated tumor cells, (c) but a sheet-like growth pattern and (d) angiocentricity are more characteristic.

Occasionally, lymphoma may present as a solitary mass and mimic a high grade glioma on imaging studies.

When lymphoma is likely, the tumor will be approached by stereotactic biopsy because aggressive resection is inappropriate and has a high morbidity.

Pathologic issues

Cytologic preparations are very useful in the evaluation of primary CNS lymphoma. Single, dyscohesive large cells with vesicular nuclei, prominent nucleoli and apoptosis are characteristic (Fig. 17.15). On FS, there is a perivascular "tree bark-" like aggregation of tumor cells, as well as brain invasion by isolated tumor cells (Fig. 17.15). Pre-operative treatment with steroids, administered to reduce raised intracranial pressure, induces marked changes including

widespread apoptosis, and at times, there is extensive lysis of neoplastic lymphocytes, leaving behind histiocytes and reactive astrocytes, changes that may be mistaken for a demyelinating disease.

Small blue cell tumors

Clinical issues

A variety of tumors, characterized by "round" or "small blue" cells, involve the CNS. All are high-grade tumors with aggressive behavior. Because treatments are varied and depend on the type of tumor, it is essential to make a specific diagnosis. As an example, medulloblastoma and supratentorial PNET require craniospinal irradiation with or without specific adjuvant chemotherapy because of the proclivity for leptomeningeal spread, whereas small cell astrocytomas are treated with irradiation to the affected compartment alone. Age and specific location help to narrow the differential diagnosis. For most of these tumors, the goal is to perform gross total resection if feasible. When resection is planned, an incisional biopsy may first be performed to confirm the provisional clinical diagnosis, followed by gross total resection.

Pathologic issues

While a specific diagnosis will eventually be needed, the purpose of IOD is to determine if sufficient diagnostic tissue has been obtained. At times, a specific diagnosis can be made intraoperatively when the pathologic findings, combined with clinical findings, point to a single diagnosis, e.g. medulloblastoma. In all other situations however, it is good enough to make a diagnosis of "small round cell malignant tumor," and to defer the specific diagnosis to permanent sections. When the surgical procedure is limited to a biopsy, the pathologist should ensure that sufficient tissue is available for ancillary studies.

Medulloblastoma is a high-grade (WHO grade IV) neoplasm that usually affects children and adolescents; by definition, this tumor arises in the cerebellum. This cellular neoplasm is composed of small oval cells with high nuclear/cytoplasmic ratio, hyperchromatic nuclei, inconspicuous nucleoli, frequent mitoses and apoptotic activity (Fig. 17.16). It is important to avoid the error of interpreting the normal granular layer of the cerebellum as medulloblastoma; the cells of the normal granular layer have uniform round nuclei and lack hyperchromasia, mitotic activity, and apoptosis. The linear arrangement of Purkinje cells is another clue to correct interpretation.

Tumors resembling medulloblastoma that occur in other areas of the CNS are termed *primitive neuroectodermal tumors* ("central neuroectodermal tumors"). Their histologic features are more varied than those of medulloblastoma and overlap with those of *small cell astrocytomas*. Although central PNETs tend to be more circumscribed, the specific diagnosis should be deferred to permanent sections. *Ewing sarcoma/peripheral primitive neuroectodermal tumors*, which have identical immunophenotypic and molecular features as their soft tissue/bone counterparts, involve the dura, or affect the lumbosacral region and may mimic meningioma on imaging. They usually occur in children and adolescents. In a very young child (<2 years of age), a small round blue cell tumor should prompt consideration of *atypical teratoid rhabdoid tumor* (ATRT) since a

significant "primitive" component is often present. Rhabdoid cells are characteristic but they may not be abundant, especially in small biopsy samples. Such tumors, characterized in part by EMA immunoreactivity and inactivating mutations of the tumor suppressor gene *INI1/SMARCB1*, are extremely aggressive and are treated differently from medulloblastoma. About half of the tumors occur in the posterior fossa, but they may also occur supratentorially. *Desmoplastic small round cell tumors* rarely affect the central nervous system; they exhibit a characteristic immunophenotype and molecular genetic profile. It is extremely rare for *lymphoma* in childhood to present as an isolated parenchymal mass.

It is often difficult to correctly classify a small round blue cell tumor intraoperatively. Fortunately, a specific diagnosis is not needed for immediate surgical management; the pathologist should ensure that there is sufficient tissue for conventional and ancillary tests such as electron microscopy (E.M.) and molecular genetic analysis.

Specific problems encountered with lesions of the spinal cord

Clinical issues

The differential diagnosis for intramedullary lesions includes ependymoma, pilocytic astrocytoma, infiltrating astrocytoma, hemangioblastoma and metastasis. One of the purposes of pre-operative imaging tests is to determine if the lesion is circumscribed and resectable, or infiltrating and non-resectable. Ependymoma, pilocytic astrocytoma, hemangioblastoma, and some metastases are circumscribed and resectable, whereas infiltrating gliomas are not, and will be subject to biopsy only. Ependymoma, which is the most common intramedullary tumor of the spinal cord, is usually suspected on clinical grounds, and the surgeon will attempt complete surgical excision because this offers the best chance of cure.[24]

Pathologic Issues

The surgeon will usually submit an incisional biopsy for IOD to confirm the provisional pre-operative diagnosis. Biopsies of the spinal cord tend to be small, and for this reason, a cytologic preparation should be performed as the initial test, and not a FS. Circumscription versus infiltrating characteristics cannot be determined on an incisional biopsy, so the imaging data should be correlated with the pathologic findings. In *ependymoma* the presence of perivascular pseudorosettes are an important clue to the

(a)

(b)

(c)

(d)

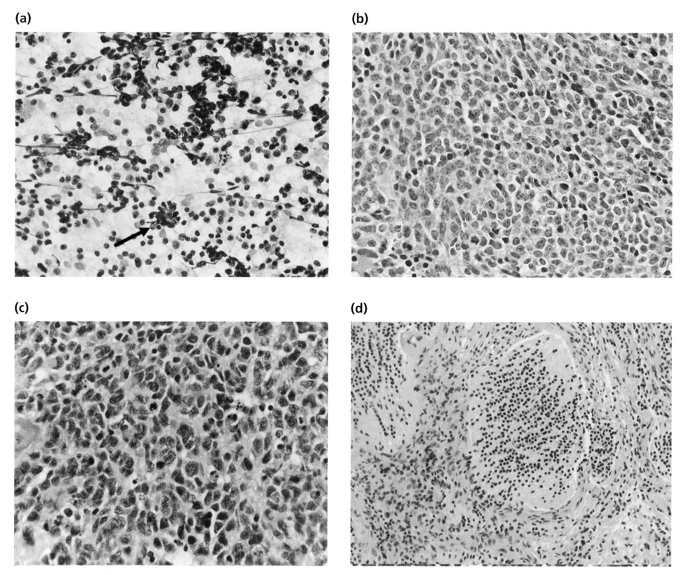

Fig. 17.16. Medulloblastoma. (a) Cytologic preparation showing isolated neoplastic cells with occasional rosettes (arrow). (b) Sheet-like growth in a classic medulloblastoma. (c) The anaplastic change is characterized by nuclear enlargement, molding, apoptotic bodies and mitoses. (d) Neuropil-rich nodules, a reflection of neuronal differentiation, is diagnostic of medulloblastoma in a small round blue cell tumor located in the posterior fossa.

diagnosis (Fig. 17.17). In addition, ependymoma cells have oval nuclei with fine chromatin and shorter processes than infiltrating astrocytomas. When ependymoma cannot be confidently distinguished from an infiltrating glioma, a piece of fresh tumor tissue should be placed in gluteraldehyde because the diagnosis can be made with confidence on E.M. *Myxopapillary ependymoma* occurs almost exclusively in the distal spinal cord and/or filum terminale region. The mucoid stroma with cuff of neoplastic cells surrounding vessels is characteristic of this tumor. *Schwannoma* and *paraganglioma* also enter into consideration. *Chordoma* enters the differential diagnosis, but it involves bone and rarely the spinal epidural space; histologicaly, it has a lobular growth pattern and has physaliferous

cells without perivascular cuffing. *Extramedullary* tumors include meningiomas, nerve sheath tumors, and paraganglioma of the filum terminale.

Evaluation of margins

Unlike in other areas in surgical pathology, the evaluation of resection margins plays a limited role in tumors of the CNS. For most tumors, including diffuse astrocytomas and metastases, the evaluation of margins is neither practical nor necessary. Some examples where evaluation of margins may be required include ependymoma, meningiomas at the base of the skull, and malignant peripheral nerve sheath tumors.

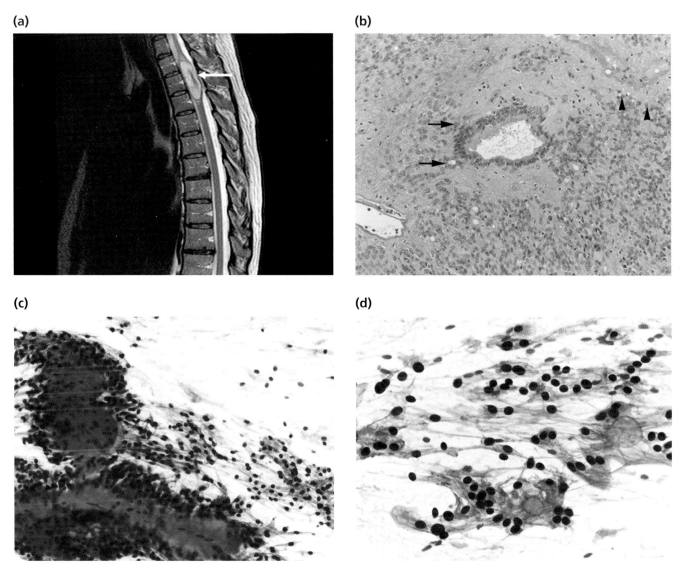

(a) **(b)**

(c) **(d)**

Fig. 17.17. (a) Ependymoma of the spinal cord, forming a solid circumscribed mass. (b) The histologic hallmarks of ependymoma are perivascular pseudorosettes (arrowheads) and true ependymal rosettes with lumens (arrows). (c) Perivascular pseudorosettes are readily seen in smears. (d) Mucoid material and small cell nests are present in myxopapillary ependymoma, and should not be confused for carcinoma.

Lesions of the sellar region

Clinical issues

A variety of neoplasms occur in the sellar region (Table 17.5), and approximately 90% are adenomas of the pituitary gland. The differential diagnosis is often narrowed by clinical history, imaging techniques, and serum tests for endocrine function. The majority of surgically treated pituitary tumors are approached by the trans-sphenoidal approach, but a craniotomy is sometimes performed for large tumors that extend outside the sella. Tumors of non-pituitary origin are approached in the same way. An attempt is made to resect the lesion entirely, but when this is not possible, the tumor is debulked and the residual tumor is treated with radiation, chemotherapy or other pharmacologic agents, depending on the type of neoplasm.

The surgeon may have a firm clinical diagnosis in the case of functioning pituitary tumors, or a limited differential diagnosis based on clinical and imaging data.

A biopsy or curettage specimen will be sent for IOD for tumors approached trans-sphenoidally, most often to confirm a nearly certain clinical diagnosis. In other situations, a biopsy sample will be submitted and the surgeon will depend on the pathologist's diagnosis to guide the extent of surgical resection. Mass lesions that are approached by craniotomy will first be subjected to an incisional biopsy, and depending on the diagnosis and the surgical findings, the mass will be completely excised or debulked.

Pathologic issues

Pituitary adenomas show cellular monomorphism, in contrast to normal pituitary tissue that is polymorphous (Fig. 17.18). The dominant cell type may vary but this is of no consequence for intraoperative management. The term *atypical adenoma* is used when mitoses are readily identified. Pituitary carcinomas are very rare and are characterized by metastases or leptomeningeal dissemination. Normal *posterior hypophysis* may be confused with a glioma but the cells lack nuclear atypia; in addition, Herring bodies are usually present.

Craniopharyngiomas occur in two different forms, adamantinomatous and papillary. The former is characterized by complex epithelium and "wet keratin" which is diagnostic, even in the absence of tumor elements. Papillary craniopharyngioma is composed of uniform, mature squamous epithelium which upon dehiscence of tissue forms a pseudopapillary pattern.

Other common entities that may be encountered in the sellar or suprasellar region include Rathke cleft cysts, gliomas, Langerhans cell histiocytosis, meningioma, granular cell tumor, and metastases. Pituicytoma and spindle cell oncocytoma are two less common neoplasms; both have a favorable prognosis.[21]

Germ cell tumors occur in the sella and the majority are germinomas resembling seminoma. Embryonal carcinomas, yolk sac tumors, and mixed germ cell tumors are only rarely encountered.

Table 17.5. *Tumors of the sellar region other than pituitary adenomas*

	Key features
Craniopharyngioma	Palisading epithelium and wet keratin (adamantinomatous variant); well formed squamous epithelium and papillary architecture, involvement of third ventricle, young adults (papillary variant).
Granular cell tumor	Round to polygonal cells with granular cytoplasm
Pituicytoma	Bipolar spindle cells arranged in fascicles
Spindle cell oncocytoma	Spindle to epithelioid cells with granular cytoplasm; mitotic activity scant
Germ cell tumors	Germinoma most common; large cells with bar shaped nucleolus and lymphocytes
Langerhans cell histiocytosis	Large multilobated cells, eosinophils
Miscellaneous	Meningioma, pilocytic and diffuse astrocytomas, ependymoma, chordoma, paraganglioma, and metastases may extend to the sellar region

Tumors in the pineal region

Pineal neoplasms are relatively rare and biopsies from this region are often small. The supracerebellar approach often permits little more than a biopsy, even in experienced hands.

Pineal neoplasms include pineal parenchymal tumors, the recently described papillary tumor of the pineal region, and gliomas primarily affecting or extending into the pineal gland.

(a)   **(b)**

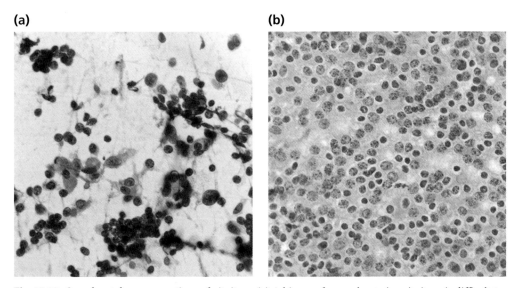

Fig. 17.18. Squash cytology preparations of pituitary. (a) A biopsy of normal anterior pituitary is difficult to smear, and is characterized by a variety of cell types. (b) In contrast, pituitary adenomas are easier to smear and consist of a monomorphic population of cells.

Pineal parenchymal tumors include the favorable *pineocytoma*, characterized by large pineocytomatous rosettes and minimal proliferation, *pineal parenchymal tumor of intermediate differentiation*, with bland cytology but increased mitotic activity, and *pineoblastoma*, a small round blue cell tumor that resembles PNET in other locations. *Pineal cysts* are occasionally biopsied and may be misdiagnosed as neoplasms; the three-layered architecture – leptomeninges, pineal parenchyma, reactive astrocytes- is characteristic.

Biopsies for medical diseases

Clinical issues

Biopsies of non-neoplastic disorders of the CNS are performed when the diagnosis is unclear in patients with progressive neurologic decline. The differential diagnosis includes a variety of encephalitides, infections, vasculitides, and some demyelinating diseases.

Pathologic issues

The main purpose of the intraoperative evaluation is to confirm that the biopsy specimen is adequate. Adequate precautions should be taken when handling these biopsies, especially if prion diseases are in the differential diagnosis, and protocols for handling these biopsies should be consulted before handling the specimen. A detailed discussion of medical diseases is beyond the scope of this chapter; the reader is directed to authoritative texts on the subject.[25,26]

REFERENCES

1. Berman JI, Berger MS, Chung SW, *et al*. Accuracy of diffusion tensor magnetic resonance imaging tractography assessed using intraoperative subcortical stimulation mapping and magnetic source imaging. *J Neurosurg* 2007; **107**: 488–494.

2. Law M, Oh S, Johnson G, *et al*. Perfusion magnetic resonance imaging predicts patient outcome as an adjunct to histopathology: a second reference standard in the surgical and nonsurgical treatment of low-grade gliomas. *Neurosurgery* 2006; **58**: 1099–1107; discussion 1099–1107.

3. Boulton M, Bernstein M. Outpatient brain tumor surgery: innovation in surgical neurooncology. *J Neurosurg* 2008; **108**: 649–654.

4. Serletis D, Bernstein M. Prospective study of awake craniotomy used routinely and nonselectively for supratentorial tumors. *J Neurosurg* 2007; **107**: 1–6.

5. Keles GE, Lundin DA, Lambown KR, *et al*. Intraoperative subcortical stimulation mapping for hemispherical perirolandic gliomas located within or adjacent to the descending motor pathways: evaluation of morbidity and assessment of functional outcome in 294 patients. *J Neurosurg* 2004; **100**: 369–375.

6. Shinoda J, Yano H, Yo Shimura S, *et al*. Fluorescence-guided resection of glioblastoma multiforme by using high-dose fluorescein sodium. Technical note. *J Neurosurg* 2003; **99**: 597–603.

7. Kuhn MJ, Picozzi P, Maldjian JA, *et al*. Evaluation of intraaxial enhancing brain tumors on magnetic resonance imaging: intraindividual crossover comparison of gadobenate dimeglumine and gadopentetate dimeglumine for visualization and assessment, and implications for surgical intervention. *J Neurosurg* 2007; **106**: 557–566.

8. Hirschberg H, Wu GN, Madsen SJ. Evaluation of Motexafin gadolinium (MGd) as a contrast agent for intraoperative MRI. *Minim Invasive Neurosurg* 2007; **50**: 318–323.

9. Stupp R, Mason WP, van den Bent WP, *et al*. Radiotherapy plus concomitant and adjuvant temozolomide for glioblastoma. *N Engl J Med* 2005; **352**: 987–996.

10. Nwokedi EC, di Base SJ, Jabbour S, *et al*. Gamma knife stereotactic radiosurgery for patients with glioblastoma multiforme. *Neurosurgery* 2002; **50**: 41–46; discussion 46–47.

11. Shaw EG, Berkey B, Coons SW, *et al*. Recurrence following neurosurgeon-determined gross-total resection of adult supratentorial low-grade glioma: results of a prospective clinical trial. *J Neurosurg* 2008; **109**: 835–841.

12. Burger PC, Nelson JS, Boyko OB. Diagnostic synergy in radiology and surgical neuropathology: neuroimaging techniques and general interpretive guidelines. *Arch Pathol Lab Med* 1998; **122**: 609–619.

13. Osborn A. *Diagnostic Imaging: Brain*. Salt Lake City: AMIRSYS, 2004.

14. Savargaonkar P, Farmer PM. Utility of intra-operative consultations for the diagnosis of central nervous system lesions. *Ann Clin Lab Sci* 2001; **31**: 133–139.

15. Tilgner J, Herr M, Ostertag C, *et al*. Validation of intraoperative diagnoses using smear preparations from stereotactic brain biopsies: intraoperative versus final diagnosis – influence of clinical factors. *Neurosurgery* 2005; **56**: 257–265; discussion 257–265.

16. Firlik, KS, Martinez AJ, Lunsford LD. Use of cytological preparations for the intraoperative diagnosis of stereotactically obtained brain biopsies: a 19-year experience and survey of neuropathologists. *J Neurosurg*, 1999; **91**(3): pp. 454–458.

17. Bleggi-Torres LF, de Noronha L, Schneider Gugelmin E, *et al*. Accuracy of the smear technique in the cytological diagnosis of 650 lesions of the central nervous system. *Diagn Cytopathol* 2001; **24**: 293–295.

18. Burger PC, Nelson JS. Stereotactic brain biopsies: specimen preparation and evaluation. *Arch Pathol Lab Med* 1997; **121**: 477–480.

19. Burger PC, Scheithauer BW. *Tumors of the Central Nervous System. AFIP Atlas of Tumor Pathology*. Washington, DC: American Registry of Pathology, 2007.

20. Cairncross JG, Ueki K, Zlatscu MC, *et al*. Specific genetic predictors of chemotherapeutic response and survival in patients with anaplastic oligodendrogliomas. *J Natl Cancer Inst* 1998; **90**: 1473–1479.

21. Louis D, Ohgaki H, Wiestler O, *et al*. *WHO Classification of Tumours of the Central Nervous System*. 4th edn. Lyon, France: IARC Press, 2007.

22. Tihan T, Fisher PG, Kepner JL *et al*. Pediatric astrocytomas with monomorphous pilomyxoid features and a less favorable outcome. *J Neuropathol Exp Neurol* 1999. **58**: 1061–1068.

23. Marks JE, Wong J. The risk of cerebral radionecrosis in relation to dose, time and fractionation. A follow-up study. *Progr Exp Tumor Res* 1985; **29**: 210–218.

24. Schwartz TH, McCormick PC. Intramedullary ependymomas: clinical presentation, surgical treatment strategies and prognosis. *J Neurooncol* 2000; **47**: 211–218.

25. Ellison D, Love S, Chimelli L, *et al*. *Neuropathology: A Reference Text of CNS Pathology*. 2nd edn. 2003: Mosby, 800pp.

26. Love S, Louis DN, Ellison DW. *Greenfield's Neuropathology*. 8th edn. 2008: Oxford University Press, USA, 2400pp.

18 SOFT TISSUE

Jesse K. McKenney, Raffi S. Avedian, and Richard L. Kempson

INTRODUCTION

The majority of soft tissue neoplasms are benign and can be managed in non-specialized medical centers. However, a significant number of soft tissue neoplasms pose diagnostic and management challenges for the following reasons:

- Sarcomas are relatively uncommon in non-specialized hospitals, and as a result, most general surgical pathologists have limited experience with the morphologic diversity of soft tissue tumors.[1]
- Changes in nomenclature, descriptions of new variants of old tumors, and descriptions of new soft tissue neoplasms make it challenging for general surgical pathologists to maintain expertise in the diagnosis of soft tissue tumors, especially on small incisional biopsies and needle core biopsies.
- There is a good deal of histologic overlap between benign and malignant neoplasms. Some sarcomas (e.g., low grade fibromyxoid sarcoma) and locally aggressive mesenchymal neoplasms (e.g., desmoid fibromatosis) have deceptively bland histological features so that they may be mistaken for benign lesions. Conversely, some benign lesions mimic malignancies because they are disturbingly cellular (e.g., cellular schwannoma), show brisk mitotic activity (e.g., fasciitis), or show significant nuclear atypia (e.g., pleomorphic lipoma).
- Some sarcomas (e.g. myxofibrosarcoma) may show a wide range of cellularity, mitotic activity and atypia within the same neoplasm. A small sample can be mistaken for a benign neoplasm if the biopsy includes only the bland appearing myxoid component.
- Carcinomas and melanomas that metastasize to soft tissue may mimic primary epithelioid and spindle cell soft tissue sarcomas.

- The vast majority of small neoplasms are benign, and the diagnosis of sarcoma should be made with reluctance if the lesion is <2–3 cm in maximum dimension. However, exceptions occur: many epithelioid sarcomas and some synovial sarcomas, in particular, may be small enough for the entire neoplasm to fit into a few blocks.[2,3] Small size, therefore, does not exclude sarcoma.
- Multiple therapeutic options may be available for managing a given subtype of sarcoma, and these options cannot be discussed with the patient without first establishing a definitive diagnosis. Optimal management usually requires careful deliberation after all of the information is available. This includes a definitive diagnosis based on permanent sections.
- Limb-sparing surgical resection along with adjuvant or neoadjuvant chemotherapy and/or radiation is now the standard of practice for many soft tissue malignancies. These therapeutic options can only be offered to the patient after correct management at every step, including an accurate diagnosis. In general, the role of frozen section (FS) is to confirm that diagnostic tissue has been obtained. Definitive treatment should be carried out only after a firm pathologic diagnosis has been rendered on permanent sections. Definitive surgical treatment should not be based on a FS diagnosis.

GENERAL CLINICAL ISSUES

Pre-treatment evaluation of soft tissue tumors

The surgeon who manages a soft tissue neoplasm has to decide whether to perform an excisional biopsy as the initial surgical procedure, or adopt a staged approach, first with a needle or incisional biopsy for the purpose of

Intraoperative Consultation in Surgical Pathology, ed. Mahendra Ranchod. Published by Cambridge University Press.
© Cambridge University Press 2010.

obtaining a specific pathologic diagnosis, followed by definitive surgical resection. This decision is crucial because an incorrect initial surgical approach to a sarcoma may seriously compromise subsequent patient care (i.e. the possibility of a more conservative resection). On the other hand, there is no need for a two-step approach for clearly benign neoplasms. The choice of surgical procedure is partly dependent on the following factors.

- *Duration of the lesion.* Long history and slow growth favor a benign lesion, but the converse is not necessarily true: benign lesions such as nodular fasciitis may grow rapidly – so rate of growth has to be taken in the context of the entire clinical picture.
- *Anatomic compartment.* Most sarcomas are deep-seated, mainly in the muscles of the limbs or in the retroperitoneum. In contrast, most soft tissue masses in the subcutaneous compartment are benign although some sarcomas do occur in this compartment (e.g., dermatofibrosarcoma protuberans and epithelioid sarcoma). As a general rule therefore, deeply located soft tissue masses are first subjected to a diagnostic biopsy, and definitive surgical resection is undertaken after a firm diagnosis has been established on permanent sections. In contrast, clinically benign subcutaneous masses are treated with a one-step excision that is both diagnostic and therapeutic.
- *Size of the mass.* Although there are exceptions, most sarcomas are large at the time of diagnosis. A large, deeply located mass is therefore, a sarcoma until proven otherwise.
- *Imaging studies.* CT scans, MRI and PET-CT scans are performed whenever there is suspicion that the lesion is a locally aggressive neoplasm or sarcoma. A large soft tissue mass that wraps around major neurovascular structures is almost certainly malignant, but circumscription should not be misconstrued as evidence of a benign neoplasm, as many sarcomas are well circumscribed. In addition, variations in density on CT scans and MRI may suggest necrosis, cystic change or histologic heterogeneity (e.g., de-differentiation in a well-differentiated retroperitoneal liposarcoma). With respect to heterogenous tumors, three dimensional imaging is helpful in directing the surgeon's biopsy to areas that will provide the most information. Finally, imaging is relatively specific for fat density, so a large adipocytic mass may be resected without biopsy if there are no radiographic changes to suggest de-differentiation.

Biopsy procedures

The biopsy procedure that is employed to make a diagnosis will depend on the provisional clinical diagnosis and location of the mass.

- *Fine needle aspiration biopsy (FNA)* is the least invasive, but has a limited role in the evaluation of soft tissue neoplasms. Most mesenchymal neoplasms yield scanty cellular material, and in addition, FNA is not ideal for evaluating architectural features. FNA however, is useful for evaluating cellular, non-mesenchymal neoplasms such as metastatic carcinoma, melanoma, lymphoma and other cellular small cell malignancies, and a specific diagnosis may be made with the help of immunohistochemical stains if sufficient material is obtained for preparation of a cell block.[4]
- *Needle core biopsy* is superior to FNA because of the larger sample and preservation of tissue architecture. Needle core biopsy, with or without CT guidance, has a high diagnostic yield and a high accuracy rate.[5–8] Core biopsies are especially useful in evaluating masses in deep sites such as the retroperitoneum because the alternative is to perform a major abdominal procedure with increased morbidity and the risk of contaminating surrounding tissues.
- *Incisional biopsy* is the ideal approach for obtaining diagnostic tissue, especially for deeply seated sarcomas of the limbs and trunk. The placement of the incision has to be carefully planned because the incision site and biopsy track have to be included in the subsequent resection if the lesion is malignant.[9] This is why it is preferable for the same surgeon to perform the initial incisional biopsy and the definitive surgical procedure.
- *Excisional biopsy* is used primarily for subcutaneous masses or very small deep masses that are benign by clinical evaluation. The procedure is intended to be both diagnostic and therapeutic. Excisional biopsies should not be performed on sarcomas because of the risk of contaminating the operative field with malignant cells, thus depriving the patient of the benefits of limb-sparing surgery.

Managerial classification of soft tissue neoplasms

Soft-tissue neoplasms show great diversity in clinical behavior, and the binary approach to classifying soft tissue neoplasms as benign and malignant is no longer tenable.

Table 18.1. Managerial categories

Group	Outcome	Usual therapy	Examples
Clinically benign			
Ia	Local excision almost always curative; metastasis never occurs	Local excision	Nodular fasciitis; dermatofibroma
Ib	Recurrence occurs, but are non-destructive; never metastasizes	Local excision; treat recurrences if they occur	Superficial angiomyxoma; fibroma of tendon sheath
Clinically indeterminate			
IIa	Local recurrence very common and may be destructive; never metastasizes	Local excision with attention to margins	Desmoid fibromatosis
IIb	Local recurrence very common; metastasis vanishingly rare unless de-differentiation to group III occurs	Local excision with attention to margins; adjuvant therapy not warranted	Atypical lipomatous tumor
IIc	Local recurrence common; metastasis can rarely occur without de-differentiation	Local excision with attention to margins; adjuvant therapy usually not warranted	Plexiform fibrohistiocytic tumor
Clinically sarcoma			
III	Local recurrence and metastasis common	Local excision with attention to margins; consideration given to adjuvant therapy	Myxoid liposarcoma; Malignant peripheral nerve sheath tumor
IV	Systemic disease assumed at diagnosis	Adjuvant therapy usual	Alveolar rhabdomyosarcoma; Ewing sarcoma

Kempson and Hendrickson have proposed six managerial categories in an attempt to match biologic behavior with treatment (Table 18.1).[10]

Surgical procedures for treating soft tissue tumors

- *Intralesional excision* refers to piece-meal removal of a tumor. There is no role for intralesional excisions in the treatment of soft tissue neoplasms.
- *Marginal excision* refers to complete removal of a neoplasm using the "capsule" (interface of tumor with normal tissue) as a guide for the plane of resection. Marginal excisions are ideal for benign neoplasms such as lipomas.
- *Wide resection* is the removal of the tumor with a cuff of normal tissue as the surgical margin. The tumor is never visualized or exposed when performing a wide resection.
- *Radical resection* involves removal of the entire musculofascial compartment containing the tumor, and is performed only after a definitive diagnosis of sarcoma has been established.
- *Amputations* are reserved for sarcomas that invade vital structures and cannot be resected without significantly compromising function, or for uncontrolled local recurrence. The excision margins in amputation specimens are usually generous.

INDICATIONS FOR INTRAOPERATIVE CONSULTATION

1. Evaluation of an incisional biopsy specimen to ensure that sufficient lesional tissue is present.
2. Evaluation of an incisional biopsy or excision specimen to procure tissue for ancillary studies.
3. Evaluation of a resection specimen to evaluate margins for completeness of excision.
4. Evaluation of an incisional biopsy to render a diagnosis for a readily recognized, common benign entity that will allow the surgeon to proceed with conservative marginal excision.

INFORMATION NEEDED BEFORE AND DURING INTRAOPERATIVE CONSULTATION

The pathologist should be familiar with the clinical aspects of the case before rendering an intraoperative diagnosis (IOD). Familiarity with the clinical history will help to make the correct diagnosis as well as help to avoid some of the pitfalls in diagnosis. The following information should be gathered before rendering an IOD:

- *Patient's age.* The spectrum of soft tissue neoplasms in children is generally more limited than in adults, and the differential diagnosis may be different for a given anatomic site (e.g. fibrous hamartoma of infancy would not be considered in the differential diagnosis of fibromatosis in an adult). It is essential to know the age of the patient before performing a FS because this may narrow the diagnostic considerations considerably.

- *Location of the lesion.* Some neoplasms have a propensity for certain anatomic locations. For example, it is helpful to know if the lesion is in the proximal limb or whether it is juxta-articular, acral, or retroperitoneal in location.

- *Familiarity with imaging studies.* Imaging studies of the lesion should be reviewed, either with a radiologist prior to surgery or with the surgeon during the surgical procedure. Radiologic images can offer helpful information in terms of size, anatomic compartment and characteristics of the lesion, and thus provide a context for the FS findings.

- *History of prior malignancy.* It is always worth soliciting a history of prior malignancy because this information is not always forthcoming. Metastases to soft tissues are uncommon but when they occur, they may mimic primary sarcomas. If a metastasis is under serious consideration pre-operatively, FNA or needle core biopsy should be the first diagnostic approach; however, this may not have been done and the lesion may be subjected to an incisional biopsy for FS evaluation.

- *Familiarity with surgeon's operative plan.* Familiarity with the surgeon's operative plan ensures that the surgeon and pathologist are in agreement about the goal of IOD. The pathologist's mettle will be tested if she discovers that the surgeon plans to proceed with a major resection on the basis of a FS diagnosis. If the pathologist is not an expert in soft tissue pathology, and the case has not been evaluated in a multidisciplinary fashion pre-operatively, the surgeon should be persuaded to defer definitive resection until a firm diagnosis is made on permanent sections.

GENERAL PATHOLOGIC ISSUES

- Sarcomas sometimes evoke reactive changes at the periphery of the neoplasm, and infrequently, this will include bone formation. If exposure of the lesion is limited, the first biopsy may be superficial and show reactive changes only. It is important to make a distinction between lesional tissue and secondary reactive changes; the non-diagnostic nature of the biopsy will be apparent if the pathologist is familiar with the clinical and imaging findings. When a sampling problem is suspected, there should be no hesitation to request a deeper biopsy.

- Cytological preparations are of limited value in evaluating mesenchymal lesions but a cytoscrape preparation should be made if the neoplasm is cellular, judging by its color and consistency. Cytologic preparations are helpful in recognizing metastatic carcinoma, melanoma, and lymphoma but they are also suitable for evaluating the degree of cytologic atypia in spindle cell lesions. However, a FS should always be performed on an incisional biopsy specimen for evaluating specimen adequacy; cytologic preparations are supplementary and not a substitute for FS in the intraoperative evaluation of soft tissue masses.

- When an incisional biopsy is submitted for tissue adequacy, the pathologist should ensure that the specimen is large enough for intraoperative evaluation as well as permanent sections and ancillary studies. Additional tissue should be requested if there is any uncertainty about the adequacy of the specimen.

- *Sampling issues.* It is not always easy to decide if the lesional tissue in an incisional biopsy is representative of the neoplasm. Some neoplasms show significant histologic heterogeneity (e.g., admixture of a low-grade myxoid component and high grade sarcoma in myxofibrosarcoma, or focal de-differentiation in a well-differentiated liposarcoma), making it difficult to decide if the specimen is adequate when the FS shows only low grade sarcoma. There is no easy solution to this dilemma but clinicopathologic correlation and close collaboration with the surgeon will go a long way towards obtaining a representative sample.

- Concept of a "good enough" diagnosis. The purpose of IOD on an incisional biopsy is to determine if the specimen contains diagnostic tissue. A diagnosis of "sarcoma, defer to permanent sections," "spindle cell neoplasm", or "small round cell neoplasm" is good enough for intraoperative purposes. There is no reason to commit to a specific diagnosis if that is likely to be overturned on permanent sections.

- Evaluation of margins. See discussion of margins on page 301.

HANDLING SPECIMENS INTRAOPERATIVELY

It is our experience that sometimes the first incisional biopsy specimen is relatively small, but is followed by additional samples that contain enough lesional tissue. It is important to know in advance that there will be no problem in procuring adequate tissue because this may influence the way the initial biopsy is handled. This is why discussion of the case with the surgeon prior to surgery is so important. If there are technical reasons why only a limited sample will be submitted, then the pathologist should limit the amount of tissue subjected to FS. Furthermore, to conserve non-frozen tissue, the FS block can be saved in the frozen state until the permanent sections are available for examination. If the non-frozen tissue is adequate in quantity, then the tissue in the FS block can be used for ancillary studies – if necessary. If the non-frozen tissue is not adequate, then the tissue in the FS block should be processed for conventional histologic examination.

Saving fresh tissue for ancillary studies will depend on the provisional diagnosis and whether the patient will be enrolled in a research protocol. If the patient is likely to be enrolled in a research protocol, fresh and or frozen tissue should be saved as directed by that protocol. This is particularly important for pediatric sarcomas. Some pathology departments routinely bank tumor tissue under IRB protocols, and in this situation, a sample of fresh tumor tissue should be snap frozen and stored in a −70 °C freezer – if there is sufficient tissue for this purpose.

We recommend the following approach if the patient is not part of a protocol study, and if there is no requirement to bank fresh frozen tissue.

- In pediatric patients with a malignant small round cell tumor, a sample of fresh tumor should be placed in tissue culture medium for cytogenetics. This is recommended because cytogenetic studies can provide a high level of specificity in diagnosis; furthermore, cytogenetic abnormalities now play a large role in the classification of many hematopoietic neoplasms, particularly acute leukemias. Tissue should also be sent for flow cytometric analysis, and a sample can be frozen for potential use to be guided by the final diagnosis (e.g., the Biology Studies Protocol of the Children's Oncology Group prefers frozen tissue for N-Myc studies in neuroblastoma).

- We do not routinely save fresh tissue for cytogenetics in adult-type sarcomas. Paraffin embedded tissue is generally adequate for FISH studies if that becomes necessary. However, if a small round cell tumor is found on FS, tissue should be procured for appropriate lymphoma protocol studies (i.e., flow cytometry and cytogenetics).

Resection specimens are usually submitted for evaluation of surgical margins. The orientation of specific margins should be confirmed with the surgeon if they are not clearly labeled. One significant challenge with evaluating margins is that tissue retracts after cutting the specimen. The retraction of the inked non-neoplastic tissue away from the underlying tumor mass makes it difficult to prepare sections that include the tumor and the closest inked margin. One way around this problem is to immerse the inked specimen into a bath of cold liquid (liquid nitrogen or cold isopentane) for 30–60 seconds. This will temporarily "fix" the outer surface of the specimen and prevent retraction after sectioning. The specimen can then be cut in the usual way to evaluate margins.

SPECIFIC CLINICOPATHOLOGIC ISSUES

The following discussion refers to soft tissue lesions that may present challenges at the time of IOD. This discussion is not meant to be exhaustive but includes diagnostic problems that we encounter in our practice.

Reactive lesions that simulate malignancy

Clinical issues
Small, rapidly growing lesions in the subcutaneous compartment may be alarming because of their growth rate, but they are usually benign reactive processes such as nodular fasciitis. Most reactive lesions are <5 cm in size although some may be large at the time of presentation (e.g., massive localized lymphedema may exceed 10 cm).

Pathologic issues
There is significant histologic overlap between benign proliferative lesions (e.g., nodular, proliferative and ischemic fasciitis) and a subset of low-grade sarcomas (e.g., low grade myxofibrosarcoma, low grade fibromyxoid sarcoma,

(a)

(b)

(c)

(d)

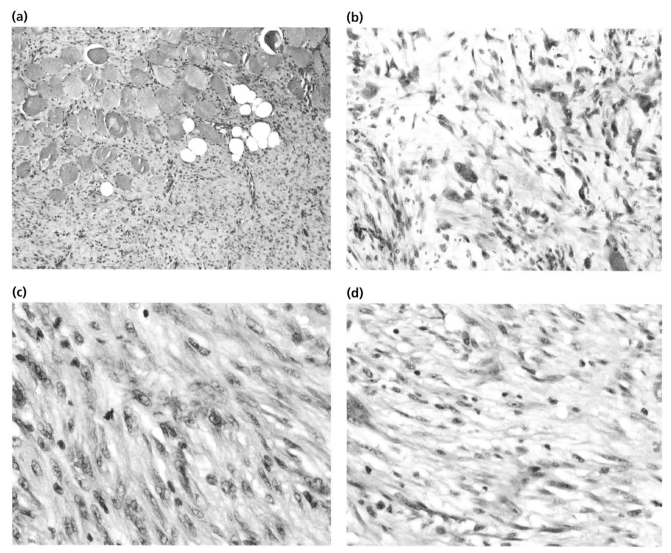

Fig. 18.1. (a) Nodular fasciitis. Myofibroblasts in nodular fasciitis or proliferative fasciitis may infiltrate skeletal muscle fibers; therefore, this feature alone does not indicate malignancy. (b) Scattered ganglion-like myofibroblasts, characterized by abundant eosinophilic cytoplasm and eccentric nuclei, may also be identified in fasciitis. These may be rare or may comprise a majority of the lesion, particularly in children. (c) Mitotic activity in cellular nodular fasciitis is expected. (d) The individual myofibroblasts may have variation in nuclear size, and nucleoli may be prominent.

and low grade myofibroblastic sarcoma). This overlap is compounded by limitations and artifacts of the FS technique. Size is a helpful guideline; a lesion is unlikely to be a sarcoma if the entire lesion can fit into one or two cassettes. Sarcomas are typically large, measuring many centimeters in dimension.

Nodular fasciitis and related lesions may be difficult to diagnose intraoperatively because characteristic architectural features such as tissue cracking and a loose fascicular arrangement may be misinterpreted as FS artifact. Brisk mitotic activity, prominent nucleoli, infiltrative margins, large epithelioid cells (ganglion-like cells) and intravascular growth may cause alarm, but they should be viewed in

context as all these features may be present in fasciitis (Fig. 18.1). If the lesion is small and superficial in location, the surgeon will excise the mass and submit the specimen for FS diagnosis. If the diagnosis of fasciitis is confirmed on FS, excision of the grossly visible lesion is sufficient; there is no reason to obtain clear margins by microscopic examination as these lesions are reactive in nature. If, on the other hand, a confident distinction cannot be made between fasciitis and low grade sarcoma, a provisional diagnosis of "spindle cell proliferation" should be made and the diagnosis deferred to permanent sections.

Ischemic fasciitis (atypical decubital fibroplasia) may mimic a sarcoma.[11–13] This reactive process may occur in

(a)

(b)

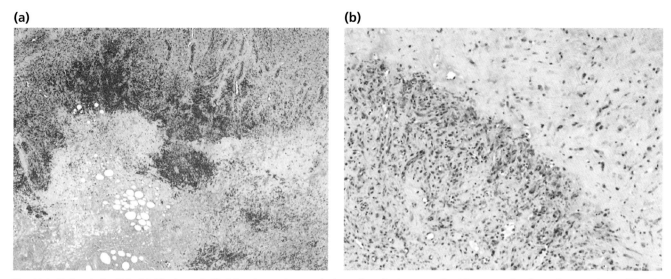

Fig. 18.2. Ischemic fasciitis. (a) The lower half of the photomicrograph shows liquefactive necrosis with an associated reactive vascular proliferation (upper half). (b) Reactive vascular proliferation has a sharp line of demarcation from the adjacent stroma, a characteristic feature of ischemic fasciitis.

any location, but often overlies bony prominences. The presence of benign reactive myofibroblasts and ganglion cell-like fibroblasts with nuclear enlargement and prominent nucleoli may suggest malignancy. Foci of zonal vascular proliferation surrounding areas of fibrinoid necrosis are characteristic of this lesion (Fig. 18.2), but if this feature is absent and the reactive nature of the lesion is not clear, the diagnosis should be deferred to permanent sections. If a definite diagnosis of ischemic fasciitis can be made on FS, the lesion may be debulked without an attempt to achieve clear surgical margins.

Massive localized lymphedema may mimic sarcoma clinically.[14] These pendulous masses are caused by localized lymphatic obstruction in patients with morbid obesity. The expansion of the septa between lobules of subcutaneous adipose tissue may simulate an atypical lipomatous tumor. The absence of significant atypia as well as sharply defined areas of vascular proliferation at the interface of fat and fibrous septae is characteristic of this lesion (Fig. 18.3). Confirmation of the diagnosis on FS will allow the surgeon to conservatively excise only the excess tissue that needs to be excised; however, distinction from atypical lipomatous tumor/well-differentiated liposarcoma may be difficult on FS if secondary changes such as fat necrosis are present.

Benign neoplasms that simulate malignancy

Most benign neoplasms are circumscribed. Occasionally, however, large benign neoplasms evoke secondary reactive changes that on imaging impart an infiltrative appearance

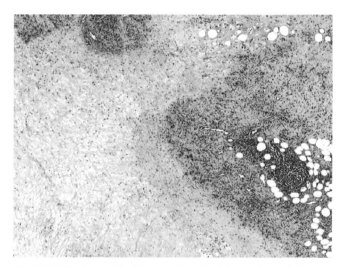

Fig. 18.3. Massive localized lymphedema. This lesion has a similar reactive vascular proliferation to ischemic fasciitis, but with stromal edema or fibrosis instead of necrosis in the intervening tissue. The sharp line of demarcation or lobular configuration of the proliferating vessels is a key feature of a reactive process.

(Fig. 18.4). The relevance of this point is that the surgeon may perform multiple biopsies and not be content with a diagnosis of benign neoplasm.

Cellular schwannoma may mimic sarcoma in a small biopsy specimen. The intersecting fascicles and high cellularity are reminiscent of synovial sarcoma (Fig. 18.5). The diagnosis of cellular schwannoma should always be considered when a cellular spindle cell neoplasm is encountered in the mediastinum or paraspinal soft tissue, the favored sites for this neoplasm. The pathologist should

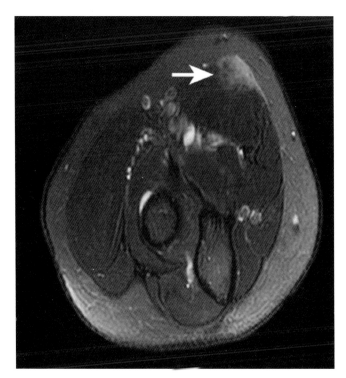

Fig. 18.4. CT scan showing a soft tissue mass with an irregular infiltrative appearance (arrow). The excision specimen revealed nodular fasciitis.

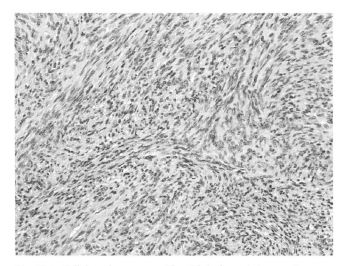

Fig. 18.5. Cellular schwannoma. The tightly formed, intersecting cellular fascicles of a cellular schwannoma may closely mimic a sarcoma, such as synovial sarcoma, on frozen section.

exercise extreme caution in rendering a diagnosis of sarcoma in this clinical setting and a diagnosis of "cellular spindle cell neoplasm" is usually appropriate. When the diagnosis is uncertain, the extent of surgical resection will depend on the size of the tumor and the nature of the surrounding tissues. Most surgeons will perform a

marginal excision (excisional biopsy) if the tumor is relatively small and if this procedure will have minimal morbidity. In this specific scenario, schwannomas often have characteristic MRI findings, so the surgeon will have a high degree of certainty that the lesion is benign and that it can be safely treated by marginal resection. The diagnosis of cellular schwannoma can be made with confidence on permanent sections; less cellular areas characteristic of schwannoma are usually present, and diffuse S-100 protein reactivity will confirm the diagnosis.

Schwannomas with degenerative atypia, so-called ancient change, may mimic malignancy on FS. The presence of scattered cells with pleomorphic, hyperchromatic nuclei may make the lesion indistinguishable from neoplasms such as myxofibrosarcoma (Fig. 18.6), especially in a small biopsy specimen that lacks the characteristic features of schwannoma (i.e., nuclear palisading, hyalinized vessels, admixed foamy histiocytes, abrupt variation in cellularity). Schwannoma with atypia illustrates the point that a FS diagnosis of sarcoma should not be based only on the presence of scattered atypical cells.

Bland appearing malignancies

A variety of sarcomas may have clinical, radiographic, and pathologic features that overlap with benign neoplasms or reactive proliferative processes.

Low grade fibromyxoid sarcoma is one of the most difficult neoplasms to recognize because of its bland appearance in the majority of cases. The innocuous appearance of this neoplasm in a biopsy specimen may suggest fibromatosis, neurofibroma, or perineurioma. Histologic clues to the diagnosis include the abrupt transition from collagenized to myxoid foci and/or the presence of perivascular epithelioid cells or rosettes (Fig. 18.7). However, it is difficult to make these distinctions on FS and it is appropriate to defer the diagnosis to permanent sections. On permanent sections, immunohistochemistry and molecular studies for the characteristic translocation involving the FUS gene will help in difficult cases.

It is often difficult to classify *cellular myofibroblastic lesions* such as inflammatory myofibroblastic tumor, fasciitis, and low grade myofibroblastic sarcoma on FS because of their rarity, and because the criteria for the diagnosis of low grade myofibroblastic sarcoma are not well defined. The admixture of spindle cells, plasma cells and lymphocytes as well as location in characteristic sites

(a)

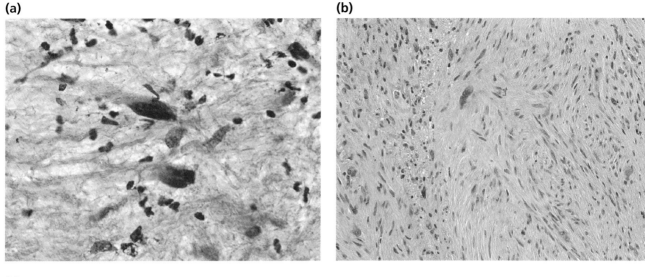

(b)

(c)

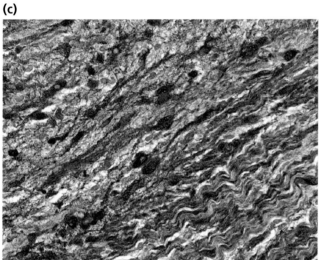

Fig. 18.6. Schwannoma with ancient change. (a) Original frozen section showing scattered large cells with multilobated, hyperchromatic nuclei. This feature alone should not prompt a diagnosis of malignancy. (b) The corresponding permanent section confirmed scattered atypical cells consistent with so-called "ancient change." (c) The diffuse S-100 protein immunoreactivity confirmed the diagnosis of schwannoma.

such as lung, may aid the recognition of inflammatory myofibroblastic tumor (Fig. 18.8). A diagnosis of "spindle cell neoplasm" may be all that can be offered intraoperatively; the definitive diagnosis should be deferred to permanent sections. If the diagnosis is entertained in intra-parenchymal sites such as the lung, complete excision (e.g., lobectomy) is appropriate.

The distinction of *myxoid liposarcoma* and *low grade myxofibrosarcoma* from *intramuscular myxoma* may be challenging (see section on myxoid neoplasms below).

Monophasic synovial sarcoma (or any sarcoma with fibrosarcoma-like pattern) may be mistaken for a benign process because of the relative uniformity of the neoplastic cells. However, the cellularity and the well-formed sharply intersecting fascicular architecture should be a clue to the diagnosis (Fig. 18.9). In most cases, the

appropriate recommendation is to obtain sufficient tissue for diagnosis and defer the diagnosis to permanent sections.

Tumor heterogeneity: Low grade and high grade sarcoma

There are two main patterns of tumor heterogeneity: low grade sarcomas with focal de-differentiation to a morphologically distinctive high grade sarcoma, and sarcomas of one cell type that show gradations of low grade to high grade sarcoma within the same lesion (Table 18.2).

Well-differentiated liposarcoma, especially tumors located in the retroperitoneum, may show focal de-differentiation to high-grade sarcoma. The de-differentiated component

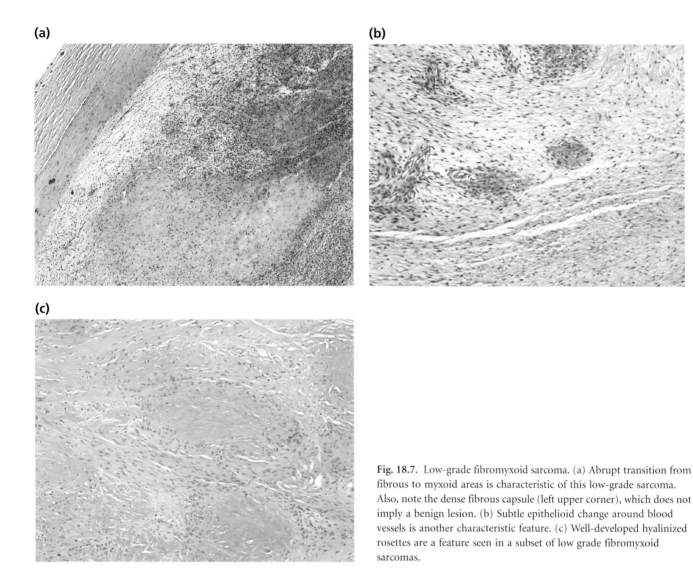

Fig. 18.7. Low-grade fibromyxoid sarcoma. (a) Abrupt transition from fibrous to myxoid areas is characteristic of this low-grade sarcoma. Also, note the dense fibrous capsule (left upper corner), which does not imply a benign lesion. (b) Subtle epithelioid change around blood vessels is another characteristic feature. (c) Well-developed hyalinized rosettes are a feature seen in a subset of low grade fibromyxoid sarcomas.

may resemble high grade myxofibrosarcoma or a pleomorphic undifferentiated sarcoma. A management problem is created if the biopsy includes only the low grade sarcomatous component. CT scans and MRI may show heterogeneity in density suggestive of de-differentiation, and one of the benefits of reviewing imaging studies pre-operatively is that this may raise the issue of tumor heterogeneity and influence the site of the biopsy.

Some sarcomas especially myxofibrosarcomas, may show low grade and high grade components in the same tumor. If a small incisional biopsy includes only the low grade component, the surgeon should be informed of the limitations of sampling, and that other parts of the mass may show higher grade sarcoma. This is a problem when stratifying patients for neoadjuvant

therapy prior to resection, but there is currently no solution to this problem.

Tumors that recur, especially the neoplasms listed in Table 18.2, may de-differentiate when they recur. Awareness of this phenomenon will guard against interpreting the recurrence as a new malignancy.

Myxoid neoplasms

Many low grade myxoid sarcomas are well circumscribed on radiographic studies, suggesting a benign neoplasm (Fig. 18.10). This may pose a problem because the surgeon may approach the case as a benign tumor and attempt a marginal excision. There is a danger to doing this: highly myxoid sarcomas rupture easily, leading to tumor spillage into the wound, an event that may place the patient at increased risk for local recurrence.

Low grade sarcomas with focal or diffuse myxoid stroma include low-grade myxofibrosarcoma, low-grade fibromyxoid sarcoma, and myxoid liposarcoma. These neoplasms typically lack nuclear pleomorphism and mitotic activity (Fig. 18.11). In a small incisional biopsy, it may be difficult to distinguish these sarcomas from benign myxoid lesions such as intramuscular myxoma and juxta-articular myxoma. Intramuscular myxomas

Table 18.2. Sarcomas with low and high grade components

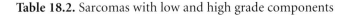

Low grade sarcoma	High grade sarcoma
Atypical lipomatous tumor/Well diff. liposarcoma	De-differentiated liposarcoma
Myxoid liposarcoma	Round cell liposarcoma
Low grade myxofibrosarcoma	High grade myxofibrosarcoma

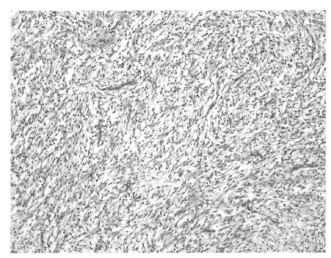

Fig. 18.8. Classic morphology of inflammatory myofibroblastic tumor with elongated spindled cells arranged into well-formed or loose fascicles, bland cytologic features, and an intimately admixed lymphocytic infiltrate. The organization of the spindle cells into fascicles can closely mimic a sarcoma in some cases.

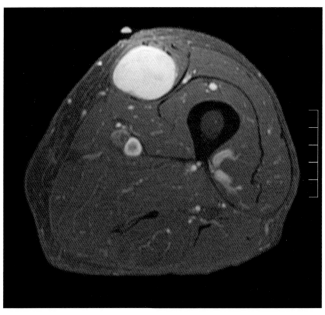

Fig. 18.10. CT scan showing a soft tissue mass with a well-delineated circumscribed margin. Circumscription of sarcomas can be misleading, and incorrectly interpreted as evidence of a benign neoplasm. The diagnosis at resection in this case was myxoid liposarcoma.

(a)   **(b)**

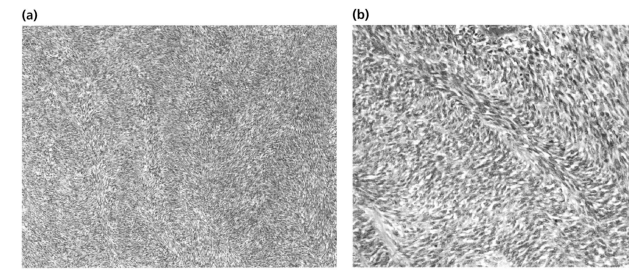

Fig. 18.9. Synovial sarcoma. (a) Despite the monomorphic cell population, the cellular intersecting fascicles are characteristic of synovial sarcoma. (b) At higher power, the organization of the fascicles into a "herring-bone pattern" is striking and subtle intercellular collagen deposition is also seen, another characteristic feature of synovial sarcoma.

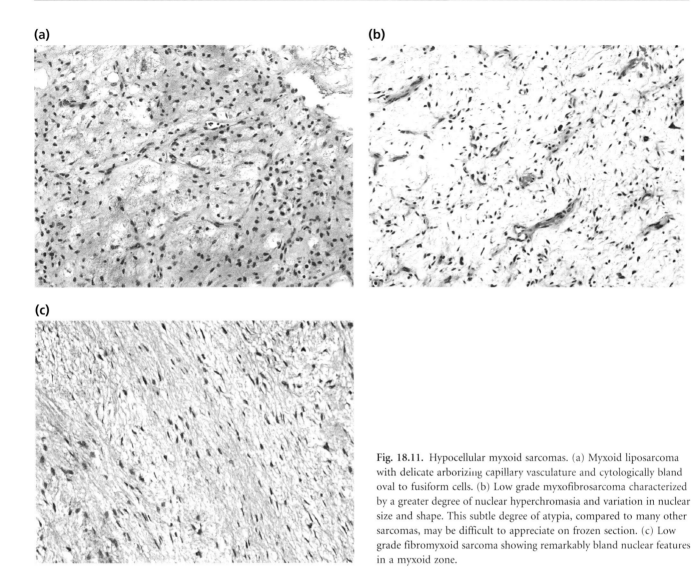

(a)

(b)

(c)

Fig. 18.11. Hypocellular myxoid sarcomas. (a) Myxoid liposarcoma with delicate arborizing capillary vasculature and cytologically bland oval to fusiform cells. (b) Low grade myxofibrosarcoma characterized by a greater degree of nuclear hyperchromasia and variation in nuclear size and shape. This subtle degree of atypia, compared to many other sarcomas, may be difficult to appreciate on frozen section. (c) Low grade fibromyxoid sarcoma showing remarkably bland nuclear features in a myxoid zone.

may have foci with increased cellularity and vascularity that closely mimic low grade myxofibrosarcoma but they lack the arching vessels characteristic of the latter.[15,16] The diagnosis of "myxoid spindle cell neoplasm" or "myxoid mesenchymal neoplasm" is usually sufficient in this setting.

Smooth muscle neoplasms

Smooth muscle neoplasms of deep soft tissue may be very well-circumscribed and mimic a benign neoplasm or cyst on clinical examination. This circumscription may lead to an inappropriate attempt at marginal excision of a leiomyosarcoma.

Criteria for the diagnosis of leiomyosarcoma vary by anatomic site, i.e. subcutaneous locations, deep soft tissue

and retroperitoneum.[17] In high grade leiomyosarcoma, the smooth muscle nature of the neoplasm may not be obvious on FS but its malignant nature will be. A diagnosis of pleomorphic sarcoma should be made and the final classification deferred to permanent sections. The diagnosis of leiomyosarcoma may be more challenging when cellularity, mitotic activity and atypia are not readily apparent on a small biopsy specimen (Fig. 18.12). Sufficient tissue should be obtained for permanent sections and the diagnosis should be deferred. Most smooth muscle neoplasms of deep somatic soft tissue are malignant.

One of the main problems with evaluating smooth muscle tumors of the soft tissue is their distinction from other mesenchymal neoplasms. It is prudent therefore, to confirm that neoplastic tissue is present

(a)
(b)

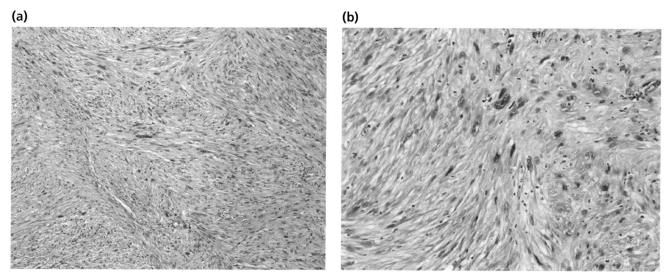

Fig. 18.12. Leiomyosarcoma of deep soft tissue. (a) The spindled cells arranged into tight bundled fascicles with obvious cytoplasmic eosinophilia are characteristic of a smooth muscle tumor. (b) In this field, scattered large hyperchromatic cells are present. Other fields showed more obvious nuclear pleomorphism. This heterogeneity within the same tumor underscores the importance of not classifying relatively bland deep smooth muscle tumors as leiomyoma on frozen section.

in the incisional biopsy, and to defer the diagnosis to permanent sections.

Leiomyomas of deep soft tissue are rare and this diagnosis should not be made on FS because this is a diagnosis of exclusion.[18] If a bland appearing smooth muscle neoplasm is encountered in the deep soft tissue, a diagnosis of "smooth muscle neoplasm, defer to permanent sections" is appropriate.

Undifferentiated malignant spindle cell neoplasm in superficial anatomic locations

When a spindle cell malignancy is encountered in the dermis and subcutaneous tissue, the differential diagnosis includes primary cutaneous malignancies such as squamous cell carcinoma, spindle cell melanoma as well as sarcoma. The distinction between these neoplasms almost always requires immunohistochemical studies on permanent sections. The initial biopsy is usually an incisional biopsy although an excision may be the first attempt at diagnosis. A diagnosis of "spindle cell neoplasm" or "malignant spindle cell neoplasm" should be rendered and the diagnosis deferred to permanent sections.

Neoplasms with a mature lipomatous component

The vast majority of lipomatous tumors in the subcutaneous compartment are lipomas. These are usually correctly diagnosed pre-operatively and excised by marginal excision.

Atypical lipomatous tumors in the subcutaneous compartment are clinically indistinguishable from lipomas and are likely therefore, to be treated like lipomas, i.e., marginal excision without a request for IOD. Although marginal excision is not optimal, it is reasonable to perform wide re-excision only after there is a local recurrence.

The adipocytic nature of deep seated lipomatous neoplasms can be recognized on imaging studies; the surgeon and pathologist are thus presented with a very narrow differential diagnosis. Unlike lipomatous neoplasms in the subcutaneous tissue, deep seated tumors are more likely to be atypical lipomatous tumor/well-differentiated liposarcoma. Histologic clues to the diagnosis of atypical lipomatous tumor/well-differentiated liposarcoma include marked variation in the size of individual adipocytes and delicate bands of fibrous tissue that entrap adipocytes. These features should prompt careful high power evaluation for the diagnostic atypical stromal cells. Chronic inflammatory infiltrates, myxoid change, and spindle cell may also be present. Atypical lipomatous tumors are difficult to evaluate intraoperatively for the following reasons:

- It is difficult to obtain good quality frozen sections of fatty tissue;
- These neoplasms are usually large and diagnostic changes may be focal;

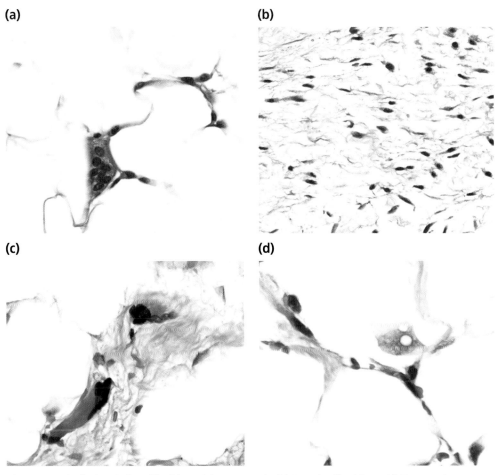

Fig. 18.13. Histologic mimics of lipoblasts: (a) Fat necrosis. (b) Reactive fibroblasts. (c) Entrapped degenerating skeletal muscle fibers, (d) Normal adipocytic nuclei with intranuclear vacuoles (Lockhern cells).

If atypical cells are present, they may be difficult to distinguish from histiocytes of fat necrosis, reactive fibroblasts, entrapped atrophic skeletal muscle fibers, and adipocytes with intranuclear vacuoles (Lockhern cells) (Fig. 18.13).

Unless there is convincing atypia, an intraoperative diagnosis of "mature adipocytic neoplasm" should be made, with deferral to permanent sections.

The pathologist should be careful not to interpret a neoplasm as lipomatous simply because it contains fat. Other types of sarcomas that infiltrate fat may closely mimic atypical lipomatous tumor/well differentiated liposarcoma, and permanent sections are usually necessary to make this distinction. In addition, angiomyolipomas may present in the retroperitoneum and may be lipid-rich, closely mimicking an adipocytic neoplasm.

Spindle cell neoplasms in parenchymal organs

Malignant spindle cell neoplasms of parenchymal organs are more likely to be spindle cell carcinomas than sarcomas. The diagnosis of primary sarcoma is made only after spindle cell carcinoma has been excluded. In most cases, the diagnosis would have been made on prior needle biopsy or the specimen that is submitted for FS is an organ or part of an organ that represents the definitive resection as well (e.g., pulmonary lobectomy). There is usually little at stake at the time of FS. If an incisional biopsy is submitted, a diagnosis of "malignant spindle cell neoplasm" should be made and the diagnosis deferred to permanent section – unless an obvious carcinomatous component is present.

Evaluation of surgical margins in sarcomas

The optimal treatment of sarcomas is surgical resection with wide margins. The definition of an adequate margin is controversial, but a "wide" margin is generally defined as greater than 2 cm.[19,20] In some regions, anatomic constraints preclude obtaining wide margins (e.g., retroperitoneum or if the tumor is adjacent to vital structures such as major vessels). Post-operative adjunctive therapy may be offered when wide margins are not achieved.

(a)   **(b)**

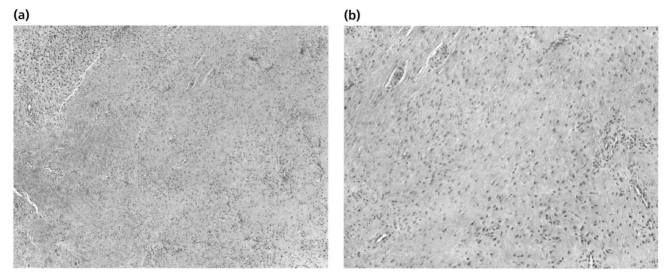

Fig. 18.14. Reactive changes in prior biopsy site. (a) Fibro/myofibroblastic proliferations in areas of previous biopsy may be indistinguishable from fibromatosis when taken out of context. This tissue from the margins of a sarcoma shows a hypocellular, cytologically bland proliferation arranged in fascicles. (b) The high-power photomicrograph shows a population of reactive spindle cells with a close resemblance to fibromatosis. It should be clear therefore, that the FS evaluation of surgical margins in fibromatosis may be impossible, especially in a re-excision specimen.

Because of the extensive surface area in large resection specimens, the challenge is to determine which margins to sample for FS. There are three possible approaches.

- The surgeon performs the definitive resection and then submits separate biopsies from the tumor bed for margin evaluation. These biopsies are usually small and should be totally embedded for FS; tumor anywhere in the specimen should be interpreted as a positive margin. If there is any doubt about the status of a margin, multiple levels should be prepared, and if necessary, sections should be cut through the block to confidently evaluate that margin. There is no reason to intentionally spare tissue for permanent sections.
- The surgeon places sutures on the surface of the resected specimen in areas of concern. The specimen is inked, and sections are taken perpendicular to the inked margin in the areas marked by sutures. The specimen should then be sectioned serially to evaluate other margins by gross examination.
- If a large resection is submitted without any direction from the surgeon, the specimen should be palpated and sectioned in a plane that will include areas where the tumor is closest to the margin. Margins that are clear by >2 cm can be reported as negative by gross examination. Margins that are 1 cm or less should be evaluated by FS, with sections taken perpendicular to the inked margin. If the margin is negative by FS

evaluation, the distance of sarcoma from the margin should be reported in mm. If many areas of the sarcoma are within <1 cm of the margin, and if additional marginal tissue cannot be excised, the surgeon should be forewarned of the limitations of evaluating margins intraoperatively, and the risk of false negative diagnosis.

Even if the surgeon cannot resect additional tissue, pathologists at some centers evaluate margins by FS to facilitate decisions for immediate intraoperative radiation therapy.

Evaluation of surgical margins in histologically bland, locally aggressive neoplasms

A variety of locally aggressive soft tissue neoplasms, including desmoid-type fibromatosis and dermatofibrosarcoma protuberans, extend beyond the grossly visible and palpable confines of the neoplasm. As a result, the initial excision may be incomplete, requiring re-excisions. Frozen section evaluation of the initial excision is less challenging than re-excisions performed days or a few weeks after initial surgery because of the difficulty of distinguishing neoplastic cells from reactive fibrous tissue at the margins of the lesion (Fig. 18.14). The distinction may not be possible on FS; the diagnosis may have to be deferred to permanent sections when immunohistochemical stains can be employed to make a more confident diagnosis (e.g., CD34 for DFSP and beta catenin for fibromatosis).

Low-grade angiosarcoma is often indistinguishable from reactive vascular tissue on FS. This is a problem especially when re-excision is performed soon after a prior attempted excision, because cellular granulation tissue may be present at the margins of the specimen. If the surgeon's goal is to obtain negative margins during this procedure, a rim of completely normal tissue – without reactive changes – will have to be excised if the pathologist is expected to make a confident diagnosis of clear margins.

REFERENCES

1. Arbiser ZK, Folpe AL, Weiss SW. Consultative (expert) second opinions in soft tissue pathology. Analysis of problem-prone diagnostic situations. *Am J Clin Pathol* 2001; **116**: 473–476.
2. Enzinger FM. Epitheloid sarcoma. A sarcoma simulating a granuloma or a carcinoma. *Cancer* 1970; **26**: 1029–1041.
3. Michal M, Fanbury-Smith JC, Lasota J, *et al.* Minute synovial sarcomas of the hands and feet: a clinicopathologic study of 21 tumors less than 1 cm, *Am J Surg Pathol* 2006; **30**: 721–726.
4. Singh HK, Kilpatrick SE, Silverman JF. Fine needle aspiration biopsy of soft tissue sarcomas: utility and diagnostic challenges. *Adv Anat Pathol* 2004; **11**: 24–37.
5. Heslin MJ, Lewis JJ, Woodruff JM, *et al.* Core needle biopsy for diagnosis of extremity soft tissue sarcoma. *Ann Surg Oncol* 1997; **4**: 425–431.
6. Ogilvie CM, Torbet JT, Finstein JL, *et al.* Clinical utility of percutaneous biopsies of musculoskeletal tumors. *Clin Orthop Relat Res* 2006; **450** 95–100.
7. Puri A, Shingade VU, Agarwal MG, *et al.* CT-guided percutaneous core needle biopsy in deep seated musculoskeletal lesions: a prospective study of 128 cases. *Skeletal Radiol* 2006; **35**: 138–143.
8. Ray-Coquard I, Ranchire Vince D, Thiesse P, *et al.* Evaluation of core needle biopsy as a substitute to open biopsy in the diagnosis of soft-tissue masses. *Eur J Cancer* 2003; **39**: 2021–2025.
9. Mankin HJ, Lange TA, Spanier SS. THE CLASSIC: The hazards of biopsy in patients with malignant primary bone and soft-tissue tumors. *J Bone Joint Surg* 1982; **64**: 1121–1127.
10. Kempson RL, Hendrickson MR. An approach to the diagnosis of soft tissue tumors, in *Soft Tissue Tumors*, SW Weiss and JJ Brooks, edrs. Baltimore: Williams & Wilkins; 1996.
11. Liegl B Fletcher CD. Ischemic fasciitis: analysis of 44 cases indicating an inconsistent association with immobility or debilitation. *Am J Surg Pathol* 2008; **32**: 1546–1552.
12. Montgomery EA, Meis JM, Mitchell MS, *et al.* Atypical decubital fibroplasia. A distinctive fibroblastic pseudotumor occurring in debilitated patients. *Am J Surg Pathol* 1992; **16**: 708–715.
13. Perosio PM Weiss SW. Ischemic fasciitis: a juxta-skeletal fibroblastic proliferation with a predilection for elderly patients. *Mod Pathol* 1993; **6**: 69–72.
14. Farshid G, Weiss SW. Massive localized lymphedema in the morbidly obese: a histologically distinct reactive lesion simulating liposarcoma. *Am J Surg Pathol* 1998; **22**: 1277–1283.
15. Nielsen GP, O'Connell JX, Rosenberg AE. Intramuscular myxoma: a clinicopathologic study of 51 cases with emphasis on hypercellular and hypervascular variants. *Am J Surg Pathol* 1998; **22**: 1222–1227.
16. van Roggen JF, McMenamin ME, Fletcher CD. Cellular myxoma of soft tissue: a clinicopathological study of 38 cases confirming indolent clinical behaviour. *Histopathology* 2001; **39**: 287–297.
17. Honick JL, Fletcher CD. Criteria for malignancy in nonvisceral smooth muscle tumors. *Ann Diagn Pathol* 2003; **7**: 60–66.
18. Billings SD, Folpe AL, Weiss SW. Do leiomyomas of deep soft tissue exist? An analysis of highly differentiated smooth muscle tumors of deep soft tissue supporting two distinct subtypes. *Am J Surg Pathol* 2001; **25**: 1134–1142.
19. Reith JD. Protocols for the examination and reporting of bone and soft tissue tumors. *Arch Pathol Lab Med* 2007; **131**: 680–681; author reply 681–682.
20. Rubin BP. Protocol for the examination of specimens from patients with soft tissue tumors of intermediate malignant potential, malignant soft tissue tumors, and benign/locally aggressive and malignant bone tumors. *Arch Pathol Lab Med* 2006; **130**: 1616–1629.

19   BONE AND JOINT

Andrew E. Horvai, Richard J. O'Donnell, and Richard L. Kempson

INTRODUCTION

Requests for intraoperative diagnosis (IOD) are made on a wide variety of lesions that occur in bones and joints. The diagnosis in many cases is relatively straightforward, especially if the clinical and imaging findings are characteristic. However, IOD on bone lesions can be challenging for the following reasons.

- Bone tumors, especially primary malignant neoplasms, are uncommon, and as a result, pathologists in non-specialized centers have limited exposure to the range of morphologic changes that occur in some bone lesions.
- A single type of neoplasm, e.g., osteogenic sarcoma, may have a wide range of appearances – from variants that may be misinterpreted as benign to variants that mimic other types of primary bone malignancies.
- Some reactive processes (e.g., florid reactive periostitis) may be atypical enough to simulate a malignancy.
- Secondary changes such as aneurysmal bone cyst and pathologic fracture may mask an underlying neoplasm or confound the histologic changes in the limited sample submitted for intraoperative diagnosis.
- Evaluation of imaging studies is integral to the evaluation of bone neoplasms, and there are cases where expert interpretation of roentgenograms is necessary to reach the correct diagnosis. Pathologists who do not have access to an expert bone radiologist are at a significant disadvantage. This is not meant to disparage radiologists but general radiologists have the same limitations as general surgical pathologists with regard to uncommon bone tumors.

There have been major changes in the management of primary malignancies of bone, in particular the use of adjuvant chemotherapy and limb-sparing surgery. Providing optimal care often means management by a multi-specialty group of physicians who have expertise in tumors of bone, and as a result, patients with suspected primary bone malignancies are often referred to specialized medical centers. However, primary malignancies are still treated at non-specialized centers and general surgical pathologists have to be familiar with management of these neoplasms.

There are a limited number of bone tumor centers where primary bone malignancies are resected on the basis of a frozen section (FS) diagnosis. However, this approach is NOT appropriate in non-specialized centers. When a general surgical pathologist encounters a potential primary bone malignancy, the purpose of IOD is to confirm that diagnostic tissue is present. Definitive surgical treatment should be deferred until the diagnosis is confirmed on permanent sections. This situation has much at stake; the pathologist should not give the surgeon license to perform a major resection based on a FS diagnosis. The converse is also true: interpretation of a primary malignancy as benign can have disastrous results if the surgeon proceeds with curettage and potential tumor contamination of the operative field. This is why clinico-pathologic correlation is so important. A pathologist should NOT render IOD on a bone lesion without being fully familiar with the clinical findings, imaging studies and the surgeon's management algorithm.

This chapter is written primarily for the general surgical pathologist.

GENERAL CLINICAL ISSUES

The approach to making a diagnosis

Orthopedic surgeons use all the information they can muster to make a pre-operative diagnosis or generate a

Intraoperative Consultation in Surgical Pathology, ed. Mahendra Ranchod. Published by Cambridge University Press.
© Cambridge University Press 2010.

limited differential diagnosis. Clinical history, physical examination, and laboratory data can sometimes point to the correct diagnosis, but the surgeon is highly dependent on imaging studies. Imaging studies for the orthopedic surgeon are analogous to gross examination for the pathologist: they are critical to making a diagnosis. Imaging studies are often characteristic enough to be diagnostic but there are times when the changes are not specific and the surgeon has to proceed with only a differential diagnosis in hand. Although newer techniques provide a great deal of information, conventional roentgenograms remain the cornerstone for evaluating lesions of bone. CT scans, MRI, PET scans and angiograms are helpful for identifying details within a lesion and for planning surgical management but they are not a substitute for conventional radiographs.[1,2]

Types of procedures for diagnosis and treatment

CT-guided FNA and needle core biopsy are useful for evaluating cellular lesions such as metastases, lymphoma, myeloma and recurrences of known malignancies, especially in deep sites such as the spine and pelvis. FNA however, is not suitable for evaluating primary mesenchymal neoplasms. Specific diagnoses can be made on needle core biopsy but this test has a limited role in evaluating primary mesenchymal neoplasms because of limitations of sampling.

Incisional biopsies are performed in two situations.

- It is the most common procedure for making an initial diagnosis on suspected primary malignancies of bone. The purpose of the biopsy is to confirm that sufficient diagnostic tissue has been obtained, and further management is planned after a definite pathologic diagnosis has been made on permanent sections.
- An incisional biopsy is also performed when the nature of the lesion is uncertain based on clinical and imaging studies. If a specific benign diagnosis can be made on FS, the surgeon will proceed with curettage. However, the pathologist should defer to permanent sections if there is any doubt about the diagnosis. An incorrect diagnosis of benign neoplasm can have dire consequences if a primary malignancy is treated by curettage, as this may disqualify the patient from having subsequent limb-sparing surgery.

Intra-lesional excision (curettage) is performed under three circumstances.

- It is the usual approach for treating benign neoplasms. The lesion is curetted, a FS is performed to confirm the diagnosis, and the defect is filled with autograft or allograft bone chips or methylmethacrylate.
- Locally aggressive bone tumors such as giant cell tumor, chondroblastoma and chondromyxoid fibroma are often treated by curettage, and this may be supplemented with cryosurgical ablation to destroy residual microscopic disease before packing the defect with bone chips and methylmethacrylate.
- Metastatic carcinoma, with or without a pathologic fracture, is usually curetted and the defect is stabilized with pins or rods.

Extra-lesional resection refers to complete resection of the neoplasm with a margin of normal tissue. This procedure is performed for selected benign neoplasms such as osteochondroma, but it is also used to treat locally aggressive neoplasms such as giant cell tumor, chondroblastoma and chondromyxoid fibroma.

Limb-sparing procedures are used to treat a variety of primary malignancies that were previously treated by amputation, such as osteosarcoma and Ewing's sarcoma. Tissue-sparing surgery requires comprehensive management by a team of experts with correct management at every step. After pathologic confirmation of the diagnosis, the tumor may be treated with chemotherapy followed by limb-sparing surgical resection.

Amputations are performed for initial and recurrent malignancies when limb-sparing surgery is not feasible.

The approach to managing bone tumors

Every step in the management of primary bone tumors is important if the patient is to be offered optimal care.[3–5] Ideally, primary malignancies of bone are managed by a multidisciplinary team consisting of one or more surgeons, radiologists, pathologists, radiation, and medical oncologists who have expertise in bone tumors. When this level of expertise is not available, it is prudent to discuss potential primary bone malignancies at the hospital's tumor board conference to allow input from multiple specialties. This also allows the opportunity to seek outside opinions if the course of management is in doubt. Unfortunately, the importance of a multidisciplinary approach is not always appreciated and the pathologist may find herself handling a bone tumor biopsy without the benefit of pre-operative discussion (see below).

INDICATIONS FOR INTRAOPERATIVE CONSULTATION (IOC)

1. To confirm a benign diagnosis, and to exclude malignancy, when the clinical and radiographic findings are typical of a benign process. A benign FS diagnosis will allow the surgeon to proceed with immediate definitive treatment (curettage or excision).
2. To determine if adequate diagnostic tissue is present in an incisional biopsy specimen of a suspected malignancy.
3. To determine if adequate lesional tissue is present in cases where only a broad differential diagnosis is possible based on clinical and imaging data.
4. To confirm malignancy in a suspected bone metastasis so that the appropriate surgical procedure can be performed to stabilize the bone (e.g., placement of a pin or rod).
5. To evaluate surgical margins of resection in locally aggressive and malignant neoplasms.
6. To procure tissue for ancillary studies (immunohistochemistry, cytogenetics, molecular genetics, flow cytometry) when appropriate.
7. To determine the presence of infection during prosthetic implant revision procedures.

INFORMATION NEEDED BEFORE AND DURING IOC

The pathologist should be familiar with the clinical history, and this includes a history of oncologic, hematologic, and endocrine conditions. Signs and symptoms, such as pain, tenderness, stiffness, mass effect, warmth, erythema, lymphadenopathy, and constitutional findings are also important. Demographic characteristics, including age and gender, are very helpful in narrowing the differential diagnosis as some lesions have a predilection for certain age groups (Table 19.1).

Consultation with an expert in skeletal radiology is the usual practice in centers that specialize in treating bone tumors, but every pathologist who handles bone lesions should be comfortable with interpreting plain radiographs, as well as be familiar with the descriptive language used by skeletal radiologists. This is particularly important in hospitals where an expert in skeletal radiology is not available. Radiologic characteristics that should be noted include: type of bone (long vs. flat); area of skeletal system involved (axial vs. appendicular); specific bone involved;

Table 19.1. Age association of common benign and malignant bone lesions

Age(yrs)	Benign	Malignant
< 10	Unicameral bone cyst Eosinophilic granuloma	Ewing's sarcoma Leukemia/lymphoma
10–20	Non-ossifying fibroma Osteoid osteoma Fibrous dysplasia Aneurysmal bone cyst Osteochondroma Osteoblastoma Chondroblastoma Chondromyxoid fibroma	Osteosarcoma Ewing's sarcoma Adamantinoma
20–40	Enchondroma Giant cell tumor	Chondrosarcoma
>40	Enchondroma	Plasmacytoma Lymphoma Metastatic malignancy Chondrosarcoma Osteosarcoma Chordoma

compartment within long bone (epiphysis, metaphysis, diaphysis or central, eccentric, parosteal); radio-opacity (sclerotic, lucent, or mixed); and aggressiveness (geographic pattern, border configuration, cortical break, periosteal reaction, soft tissue mass, or pathologic fracture). It is important to note the presence of a fracture either by history and/or radiology, as fracture callus can show proliferation of immature mesenchyme, bone, and cartilage that may be mistaken for neoplastic tissue. Table 19.2 lists common changes seen in conventional roentgenograms and examples are illustrated in Fig. 19.1.

It is essential to know the surgeon's treatment plan when rendering an IOD, a point that is particularly important if the pathologist was not involved in pre-operative discussions of the case. The pathologist should recognize high stake situations and make certain that the surgeon does not undertake major surgery based on a FS diagnosis.[6]

Surgical pathologists who work in hospitals that lack a multi-disciplinary team approach work under suboptimal conditions and often face the following situations.

- Imaging studies are not available in the hospital's radiology department because they were performed at an outside institution, and sometimes specialized studies such as MRI are available but not conventional roentgenograms. The pathologist is thus denied the opportunity to obtain a comprehensive opinion from a radiologist prior to surgery.

Table 19.2. Radiologic terms used to describe intraosseous lesions and their *usual* clinical significance

Radiologic term	Usual clinical significance
• *Opacity*	
○ Lucent: loss of radiodenisty without aggressiveness	Benign lesion
○ Lytic: destructive with no new mineral deposit	Variable significance
○ Sclerotic: new mineral deposit	Variable significance
○ Mixed: alternating lytic and sclerotic areas	Variable significance
• *Border*	
○ Marginated: Sclerotic rim, "walled off" lesion	Slowest growth
○ Circumscribed: delineated, no rim	Slow growth
○ Moth eaten: multiple punched out, ill-defined lesions	Aggressive
○ Permeative: ill-defined, difficult to draw a line around	Aggressive
• *Periosteum*	
○ Solid: thickened cortex	Aggressive
○ Elevated: Codman triangle	Aggressive
○ Spiculated: new bone at right angles to cortex	Osteosarcoma
○ Onion skin: new bone parallel to cortex	Ewing's sarcoma

- Diagnostic images are available, but the radiologists in the institution lack expertise in bone tumors. The radiologist is prepared to offer a broad differential diagnosis but is unable to make a specific diagnosis or generate a limited differential diagnosis.

- The pathologist has not been forewarned, and the first inkling of the case is the arrival of the specimen in the laboratory for FS diagnosis. This situation requires due diligence on the part of the pathologist. It is reasonable to perform the FS without all the information on hand, but a visit to the operating room is mandatory. The pathologist should obtain the clinical history, review the appropriate images with the surgeon, discuss the surgical findings, and inquire about the surgeon's operative plan before committing to a diagnosis. In our opinion, it is below the standard of care to render a FS diagnosis on a bone neoplasm without being adequately informed of the clinical and imaging data; as a consultant, the pathologist is responsible for seeking the information needed to make a diagnosis.

There are occasions when a definite diagnosis cannot be made even when all the information is available. An inconclusive diagnosis is never welcome but the surgeon should understand that even an expert in bone pathology, equipped with all the pertinent clinical, laboratory, and radiologic information, is sometimes unable to offer a definite IOD.[7,8]

GENERAL PATHOLOGIC ISSUES

There are a number of general principles that should be considered when evaluating bone biopsies.

- Many histologic changes are common to a variety of disparate lesions, creating pitfalls in diagnosis. Giant cells, new bone formation, and cartilage production may be found in reactive lesions, benign neoplasms, and malignant neoplasms.

- Secondary changes, such as fracture callus and aneurysmal bone cyst formation, may obscure an underlying neoplasm and confound interpretation of a small biopsy sample.

- Reactive processes and benign neoplasms may be cellular and show features that, if taken out of context, may be mistaken for malignancy. For example, giant cell tumor of bone can show highly cellular areas, high mitotic activity, necrosis, and even vascular invasion, but these features do not necessarily imply malignancy.

- It may not be possible to precisely classify a bone lesion on a small biopsy submitted for FS evaluation, even *with* good clinical and radiologic correlation. However, an attempt should be made to provide a managerial diagnosis, such as reactive, inflammatory/infectious or neoplastic, and if neoplastic, if it benign or malignant, as this will help the surgeon with immediate surgical management.

- Evaluation of the relationship of a lesion to surrounding native bone is essential in the evaluation of some bone tumors because the distinction between benign and malignant may not be possible when the biopsy is composed entirely of neoplastic tissue. For example, it may not be possible to distinguish an enchondroma from low grade chondrosarcoma in a small sample, and the surgeon should be warned that a seemingly benign neoplasm may be re-interpreted as a low grade sarcoma after a larger sample is examined.[2,8,9] Similarly, the histologic appearance of low grade, central osteosarcoma may be indistinguishable from fibrous dysplasia on small biopsies.

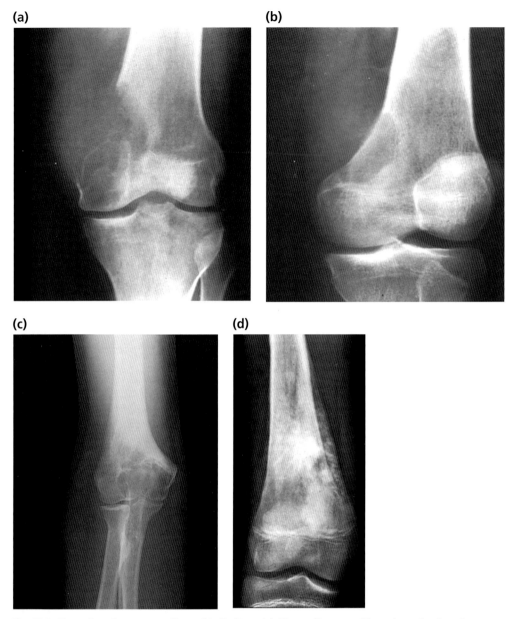

Fig. 19.1. Examples of common radiographic findings. (a) Giant cell tumor of bone is predominantly an epiphyseal lesion which may show metaphyseal and even soft tissue extension. Note that the lesion is circumscribed but not marginated, and that it largely lacks mineralization. (b) Aneurysmal bone cyst is also circumscribed and lacks mineralization but it is most commonly a metaphyseal lesion. (c) Chondroblastoma is epiphyseal and marginated with both lytic and sclerotic components. (d) Giant cell rich osteosarcoma is metaphyseal with a geographic growth pattern; note the periosteal reaction and subperiosteal new bone formation.

■ The presence of abnormal tissue does not necessarily equate to lesional tissue. The finding of fracture callus, aneurysmal bone cyst, fibrosis of the marrow space, or necrotic bone may be secondary phenomena, and when these are present in the FS sample, the pathologist should discuss the findings with the surgeon to determine if the biopsy is indeed derived from the target lesion. This is relevant because orthopedic surgeons will sometimes submit a preliminary, superficial biopsy as the first specimen as the lesion is being approached, especially when the target is difficult to reach.

■ Histologic sections of bone lesions/tumors should not be examined in isolation. This point cannot be emphasized enough. There *are* lesions that can be diagnosed without the help of clinical history and imaging studies but serious errors will be made if the pathologist does not make a habit of taking clinical and imaging data into consideration before making a diagnosis.

- Proper handling of the specimen is of paramount importance. The operating room staff should be educated about how to submit specimens for IOD as well as for ancillary studies.

- Only limited information can be obtained from specimens composed entirely of cortical bone. Touch or cytoscrape preparations should be prepared but the yield is likely to be low. There are reports of "rapid" microwave decalcification of tissue for intraoperative diagnosis,[10] but this procedure is not available in most pathology laboratories.

- Cytologic preparations should be made if the specimen is composed of cancellous bone or if there is an admixture of bone and soft tissue. Cytologic preparations will often yield sufficient material for diagnosis if the lesion is non-mesenchymal in nature, e.g., metastatic carcinoma, melanoma, myeloma, etc. If cytologic preparations do not yield a diagnosis, the softest portions of the specimen should be submitted for FS. There should be no hesitation to cut FSs on cancellous bone with small bony fragments as surprisingly good sections can be obtained. And if the process is unsuccessful, little is lost: modern cryostats have disposable blades that are readily replaced if the blade is dulled or nicked from cutting bony specimens.[13]

- When appropriate, approximately 1 ml^3 of fresh tissue should be snap frozen and stored at -80 °C for molecular studies. A similar amount of viable tissue should be placed in cell culture medium (e.g., RPMI) for cytogenetic studies or flow cytometry, as dictated by the intraoperative findings.

SPECIFIC CLINICO-PATHOLOGIC ISSUES

A discussion of all the specific diagnostic issues that may be encountered intraoperatively is beyond the scope of this chapter. The sections below address the most important issues that are likely to be encountered.

Giant cell-rich lesions

Clinical issues

Osteoclast giant cells are common in a variety of bone lesions. However, the most common lesions in which giant cells dominate the histologic picture are giant cell tumor,

chondroblastoma, aneurysmal bone cyst (including the solid variant) and giant cell rich osteosarcoma. Fortunately, these entities can often be distinguished by their radiologic characteristics. Giant cell tumor is a lytic epiphyseal–metaphyseal lesion that generally presents during the third and fourth decades (Fig. 19.1). Primary aneurysmal bone cyst (ABC) is most often metaphyseal, although exceptional cases involve the epiphysis. Chondroblastoma is a purely lucent epiphyseal or apophyseal lesion that occurs in early adolescence. Finally, the radiographic findings of giant cell rich osteosarcoma are those of a permeative, mixed lytic and sclerotic lesion, usually metaphyseal in location and often with a periosteal reaction.

Chondroblastoma, giant cell tumor, and aneurysmal bone cyst are treated with curettage, burring and packing of the defect with cement or bone graft. Fortunately, the clinical behavior of these three lesions is similar enough that the main purpose of intraoperative evaluation is to exclude giant cell rich osteosarcoma, or some other malignancy (Table 19.3). One might ask why intraoperative diagnosis is sought in these cases if the radiologic findings are considered diagnostic by the radiologist. This is because rarely, osteosarcoma, malignant giant cell tumor and even metastases may present with an epiphyseal lesion that mimics giant cell tumor. Furthermore, the radiographic findings of the lesions under discussion are not *always* diagnostic so that an intralesional biopsy is necessary to exclude malignancy before proceeding with the planned curettage. Giant cell rich osteosarcoma, like all high grade osteosarcomas, is treated with neoadjuvant chemotherapy followed by complete resection; curettage of this neoplasm is not appropriate and may, in fact, compromise later surgery.

Pathologic issues

The specimen characteristically consists of aggregates of red clot, pale pink soft tissue, and a minor component of cancellous bone. Since the surgeon's intention is to perform curettage, the initial biopsy specimen is usually generous and should contain enough lesional soft tissue to submit for FS.

The presence of abundant osteoclast giant cells is a secondary finding in giant cell tumor, ABC and chondroblastoma. Thus, although it is useful to pay attention to the distribution of the osteoclasts (osteoclasts are more uniformly distributed in giant cell tumors), what matters in most cases is what lies between the giant cells, i.e., the nature of the matrix and the appearance of the mononuclear cells.

Table 19.3. Summary of clinical findings of giant cell rich lesions

	Giant cell tumor	Chondroblastoma	Aneurysmal bone cyst	Giant cell rich osteosarcoma
Peak age	35–45	10–20	10–15	15–20
Sex	F≥M	M>F	M=F	M>F
Compartment	Epiphysis-metaphysis	Epiphysis	Metaphysis, mandible	Metaphysis
Symptoms	Pain, swelling, often short duration	Pain, often long duration	Pain, short duration	Pain, swelling short duration
Local Recurrence	25%	5–20%	<5%	<5%
Metastasis	2–4%	0.1%	None[a]	35%[b]
Malignancy	≪1%	None[a]	None[a]	100%
Treatment	Curettage/cement	Curettage/bone graft	Curettage/bone graft	Neo-adjuvant chemotherapy/resection

[a] Case reports of malignancy associated with chondroblastoma and conventional ABC.[11,12]

[b] Osteosarcoma is considered a systemic disease at diagnosis and is treated with chemotherapy. Mortality with surgery alone, in the absence of radiographic evidence of pulmonary metastases at diagnosis, is 80%–90%.[13]

Table 19.4. Summary of histologic findings in giant cell rich lesions

	Giant cell tumor	Chondroblastoma	Aneurysmal bone cyst	Giant cell rich osteosarcoma
Distribution of giant cells	Uniform	Heterogeneous	Heterogeneous	Heterogeneous
Matrix	Absent	"Fibrochondroid" plaques + calcification	Osteoid, sometimes abundant	Osteoid and tumor bone
Mononuclear cells	Ovoid, uniform, nuclei similar to giant cells	Ovoid, eccentric nuclei with grooves (S100+)	Spindled, fibroblastic/ "fibrohistiocytic"	Polygonal to spindled, nuclear hyperchromasia, high nuclear/cytoplasmic ratio
Mitosis	Abundant	Rare	May be abundant	Abundant, atypical
Necrosis	May be present	Absent	Absent	May be present
Atypia	Absent	Absent	Absent	Marked

Table 19.4 lists the common histological findings of these lesions, with the most useful features italicized.

ABC can occur as both a primary neoplasm and a secondary reactive process in response to other bone neoplasms. For example, ABC changes are present in ~20% of giant cell tumors and chondroblastomas.[14,15] One of the problems in ABC lesions is that of sampling; a biopsy from the metaphysis of an epi-metaphyseal lesion may only show the changes of ABC, and not include the underlying giant cell tumor or chondroblastoma located in the epiphysis (Fig. 19.2). This pitfall can be avoided if the clinical history and imaging studies are correlated with the histologic findings.

Frequently, a non-specific IOD such as "fibro-osseous lesion with abundant giant cells" is all that the pathologist is able to offer, and this should be sufficient for the surgeon to proceed with the curettage. However, the pathologist should review the radiographs, determine the exact location of biopsy (soft tissue, epiphysis, metaphysis), and

discuss the findings with the surgeon to make sure that the lesion is not an osteosarcoma.

The suspicion of malignancy, specifically giant cell rich osteosarcoma, is based on the presence of cytologic atypia in the mononuclear cell population. These cells have a high nuclear/cytoplasmic ratio, show nuclear hyperchromasia and demonstrate atypical mitotic figures (Fig. 19.3). A specific diagnosis of osteosarcoma is not required in this clinical context, but the surgeon should be informed that the biopsy findings are suspicious or diagnostic of malignancy. This provisional diagnosis will ensure the correct course of action; curettage will not be performed, and definitive treatment will be withheld until a final diagnosis is rendered on permanent sections.

Occasionally, benign giant cell tumors show necrosis, abundant mitoses and even vascular invasion, making it difficult to distinguish this lesion from a sarcoma (Fig. 19.4). If the distinction cannot be made with confidence, it is better

(a)   **(b)**   **(c)**

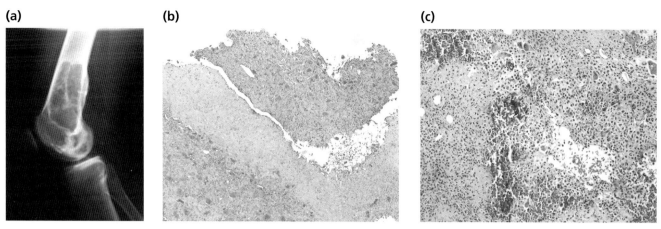

Fig. 19.2. Secondary aneurysmal bone cyst (ABC) in chondroblastoma. (a) The plain radiograph demonstrates a circumscribed lesion that involves both the epiphysis and metaphysis. Although this example is from an 18-year old, the growth plates have closed. (b) Initial material obtained from the metaphyseal component of the lesion demonstrates fibrous septae, a spindle cell proliferation, and hemorrhage and giant cells suggesting ABC. (c) A second specimen from the epiphyseal component of the same lesion demonstrates characteristic features of chondroblastoma.

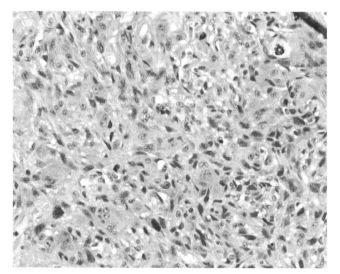

Fig. 19.3. Giant cell rich osteosarcoma demonstrates occasional multinucleated osteoclast-like giant cells. The background, however, contains osteoid associated with cytologically malignant, hyperchromatic osteoblasts.

to err on the side of caution and defer the diagnosis to permanent sections.

To reiterate, the main purpose of IOD in giant cell-rich lesions is to decide if the surgeon should proceed with curettage (for a benign diagnosis) or stop after performing an incisional biopsy (malignancy or possible malignancy). The specific diagnosis is best made after review of all the pathologic material, and after obtaining expert consultation if this becomes necessary.

Cartilaginous tumors

Most cartilaginous neoplasms can be diagnosed or suspected on clinical and imaging findings alone. High grade chondrosarcomas are readily confirmed by histologic examination, but the distinction between enchondroma and grade 1 chondrosarcoma can be challenging.

High grade chondrosarcoma

Clinical issues

Many high grade chondrosarcomas have radiographic changes that are either diagnostic or suggestive of malignancy (destructive growth, soft tissue extension, etc.). An incisional biopsy is performed and submitted for FS diagnosis. The purpose of IOD is to confirm that the biopsy contains sarcoma. After confirmation of the diagnosis on permanent sections, tissue-sparing surgical resection is the procedure of choice. Adjuvant chemotherapy is often administered to patients with grade 3 chondrosarcoma prior to surgical resection. Amputation is resorted to when limb-sparing surgery is not feasible.

MRI is used to plan the scope of limb-sparing surgical resection. For technical reasons, MRI is more accurate in determining the extent of tumor in long bones than in flat bones. At the time of definitive surgical resection, the surgeon is likely to request IOD on the surgical margins, especially on resections of flat bones such as pelvic bones.

Pathologic issues

The initial diagnosis of high-grade chondrosarcoma (grades 2 and 3) can be readily made on FS (Fig. 19.5). The purpose of IOD is to confirm that diagnostic tissue is present. A diagnosis of "high grade chondrosarcoma"

(a)

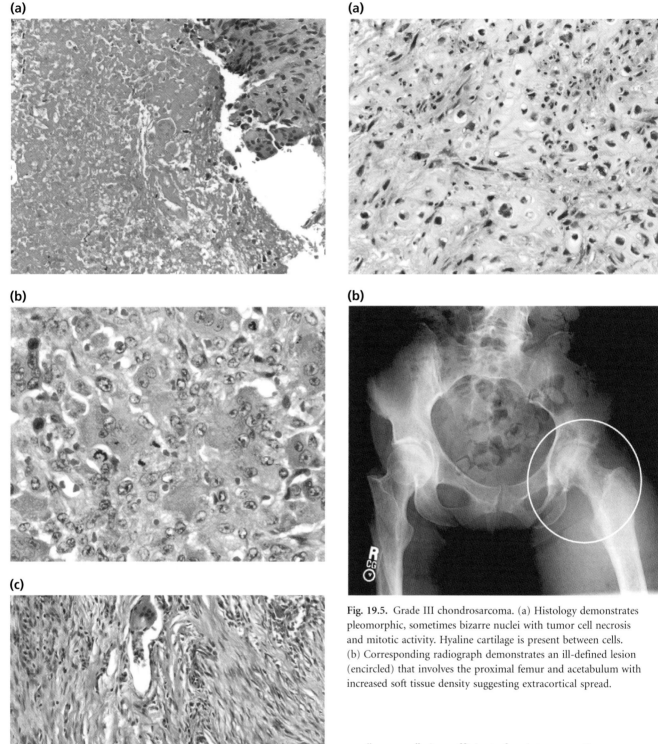

(b)

(c)

Fig. 19.4. Features of giant cell tumor that might cause confusion with sarcoma but are not diagnostic of malignancy. (a) Necrosis. (b) High mitotic rate. (c) Vascular invasion.

(a)

(b)

Fig. 19.5. Grade III chondrosarcoma. (a) Histology demonstrates pleomorphic, sometimes bizarre nuclei with tumor cell necrosis and mitotic activity. Hyaline cartilage is present between cells. (b) Corresponding radiograph demonstrates an ill-defined lesion (encircled) that involves the proximal femur and acetabulum with increased soft tissue density suggesting extracortical spread.

or "sarcoma" is sufficient for intraoperative purposes, and when a diagnosis of chondrosarcoma is made, the distinction between grade 2 and grade 3 should be deferred to permanent sections.

When the surgeon requests intraoperative evaluation of the surgical margins, the cancellous bone at the margins should be curetted and evaluated by touch preparation or FS.

Low grade chondrosarcoma and enchondroma

Clinical issues

The distinction between enchondroma and grade 1 chondrosarcoma is often difficult. Radiographic changes such as pathologic fracture, soft tissue edema and hemorrhage, periosteal reaction, cortical disruption, and cortical thickening favor chondrosarcoma, but these findings are not always present, nor are they fully diagnostic of malignancy. In spite of these limitations, clinical and radiographic findings remain the most reliable parameters for distinguishing enchondroma from low grade chondrosarcoma. As an example, anatomic location is crucial: the vast majority of cartilaginous tumors of the digits are benign, whereas the majority of cartilaginous tumors of pelvic bones are classified as grade 1 chondrosarcoma. This underscores the pivotal role of imaging in the evaluation and management of cartilaginous neoplasms.

Surgeons request IOD on suspected low grade chondrosarcomas for two reasons: (a) to confirm that the neoplasm is indeed cartilaginous in nature, and (b) to exclude the presence of an unexpected high grade chondrosarcoma masquerading as a low grade sarcoma on imaging; this is important because high grade sarcoma precludes curettage as definitive treatment. Lesions suspected to be low grade chondrosarcoma – as determined on clinical and imaging studies – are treated with curettage. The post-curettage defect is packed with methylmethacrylate.

Enchondromas may be managed conservatively and followed with periodic radiographs, but many are eventually treated by curettage, especially if they become symptomatic. The specimen is not submitted for FS diagnosis if the clinical and imaging findings are characteristic of a benign neoplasm (e.g., a small, well circumscribed, lytic lesion of a digit). Radiologically benign surface cartilaginous tumors, e.g., osteochondroma and periosteal chondroma, are treated by complete excision, and these specimens are not submitted for IOD.

Pathologic issues

Histologic examination cannot reliably distinguish between enchondroma and grade 1 chondrosarcoma because of the overlap in cellularity and cytologic atypia,[*]

---

[*] Some authors feel that grade 1 chondrosarcomas can be recognized by permeation of normal lamellar bone at the periphery of the lesion.[16] The veracity of this finding is in dispute. In addition, this requires extensive sampling as well as examination of the periphery of the neoplasm, both of which may not be possible intraoperatively.

and it follows that this distinction cannot be made intraoperatively, either by FS or cytologic examination. As stated earlier, clinical and radiographic findings are more reliable for discriminating between these two neoplasms (Fig. 19.6).[16–22]

On gross examination, the tissue is usually recognizable as cartilaginous. Touch preparations and FS are equally good for confirming the cartilaginous nature of the neoplasm but a FS should be performed as it is superior for evaluating cellularity; this is relevant because one of the goals of IOD is to rule out high grade chondrosarcoma. Because of their low fluid content, low cellularity cartilaginous neoplasms may wash off the slide during H&E staining. This slippage can be minimized by allowing the alcohol-fixed slide to air-dry for about 1 minute before taking the slide through the staining solutions.

Orthopedic surgeons who have limited experience with bone tumors may expect the pathologist to distinguish between enchondroma and grade 1 chondrosarcoma by FS examination. The pathologist should diplomatically inform the surgeon that this distinction cannot be made, and that the diagnosis is more reliably made on the basis of clinical and imaging data. The pathologist may, however, be in a position to support a diagnosis of grade 1 chondrosarcoma if the clinical and imaging studies are compelling (e.g., destructive lesion with extension into soft tissue) – especially if an expert bone radiologist has rendered a diagnosis of chondrosarcoma on the imaging studies. The inability to distinguish between enchondroma and grade 1 chondrosarcoma by FS is mitigated by the fact that both neoplasms are treated by curettage. Surgical curettage may be supplemented with cryosurgery in grade 1 chondrosarcomas, but this decision should be guided by clinical and radiographic findings and not the FS findings.

Pathologists should be particularly cautious about intraoperative evaluation of cartilaginous tumors of the hands and feet because radiographic changes such as cortical erosion may be worrisome (Fig. 19.7).[17] On FS, these neoplasms are often hypercellular, show myxoid change and nuclear atypia, and sometimes show permeation of medullary spaces – features that would be interpreted as evidence of low grade chondrosarcoma in sites such as the pelvic bones. It is worth remembering that chondrosarcomas of the hands and feet are rare, and the diagnosis should be made only if the clinical, imaging, and morphologic features are compelling. As with any unusual bone neoplasm, it would be prudent for the general surgical pathologist to seek consultation from an expert bone

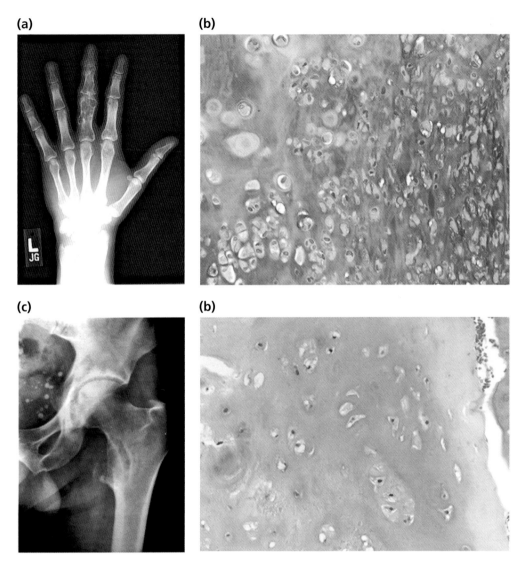

Fig. 19.6. Histologic overlap between enchondroma and grade 1 chondrosarcoma. (a) This radiograph shows multiple enchondromas of the proximal and middle phalange of the third digit; multiple enchondromas of the hand are uncommon and should raise the possibility of the Ollier's syndrome. (b) Corresponding histology of enchondroma of the phalanx. (c) The radiograph in this case of chondrosarcoma shows a mass that is circumscribed laterally but with cortical destruction and soft tissue extension medially. (d) Grade 1 chondrosarcoma of the pelvis, with *lower* cellularity than the chondroma illustrated in (b). This patient later developed pulmonary metastases.

pathologist before making the diagnosis of chondrosarcoma of the hands and feet.

Osteogenic neoplasms

Clinical issues

Osteosarcoma is the most common primary osseous malignancy in adolescents and young adults, and is the second most common primary bone malignancy in patients older than 40. Although a variety of clinically significant subtypes have been described, for practical purposes, osteosarcomas can be divided into low grade and high grade forms. Low-grade osteosarcomas include parosteal osteosarcoma and central low-grade osteosarcoma. The remaining subtypes, such as conventional intramedullary, telangiectatic, giant cell rich, and small cell osteosarcoma, are considered high grade. Low grade osteosarcomas are treated by complete surgical resection, whereas high grade osteosarcomas are treated with neoadjuvant ifosfamide-based chemotherapy followed by complete surgical resection. Periosteal osteosarcomas rarely metastasize and have a much better prognosis than other high grade osteosarcomas; treatment is tailored to the individual patient (Table 19.5).[23,24]

The radiologic appearance of most high-grade osteo-sarcomas is sufficiently destructive in appearance to warrant a pre-operative suspicion of malignancy. Most osteosarcomas show an aggressive sclerotic or mixed lytic and sclerotic appearance, periosteal reaction, periosteal elevation (Codman triangle), and a soft tissue mass (Fig. 19.8). An incisional biopsy is performed and a FS is requested to: (a) confirm the presence of diagnostic tissue; (b) to ensure that high grade sarcoma is present if the radiographs suggest a high grade malignancy; and (c) procure tissue for ancillary studies if the patient is likely to be enrolled in a clinical trial. Definitive surgical resection of high grade osteosarcomas is performed after diagnosis on permanent sections, and treatment with neoadjuvant chemotherapy.

Pathologic issues

The diagnosis of osteosarcoma requires the production of osteoid and/or mineralized bone (tumor bone) by neoplastic cells. The diagnosis can be challenging because osteoid and tumor bone formation can be focal, and may not be present in the biopsy specimen. Some experts have suggested that the diagnosis of osteosarcoma can be made in the absence of

Table 19.5. Comparison of osteosarcoma subtypes, grade and clinical management

Grade	Subtype	Management
I	Central low grade and parosteal	Local resection
II	Periosteal	Local resection, rarely adjuvant chemotherapy
III	Conventional, telangiectatic, small cell, and giant cell rich	Neoadjuvant chemotherapy, resection or amputation

osteoid if the imaging studies are typical and show bone matrix;[2] however, we recommend that the general surgical pathologist should seek consultation from a bone tumor expert before making a diagnosis of osteosarcoma in this situation.

The unifying characteristic of all high grade osteosarcomas is the presence of cytologic atypia, including irregular, hyperchromatic nuclei, anaplasia, and atypical mitotic figures (Fig. 19.9). The cells may grow in sheets or fascicles, and be admixed with newly formed cartilage or trabeculae of woven bone. The diagnosis of sarcoma, not further specified, is sufficient for the purpose of IOD.

The differential diagnosis of high grade osteosarcoma depends on the subtype. Conventional osteosarcoma may raise the possibility of some benign entities such as osteoblastoma, giant cell tumor, and chondroblastoma, depending on the presence of matrix or abundant osteoclast-like giant cells. However, the presence of nuclear hyperchromasia, variable nuclear size and shape, atypical mitotic figures and, most importantly, the radiographic findings, help to exclude these lesions. The radiographic findings and low-power architecture of telangiectatic osteosarcoma may resemble those of ABC but the presence of malignant cytologic features excludes ABC. Small cell osteosarcoma may raise the possibility of Ewing sarcoma or lymphoma, especially if no osteoid is present in the frozen section material. In such cases, a diagnosis of "malignant small round cell neoplasm" is sufficient for purposes of IOD; tissue should be procured for ancillary studies should they be needed (flow-cytometry, cytogenetics, RT-PCR and fluorescence in-situ hybridization).

In contrast, low-grade osteosarcomas have more subtle atypia that may be difficult to discern, even on permanent

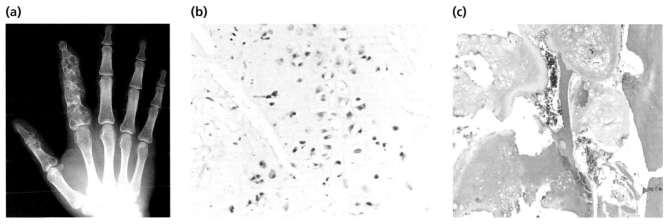

(a) **(b)** **(c)**

Fig. 19.7. Enchondromas of the hands and feet may be diagnostically challenging. (a) Radiograph of the hand showing enchondromas of the proximal and middle phalanges of the second finger. Cortical erosion is present, but this should not be taken as evidence of malignancy. (b) Hypercellularity and myxoid change are common in enchondromas of digits. (c) Enchondroma showing focal permeation of the medullary bone; however, transcortical spread (note intact cortex on the right) and spread through Haversian canals should be absent.

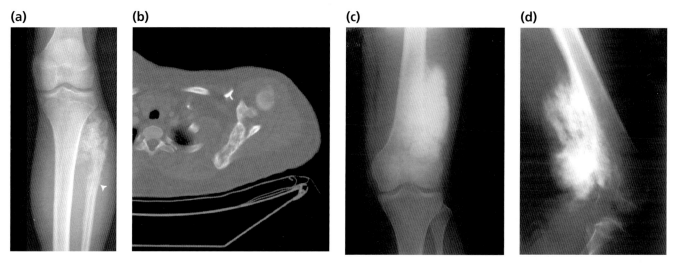

Fig. 19.8. Radiographs of osteosarcoma subtypes. (a) Conventional intramedullary osteosarcoma is permeative with calcification and periosteal reaction (arrowhead). (b) Low-grade central osteosarcoma of the scapula; the lesion is poorly marginated and predominantly sclerotic without a soft tissue mass. (c) Parosteal osteosarcoma forming a lobulated mass with broad attachment to the cortex, encircling bone but without medullary involvement. (d) Periosteal osteosarcoma that is meta-diaphyseal, with a thickened cortex and sparing of the medullary cavity.

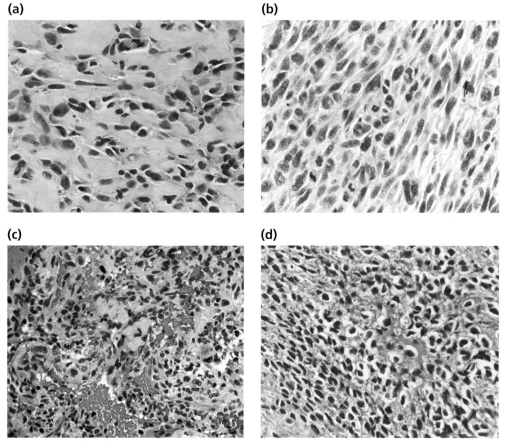

Fig. 19.9. Examples of osteosarcoma. (a) The presence of eosinophilic osteoid matrix associated with malignant cells is diagnostic of osteosarcoma. (b) Small intraoperative specimen demonstrating malignant cytologic features but lacking osteoid. (c) Telangiectatic osteosarcoma admixed with hemorrhage. (d) Small cell osteosarcoma which has to be distinguished from other small round blue cell tumors.

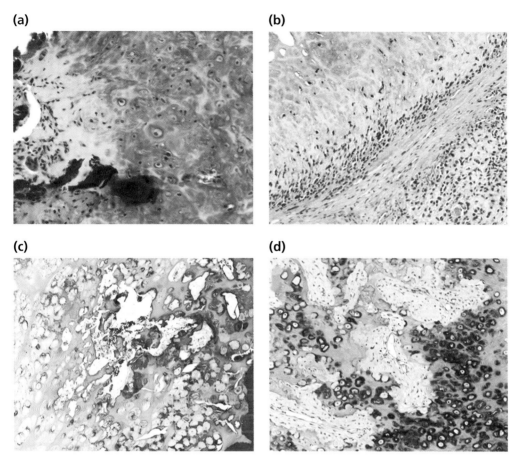

Fig. 19.10. Histologic overlap of chondro-osteoid surface lesions. (a) Bizarre parosteal osteochondromatous proliferation (Nora's lesion). (b) Periosteal osteosarcoma. (c) Chondrosarcoma arising in osteochondroma. (d) Florid reactive periostitis.

sections. The diagnosis of low grade osteosarcoma requires an assessment of the architecture, and this includes broad parallel trabeculae in the case of parosteal osteosarcoma and permeation of viable lamellar bone in low grade central osteosarcoma. As usual, the radiographic findings weigh heavily in the diagnosis of low grade osteosarcomas. At times, an IOD of "low grade osteogenic neoplasm" is all the pathologist can offer; the differential diagnosis should be discussed with the surgeon (e.g., fibrous dysplasia, desmoplastic fibroma, etc.) and the diagnosis should be deferred to permanent sections. Definitive resection should be performed only after a firm diagnosis has been made on permanent sections.

The diagnosis of surface osteogenic lesions should be deferred to permanent sections because of the difficulty in distinguishing between sarcomas and reactive conditions on FS. Florid reactive periostitis, bizarre parosteal osteochondromatous proliferation (Nora's lesion), periosteal osteosarcoma, parosteal osteosarcoma, and chondrosarcoma arising in an osteochondroma may present as surface lesions that can be confusing especially in the absence of expert radiologic interpretation (Fig. 19.10).

Small round cell neoplasms

Small round cell neoplasms of bone include small cell osteosarcoma, Ewing's sarcoma, mesenchymal chondrosarcoma, lymphoma, and rarely metastatic neuroblastoma and rhabdomyosarcoma. These neoplasms are discussed in detail in Chapter 20.

Evaluation of surgical margins

Clinical issues

Some sarcomas, especially osteosarcomas, show intramedullary spread beyond the radiographic boundaries of the lesion.[25] Modern imaging techniques, especially MR scanning, have dramatically improved the accuracy of predicting the extent of tumor but even these techniques have their limitations.[26,27] MRI may give false-negative and false-positive results, especially after treatment with

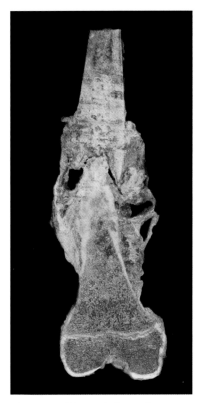

Fig. 19.11. Gross pathology of osteosarcoma involving distal femur. The hard, white-tan bone-forming mass can reliably be measured from the normal marrow margin above.

chemotherapy,[28] and for technical reasons, flat bones such as ilium and scapula are more difficult to evaluate with MRI, both with regard to extent of tumor as well as the relationship of the neoplasm to surgical margins. As a result, surgical skill and judgment are important in determining the extent of the osteotomy in flat bones such as the scapula and pelvis.

Positive surgical margins are more likely to occur in limb salvage procedures than in amputations, and surgeons will therefore request intraoperative evaluation of the margins in limb-sparing resections.

Pathologic issues
In some tumors involving long bones, the extent of the tumor and the status of surgical margins can be reliably evaluated by gross examination.[29] This is especially true of osteosarcomas and chondrosarcomas because of grossly visible tumor matrix (Fig. 19.11). However, this requires rapid bivalving of the specimen, a technique that may not be possible in all laboratories. Gross examination does, however, have its limitations: sarcomas such as Ewing sarcoma may have subtle infiltrative margins that are not

grossly visible, and while gross examination can identify tumor matrix, it cannot distinguish between viable osteosarcoma and successfully treated osteosarcoma with residual bone matrix; microscopic evaluation of the margins is required in these situations.

As discussed above, the pathologist should be aware of the surgeon's treatment plan, especially in the event of a positive margin in a limb-sparing resection; the surgical margins should be interpreted with caution if a positive margin will convert a limb-sparing procedure to amputation.

The surgical margin is evaluated by examining the cancellous bone at the margin. This can be done in two ways: the surgeon may submit a curetting of the margin or the pathologist may scrape the margin/s in the resected specimen. Samples are obtained from the proximal and distal margins of long bones and from multiple sites in flat bones. The specimen will consist of gritty medullary bone and marrow. Touch and smear preparations are generally the best way to evaluate these samples, although it is also possible to perform FS if fragments of bone >5 mm are first removed.[29] All of the submitted material should be examined intraoperatively to avoid overlooking focal involvement of the margin by sarcoma.

Osteomyelitis

Clinical issues
Osteomyelitis occurs either directly from sites of trauma or as a result of bacteremia. Acute osteomyelitis presents with systemic symptoms, leukocytosis, progressive pain and swelling, and approximately 10% of cases progress to a chronic form that can wax and wane for months. Occasionally, chronic osteomyelitis may enter a sclerotic phase. Radiographically, osteomyelitis is a "great mimicker" because of its protean appearances. It may be non-destructive and resemble eosinophilic granuloma, or have a destructive appearance mimicking malignancies such as lymphoma and Ewing's sarcoma. Whenever possible, an attempt is made to identify the causative organism to guide antibiotic therapy. Antibiotics are typically administered for 6 weeks and may be tailored empirically based on the clinical presentation (e.g., Gram positive cocci in children with suspected hematogenous osteomyelitis, *Salmonella* in patients with sickle cell anemia). Chronic osteomyelitis may require debridement of necrotic bone (sequestrum) to improve the response to antibiotic therapy.

IOD is requested to confirm the diagnosis of infection, exclude malignancy in radiologically aggressive-appearing lesions, and to procure material for culture.

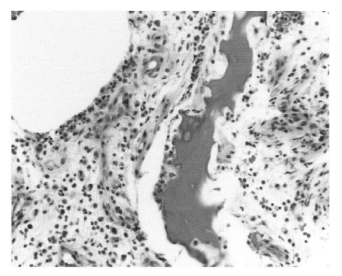

Fig. 19.12. Acute osteomyelitis demonstrates necrotic bone and a fibrinopurulent exudate.

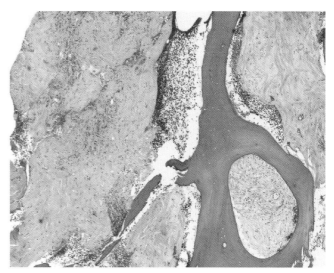

Fig. 19.13. Chronic, sclerosing osteomyelitis. Some examples demonstrate a sclerotic, vascularized stroma with only minimal chronic inflammation.

Pathologic issues

Histologically, the detection of bacterial organisms inside neutrophils is pathognomonic of osteomyelitis, but this is rarely identified on FS. It is more common to find a neutrophilic infiltrate, replacement of the marrow space by granulation tissue, and necrotic bone (Fig. 19.12). A recent fracture (<3 days old) can show similar findings so the distinction between acute osteomyelitis and recent fracture requires clinico-radio-pathologic correlation.

Chronic osteomyelitis can have a wide range of appearances so the diagnosis is often made by exclusion. An infiltrate of plasma cells accompanied by granulation tissue replacement of the marrow favors osteomyelitis. When plasma cells are abundant, flow cytometry or immunohistochemistry for kappa and lambda light chains may be necessary to exclude myeloma. When inflammation is inconspicuous, the sclerosing form of chronic osteomyelitis is difficult to distinguish from other fibro-osseous lesions such as fibrous dysplasia, central low-grade osteosarcoma and desmoplastic fibroma (Fig. 19.13). The stroma of these neoplasms is composed of cellular fascicles of spindle cells in contrast to the hypocellular vascular stroma of chronic osteomyelitis. Osteonecrosis is a clue to osteomyelitis, but it is not specific. Long standing osteomyelitis may show abundant new woven bone (involucrum), simulating neoplastic bone formation.

Infection in reimplantation arthroplasties

Clinical issues

Aseptic loosening of prosthetic implants is approximately six times more frequent than septic loosening. Aseptic loosening is secondary to inflammation initiated by wear-induced particle debris, but mechanical issues, such as stress shielding and hardware breakage, are also responsible for failure. Infection of a prosthesis may occur with or without loosening of the prosthesis. Unless the diagnosis is made very early and treated with prompt debridement, prosthetic infections usually require removal of the entire device and associated foreign material, followed by implantation of an antibiotic-impregnated cement spacer. The patient then receives 6 weeks of intravenous antibiotics, followed by 6 weeks of observation before considering implantation of a new prosthesis. The presence of persistent infection is a contraindication to proceeding with re-implantation; instead, further debridement is undertaken, antibiotic treatment is continued and re-implantation is delayed. The placement of new orthopedic hardware into an infected site may have serious consequences, and may ultimately lead to resection arthroplasty or even to amputation.[30] Accurate intraoperative diagnosis of infection is therefore, critical.

The gold-standard for the diagnosis of infection is positive culture of the same organism from multiple sites. Surgeons therefore submit biopsy material from the pseudocapsule or membrane surrounding the prosthesis as well as from tissue that appears suspicious for infection. Tissue is routinely sent to pathology for frozen section and to microbiology for culture and Gram stain. The histologic criteria for the intraoperative diagnosis of infection are based on high virulence organisms (*E. coli, Pseudomonas,*

(a)   **(b)**

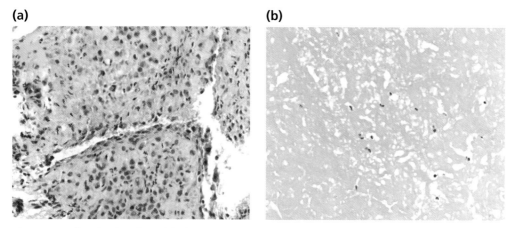

Fig. 19.14. Infected arthroplasty. (a) The presence of neutrophils in subsynovial tissue is diagnostic. (b) Neutrophils in fibrin are common in arthroplasty specimens but are *not* diagnostic of infection.

S. aureus). Controversy exists about the validity of applying these criteria to less virulent bacteria such as coagulase negative staphylococci.[31,32]

Pathologic issues

Ideally, the gross specimen should be sectioned perpendicular to the synovium or capsule, which in the normal state is smooth and glistening rather than rough. We recommend freezing the entire specimen if it fits in two blocks. Otherwise, representative sections are taken from each piece of tissue and embedded in two FS blocks. The presence of neutrophils in the synovium, subsynovial connective tissue, or granulation tissue constitutes evidence of infection, and the most cellular areas are chosen for evaluation. When counting neutrophils, polymorphonuclear leukocytes entrapped in fibrin should not be counted as this is non-specific and should not be taken as evidence of infection (Fig. 19.14).

Two different criteria are currently in use for the diagnosis of infection. The Feldman criterion[33] requires at least five neutrophils per high power field (400×) in at least five fields, and the Athanasou criterion requires 10 neutrophils in 10 high power fields (average of one neutrophil per high power field).[34] As expected, the Feldman system is more *specific* but less *sensitive* than the Athanasou method (Table 19.6).[35,36] Furthermore, the diameter of a 400× field can vary between microscopes, further confounding the significance of these findings. We recommend using the Athanasou criterion (≥10 neutrophils per 10 high power fields) as evidence of infection. When the counts are below this threshold, the pathologist should report to the surgeon that even an average of <1

neutrophil per high power field does not exclude infection. Depending on the level of clinical suspicion, the surgeon may choose to continue oral antibiotics until culture results are available.[37]

Table 19.6. Criteria for infection in reimplantation arthroplasties

	Criterion	Sensitivity	Specificity
Feldman	5 neutrophils/hpf in ≥ 5 hpf[a]	25%	98%
Athanasou	10 neutrophils/10 hpf	70%	64%

[a] hpf: 400X high power field.

REFERENCES

1. Ayala AG, Ro JY, Fanning CV, Flores JP, Yasko AW. Core needle biopsy and fine-needle aspiration in the diagnosis of bone and soft-tissue lesions. *Hematol Oncol Clin North Am* 1995; **9**: 633–651.
2. McCarthy EF. CT-guided needle biopsies of bone and soft tissue tumors: a pathologist's perspective. *Skeletal Radiol* 2007; **36**: 181–182.
3. Mankin HJ. Chondrosarcomas of digits: are they really malignant? *Cancer* 1999; **86**: 1635–1637.
4. Mankin HJ, Lange TA, Spanier SS. The hazards of biopsy in patients with malignant primary bone and soft-tissue tumors. *J Bone Joint Surg Am* 1982; **64**: 1121–1127.
5. Pollock RC, Stalley PD. Biopsy of musculoskeletal tumours – beware. *ANZ J Surg* 2004; **74**: 516–519.
6. Rubin BP, Fletcher CD, Inwards C, *et al.* Protocol for the examination of specimens from patients with soft tissue tumors of intermediate malignant potential, malignant soft tissue tumors, and benign/locally aggressive and malignant bone tumors. *Arch Pathol Lab Med* 2006; **130**: 1616–1629.
7. Estrada-Villasenor EG, Cedillo ED, Gonzalez LM, Martinez GR. Accuracy of intraoperative consultation for bone tumors: experience in an orthopedic hospital. *J Orthop Sci* 2007; **12**: 123–126.

8. Mirra JM, Brien EW, Luck JV, Jr. Intraoperative pathologic consultation (IOC) for tumors of the bone. *Chir Organi Mov* 1997; **82**: 7–31.

9. Reliability of histopathologic and radiologic grading of cartilaginous neoplasms in long bones. *J Bone Joint Surg Am* 2007; **89**: 2113–2123.

10. Weisberger EC, Hilburn M, Johnson B, Nguyen C. Intraoperative microwave processing of bone margins during resection of head and neck cancer. *Arch Otolaryngol Head Neck Surg* 2001; **127**: 790–793.

11. Kyriakos M, Hardy D. Malignant transformation of aneurysmal bone cyst, with an analysis of the literature. *Cancer* 1991; **68**: 1770–1780.

12. Kyriakos M, Land VJ, Penning HL, Parker SG. Metastatic chondroblastoma. Report of a fatal case with a review of the literature on atypical, aggressive, and malignant chondroblastoma. *Cancer* 1985; **55**: 1770–1789.

13. Fletcher CDM, Unni KK, Mertens F, eds. *Pathology and Genetics of Tumours of Soft Tissue and Bone.* Lyon: IARC Press, 2002.

14. de Silva MV, Reid R. Chondroblastoma: varied histologic appearance, potential diagnostic pitfalls, and clinicopathologic features associated with local recurrence. *Ann Diagn Pathol* 2003; **7**: 205–213.

15. Kurt AM, Unni KK, Sim FH, McLeod RA. Chondroblastoma of bone. *Hum Pathol.* 1989; **20**: 965–976.

16. Mirra JM, Gold R, Downs J, Eckardt JJ. A new histologic approach to the differentiation of enchondroma and chondrosarcoma of the bones. A clinicopathologic analysis of 51 cases. *Clin Orthop Relat Res* 1985 **201**: 214–237.

17. Geirnaerdt MJ, Hermans J, Bloem JL, *et al.* Usefulness of radiography in differentiating enchondroma from central grade 1 chondrosarcoma. *Am J Roentgenol* 1997; **169**: 1097–1104.

18. Giudici MA, Moser RP, Jr, Kransdorf MJ. Cartilaginous bone tumors. *Radiol Clin North Am* 1993; **31**: 237–259.

19. Murphey MD, Walker EA, Wilson AJ, Kransdorf MJ, Temple HT, Gannon FH. From the archives of the AFIP: imaging of primary chondrosarcoma: radiologic-pathologic correlation. *Radiographics* 2003; **23**: 1245–1278.

20. Rosenthal DI, Schiller AL, Mankin HJ. Chondrosarcoma: correlation of radiological and histological grade. *Radiology* 1984; **150**: 21–26.

21. Bjornsson J, McLeod RA, Unni KK, Ilstrup DM, Pritchard DJ. Primary chondrosarcoma of long bones and limb girdles. *Cancer* 1998; **83**: 2105–2119.

22. Wold LE, Adler C-P, Sim FH, Unni KK, eds. *Atlas of Orthopedic Pathology.* Philadelphia: Saunders, 2003.

23. Bertoni F, Boriani S, Laus M, Campanacci M. Periosteal chondrosarcoma and periosteal osteosarcoma. Two distinct entities. *J Bone Joint Surg Br* 1982; **64**: 370–376.

24. Ritts GD, Pritchard DJ, Unni KK, Beabout JW, Eckardt JJ. Periosteal osteosarcoma. *Clin Orthop Relat Res.* 1987 **219**: 299–307.

25. O'Flanagan SJ, Stack JP, McGee HM, Dervan P, Hurson B. Imaging of intramedullary tumour spread in osteosarcoma. A comparison of techniques. *J Bone Joint Surg Br* 1991; **73**: 998–1001.

26. Onikul E, Fletcher BD, Parham DM, Chen G. Accuracy of MR imaging for estimating intraosseous extent of osteosarcoma. *Am J Roentgenol* 1996; **167**: 1211–1215.

27. Sundaram M, McGuire MH, Herbold DR, Wolverson MK, Heiberg E. Magnetic resonance imaging in planning limb-salvage surgery for primary malignant tumors of bone. *J Bone Joint Surg Am* 1986; **68**: 809–819.

28. Golfieri R, Baddeley H, Pringle JS, Leung AW, Greco A, Souhami R. MRI in primary bone tumors: therapeutic implications. *Eur J Radiol* 1991; **12**: 201–207.

29. Meyer MS, Spanier SS, Moser M, Scarborough MT. Evaluating marrow margins for resection of osteosarcoma. A modern approach. *Clin Orthop Relat Res* 1999 **363**: 170–175.

30. Segawa H, Tsukayama DT, Kyle RF, Becker DA, Gustilo RB. Infection after total knee arthroplasty. A retrospective study of the treatment of eighty-one infections. *J Bone Joint Surg Am* 1999; **81**: 1434–1445.

31. Langlais F. Can we improve the results of revision arthroplasty for infected total hip replacement? *J Bone Joint Surg Br* 2003; **85**: 637–640.

32. Ure KJ, Amstutz HC, Nasser S, Schmalzried TP. Direct-exchange arthroplasty for the treatment of infection after total hip replacement. An average ten-year follow-up. *J Bone Joint Surg Am* 1998; **80**: 961–968.

33. Mirra JM, Amstutz HC, Matos M, Gold R. The pathology of the joint tissues and its clinical relevance in prosthesis failure. *Clin Orthop Relat Res* 1976; **117**: 221–240.

34. Athanasou NA, Pandey R, de Steiger R, Crook D, Smith PM. Diagnosis of infection by frozen section during revision arthroplasty. *J Bone Joint Surg Br* 1995; **77**: 28–33.

35. Athanasou NA, Pandey R, de Steiger R, McLardy Smith P. The role of intraoperative frozen sections in revision total joint arthroplasty. *J Bone Joint Surg Am* 1997; **79**: 1433–1434.

36. Della Valle CJ, Bogner E, Desai P, *et al.* Analysis of frozen sections of intraoperative specimens obtained at the time of reoperation after hip or knee resection arthroplasty for the treatment of infection. *J Bone Joint Surg Am* 1999; **81**: 684–689.

37. Bori G, Soriano A, Garcia S, Mallofre C, Riba J, Mensa J. Usefulness of histological analysis for predicting the presence of microorganisms at the time of reimplantation after hip resection arthroplasty for the treatment of infection. *J Bone Joint Surg Am* 2007; **89**: 1232–1237.

20 PEDIATRIC SURGICAL PATHOLOGY

Robert H. Byrd, Darrell L. Cass, and Megan K. Dishop

INTRODUCTION

Pediatric surgical pathology is often challenging for the general surgical pathologist. There are two reasons for this: First, the types of surgical diseases that occur in children and infants are quite different from adult patients, and second, many patients with serious pediatric diseases are referred directly to a children's hospital, thus limiting the experience for general surgical pathologists. This chapter will discuss selected pediatric diseases that the general surgical pathologist is likely to encounter, including small blue cell tumors, renal tumors, liver tumors, Hirschsprung's disease, and extrahepatic biliary atresia. Pediatric tumors of the central nervous system are discussed in Chapter 17, p. 283 and ovarian tumors are discussed in Chapter 14, p. 224).

DIFFERENCES BETWEEN PEDIATRIC AND ADULT PATIENTS

One of the major differences between pediatric and adult patients is the distribution of tumor types, as children have a predilection for embryonal tumors ("small blue cell tumors"), germ cell tumors, and lesions of bone and soft tissue. In addition, surgery for congenital lesions, developmental disorders, and malformations are almost unique to the pediatric population, and can be challenging during intraoperative consultation (IOC).[1] Neoplastic disease accounts for approximately 70% of intraoperative consultations, and non-neoplastic lesions for the remaining 30% (Fig. 20.1).[2,3] Lesions of the central nervous system account for a significant proportion of pediatric consultations, ranging from 20%–40% of cases.[4] Hirschsprung's disease is the most common non-neoplastic indication for

IOC, accounting for 12%–25% of all IOC cases at children's hospitals.[2,3]

In general, IOC is employed less frequently in pediatric patients, especially in surgical oncology. Some reasons are:

- A limited range of neoplasms occur in certain anatomic sites, and a specific or near specific diagnosis can be made on the basis of tumor site, patient age, imaging characteristics and laboratory data, allowing the surgeon to proceed with definitive surgical resection without an intraoperative diagnosis (IOD); examples include Wilms' tumor of the kidney and neuroblastoma of the adrenal gland.

- If the neoplasm is confined to the target organ by imaging studies, definitive surgical resection will remove the entire malignancy with adequate surgical margins, eliminating the need for IOD.

- Malignancies that commonly require evaluation of surgical margins in adult patients, such as breast carcinoma, cutaneous carcinomas and carcinomas that arise from mucosal sites, are rare in the pediatric population.[2]

INFORMATION NEEDED BEFORE AND DURING INTRAOPERATIVE CONSULTATION

Familiarity with the clinical history, imaging findings, and laboratory data is essential if the pathologist is to act as an informed consultant. Age and site of the neoplasm are two of the most important data points, and the differential diagnosis begins with this information. Prior biopsies should be reviewed, if applicable. The pathologist should be aware of the surgeon's operative plan, and know how the results of IOD will change the operative plan, especially if the stakes

Intraoperative Consultation in Surgical Pathology, ed. Mahendra Ranchod. Published by Cambridge University Press.
© Cambridge University Press 2010.

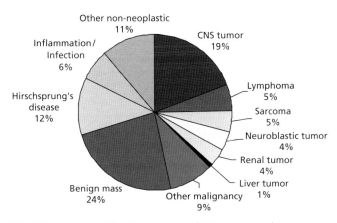

Fig. 20.1. Intraoperative diagnosis in pediatric surgery. The most common indications for pediatric intraoperative consultation are evaluation of brain tumors, lymphoma, solid tumors, benign neoplasms, benign inflammatory lesions, and Hirschsprung's disease. (*Data from Texas Children's Hospital experience, 974 IOC cases, 2004–2008.*)

Table 20.1. Differential diagnosis of primitive round cell tumors of childhood

Diagnosis	*Primary anatomic sites*
Neuroblastoma	Adrenal, paraspinal (mediastinal or retroperitoneal)
Ewing sarcoma/Primitive neuroectodermal tumor	Soft tissue, bone, other organs
Rhabdomyosarcoma	Soft tissue, extremities, head and neck, genitourinary tract, biliary tract, paratesticular, meningeal, other organs
Non-Hodgkin's lymphoma	Lymph node, mediastinum, intestine, brain, kidney, lung, other organs
Wilms tumor, blastemal	Kidney
Osteosarcoma, small cell variant	Bone
Hepatoblastoma, small cell undifferentiated	Liver
Desmoplastic small round cell tumor	Pleuroperitoneal
Rhabdoid tumor	Kidney, soft tissue, liver, brain
Medulloblastoma	Brain (cerebellum)

are high. The collection of samples for ancillary studies is often critical in pediatric neoplasms, so it is necessary to be familiar with the requirements of various pediatric protocols, should the patient be entered into such a study.

INDICATIONS FOR INTRAOPERATIVE CONSULTATION

1. To determine the adequacy of an incisional or core biopsy specimen. Examples include suspected malignancies in a variety of anatomic sites, including abdominal, soft tissue, bone, and brain, as well as for kidney biopsy for medical renal diseases.
2. To triage tissue for ancillary studies.
3. To confirm a diagnosis of malignancy prior to insertion of central venous lines.[4]
4. To distinguish inflammatory/infectious lesions from neoplastic lesions.
5. To distinguish benign and malignant lesions; as an example, if a bone biopsy shows a benign lesion, such as an aneurysmal bone cyst, the surgeon can proceed with curettage and packing, whereas management will be deferred if the frozen section (FS) is interpreted as malignant, for example, telangiectatic osteosarcoma.
6. To evaluate surgical margins in definitive resection specimens, for example, partial hepatectomy for liver tumors, and partial nephrectomy for Wilms' tumor.
7. To make specific diagnoses in non-neoplastic diseases that influence immediate surgical management (e.g., identification of ganglion cells in Hirschsprung's disease).

SPECIFIC CLINICO-PATHOLOGIC ISSUES

Small blue cell tumors of childhood

Many childhood malignancies are composed of immature-appearing primitive or undifferentiated cells, collectively called "small round blue cell tumors" and they constitute 19%–38% of pediatric cases submitted for IOC.[4,5] These neoplasms are discussed as a group because of overlapping features on conventional light microscopic examination, but each of these tumors has characteristic pathologic features when evaluated with ancillary studies, and each requires specific treatment, making it essential to render a specific diagnosis. The differential diagnosis of primitive round cell and primitive spindle cell malignancies and their usual anatomic sites are listed in Table 20.1 and Table 20.2, respectively.

Clinical issues

Clinical information, imaging studies, and laboratory data will provide information with varying degrees of specificity, and this in turn will determine the pathologist's role in IOD. The following examples illustrate this point.

- In the first situation, clinical, imaging, and laboratory data provide an almost specific diagnosis. Neuroblastoma of the adrenal gland is a case in point: if an infant

Table 20.2. Differential diagnosis of primitive spindle cell tumors of childhood

Diagnosis	Primary anatomic sites
Rhabdomyosarcoma, embryonal	Soft tissue, head and neck, viscera
Infantile fibrosarcoma	Soft tissue, extremities
Synovial sarcoma	Soft tissue, viscera
Malignant peripheral nerve sheath tumor	Soft tissue, peripheral nerves/paraspinal
Osteosarcoma	Bone
Mesenchymal chondrosarcoma	Bone, soft tissue
Congenital mesoblastic nephroma	Kidney
Fibroblastic/myofibroblastic tumors	Soft tissue, bone, viscera
Fibromatosis	Soft tissue, mesentery

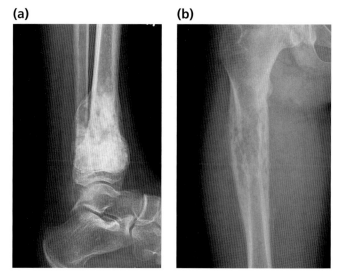

(a) **(b)**

Fig. 20.2. Diagnostic imaging features of pediatric bone tumors. Accurate diagnosis of pediatric bone tumors requires radiographic correlation during intraoperative consultation. (a) Osteosarcoma often shows a mixed lytic and sclerotic lesion with periosteal elevation (Codman's triangle), cortical destruction, and calcification within an associated soft tissue component. Pathologic features of osteosarcoma are shown in Fig. 20.3f and 20.4(d). (b) Ewing's sarcoma is typically characterized with a "moth-eaten" lytic lesion with layered periosteal reaction ("onion-skinning"). Pathologic features of Ewing's sarcoma are shown in Fig. 20.4(e).

or young child presents with an adrenal mass and elevated levels of urinary vanillylmandelic acid (VMA) and homovanillic acid (HVA), then a specific diagnosis of neuroblastomic tumor is made clinically. Neuroblastomas confined to the adrenal gland are treated primarily by surgical resection with an attempt to obtain gross total excision, and in this situation, there is no role for IOD. If, on the other hand, the neoplasm is unresectable, the surgeon will perform an incisional biopsy and submit the specimen for IOD to ensure that sufficient tissue is available for comprehensive pathologic examination before treating the patient with chemotherapy.[6]

- In the second situation, the surgeon will submit a biopsy for IOD, with the expectation that the pathologist will render a sufficiently specific diagnosis to proceed with immediate management. In the case of medulloblastoma, confirmation of the diagnosis will lead to immediate total or subtotal resection of the cerebellar mass, and in the case of mediastinal lymphoblastic lymphoma, confirmation of the diagnosis will result in surgical biopsy only, followed by post-operative chemotherapy (see Chapter 16, p. 258 and Chapter 17, p. 283 for further discussion of these two neoplasms).

- In the third scenario, the surgeon suspects a malignant neoplasm, but there is a broad differential diagnosis, and management is a two-step process: an incisional biopsy is performed to obtain tissue for diagnosis, and if the lesion is malignant, decisions about management are deferred until permanent sections have been

examined with the help of ancillary studies. A variety of small cell malignant neoplasms are managed in this way, including malignancies of soft tissue and bone. For example, Ewing's sarcoma or osteosarcoma may be the favored diagnosis for a lytic bone lesion, but the differential diagnosis may include osteomyelitis, Langerhans cell histiocytosis, non-ossifying fibroma and fibrous dysplasia. The differential diagnosis is guided by radiographic features (Fig. 20.2), but biopsy is necessary to establish the diagnosis.

Pathologic issues

INITIAL INCISIONAL BIOPSY

- The purpose of IOC on an incisional biopsy is to confirm that the biopsy contains lesional tissue compatible with the provisional clinical diagnosis, and to ensure that sufficient tissue is present for conventional microscopy and all necessary ancillary studies. Cytologic preparations should be made routinely because they often provide important information about cytodifferentiation in small blue cell tumors (Fig. 20.3). In general, the Diff Quik stain is superior for the recognition of hematopoietic malignancies, while the H&E stain is best for most other types of small blue cell

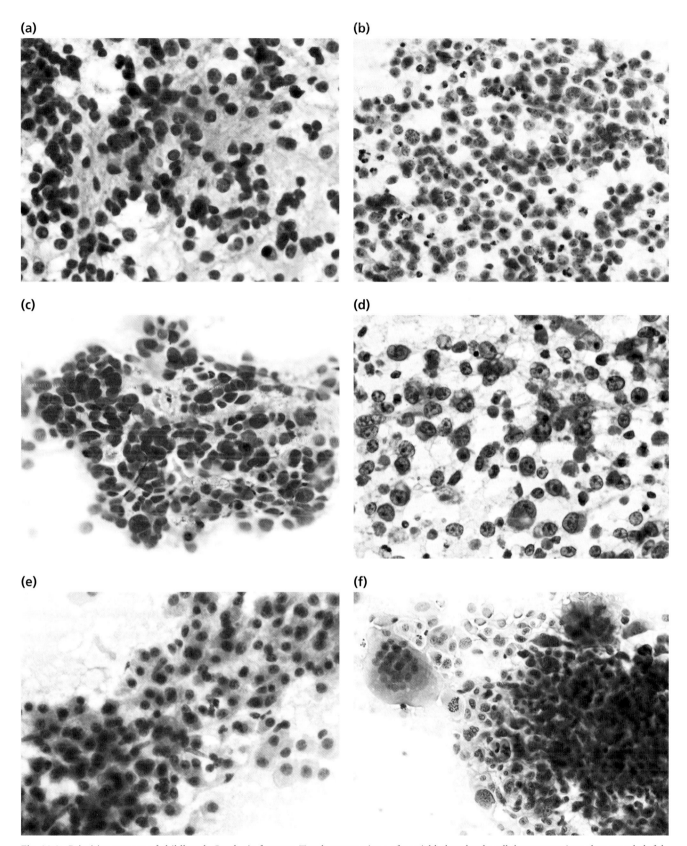

Fig. 20.3. Primitive tumors of childhood: Cytologic features. Touch preparations often yield abundantly cellular preparations that are a helpful adjunct to frozen section during intraoperative consultation. Distinguishing cytologic features often reflect areas of cytodifferentiation within the tumor. (a) Poorly differentiated neuroblastoma with neuropil production and vague Homer–Wright pseudorosettes. (b) Undifferentiated neuroblastoma with frequent karyorrhectic bodies (high mitotic-karyorrhectic index). (c) Rhabdomyosarcoma with some rhabdomyoblasts containing eosinophilic globoid cytoplasm. (d) Rhabdoid tumor with round eosinophilic cytoplasmic inclusions, eccentric nuclei, and prominent nucleoli. (e) Hepatoblastoma with epithelioid cells with eosinophilic cytoplasm, arranged in vague cords or trabeculae. (f) Osteosarcoma with pleomorphic hyperchromatic nuclei, frequent mitoses, and occasional multinucleate osteoclast-like giant cells.

tumors. Frozen section (FS) should be performed routinely, not only because it provides information about the architectural features of the neoplasm (Fig. 20.4), but because FSs are superior for evaluating the quantity of "viable" neoplastic tissue, in the event that there is extensive necrosis or fibrosis.

- There is a great deal of overlap in the cytologic and histologic appearance of small cell tumors of childhood, and it may not be possible to make a specific diagnosis intraoperatively. In this circumstance, the goal of IOD is to determine if sufficient diagnostic tissue is present in the biopsy, and to make a provisional, "good enough" diagnosis – because management is planned only after a final diagnosis is made on permanent sections. A diagnosis of "small cell malignant neoplasm" should be made, and if the lesion is compatible with the clinical diagnosis, there is no harm in adding that the biopsy changes are consistent with the surgeon's favored diagnosis. However, there should be no compulsion to make a specific diagnosis when that is not possible. Pediatric surgeons understand that a specific diagnosis usually requires ancillary studies, including immunohistochemical stains, in situ hybridization, flow cytometry, cytogenetic tests, and/or electron microscopy.

- A wider range of ancillary studies are performed more frequently in pediatric neoplasms than adult neoplasms, for both diagnosis and prognosis, and these are summarized in Table 20.3. The amount of tumor tissue required for these tests depends on the differential diagnosis, but approximately 1cm^3 of tissue is usually sufficient to complete all necessary studies.

RESECTION SPECIMENS

The intraoperative evaluation of surgical margins for pediatric malignancies is similar to adult malignancies. Depending on the clinical situation, definitive surgical resection may proceed without an initial confirmatory biopsy, or the resection may be performed after the diagnosis of malignancy is confirmed by IOD. Furthermore, surgical resection may be undertaken after adjuvant chemotherapy, in which case, the morphologic features of the neoplasm will be altered by treatment.

Intraoperative assessment of surgical margins is not required in all tumor resections; for example, in neuroblastoma, the goal of surgical management is gross total excision rather than negative microscopic margins. Similarly, the surgeon may not submit a soft tissue sarcoma resection specimen for intraoperative evaluation of surgical margins if the resection is considered adequate on clinical grounds.

When the specimen is submitted for intraoperative assessment of surgical margins, this can be done by gross examination alone or by FS, depending on the circumstances. Gross examination is sufficient for non-infiltrative tumors that have a margin of >1 cm, but the margins should be evaluated by FS if the malignancy is infiltrative or if the neoplasm is within 1cm of the margin. In the latter situation, sections should be taken perpendicular to the margin of concern.

The surgeon may request evaluation of bone margins on amputations or limb-sparing resections of malignancies such as Ewing's sarcoma. The cortical bone margins cannot be assessed intraoperatively, but the cancellous bone can be evaluated by curetting the tissue at the margin, and by examining the specimen by using touch preparations or by embedding the material for FS. Particular care should be taken when evaluating bone marrow margins in patients who have received granulocyte–macrophage colony stimulating factor (GM–CSF) therapy because myeloid hyperplasia induced by this medication may be mistaken for a small round cell malignancy.

Renal neoplasms of childhood

Clinical issues

Wilms' tumor (WT) constitutes approximately 80% of primary renal malignancies of childhood, followed by mesoblastic nephroma (MN), clear cell sarcoma (CCSK), and rhabdoid tumor (RT). The differential diagnosis of pediatric renal tumors is listed in Table 20.4.[7]

Ultrasound, CT, and MRI are used to determine the nature of renal mass lesions and to stage the tumor. Pediatric renal tumors are usually quite large, but most are amenable to primary surgical resection by nephrectomy. The usual approach to treatment in North America is as follows.

- Unilateral tumors that are resectable are removed by simple or radical nephrectomy, taking care to avoid rupture of the tumor, as rupture upstages the tumor and places the patient at high risk for local recurrence. Lymph nodes are sampled for staging. Unilateral tumors that are unresectable are biopsied and staged surgically, after which they are treated with chemotherapy; nephrectomy is performed after a suitable response to chemotherapy.

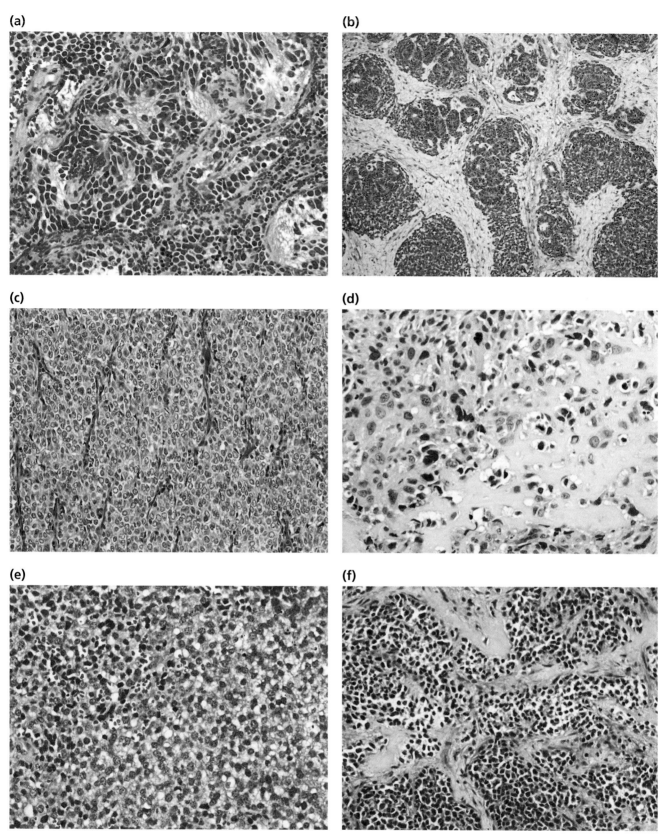

Fig. 20.4. Primitive tumors of childhood: Architectural features. Architectural features may help to distinguish the primitive tumors of childhood on frozen section. (a) Neuroblastoma with a hypervascular nested pattern and Homer-Wright pseudorosettes. (b) Wilms' tumor with triphasic pattern, including serpentine blastema, epithelial tubules, and intervening stroma. Wilms' tumor typically has a well-defined pseudocapsule at the interface to normal kidney. (c) Clear cell sarcoma of the kidney with "chickenwire" vascular pattern subdividing cells with dispersed nuclei and pale nuclear chromatin. (d) Osteosarcoma with lace-like eosinophilic osteoid matrix. (e) Ewing sarcoma with solid compact sheets of small hyperchromatic round cells with a pattern of "light and dark" nuclei due to variable pyknosis. "Light" cells may also be produced by increased cytoplasmic glycogen. Extensive necrosis is also common in Ewing sarcoma. (f) Alveolar rhabdomyosarcoma with pseudoalveolar pattern produced by cells lining fibrovascular septations. Other variants of rhabdomyosarcoma show a loose "tissue culture" pattern of spindled cells (embryonal rhabdomyosarcoma) or presence of a submucosal cambium layer (botryoid rhabdomyosarcoma). "Strap cells" with cross-striations are seen occasionally.

Table 20.3. Special studies and tissue handling in the evaluation of pediatric tumors

Special study	Recommended for	Collection Procedure
Cytogenetic analysis	All tumors	Fresh sterile tumor tissue in culture media
Fluoresence in situ hybridization (FISH)	Neuroblastic tumors (MYCN) Ewing sarcoma (EWS) Burkitt lymphoma (c-myc)	Imprint slides of fresh tumor tissue
Molecular testing (PCR)	All tumors	Frozen tumor tissue −80 °C
Electron microscopy	All tumors	Glutaraldehyde-fixed tumor tissue (1 mm³ pieces)
Flow cytometry	Lymphoma/leukemia	Fresh tumor tissue in culture media
Biology studies	Tumors for Children's Oncology Group or other research protocols	Frozen tumor and non-neoplastic tissue −80 °C Fresh tumor tissue in culture media

- 5%–10% of patients who have WT have bilateral disease, presenting difficult management issues. These patients undergo surgical exploration and staging; both tumors are biopsied to confirm the diagnosis, following which the patient is treated with chemotherapy.[8] After chemotherapy, nephron-sparing surgery will be attempted, either by bilateral partial nephrectomy or combined partial and complete nephrectomy, depending on the number, location, and size of the tumors.

Pathologic issues
- IOD on a complete nephrectomy specimen is generally not necessary and not indicated. The exception may be confirmation of the diagnosis of WT in order to place a central line, for example, in young infants for whom the differential diagnosis includes both benign neoplasms, such as classical mesoblastic nephroma and malignant neoplasms, such as Wilms' tumor and rhabdoid tumors (Fig. 20.5).
- Intraoperative evaluation of surgical margins is usually not requested for stage I and stage II tumors* because the surgeon is able to remove the entire neoplasm with clear margins without the help of IOD.

Table 20.4. Differential diagnosis of renal tumors of childhood

Wilms' tumor
  Favorable histology
  Unfavorable histology (anaplastic)
Mesoblastic nephroma (classic/cellular/mixed)
Rhabdoid tumor
Clear cell sarcoma of the kidney
Renal cell carcinoma
Metanephric adenoma
Cystic nephroma
Angiomyolipoma
Oncocytoma
Ossifying tumor of the infantile kidney
Renal medullary carcinoma
Juxtaglomerular cell tumor
Other (lymphoma, NB, PNET, synovial sarcoma, metastasis)

- Incisional biopsies that are performed on unresectable tumors are usually submitted for FS diagnosis to assess specimen adequacy and to allow triage of the specimen for ancillary studies.
- In the uncommon setting of bilateral (stage V) WT pre-treated with chemotherapy, partial nephrectomies may be submitted for evaluation of surgical margins. These cases can be challenging so the pathologist should be familiar with the clinical details and the surgeon's goals. One of the challenges is to distinguish a hyperplastic nephrogenic rest from a small WT, a distinction that requires assessment of the architecture of the lesion; nephrogenic rests are often wedge-shaped and interdigitate with normal renal tubules, whereas small WTs are spherical and have a tumor pseudocapsule.

When handling a partial nephrectomy specimen, the surgical margins should be inked, and the margins should be evaluated either with an en face section or a representative perpendicular section, depending on the gross findings. Microscopic nephrogenic rests are common in patients with bilateral tumors, and these should not be over-interpreted as a positive margin.

* Stage I: Tumor is limited to the kidney and completely resected.
Stage II: Tumor extends beyond the kidney but completely resected; extension is either by capsular invasion with negative margin, or by vascular invasion in the renal sinus or outside of the kidney.

(a)

(b)

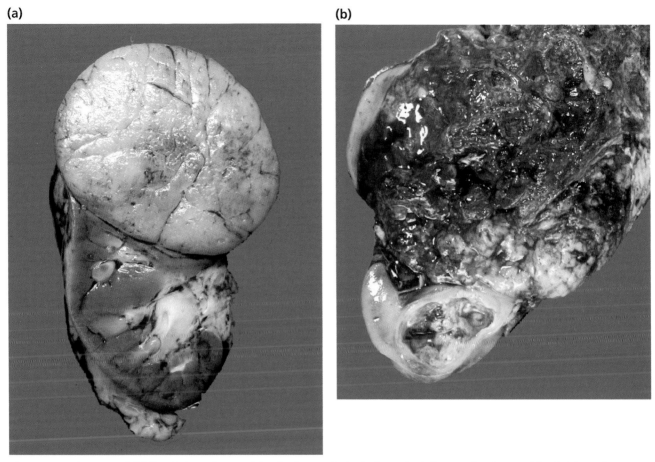

Fig. 20.5. Renal tumors of childhood: Gross features. (a) Wilms' tumor is classically a spherical encapsulated mass with a bulging soft tan cut surface. In contrast, congenital mesoblastic nephroma typically has a more whorled "fibrous" gross appearance and has a more infiltrative border with the adjacent kidney parenchyma. (b) This example of a rhabdoid tumor shows more aggressive features with extensive hemorrhage, necrosis, and extension beyond the renal capsule.

Hepatic tumors of childhood

Clinical issues

The differential diagnosis of hepatic masses in the pediatric age group is shown in Table 20.5.[9] The clinical presentation of hepatic neoplasms is generally non-specific and related to mass effect. Elevated serum alpha-fetoprotein (AFP) levels, in the range of 100 000 – 1 000 000 units, suggest the diagnosis of hepatoblastoma (HB) or hepatocellular carcinoma (HCC), although mildly elevated levels may also occur in non-neoplastic liver disease. Not all HBs and HCCs have markedly elevated levels of alpha fetoprotein at the time of diagnosis, but when elevated, it serves as a useful marker for monitoring tumor regression and recurrence.

Imaging studies, including ultrasound, CT and MRI, provide little help in the distinction of HB and HCC, but imaging is helpful in staging the neoplasm and determining its resectability. The diagnosis is usually established by pre-operative needle core biopsy.[10]

Surgical resection is the primary treatment for all neoplasms of the liver that are amenable to resection. Because of their large size and anatomic location within the liver, approximately 70% of hepatoblastomas are treated with neoadjuvant chemotherapy to shrink the tumor before surgical resection. Extra-hepatic venous invasion is not a contraindication for partial hepatectomy if the area of venous invasion can also be resected. Orthotopic liver transplantation is an option for patients with multifocal tumors, and for tumors that are unresectable by partial hepatectomy, for example, central tumors that involve hilar vessels.[10]

Pathologic issues

IOC is usually requested for evaluation of surgical margins, rather than confirmation of the diagnosis. If the surgeon is

Table 20.5. Differential diagnosis of hepatic masses in children

Hepatoblastoma

Epithelial type
Pure fetal pattern
Embryonal and fetal pattern
Macrotrabecular pattern
Small cell undifferentiated pattern

Mixed epithelial and mesenchymal type
Primitive spindled mesenchyme, osteoid, cartilaginous, skeletal muscle
Teratoid features (squamous, mucinous, neuroectodermal, melanin)

Hepatocellular carcinoma

Conventional
Fibrolamellar variant

Infantile hemangioendothelioma

Focal nodular hyperplasia

Mesenchymal hamartoma

Undifferentiated embryonal sarcoma

Nodular regenerative hyperplasia

Hepatocellular adenoma

Angiosarcoma

Embryonal rhabdomyosarcoma of biliary tree

Other (leukemia/lymphoma; metastasis from neuroblastoma or gastrointestinal tract tumors)

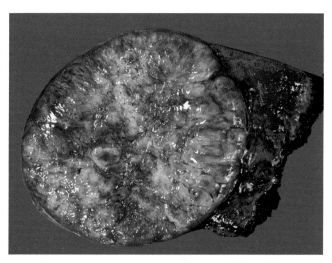

Fig. 20.6. Hepatoblastoma: gross features. Assessment of margins requires inking of the parenchymal margin and perpendicular sectioning to assess proximity of the mass to the surgical margin. This solitary hepatoblastoma showed grossly clear margins and frozen section was not performed during intraoperative consultation in this case.

concerned about a particular area of the margin (e.g. a vascular structure), this area will be identified separately. The pathologist should have a clear understanding of the surgeon's concerns about surgical margins before inking and sectioning the specimen, and the best way to do this is to have a direct discussion with the surgeon in the operating room.

The surgical margin should be inked prior to sectioning and care should be taken to minimize "bleeding" of ink into the uneven surfaces of the parenchymal margin. The specimen should be sectioned serially at close intervals, in a plane perpendicular to the surgical margin (Fig. 20.6), and the proximity of the neoplasm to the margin will determine the next step.[11] If the tumor margin is clearly positive or clearly negative by gross examination, then FS during IOC may not be necessary; if, however, the margins are close (for example, <1 cm by gross examination), then one or more sections should be taken perpendicular to the margin from areas where the tumor is closest to that margin. Pre-operative chemotherapy of HB may produce extensive necrosis of the tumor but this should not compromise evaluation of the margins. HB shows a range of histologic patterns and these are listed in Table 20.5 and illustrated in Fig. 20.7.[9,12]

Hirschsprung's disease

Clinical issues

Hirschsprung's disease (HD) is a developmental disorder of the enteric nervous system in which there is incomplete migration of ganglion cells from proximal to distal intestine, resulting in aganglionosis of the rectum and a variable length of more proximal intestine. Aganglionosis is limited to the rectum in 30% of cases and to the rectosigmoid in about 45% of cases. Total colonic aganglionosis occurs in less than 10% of cases, and involvement of the terminal ileum is rare. Ultra-short segment disease refers to aganglionosis limited to the lower half of the rectum, approximately 2–4 cm above the mucocutaneous line.[13]

Hirschsprung's disease is suspected in neonates who have delayed passage of meconium, and in older children and adolescents with chronic constipation. Contrast enema shows a normal caliber or narrow distal segment, a funnel-shaped dilation at the transition zone, and marked dilation of the more proximal normally-ganglionated bowel. Anorectal manometry is sometimes used to identify an absence of normal rectoanal reflexes. Definitive diagnosis requires the demonstration of aganglionosis and hypertrophic nerve fibrils in a rectal biopsy, a procedure with a sensitivity of 93% and specificity of 98%.[14] Most initial rectal biopsies are submucosal suction biopsies, which are less invasive than operative biopsies and can be performed at the bedside. These biopsies should be obtained 3 cm or

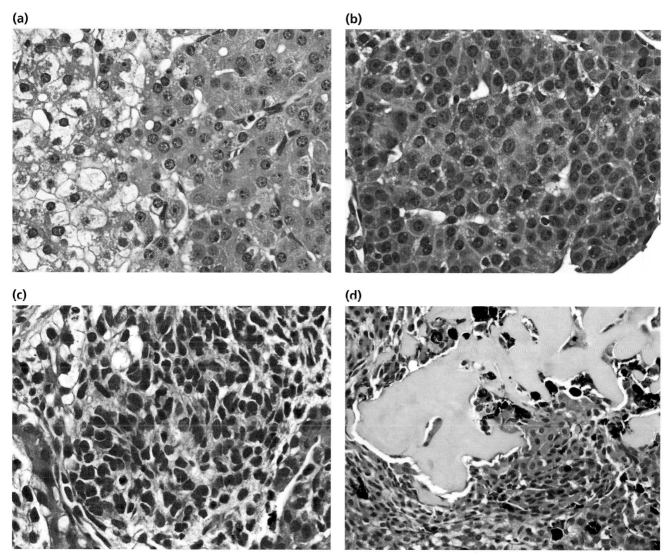

Fig. 20.7. Hepatoblastoma: Microscopic features. Microscopic patterns in hepatoblastoma include: (a) Fetal epithelial pattern with abundant eosinophilic cytoplasm and frequent glycogenation. (b) Embryonal epithelial pattern with higher nuclear-cytoplasmic ratio and lack of glycogenation. (c) Small cell undifferentiated pattern resembling other small blue cell tumors. (d) Osteoid and melanin in a teratoid hepatoblastoma.

more from the dentate line, in order to avoid the normal hypoganglionic zone immediately adjacent to the anus, and multiple biopsies are often obtained to ensure adequacy of tissue. These diagnostic biopsies are received in formalin, processed routinely, and interpreted on permanent sections, as there are significantly higher error rates for initial diagnosis of HD by FS.[15] Seromuscular biopsy of the rectum is rarely performed for initial diagnosis, but may be used when multiple suction biopsies have been unsatisfactory or in the event of emergent abdominal exploration due to perforation, warranting an open biopsy for exclusion of HD.[13]

After the diagnosis of HD is established, surgical treatment consists of a pull-through procedure, during which the aganglionic intestine and transition zone are removed, and the normal ganglionic bowel is pulled down and anastomosed to a cuff of rectal muscle. In an attempt to conserve intestinal tissue, the surgeon will submit a biopsy for FS from the distal-most level of the colon thought to be normally innervated. Multiple sequential biopsies may be necessary, each more proximal than the previous, in an attempt to find the correct level of normally ganglionic intestine for the pull through procedure ("leveling procedure").[16] Definitive surgical correction may be performed as either a one-stage or two-stage procedure (Fig. 20.8). The one-stage procedure ("primary pull-through") involves a leveling procedure with FS guidance, followed by immediate pull-through and resection of the abnormal aganglionic

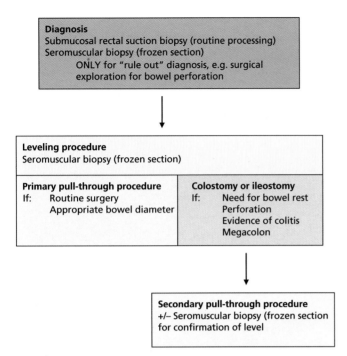

Fig. 20.8. Algorithm for surgical management of Hirschsprung's disease.

intestine during the same operation. The two-stage procedure involves a leveling procedure for creation of an ostomy during the first operation, followed by the definitive pull-through procedure during a second operation after a period of bowel rest. The primary pull-through procedure has been performed increasingly in recent years, although the two-step procedure is typically chosen for older children with markedly overdistended colons and in patients with HD-associated enterocolitis. Both the one-stage and two-stage approaches require the surgeon to identify the most distal, normally innervated segment of intestine for the pull through procedure, and this requires FS guidance.

Pathologic issues
Frozen section evaluation of colonic biopsies for ganglion cells represents more than 15% of all FSs performed in large pediatric medical centers,[2] and errors in FS diagnosis. occur in approximately 3% of cases,[17] either because of technical factors, or incorrect interpretation of immature ganglion cells. The biopsy submitted for FS typically occurs during a leveling procedure, and is a seromuscular or full-thickness biopsy, which allows for the evaluation of ganglion cells in the myenteric plexus where ganglion cells are more abundant. An attempt should be made to embed the specimen with proper orientation to allow for optimal assessment of the myenteric plexus. Multiple levels should be prepared routinely (for example, a few

sections on each of two or three slides), and more levels may be needed if the specimen has not been embedded in an optimal fashion. In addition to H&E stained sections, some pathologists use toluidine blue, Giemsa or Diff Quik stains to highlight the cytoplasm of ganglion cells. Rapid staining techniques for acetylcholinesterase have been developed for intraoperative diagnosis, but are not used in most institutions, and are not necessary for accurate interpretation.

Assessment of ganglion cells is a critical step in the management of HD and can be an anxiety-producing process for general surgical pathologists who interpret these cases infrequently. The following points should be kept in mind:

- Immature ganglion cells in premature or term neonates may be difficult to recognize. Immature ganglion cells are smaller than adult ganglion cells, have scanty cytoplasm and inconspicuous nucleoli compared to adult ganglion cells (Fig. 20.9), and they may be mistaken for reactive endothelial cells, fibroblasts, or small mononuclear cells (Fig. 20.10).

- It is important to recognize when a biopsy has been taken from the transition zone because this level of the colon is not normally innervated, and the surgeon should be directed to seek a more proximal level. The transition zone can be recognized by a paucity of ganglion cells and/or ganglion cells associated with hypertrophic nerve fibrils (Fig. 20.10[b]). Normally ganglionated bowel typically has large clusters of ganglion cells, so the presence of only rare individual ganglion cells in the myenteric plexus should alert the pathologist that the biopsy may be from the transition zone. An infiltrate of eosinophils in the myenteric plexus is another clue that the biopsy may be from the transition zone.

- When there is uncertainty about the presence of ganglion cells, it is better to err on the side of caution by making a "false-negative" diagnosis. This will prompt the surgeon to submit another biopsy from a level a few centimeters more proximally, with very little disadvantage to the patient, in contrast to a "false-positive" diagnosis that would lead to a pull-through procedure with intestine that has poor motility because of absent or insufficient ganglion cells. Of course, repeated failure to recognize immature ganglion cells would lead to an escalation in the amount of intestine that is resected, and this too can have serious consequences.

(a)

(b)

(c)

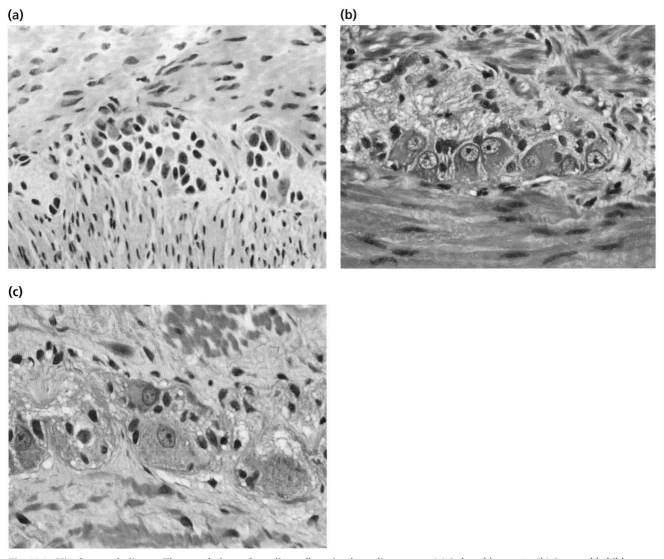

Fig. 20.9. Hirschsprung's disease. The morphology of ganglion cells varies depending on age. (a) 3-day-old neonate. (b) 2-year-old child. (c) 15-year-old adolescent.

■ The appendix is notoriously unreliable for evaluating total colonic aganglionosis, as ganglionation of the appendix may not correlate with the presence or absence of ganglion cells in the adjacent cecum.

Extrahepatic biliary atresia

Clinical issues

Biliary atresia (BA) is an important cause of conjugated hyperbilirubinemia in the newborn period, typically presenting with persistent jaundice and/or acholic stools, although some infants are not appreciably jaundiced and appear well at diagnosis. The entire extrahepatic biliary tree, including the gallbladder, may be atretic, or there may be segmental atresia of only proximal or distal segments, with or without involvement of the gallbladder. As the disease progresses, there may be involvement of the intrahepatic ducts as well. Untreated BA progresses rapidly to hepatic fibrosis and biliary cirrhosis, with hepatic failure and death occurring within months.

Liver biopsy is performed prior to intraoperative exploration in order to exclude non-surgical causes of neonatal cholestasis, such as neonatal viral hepatitis, alpha-1-antitrypsin deficiency, galactosemia, cystic fibrosis, and other biliary tract disorders.[18] Once it is determined that the clinical, imaging, and histologic findings are consistent with extrahepatic biliary obstruction, the pediatric surgeon will explore the biliary tract and perform an intraoperative cholangiogram. If these findings support the

(a)

(b)

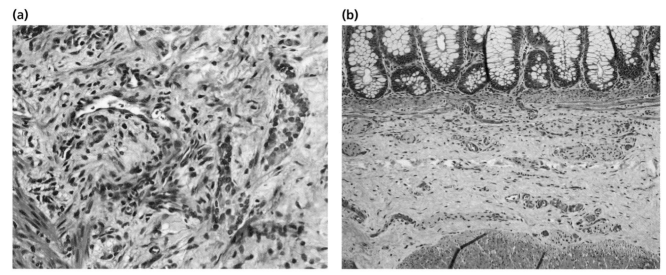

Fig. 20.10. Hirschsprung's disease. (a) The small size and high nuclear to cytoplasmic ratio of immature ganglion cells (right) may mimic plump endothelial cells and fibroblasts (left) on frozen section. Clustering and proximity to nerve fibrils can be helpful in correct identification of "baby" ganglion cells. (b) Hypertrophic nerve fibrils in the submucosa and myenteric plexus are typical of the aganglionic intestine in Hirschsprung's disease, and may also be seen with ganglion cells in the transition zone (submucosal plexus).

diagnosis of extrahepatic biliary atresia, a Kasai procedure (hepatic portoenterostomy) is performed, with excision of the extra-hepatic biliary tree and creation of a conduit for drainage of bile from the porta hepatis to the small intestine via a Roux-en-Y loop of jejunum.

Success of the Kasai procedure depends on the flow of bile from the tiny residual ducts in the fibrous remnant of the porta hepatis. Frozen section diagnosis may be requested at the time of the Kasai procedure to assess the adequacy of the diameter of these bile duct profiles, although this practice is controversial and has generally fallen out of favor. Duct diameters greater than 150 microns have been thought to indicate a greater likelihood of successful post-operative function,[19,20] but there is no evidence that more aggressive dissection to identify larger, more proximal ducts is advantageous; the most important indicator of operative success appears to be the severity of intrahepatic biliary disease and liver injury.[21] As a result, most pediatric surgeons no longer request FS guidance during the Kasai procedure, and instead, resect the portal plate flush with the liver interface to achieve adequate bile flow. The outcome of the Kasai procedure is best if performed within the first 60 days of life. The Kasai procedure provides successful long-term bile drainage in less than 20% of patients, and approximately 50% of patients develop progressive liver fibrosis and portal hypertension 4–5 years after the procedure.[21] Patients older than 4 months of age with cirrhosis may be candidates for primary liver transplantation.[21]

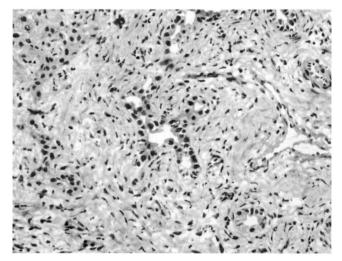

Fig. 20.11. Kasai procedure. Frozen section diagnosis has been used historically to assess adequacy of the portal plate bile ducts. Presence of patent epithelial-lined ducts is demonstrated, with a desired duct diameter of approximately 150 microns or greater. In current surgical practice, intraoperative consultation is requested uncommonly during Kasai procedure.

Pathologic issues

In the past, IOC was used to confirm the presence of bile ducts in the newly created porta hepatis margin prior to anastomosis (Fig. 20.11), and the presence of bile ducts with a minimum diameter of 150 microns was reported to correlate with increased post-operative bile flow compared to the smaller ductules.[20,22] There are two problems with the FS evaluation of tissue from the porta hepatis: first, loss of epithelium may impair recognition of bile ducts in the portal plate, and second, dilated peribiliary glands and duct-like structures, neither of which communicate with the intrahepatic biliary tree, can be mistaken for functional bile ducts on FS. Considerable doubt has been cast on the value of FSs to determine the adequacy of the bile ducts in the portal plate[23] and it is now generally accepted that bile duct diameter does not determine long-term success of the portoenterostomy. FS is no longer performed at most centers.[4,24]

REFERENCES

1. Coffin CM. Pediatric surgical pathology: Pitfalls and strategies for error prevention. *Arch Pathol Lab Med* 2005; **130**: 610–612.
2. Coffin CM, Spilker K, Zhou H, Lowichik A, Pysher TJ. Frozen section diagnosis in pediatric surgical pathology: a decades' experience at a children's hospital. *Arch Pathol Lab Med* 2005; **129**: 1619–1625.
3. Fisher JE, Burger PC, Perlman EJ, *et al*. The frozen section yesterday and today: pediatric solid tumors – crucial issues. *Pediatr Dev Pathol* 2001; **4**: 252–266.
4. Preston HS, Bale PM. Rapid frozen section in pediatric pathology. *Am J Surg Pathol* 1985; **9**: 570–576.
5. Wakely PE, Frable WJ, Kornstein MJ. Role of intraoperative cytopathology in pediatric surgical pathology. *Hum Pathol* 1993; **24**: 311–315.
6. La Quaglia MP, Rutigliano DN. 'Neuroblastoma and other adrenal tumors.' In *The Surgery of Childhood Tumors*, Carachi, R Grosfeld, JL Azmy, AF (eds.) 2nd edn. Springer-Verlag: Berlin, 2008, pp. 201–225.
7. Parham DM. 'Renal neoplasms.' In *Pediatric Neoplasia: Morphology and Biology*, DM Parham (ed.) Philadelphia: Lippincott-Raven; 1996, pp. 33–64.
8. Shamberger RC. 'Renal tumors'. In *The Surgery of Childhood Tumors*, Carachi, R Grosfeld, JL Azmy, AF (eds.) 2nd edn. Berlin: Springer-Verlag; 2008, pp. 171–199.
9. JT Stocker, RM Conran, DM Selby. Tumors and pseudotumors of the liver. In *Pathology of Solid Tumors in Children*. Stocker JT, Askin, FB (eds.) New York: Chapman and Hall; 1998, pp. 83–110.
10. Grosfeld JL, Otte J-B. Liver tumors in children. In *The Surgery of Childhood Tumors*, Carachi, R Grosfeld, JL Azmy, AF, (eds.) 2nd edn. Springer-Verlag: Berlin, 2008. pp. 227–260.
11. Stocker JT. An approach to handling pediatric liver tumors. *Am J Clin Pathol* 1998; **209** (Suppl 1): S67–S72.
12. K Patterson. Liver tumors and tumorlike masses. In: DM Parham, ed. *Pediatric Neoplasia: Morphology and Biology*. Philadelphia: Lippincott-Raven; 1996. pp. 331–362.
13. A Holschneider, BM Ure. Hirschsprung's disease. In *Pediatric Surgery*, Ashcraft, KW (ed.) 4th edn. Philadelphia: Elsevier Saunders; 2005. pp. 477–495.
14. De Lorijn F, Kremer LCM, Reitsma JB, Benninga MA. Diagnostic tests in Hirschsprung disease: a systematic review. *J Pediatr Gastroenterol Nutr* 2006; **42**: 496–505.
15. Maia DM. The reliability of frozen-section diagnosis in the pathologic evaluation of Hirschsprung's disease. *Am J Surg Pathol* 2000; **24**: 1675–1677.
16. Kapur RP. Hirschsprung disease and other enteric dysganglionoses. *Crit Rev Clin Lab Sci.* 1999; **36**: 225–273.
17. Shayan K, Smith C, Langer JC. Reliability of intraoperative frozen sections in the management of Hirschsprung's disease. *J Pediatr Surg* 2004; **39**: 1345–1348.
18. Portmann BC, Roberts EA. Extrahepatic biliary atresia. In *MacSween's Pathology of the Liver*, Burt AD, Portmann BC, Ferrell LD, (eds.) 5th edn. Philadelphia: Churchill Livingston Elsevier, 2007, pp. 153–159.
19. Gautier M, Jehan P, Odievre M. Histologic study of biliary fibrous remnants in 48 cases of extrahepatic biliary atresia: Correlation with postoperative bile flow restoration. *J Pediatr* 1976; **89**: 704–709.
20. Chandra RS, Altman RP. Ductal remnants in extrahepatic biliary atresia: a histopathologic study with clinical correlation. *J Pediatr* 1978; **93**: 196–200.
21. DL Sigalet. Biliary tract disorders and portal hypertension. In *Pediatric Surgery*, Ashcraft KW, (ed.) 3rd edn. Philadelphia: WB Saunders, 2000, pp. 580–596.
22. Ohi R, Shikes RH, Stellin GP, Lilly JR. In biliary atresia duct histology correlates with bile flow. *J Pediatr Surgery* 1984; **19**: 467–470.
23. Tan EL, Davenport M, Driver M, Howard ER. Does the morphology of the extrahepatic biliary remnants in biliary atresia influence survival? A review of 205 cases. *J Pediatr Surg* 1994; **29**: 1459–1464.
24. Dolgin SE. Answered and unanswered controversies in the surgical management of extrahepatic biliary atresia. *Pediatr Transplant* 2004; **8**: 628–631.

INDEX